Sepsis and Septic Shock: An Issue of Critical Care Clinics

Sepsis and Septic Shock: An Issue of Critical Care Clinics

Editor: Claudia Lance

AMERICAN
MEDICAL PUBLISHERS
www.americanmedicalpublishers.com

AMERICAN
MEDICAL PUBLISHERS
www.americanmedicalpublishers.com

Cataloging-in-Publication Data

Sepsis and septic shock : an issue of critical care clinics / edited by Claudia Lance.
p. cm.
Includes bibliographical references and index.
ISBN 978-1-63927-107-8
1. Septicemia. 2. Septic shock. 3. Critical care medicine. 4. Emergency medicine. I. Lance, Claudia.
RC182.S4 S47 2021
616.944--dc23

American Medical Publishers,
41 Flatbush Avenue,
1st Floor, New York,
NY 11217, USA

ISBN 978-1-63927-107-8 (Hardback)

Contents

Preface

This book has been a concerted effort by a group of academicians, researchers and scientists, who have contributed their research works for the realization of the book. This book has materialized in the wake of emerging advancements and innovations in this field. Therefore, the need of the hour was to compile all the required researches and disseminate the knowledge to a broad spectrum of people comprising of students, researchers and specialists of the field.

Shock is caused by the decreased flow of blood to the body tissues due to circulatory system related problems. Sepsis refers to a life-threatening condition where the body causes injury to its own organs and tissues in response to an infection. When sepsis lowers the blood pressure to the extent where it does not improve after fluid replacement, it is known as septic shock. Sepsis happens due to an inflammatory immune response which is triggered by an infection. Septic shock is usually caused by bacteria but it can also be caused by fungi, parasites or viruses. It generally affects the lungs, urinary tract, brain or skin. Fever, increased breathing and heart rate, and confusion are some of its common signs and symptoms. Severe sepsis results in organ dysfunction and poor blood flow. This book provides significant information to help develop a good understanding of sepsis and septic shock. Different approaches, evaluations, methodologies and advanced studies have been included herein. Those in search of information to further their knowledge will be greatly assisted by this book.

At the end of the preface, I would like to thank the authors for their brilliant chapters and the publisher for guiding us all-through the making of the book till its final stage. Also, I would like to thank my family for providing the support and encouragement throughout my academic career and research projects.

Editor

1

Prognostic value of PCT in septic emergency patients

Nicolas Peschanski[1], Camille Chenevier-Gobeaux[2*], Lynda Mzabi[3], Rémy Lucas[1], Siham Ouahabi[4], Vianney Aquilina[1], Valéry Brunel[5], Guillaume Lefevre[4] and Patrick Ray[3,6]

Abstract

Background: An accurate assessment of septic patients at risk for poor clinical outcomes is challenging for clinicians in the emergency department (ED).

Objectives: We aimed to evaluate the prognostic value of procalcitonin (PCT) in septic patients in the ED for predicting death.

Results: In a retrospective study, 188 septic patients (median age 63 [IQR 51–80]) of two French university hospitals were included. Patients who deceased within 30 days (20 %, $n = 37$) presented higher PCT value at admission (median 34.0 µg/L [5.0–71.9]) in comparison with the survivals (median 6.4 µg/L [4.1–13.1], $p = 0.0005$). ROC curve analysis indicated a moderate AUC of 0.686 [95 % CI 0.613–0.752] and an optimal PCT threshold value at 32.5 [95 % CI 21.8–43.3] µg/L that was associated with a 51 % [34–67] sensitivity, a 96 % [90–98] specificity, a 73 % [52–88] positive predictive value, and a 89 % [83–93] negative predictive value for death. Only 26 patients (14 %) had PCT values above this threshold (19 in the deceased group vs 7 in survival group, $p < 0.0001$). By multivariate analysis, only three variables remained significantly predictive of the death: personal history of cardiovascular disease (OR 3.1 [1.0–9.4], $p = 0.046$), the presence of severe sepsis/septic shock in the ER (OR 4.4 [1.3–12.3], $p = 0.013$), and a PCT level >32.5 µg/L (OR 36.0 [10.0–128.4], $p < 0.0001$). Similar results were obtained when considering the combined outcome death and/or admission in ICU.

Conclusion: Elevated value of PCT at admission has moderate accuracy to identify poor outcome in ED septic patients in daily practice.

Keywords: Procalcitonin, Sepsis, Emergency department, Prognostic

Background

Sepsis is a life-threatening condition that arises when the host's response to an infection injures its own tissues and organs [1]. The accurate identification of sepsis is one of the main challenges in emergency medicine. Despite advances in antibiotic therapy and modern life support, fatality rate of patients with sepsis has remained high worldwide (>30 %) [1, 2].

Early identification of patients at high risk of dying from sepsis may help initiate rapid and appropriate therapeutic interventions. However, signs of organ dysfunction may not be obvious for the physician's at the time of presentation [3]. Thus, an accurate assessment of patients at risk for poor clinical outcomes is challenging for clinicians in the emergency department (ED).

Procalcitonin (PCT), the pro-hormone of calcitonin, is synthesized by thyroid cells. During sepsis, many tissues and immune cells become able to secrete PCT. The enhanced specificity of PCT along with the publication of numerous clinical and interventional studies has contributed to the growing interest and implementation of PCT in the ED as a biomarker of the systemic host response to bacterial invasion [3, 4]. Several studies have demonstrated that PCT may confer prognostic information in PAC [5] and in sepsis [6], and some have suggested the

*Correspondence: camille.gobeaux@cch.aphp.fr
[2] Department of Automated Biological Diagnosis, Hôpitaux Universitaires Paris Centre (HUPC) – Hôpital Cochin, Assistance Publique des Hôpitaux de Paris (AP-HP), Paris, France
Full list of author information is available at the end of the article

same in an ED. Recently, PCT-based sepsis diagnosis was demonstrated to be more reliable and discriminating than clinical sepsis diagnosis [7]. Furthermore, lactate and PCT might be complementary biomarkers for the risk stratification of ED patients evaluation [3]. Thus, PCT might be a good candidate to accurately identify ED septic patients with poor outcome.

Therefore, we aimed to evaluate the prognostic value of PCT in septic patients in the ED.

Patients and methods

It was a retrospective study, which took place in the EDs of two university hospitals (Tenon hospital in Paris and Rouen), from July 2011 to December 2011. Both were urban adult ED and teaching hospitals with, respectively, 45,000 and 82,000 annual new patient attendances. Because of the observational design of the study, the ethical committee (CPP Ile-de-France Paris VI, Paris, France) authorized a waiver of informed consent. In these two hospitals, PCT is widely used by physicians' in charge, for patients with suspected or confirmed infections, especially in suspicion of lower respiratory tract infections. However, no real guideline is associated with the result of PCT.

Studied population

Patients ≥18 years old were included if they presented with a confirmed diagnosis of infection, and had a PCT measurement blood sampled routinely performed in the ED with a level ≥2 µg/L. This PCT threshold was chosen upon previous studies observations, where ED patients with PCT ≥2 µg/L were suggested as having a sepsis and high risk of development of organ dysfunction [4, 8]. For each patient, ED electronic file and recorded admission data (including initial vital variables, routine biological data, and admitting diagnosis in ED) were collected, as well as outcome (discharge, admission to a medical ward or ICU, in-hospital mortality) and final diagnosis, i.e., each patient had a confirmation of sepsis suspected in the ED (based on all medical charts and available microbiological data). The presence of systemic inflammatory response syndrome (SIRS), sepsis, or severe sepsis/septic shock criteria [9] was also recorded, either at ED admission or during follow-up. For this study, hyperlactatemia (>2 mmol/L) was used as a severe sepsis criterion (although not specific) [10]. However, patients with other causes of high lactate levels were not excluded.

Patients were further categorized according to two different outcomes: death at day 30, or a combined outcome of death and/or admission to ICU during the follow-up of day 30.

PCT measurement

In Tenon hospital, PCT concentrations were analyzed using a sandwich immunoassay based on time-resolved amplified cryptate emission (TRACE) measurement (Kryptor analyzer; B.R.A.H.M.S. Thermo Fischer, Germany). In our laboratory, coefficients of variation (CV) for PCT were found to be <10 % at 0.28 and 10.8 µg/L. In Rouen hospital, procalcitonin concentrations were analyzed using an electrochemiluminescent immunoassay (ELECSYS BRAHMS procalcitonin, Hennigsdorf, Germany), performed on a Cobas e601 analyzer (Roche Diagnostics, Meylan, France). In our laboratories, coefficients of variation for procalcitonin were <4 % at 2 concentrations during the study period. Both methods are correlated [11]. In our laboratories, correlation coefficient was $R^2 = 0.964$ (slope: 1.04, intercept: −0.73), and we observed 96.4 % of concordance between the two methods (data not shown). Median bias observed between the two methods was 11 %, which is acceptable [12]. The upper reference limit (URL) announced by the manufacturer was 0.046 µg/L.

Statistical analysis

Results were expressed as medians [interquartile range, IQR] for continuous variables and numbers (percentage) for discrete variables. Data were compared using the Kruskal–Wallis test for continuous variables, and the Chi-square for differences in frequencies.

Receiver operating characteristic (ROC) analysis was performed in order to determine the best thresholds for PCT (or the combination of PCT + lactate after log transformation) which would be predictive of the outcome. Because of the possible impact of sample size on threshold value, a bootstrap analysis (1000 random samples with replacement) was performed to obtain a calculation of the optimal threshold of PCT and its 95 % confidence interval [13]. We assessed the sensitivity and specificity, positive (PPV) and negative predictive value (NPV) (all with their 95 % confidence intervals [95 % CI], calculated with the Wilson's score with correction of continuity) for thresholds.

As the ROC curve is recognized to be potentially insensitive, the net reclassification index (NRI) method was used, as described [13]. For tests with binary outcomes, NRI is the same as the gain in certainty of the first test minus the gain in certainty of the second test, or alternatively stated, the differences in the sum of the sensitivity and specificity:

$$NRI_{\text{second test vs first test}} = (\text{Sensitivity} + \text{Specificity})_{\text{second test}} - (\text{Sensitivity} + \text{Specificity})_{\text{first test}}$$

Since NRI is a powerful statistical tool, significant results might only have a poor clinical impact. In order to illustrate the improvement given by lactate in association with PCT, we provide a reclassification table that enables us to quantify the benefit of the association in terms of number of patients correctly reclassified. Furthermore, the reclassification table offers a practical representation of both the relationship between false positive and false negative, and the magnitude of the gain of predictability in quantitative terms (number of patients).

We further evaluated PCT and lactate combination using the best linear combination (BLC) method [14]. Briefly, this method relies on the creation of a formula in which PCT and lactate are moderated by their coefficient of covariance in the studied population. The obtained combination gives a score for each patient that can be studied as a biomarker by itself and submitted to ROC analysis and logistic regression.

A forward logistic regression was performed to assess variables associated with outcome. For this analysis, PCT levels were evaluated as categorical variables based on the optimum cutoff point previously determined by ROC curve. We adopted a conservative approach and only included significant preoperative variables in the univariate analysis (p value of entry <0.10). The discriminate power of the logistic regression was evaluated by the c-statistic (concordance index) and the goodness of fit of the model by the Hosmer–Lemeshow test.

The results were analyzed using Med Calc 3.4.2.0 for Windows (MedCalc Software, Mariakerke, Belgium). All tests were two-tailed. A p value <0.05 was considered to be statistically significant.

Results

Main characteristics of the studied population ($n = 188$) are presented in Table 1. As expected, main sources of sepsis were pulmonary and urinary infections. Forty-three percent of patients had a severe sepsis/septic shock, and 28 % were transferred in ICU. Briefly, patients who deceased within 30 days (20 %; $n = 37$) were older, presented an initial higher cardiac rate and respiratory rate, had more comorbidity, had more frequently severe sepsis or septic shock, and presented higher lactate levels than survivals. Of note, there was no difference in age values between recruitment sites ($p = 0.337$). Ninety-one percent of patients were admitted to the hospital.

Patients with severe sepsis/septic shock had higher cardiac rate (110 [94–125] vs. 96 [84–110], $p = 0.001$) and respiratory rate (30 [24–38] vs. 20 [18–26], $p = 0.003$), higher lactate (2.4 [1.7–3.6] vs. 1.9 [1.5–2.8] mmol/L, $p = 0.053$), and lower diastolic blood pressure (62 [51–75] vs. 76 [64–84], $p < 0.0001$), lower systolic blood pressure (99 [88–119] vs. 129 [107–148], $p < 0.0001$), and higher SpO_2 (96 [94–98] vs. 94 [91–98] %, $p = 0.041$), than those without severe sepsis/septic shock. Furthermore, patients admitted to ICU were younger (60 [49–81] vs. 69 [52–83] years, $p = 0.011$), had lower diastolic blood pressure (62 [50–76] vs. 73 [61–81] mm Hg, $p = 0.005$), lower systolic blood pressure (100 [90–126] vs. 120 [100–139] mm Hg, $p = 0.005$), higher respiratory rate (32 [27–39] vs. 24 [20–32], $p = 0.010$), higher lactate (2.5 [2.0–3.4] vs. 2.1 [1.5–2.9] mmol/L, $p = 0.039$), and presented more frequently severe sepsis/septic shock (68 vs. 38 %, $p = 0.001$), than patients not admitted to ICU.

The median PCT value was higher in the deceased group (median [interquartile range, IQR]) (34.0 µg/L [5.0–71.9]) in comparison with the survivals (6.4 [4.1–13.1] µg/L, $p = 0.0005$) (Fig. 1). However, PCT values were not significantly higher in patients admitted to ICU in comparison with the others (9.6 [4.1–18.2] vs. 6.1 [3.9–14.1] µg/L, $p = 0.145$); same observation was done when comparing PCT values between patients with severe sepsis/septic shock versus others (8.6 [4.9–23.7] vs. 6.2 [3.6–12.3] µg/L, $p = 0.064$). Of note, there was no difference in PCT values between recruitment sites ($p = 0.674$).

ROC analysis

The ROC curve analysis indicated a moderate accuracy, with an AUC at 0.686 [95 % CI 0.613–0.752] ($p = 0.002$) for PCT to predict 30-day mortality (Fig. 2a). Defined by the ROC curve, the optimal threshold value was 32.5 [95 % CI 21.8–43.3] µg/L and was associated with a 51 % [34–67] sensitivity, a 96 % [90–98] specificity, a 73 % [52–88] PPV, and a 89 % [83–93] NPV. Only 26 patients (14 %) had PCT values above this threshold. The proportion of patients with PCT > 32.5 µg/L in the deceased group was significantly higher (51 %, $n = 19$) than in the survival group (5 %, $n = 7$) ($p < 0.0001$). However, the proportion of patients with PCT > 32.5 µg/L in the severe sepsis/septic shock (19 %, $n = 16$) was not significantly different from the proportion of patients with PCT > 32.5 µg/L in patients without severe sepsis/septic shock (10 %, $n = 12$) ($p = 0.123$).

The ROC curve analysis indicated a moderate accuracy for PCT to predict death and/or admission in ICU, with an AUC at 0.644 [0.571–0.712] ($p = 0.007$), with an optimal threshold value at 9.9 µg/L (Fig. 2b). This threshold was associated with a 54 % [42–65] sensitivity, a 73 % [63–90] specificity, a 70 % [61–78] PPV, and a 57 % [45–68] NPV.

When patients were classified according to PCT categories (arbitrarily defined as PCT < 5 µg/L, PCT between 5 and 19.9 µg/L, PCT between 20 and 31.9 µg/L, and PCT $\geq$ 32 µg/L), we observed that mortality raised dramatically only in patients with PCT $\geq$ 32 µg/L, while ICU transfer was not affected by PCT value (Fig. 3).

Table 1 Characteristics of the studied population

	All patients	Deceased at 30 days	Survival	p*
n	188	37	151	
Patients of Rouen [n (%)]	97 (52)	21 (57)	76 (50)	0.605
Patients of Tenon [n (%)]	91 (48)	16 (43)	75 (50)	vs Tenon
Age (years)	63 (51–80)	78 (63–83)	64 (46–78)	0.001
Men [n (%)]	101 (54)	22 (59)	79 (52)	0.551
Temperature (°C)	38.1 (37.1–39.0)	38.2 (37.1–39.8)	38.1 (37.0–38.8)	0.321
Systolic blood pressure (mmHg)	113 (96–137)	113 (93–136)	116 (97–137)	0.524
Diastolic blood pressure (mmHg)	70 (57–80)	65 (52–81)	72 (59–80)	0.260
Cardiac rate, in bpm	100 (87–118)	110 (95–129)	99 (85–116)	0.051
Respiratory rate (RR) ($n = 74$)	26 (20–34)	32 (29–40)	25 (20–32)	0.009
SpO_2 in %	95.0 (92.5–98.0)	95.0 (91.0–97.5)	95.0 (93.0–98.0)	0.636
Personal history of:				
Cardiovascular disease [n (%)]	94 (50)	24 (65)	70 (46)	0.052
Respiratory disease [n (%)]	43 (23)	13 (35)	30 (20)	0.063
Other (chronic) [n (%)]	51 (27)	5 (14)	46 (30)	0.099
Immunosuppressors, corticoids, or chemotherapy [n (%)]	29 (15)	5 (14)	24 (16)	0.677
Bacterial infection [n (%)]	139 (74)	27 (73)	112 (74)	0.159
Pulmonary infection [n (%)]	59 (31)	7 (19)	52 (34)	0.085
Urinary infection [n (%)]	30 (16)	5 (14)	25 (17)	0.914
Abdominal infection [n (%)]	21 (11)	7 (19)	14 (9)	0.169
Skin/tissue infection [n (%)]	8 (4)	3 (8)	5 (3)	0.361
Meningitis [n (%)]	2 (1)	1 (3)	1 (1)	0.828
Several sites[a]	12 (6)	1 (3)	11 (7)	0.526
Other site[b]	7 (4)	3 (8)	4 (3)	0.264
Viral infection [n (%)]	3 (2)	1 (3)	2 (1)	0.835
Other infection [n (%)][c]	46 (24)	9 (24)	37 (25)	0.669
Severe sepsis/septic shock [n (%)]	81 (43)	22 (59)	59 (39)	0.040
Median lactate (mmol/L) ($n = 103$)	2.2 (1.5–3.2)	3.1 (2.2–4.4)	2.1 (1.5–2.8)	0.003
Median white blood cells (G/L)	12.1 (7.9–18.4)	12.1 (9.0–17.4)	12.0 (7.5–18.7)	0.966
Hospital admission [n (%)]	172 (91)	33 (89)	139 (92)	0.818
Admission in ICU [n (%)]	52 (28)	14 (38)	38 (25)	0.181
Length of hospitalization (days)	9 (5–14)	5 (2–10)	10 (6–16)	<0.0001

Results are in mean ± SD, median (25th–75th percentile), or number (percentage)

* Between patients deceased and survival

[a] Mainly pulmonary and urinary concomitant bacterial infection

[b] Bacterial infection (ENT, blood stream infection from unknown origin)

[c] Non-bacterial infection (i.e., parasitic, fungic, or mycobacterium infection)

Analysis of subgroup in patients with available lactate measurement

When considering patients with available lactate measurement ($n = 103$), patients with PCT > 32.5 μg/L presented higher median lactate values (3.3 [1.9–4.3] mmol/L), in comparison with patients with lower PCT (2.1 [1.5–3.0] mmol/L, $p = 0.0347$).

When combining PCT and lactate log-transformed values, the ROC curve analysis indicated an AUC at 0.692 [95 % CI 0.594–0.780] for the prediction of 30-day mortality. This was significantly higher than PCT alone in this subgroup ($p = 0.020$). However, sensitivity (50 %) and specificity (96 %) were similar to those obtained with PCT alone. Alternatively, using the BLC method, we obtained the following combination: PCT (in μg/L) + 0.025 × lactate (in mmol/L). This combination gives a score for each patient and was tested in ROC analysis. Unfortunately, it failed to maximize ROC curve (AUC = 0.633 [0.533–0.726] vs. PCT alone, $p = 0.061$).

Patients with both PCT > 32.5 μg/L and lactate >2.2 mmol/L (i.e., above ROC thresholds) presented the worse outcome if considering death at day 30 ($p < 0.0001$)

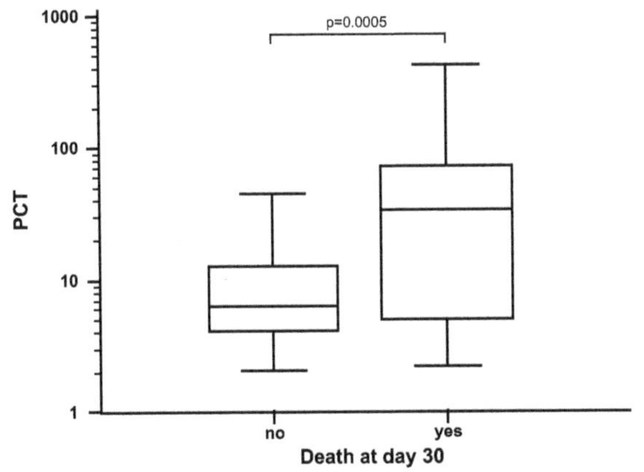

Fig. 1 PCT values according to 30-day mortality

(Fig. 4). Using these thresholds, a table of contingency was built (Table 2), and NRI was calculated. The NRI was 0.8 % ($p = 0.980$), indicating that patients were not significantly better identified as at risk of death using lactate on top of PCT alone.

When considering the prediction of death and/or admission in ICU, the combination of PCT and lactate indicated an AUC at 0.677 [95 % CI 0.578–0.765], which was significantly higher than PCT alone in this subgroup ($p = 0.012$). However, sensitivity (50 %) and specificity (73 %) were similar to those obtained with PCT alone.

Multivariate analysis

Multivariate analysis was performed on the entire study group and is presented in Table 3. Three variables remained independently and significantly predictive of death at day 30: previous history of cardiovascular disease, the presence of severe sepsis/septic shock, and a PCT > 32.5 μg/L, which remained the strongest predictor of death. If considering prediction of death and/or admission to ICU, a PCT value >32.5 μg/L also remained the strongest independent and significant predictor, with an OR value at 6.4 [2.3–17.9] ($p = 0.0004$), with the presence of severe sepsis/septic shock (OR 4.4 [2.2–8.9]).

If considering prediction of death and/or admission to ICU, the PCT + lactate score remained the only independent and significant predictor of death, with an OR value at 6.0 [95 % CI 1.3–28.5] ($p = 0.024$).

Discussion

We aimed to evaluate in the emergency setting the prognostic value of PCT in septic patients. Our results demonstrated that PCT is a potential tool by itself for early identification of ED septic patients with poor outcome (death at day 30). However, its prognostic accuracy is not useful enough, to be used in daily practice.

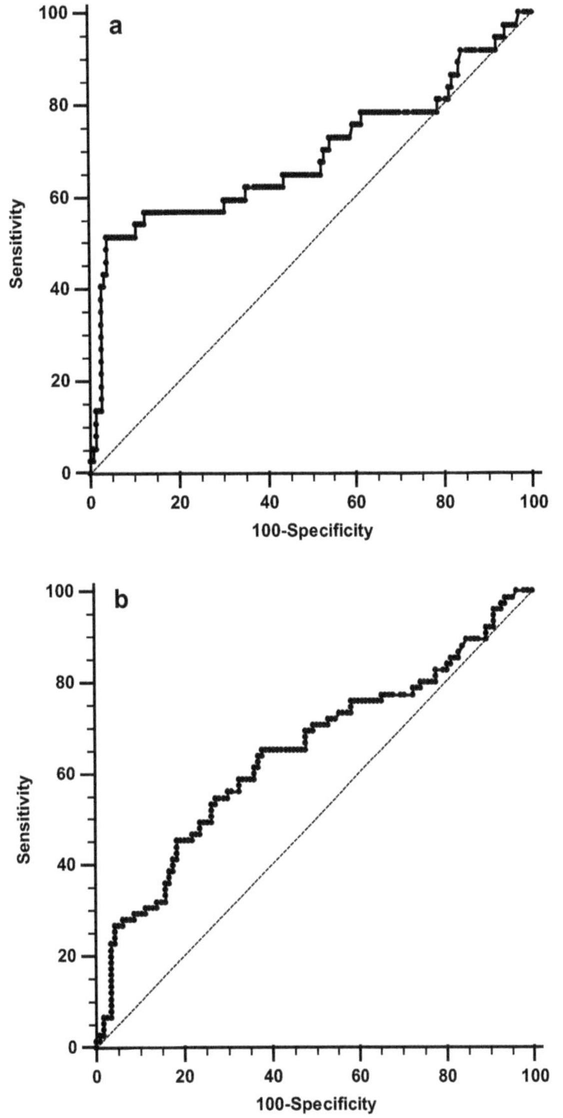

Fig. 2 AUC of PCT to predict 30-day mortality (**a**) or to predict death and/or admission in ICU (**b**)

A recent meta-analysis indicated that elevated PCT concentrations are associated with all-cause mortality in septic patients. However, studies are still lacking to define the optimal cutoff point, especially in ED patients [1]. This previous meta-analysis pointed out the heterogeneity of the results observed in the studies. In the specific field of ED patients, there are few studies that report association of PCT level with mortality [15–17]. Authors present heterogeneity in methodologies (fully automated or semiquantitative assays), in reported cutoffs (from 0.9 to 10 μg/L), and in testing time (day 0, 1 or 5). In addition to these data, the study of Freund et al. [3] indicated, with another fully automated method for PCT (Kryptor

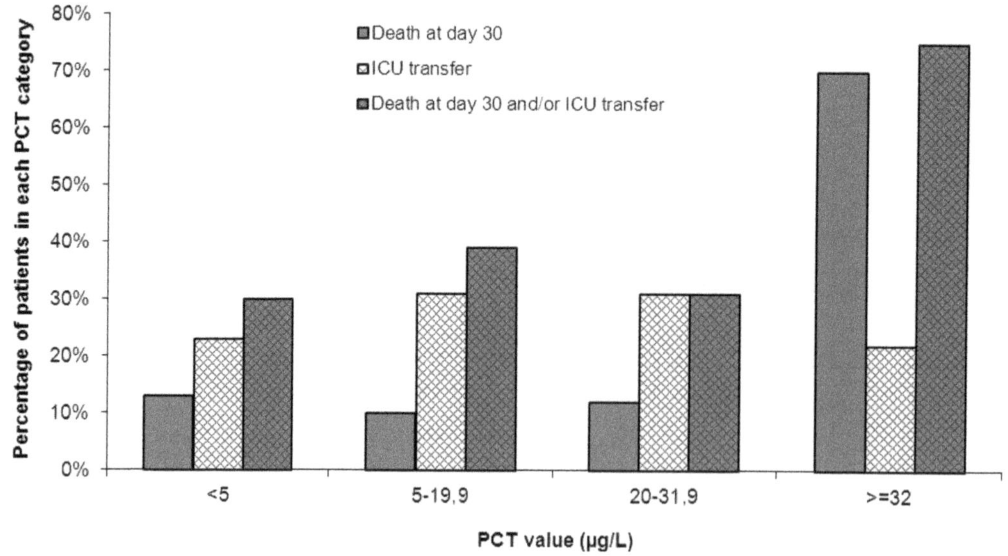

Fig. 3 Outcomes (30-day mortality and/or combination of ICU transfer) according to levels of PCT

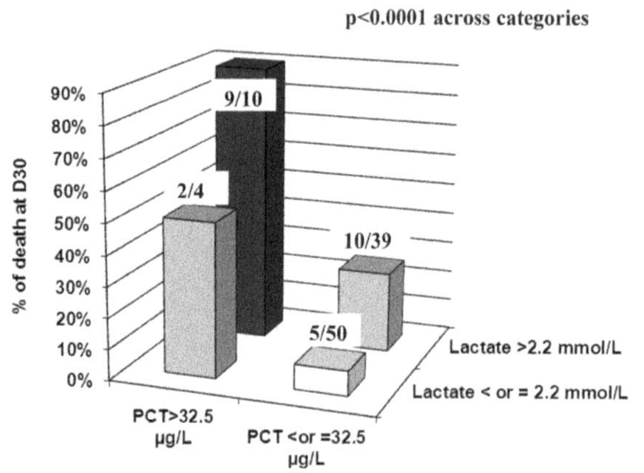

Fig. 4 Outcome according to PCT and lactate thresholds. PCT and lactate thresholds were given by ROC analysis. *Ratio* indicates number of deceased patient at day 30 over number of patients in each category

Brahms), a cutoff at 0.8 µg/L for identification of severe outcome in the ED. Thus, relationship between PCT and prognosis required further study.

To our knowledge, our study is the first to focus on patients with high-PCT values (above 2 µg/L) in emergency septic patients. Our results suggest a moderate relation between PCT level and outcome, in the specific population of septic patients with high PCT. As expected, we find a higher cutoff than previous studies performed in ED [3, 15–17], but we also had a better specificity. In terms of patients' recruitment, our results should be compared to those of Hur et al. [7] who investigated the diagnostic and prognostic utility of PCT in critically ill patients with suspected sepsis in ED and ICU, for whom sepsis was diagnosed clinically or on PCT concentrations. Thus, our results are in accordance with those of Hur et al. [7], as we found similar PCT values in non-survivors (mean PCT at admission around 32 µg/L).

When considering our ROC curve analysis for death prediction, our results are similar to those of Zhao et al. [18] and to those of Wang et al. [19], but with a higher cutoff. In our population, we observe similar performances with the solely PCT, in comparison with that of Zhao when using MEDS score +PCT [18], or to that of Wang using PCT alone [19]. Wang et al. [19] found a 28-day mortality cutoff at 4.3 µg/L, which is lower than ours, but they included both septic patients and SIRS patients without infection. MEDS score has been suggested as a score system with high ability to predict the 28-day outcome of ED patients with systemic inflammatory response syndrome (SIRS), sepsis, or severe sepsis [20–22]. However, some studies indicated that MEDS score is not suitable for patients with severe sepsis or septic shock [23, 24].

We found that PCT is a moderate predictor of 30-day mortality but also for the prediction of death and/or admission in ICU in confirmed septic ED patients. Our results are in accordance with most of the previous studies [4, 7, 15–18]. However, some studies also failed to demonstrate any prognostic value of PCT [19]. In our septic population, the PCT value for predicting 30-day mortality is higher (32.5 vs 4.3 µg/L), with a better specificity (96 vs 84 %) than previously observed [19]. However, this strategy allows to target a small number of patients in our population ($n = 19$ deceased patients with

Table 2 Net reclassification table of patients according to PCT and lactate values

	Death at 30 days (*n*)	Alive (*n*)	Total (*n*)
PCT>32.5 μg/L / PCT and/or lactate above threshold[a]	11 / 21	3 / 32	14 / 53
PCT<32.5 μg/L / PCT and lactate below thresholds[a]	15 / 5	74 / 45	89 / 50
Total	26	77	103

NB. This is the practical representation of both the relationship between false positive and false negative (gray zones), and the magnitude of the gain of predictability in quantitative terms (number of patients): here, the strategy PCT + lactates provokes a decrease in false negative (from 15 to 5) but a concomitant increase in false positives (from 3 to 32). The consequence is that sensitivity is improved (from 11/26 = 42.3 % to 21/26 = 80.8 %), but consequently specificity is dramatically decreased (from 74/77 = 96.1 % to 45/77 = 58.4 %)

Thus, the NRI calculation is: NRI = (80.8 + 58.4) − (42.3 + 96.1) = 0.8 %

[a] 32.5 μg/L for PCT, 2.2 mmol/L for lactate

Table 3 Univariate and multivariate analysis for independent prediction of death at 30 days

	Univariate analysis OR [95 % CI]	*p*	Multivariate analysis OR [95 % CI]	*p*
Age	1.04 [1.01–1.06]	0.0015	/	
Heart rate	1.02 [1.00–1.03]	0.047	/	
Personal history of:				
Cardiovascular diseases	2.5 [1.1–5.7]	0.024	3.1 [1.0–9.4]	0.0462
Respiratory disease	2.4 [1.05–5.2]	0.036	/	
"Other" chronic diseases	0.4 [0.1–1.0]	0.052	/	
Severe sepsis/septic shock	2.3 [1.1–4.8]	0.027	4.0 [1.3–12.3]	0.0130
PCT > 32.5 μg/L	21.7 [8.0–58.8]	<0.0001	36.0 [10.0–128.4]	<0.0001

As data were partially collected for lactate and respiratory rate, these parameters could not be included in the analysis

a PCT above 32.5 μg/L, corresponding to 51 % of the deceased patients but only 10 % of the whole study population), and thus the interest of its use in routine might be limited.

Furthermore, when considering the ROC curve analysis for the prediction of death and/or admission in ICU, prognostic performances were lower, and we did not find any significant difference in PCT values between patients admitted to ICU versus the others. This latest observation was somehow expected as many other factors (such as comorbidities including dementia, functional status, and bed availability…) are used in the decision to admit a patient in ICU. The weight of biological (as PCT) or physiological data is probably relatively low compared to other variables in the decision of ICU transfer, as reflected by our Fig. 3.

In our subgroup analysis, we did not observe any additional performance when combining lactate to PCT, for the prediction of 30-day mortality or for the prediction of death and/or admission in ICU. This is not in accordance with results obtained by Freund et al. [3], who—in a larger sample of ED patients—considered a combined outcome (death and/or ICU admission and/or terminal patients with therapy limitations). However, our patients with both PCT > 32.5 µg/L and lactate >2.2 mmol/L presented the worst outcome, which suggests the potential complementary role of both biomarkers in identifying very high-risk patients. Unfortunately, using NRI and BLC methods, we failed in finding strong additional information in the association PCT + lactate. This might be because of the small subgroup number of patients and should be specifically investigated in a larger cohort.

Limitations

Some limitations merit consideration in this study. Firstly, this is a bicentric retrospective, non-blind study, including a somehow limited number of patients. Secondly, we did not use severity score systems (MEDS, SOFA, etc.) to compare with, or in addition to PCT. Thirdly, the dynamic changes in biomarkers were not evaluated. Fourthly, we do not have data on previous antibiotherapy or antibiotics given in the ER or after. Thus, we do not have information on their adequacy. Fifthly, lactate was not measured systematically to all patients. Therefore, this variable could not be fully investigated and included in our multivariate analysis. Finally, two different methods were used to assay PCT. However, the two methods are known to be highly correlated [11, 12], and a minimal bias was observed in our population.

Conclusion

Elevated value of PCT at admission has moderate accuracy to identify poor outcome in ED septic patients. We suggest that the measurement of PCT in ED septic patients should not be routinely performed to assess prognostic information, before other evaluation of its added value in further studies.

Authors' contributions

NP and PR designed the study and contributed substantially to patients' recruitment, analysis of data, and drafting the manuscript. CCG performed analysis of data and wrote the manuscript. LM, NP, RL, and VA contributed substantially to patients' recruitment and were actively involved in the acquisition of data. VB and GL performed measurements and contributed substantially to analysis and interpretation of data. All authors read and approved the final manuscript.

Author details

[1] Department of Emergency Medicine, Centre Hospitalo-universitaire de Rouen, 1 rue de Germont, 76000 Rouen, France. [2] Department of Automated Biological Diagnosis, Hôpitaux Universitaires Paris Centre (HUPC) – Hôpital Cochin, Assistance Publique des Hôpitaux de Paris (AP-HP), Paris, France. [3] Department of Emergency Medicine, Hôpitaux Universitaires Est Parisien - Hôpital Tenon, Assistance Publique des Hôpitaux de Paris (AP-HP), 4 rue de la Chine, 75020 Paris, France. [4] Department of Biochemistry and Hormonology, Hôpitaux Universitaires Est Parisien - Hôpital Tenon, Assistance Publique des Hôpitaux de Paris (AP-HP), 4 rue de la Chine, 75020 Paris, France. [5] Department of Biochemistry, Clinical Biology Institut, Centre Hospitalo-universitaire de Rouen, 1 rue de Germont, 76000 Rouen, France. [6] Sorbonne Universités UMPC Université Paris 06, DHU Fighting Aging and Stress (FAST), Paris, France.

Competing interests

The authors declare that they have no competing interests.

References

1. Liu D, Su L, Han G, Yan P, Xie L. Prognostic value of procalcitonin in adult patients with sepsis: a systematic review and meta-analysis. PLoS One. 2015;5(10):e0129450.
2. Dellinger RP, Levy MM, Rhodes A, Annane D, Gerlach H, Opal SM, et al. Surviving sepsis campaign: international guidelines for management of severe sepsis and septic shock: 2012. Crit Care Med. 2013;41:580–637.
3. Freund Y, Delerme S, Goulet H, Bernard M, Riou B, Hausfater P. Serum lactate and procalcitonin measurements in emergency room for the diagnosis and risk-stratification of patients with suspected infection. Biomarkers. 2012;17:590–6.
4. Hausfater P, Juillien G, Madonna-Py B, Haroche J, Bernard M, Riou B. Serum procalcitonin measurement as diagnostic and prognostic marker in febrile adult patients presenting to the emergency department. Crit Care. 2007;11:R60.
5. Huang DT, Weissfeld LA, Kellum JA, Yealy DM, Kong L, Martino M, et al. Risk prediction with procalcitonin and clinical rules in community-acquired pneumonia. Ann Emerg Med. 2008;52:48–58.
6. Garnacho-Montero J, Huici-Moreno MJ, Gutiérrez-Pizarraya A, López I, Márquez-Vácaro JA, Macher H, et al. Prognostic and diagnostic value of eosinopenia, C-reactive protein, procalcitonin, and circulating cell-free DNA in critically ill patients admitted with suspicion of sepsis. Crit Care. 2014;18:R116.
7. Hur M, Kim H, Lee S, Cristofano F, Magrini L, Marino R, et al. Diagnostic and prognostic utilities of multimarkers approach using procalcitonin, B-type natriuretic peptide, and neutrophil gelatinase-associated lipocalin in critically ill patients with suspected sepsis. BMC Infect Dis. 2014;14:224.
8. Meisner M. Procalcitonin—biochemistry and clinical diagnosis. 1st ed. Bremen: UNI-MED; 2010.
9. Levy MM, Fink MP, Marshall JC, Abraham E, Angus D, Cook D, et al. 2001 SCCM/ESICM/ACCP/ATS/SIS international sepsis definitions conference. Intensive Care Med. 2003;29:530–8.
10. Singer M, Deutschman CS, Seymour CW, Shankar-Hari M, Annane D, Bauer M, et al. The Third International Consensus definitions for sepsis and septic shock (Sepsis-3). JAMA. 2016;315(8):801–10.
11. de Wolf HK, Gunnewiek JK, Berk Y, van den Ouweland J, de Metz M. Comparison of a new procalcitonin assay from roche with the established method on the brahms kryptor. Clin Chem. 2009;55:1043–4.
12. Dipalo M, Guido L, Micca G, Pittalis S, Locatelli M, Motta A, et al. Multicenter comparison of automated procalcitonin immunoassays. Pract Lab Med. 2015;2:2–28.
13. Ray P, Le Manach Y, Riou B, Houle TT. Statistical evaluation of a biomarker. Anesthesiology. 2010;112:1023–40.
14. Su JQ, Liu JS. Linear combinations of multiple diagnostic markers. J Am Stat Assoc. 1993;88:1350–5.
15. Yin Q, Liu B, Chen Y, Zhao Y, Li C. The role of soluble thrombomodulin in the risk stratification and prognosis evaluation of septic patients in the emergency department. Thromb Res. 2013;132:471–6.
16. Magrini L, Travaglino F, Marino R, Ferri E, De Berardinis B, Cardelli P, et al. Procalcitonin variations after Emergency Department admission are highly predictive of hospital mortality in patients with acute infectious diseases. Eur Rev Med Pharmacol Sci. 2013;17:133–42.
17. Kenzaka T, Okayama M, Kuroki S, Fukui M, Yahata S, Hayashi H, et al. Use of a semiquantitative procalcitonin kit for evaluating severity and predicting mortality in patients with sepsis. Int J Gen Med. 2012;5:483–8.
18. Zhao Y, Li C, Jia Y. Evaluation of the Mortality in Emergency Department Sepsis score combined with procalcitonin in septic patients. Am J Emerg Med. 2013;31:1086–91.
19. Wang M, Zhang Q, Zhao X, Dong G, Li C. Diagnostic and prognostic value of neutrophil gelatinase-associated lipocalin, matrix metalloproteinase-9, and tissue inhibitor of matrix metalloproteinases-1 for sepsis in the Emergency Department: an observational study. Crit Care. 2014;18:634.
20. Sankoff JD, Goyal M, Gaieski DF, Deitch K, Davis CB, Sabel AL, et al. Validation of the Mortality in Emergency Department Sepsis (MEDS) score in

patients with the systemic inflammatory response syndrome (SIRS). Crit Care Med. 2008;36:421–6.
21. Lee CC, Chen SY, Tsai CL, Wu SC, Chiang WC, Wang JL, et al. Prognostic value of mortality in emergency department sepsis score, procalcitonin, and C-reactive protein in patients with sepsis at the emergency department. Shock. 2008;29:322–7.
22. Chen CC, Chong CF, Liu YL, Chen KC, Wang TL. Risk stratification of severe sepsis patients in the emergency department. Emerg Med J. 2006;23:281–5.
23. Jones AE, Saak K, Kline JA. Performance of the Mortality in Emergency Department Sepsis score for predicting hospital mortality among patients with severe sepsis and septic shock. Am J Emerg Med. 2008;26:689–92.
24. Nguyen HB, Banta JE, Cho TW, Van Ginkel C, Burroughs K, Wittlake WA, et al. Mortality predictions using current physiologic scoring systems in patients meeting criteria for early goal-directed therapy and the severe sepsis resuscitation bundle. Shock. 2008;30:23–8.

2

Erythrocyte superoxide dismutase as a biomarker of septic acute kidney injury

Nara Aline Costa[1], Ana Lúcia Gut[1], Paula Schmidt Azevedo[1], Suzana Erico Tanni[1], Natália Baraldi Cunha[1], Eloá Siqueira Magalhães[1], Graziela Biude Silva[2], Bertha Furlan Polegato[1], Leonardo Antonio Mamede Zornoff[1], Sergio Alberto Rupp de Paiva[1], André Luís Balbi[1], Daniela Ponce[1] and Marcos Ferreira Minicucci[1*]

Abstract

Background: Oxidative stress is a key feature of sepsis and could be a common pathophysiological pathway between septic shock and acute kidney injury (AKI) Our objective was to evaluate the erythrocyte superoxide dismutase (SOD1) activity as predictor of AKI in patients with septic shock.

Methods: This is a prospective observational study that evaluated 175 consecutive patients over the age of 18 years with septic shock upon intensive care unit (ICU) admission. However, 43 patients were excluded (27 due to AKI at ICU admission). Thus, 132 patients were enrolled in the study. At the time of the patients' enrollment, demographic information was recorded. Blood samples were taken within the first 24 h of the patient's admission to determine the erythrocyte SOD1 activity. All patients were followed throughout the ICU stay, and the development of AKI was evaluated. In addition, we also evaluated 17 control subjects.

Results: The mean age of patients with septic shock was 63.2 ± 15.7 years, 53 % were male and the median ICU stay was 8 days (4–16). Approximately 50.7 % developed AKI during the ICU stay. The median erythrocyte SOD1 activity was 2.92 (2.19–3.92) U/mg Hb. When compared to control subjects, septic shock patients had a higher serum malondialdehyde concentration and lower erythrocyte SOD1 activity. In univariate analysis, erythrocyte SOD1 activity was lower in patients who developed AKI. The ROC curve analysis revealed that lower erythrocyte SOD1 activity was associated with AKI development (AUC 0.686; CI 95 % 0.595–0.777; $p < 0.001$) at the cutoff of <3.32 U/mg Hb. In the logistic regression models, SOD1 activity higher than 3.32 U/mg Hb was associated with protection of AKI development when adjusted by hemoglobin, phosphorus and APACHE II score (OR 0.309; CI 95 % 0.137–0.695; $p = 0.005$) and when adjusted by age, gender, chronic kidney disease, admission category (medical or surgery) and APACHE II score (OR 0.129; CI 95 % 0.033–0.508; $p = 0.003$).

Conclusions: In conclusion, our data suggest that erythrocyte SOD1 activity could play a role as an early marker of septic AKI and could be seen as a new research avenue in the field of biomarker in AKI. However, our study did not show a strong correlation between SOD activity and AKI. Nevertheless, these original data do warrant further research in order to confirm or not this hypothesis.

Keywords: Superoxide dismutase, Acute kidney injury, Sepsis, Oxidative stress

Background

Acute kidney injury (AKI) is one of the most serious and frequent complications of sepsis in critically ill patients [1]. It is estimated that AKI develops within the first 24 h in 51–64 % of patients with sepsis with hypotension [2]. Septic shock is the major cause of death in the intensive care unit (ICU), and the presence of AKI in these patients leads to an increase in mortality [3].

The diagnosis of AKI is usually based on either an elevation of serum creatinine or the detection of oliguria [4]. However, these tests have limited sensitivity and

*Correspondence: minicucci@fmb.unesp.br
[1] Department of Internal Medicine, Botucatu Medical School, UNESP – Univ Estadual Paulista, Rubião Júnior s/n, Botucatu, SP CEP: 18618-970, Brazil
Full list of author information is available at the end of the article

specificity for the detection of renal dysfunction [5]. In this way, the development of biomarkers for the early detection of AKI is a research priority [6]. Some AKI markers are currently being intensely studied in several different clinical situations, mainly in critically ill patients [7–11]. However, some of these markers could be influenced by systemic inflammation and infections, and early AKI predictors in patients with sepsis are still lacking.

A barrier to uncovering new specific biomarkers for sepsis-induced AKI is a lack of understanding of its pathophysiology. It is known that the oxidative stress caused by sepsis is one factor responsible for its development [12, 13]. Oxidative stress is regulated by a balance between the rates of reactive oxygen species (ROS) generation and antioxidant systems, including superoxide dismutase (SOD), catalase, glutathione peroxidase, thioredoxin and vitamins [14]. SOD is considered to be the first line of defense against ROS because it catalyzes the dismutation of superoxide radicals to a less reactive product, hydrogen peroxide. Increased ROS production or an impaired antioxidant system will lead to oxidative damage to proteins, lipids and DNA. There is no ideal marker for oxidative stress; however, with regard to lipid peroxidation, malondialdehyde (MDA) is one of the most commonly used markers for the determination of oxidative stress in humans [15].

Experimental and clinical studies of chronic kidney disease showed that SOD levels were reduced and markers of oxidative damage were increased in this scenario [16–18]. In addition, strategies to increase SOD activity with recombinant SOD molecules and gene transfer led to reduced inflammation and oxidative stress in experimental models of ischemia–reperfusion and contrast-induced AKI [19–21]. It is also interesting to observe that in patients submitted to kidney transplantation, MDA levels were predictors of graft dysfunction [22, 23]. Despite the importance of oxidative stress, SOD1 activity has not yet been evaluated as predictor of AKI in patients with septic shock.

Therefore, the aim of our study was to evaluate the erythrocyte SOD1 activity as predictor of AKI in patients with septic shock.

Methods

This prospective observational study was conducted from May 2014 to June 2015 with patients admitted to the intensive care unit of our hospital. The protocol was approved by the ethics committee of our institution (30457414.7.0000.5411). Written informed consent was obtained from all patients or relatives prior to their inclusion in the study.

This study was a subanalysis of a larger unpublished study, which evaluated the relationship between oxidative stress and mortality in patients with septic shock. The sample size was calculated using the Fisher and Belle formula, with the following variables: mortality rate of septic shock 40–60 %, 95 % confidence interval and 10 % sample error. The result was a minimum sample size of 96 patients.

Patients were eligible for enrollment if they were 18 years or older and had septic shock on ICU admission. Exclusion criteria were patients with AKI at ICU admission, patients with stage 4 or 5 chronic kidney disease (CKD) (creatinine clearance lower than 30 mL/min/1.73 m^2), a delay in septic shock diagnosis (longer than 24 h), pregnant women, patients with confirmed brain death, patients in palliative care, and those who used vasoactive drugs for <24 h.

At the time of the patients' enrollment, demographic information, the Acute Physiology and Chronic Health Evaluation (APACHE II) score and the Sequential Organ Failure Assessment (SOFA) score were recorded. Blood samples were taken within the first 24 h of the patient's admission, after hemodynamic stabilization, to determine the erythrocyte SOD1 activity. All patients were followed during their ICU stay, and the development of AKI was evaluated. Mortality rate and the length of the ICU stay were also recorded.

Septic shock was defined according to Survival Sepsis guidelines [24], and AKI was defined according to Kidney Disease Improving Global Outcomes (KDIGO) criteria, using the increase in serum creatinine $\geq$0.3 mg/dL within 48 h or increase in serum creatinine $\geq$1.5 times baseline within 7 days [25]. Classification of AKI remains challenging because serum creatinine measurements, before the inciting illness, are often missing. In the absence of a standard method to accommodate missing values, investigators have used a variety of surrogate measures. One of these methods is to use the baseline creatinine as the lowest creatinine value in the last 6 months before AKI or, for those without this measurement, the lowest value achieved during hospitalization in the absence of dialysis [26, 27]. This was the definition we used of baseline creatinine in our study. CKD was defined as glomerular filtration rate lower than 60 mL/min/1.73 m^2 using baseline creatinine and CKD Epidemiology Collaboration equation (CKD-EPI) (GFR $= 141 \times \min(Scr/\kappa, 1)\alpha \times \max(Scr/\kappa, 1) - 1.209 \times 0.993$ Age $\times$ 1.018 [if female] _ 1.159 [if black], where Scr is serum creatinine, κ is 0.7 for females and 0.9 for males, α is -0.329 for females and -0.411 for males, min indicates the minimum of Scr/κ or 1, and max indicates the maximum of Scr/κ or 1) [28].

To understand the behavior of erythrocyte SOD1 activity in our patients with septic shock, we also evaluated these variables in 17 control subjects (non-hospitalized individuals without any acute disease).

Laboratorial analysis

Total serum levels of sodium, potassium, phosphorus, C-reactive protein (CRP), albumin, creatinine and urea were measured using the dry chemistry method (Ortho-Clinical Diagnostics VITROS 950®, Johnson & Johnson), and lactate was measured using a Roche OMNI® S Blood Gas Analyzer. Hemograms were performed with a Coulter STKS hematologic autoanalyzer (Luton/Bedfordshire, UK).

Serum MDA concentration

Serum MDA levels were analyzed based on the reaction with thiobarbituric acid by high-performance liquid chromatography (HPLC) according to a method developed by Katepe [29]. UV detection was performed at 532 nm.

Erythrocyte SOD1 activity

The SOD enzyme activity in erythrocytes was determined in a Lyasis biochemical analyzer according to methodology recommended by the manufacturer (Ransod kit; Randox Laboratories Ltd., Crumlin, Antrim, UK) [30].

Statistical analysis

Data are expressed as the mean ± SD, the median (including the lower and upper quartiles) or percentage. Comparisons between two groups for continuous variables were made using Student's t test or the Mann–Whitney U test. Comparisons between two groups for categorical variables were made using the χ^2 test or Fisher's exact test. Comparisons between continuous variables were made using Spearman correlation test. Receiver operating characteristic (ROC) curve analysis was performed to determine the performance of erythrocyte SOD1 activity to predict AKI development. A logistic regression model was used to predict AKI. We constructed two regression models. Erythrocyte SOD1 activity was tested as a categorical variable (>3.32 U/mg Hb, cutoff obtained by ROC curve). In the first model, erythrocyte SOD1 activity was adjusted with parameters that exhibited significant differences in the univariate analysis. The only exceptions were variables with high collinearity among them (urea, creatinine, potassium, MDA, CKD and SOFA score). In the other, SOD1 was adjusted by age, gender, CKD, admission category (medical or surgery) and APACHE II score. Data analysis was performed using SigmaPlot software for Windows v12.0 (Systat Software Inc., San Jose, CA, USA). p values lower than 0.05 were considered statistically significant.

Results

During the study, 175 consecutive patients were admitted with a diagnosis of septic shock in the ICU; however, 43 patients were excluded (presence of AKI at ICU admission: 27 patients; delay in septic shock diagnosis: 12 patients; presence of advanced chronic kidney disease: 4 patients). Thus, we evaluated 132 patients (Fig. 1). The mean age was 63.2 ± 15.7 years, 53 % were male and the median length of ICU stay was 8 days (4–16). The mortality rate during the ICU stay was 65.9 %. Median erythrocyte SOD1 activity was 2.92 (2.19–3.92) U/mg Hb.

Among those patients with septic shock, 50.7 % developed AKI during the ICU stay. We have baseline serum creatinine levels in 37 patients of 67 patients who developed AKI, and in 30 patients, we used the lowest value achieved during hospitalization in the absence of dialysis. Regarding KDIGO stages, 17.9 % were classified as KDIGO 1, 19.4 % as KDIGO 2 and 62.7 % as KDIGO 3. The median time for AKI diagnosis based on KDIGO criteria was 2.3 days after admission. Among patients who developed AKI, 24.5 % needed dialysis during the ICU stay. The APACHE II and SOFA scores were also higher in patients in the AKI group. The mortality rate increased more than 30 % in patients with AKI. There were no differences between groups in the other demographic and clinical data (Table 1).

The laboratory data are presented in Table 2. Patients who developed AKI had higher levels of potassium, phosphorus, MDA, urea and creatinine and lower levels of hemoglobin at baseline than patients without renal injury.

Erythrocyte SOD1 activity was lower in patients who developed AKI [non-AKI: 3.62 (2.59–4.34) vs AKI: 2.62 (2.02–3.63) U/mg Hb; $p = 0.001$; Fig. 2]. It is also important to observe that, although creatinine levels at ICU admission were higher in patients who developed AKI during ICU stay, erythrocyte SOD1 activity was not correlated with serum creatinine at ICU admission (Fig. 3). Our patients with septic shock had higher levels of serum MDA concentration [septic shock (n:132): 1.43 (0.77–2.19) μmol/L; controls (n:17): 0.86 (0.49–1.07) μmol/L; $p = 0.003$] and lower erythrocyte SOD1 activity [septic shock (n:132): 2.92 (2.19–3.92) U/mg Hb; controls (n:17): 4.35 (3.32–4.68) U/mg Hb; $p = 0.001$] when compared to control subjects.

The ROC curve analysis revealed that lower erythrocyte SOD1 activity was associated with AKI development (AUC 0.686; CI 95 % 0.595–0.777; $p < 0.001$) at the cut-off of <3.32 U/mg Hb [sensibility: 68.7 % (CI 95 % 57.6–79.8 %); specificity: 55.4 % (CI 95 % 43.3–67.5 %); positive predictive value: 61.3 % (CI 95 % 50.3–72.3 %); negative predictive value: 63.2 % (CI 95 % 50.7–75.7 %)] (Table 3; Fig. 4).

In the logistic regression models, SOD1 activity higher than 3.32 U/mg Hb was associated with protection of AKI development when adjusted by hemoglobin, phosphorus and APACHE II score (OR 0.309; CI 95 %

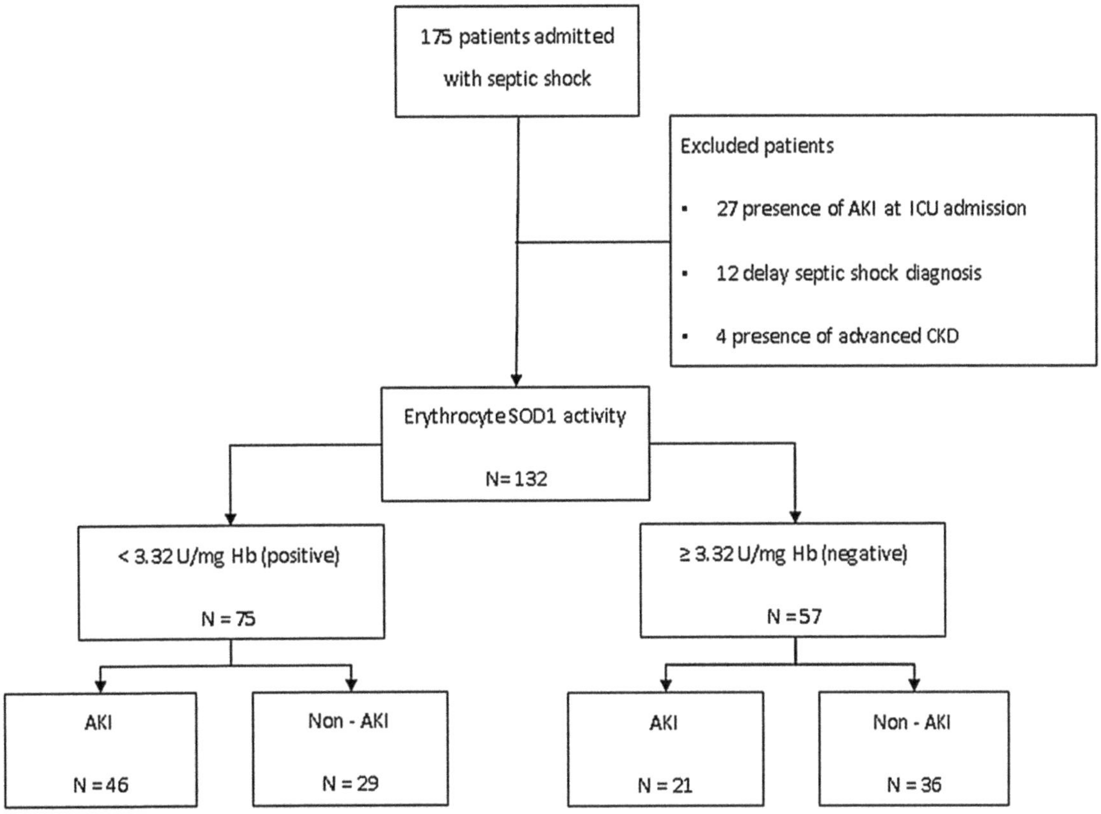

Fig. 1 Flow diagram of studied patients with septic shock

0.137–0.695; $p = 0.005$) and when adjusted by age, gender, CKD, admission category (medical or surgery) and APACHE II (OR 0.129; CI 95 % 0.033–0.508; $p = 0.003$; Table 4).

Discussion

The objective of our study was to evaluate the erythrocyte SOD1 activity as marker of AKI in patients with septic shock. Although our study is a preliminary data, it showed for the first time in septic shock patients that erythrocyte SOD1 activity plays a role as a biomarker of AKI.

Sepsis is defined as the presence (probable or documented) of infection together with a systemic inflammatory response [24]. Septic shock is defined as sepsis-induced hypotension that persists despite adequate fluid resuscitation [24]. Regardless of the creation of international guidelines for the early diagnosis and treatment of septic shock, its mortality remains high. This mortality rate is even higher when septic shock is associated with AKI. In our study, the mortality rate increased more than 30 % in patients with AKI. Thus, the early detection and treatment of patients who develop AKI are extremely important.

Several studies were performed in different clinical settings to identify biomarkers for AKI prediction, most of them in critically ill patients [5–8, 10, 11]. Until now, there have been four major categories of biomarkers for AKI in these patients: functional markers, such as serum creatinine; up-regulated proteins, such as NGAL and IL-18; low molecular weight proteins, such as urine cystatin C; and enzymes, such as alpha-glutathione *s*-transferase and pi-glutathione *s*-transferase [10]. Recently, the combination of urine tissue inhibitor of metalloproteinase 2 and insulin-like growth factor binding protein 7, known as TIMP-2 × IGFBP7, was allowed for marketing by the US Food and Drug Administration [11]. Up-regulation of these markers in patients with AKI has been proposed to reflect their growth-inhibitory function due to G1 cell-cycle arrest, a known consequence of AKI [11]. Despite all of these new markers, the prediction of AKI in patients with septic shock is still challenging. A barrier to uncovering new biomarkers for this scenario is a lack of understanding of the pathophysiology of sepsis-induced AKI [12, 13]. However, oxidative stress is a key feature of sepsis and could be a common pathophysiological pathway between septic shock and AKI [31].

Table 1 Demographic and clinical data of 132 patients with septic shock

Variable	Acute kidney injury		*p* value
	Yes (*n* = 67)	No (*n* = 65)	
Age (years)	67.0 (59.0–75.0)	64.0 (50.5–72.5)	0.20
Male, *n* (%)	35.0 (52.2)	35 (53.8)	0.99
APACHE II score	18.7 ± 6.0	16.0 ± 6.4	<0.001
SOFA score	10.0 (8.0–12.0)	8.0 (7.0–9.5)	<0.001
RBC transfusions, *n* (%)	36 (53.7)	29 (44.6)	0.38
Steroids, *n* (%)	38 (56.7)	30 (46.2)	0.30
Admission category, *n* (%)			
Medical	18 (26.9)	27 (41.5)	0.11
Surgery	49 (73.1)	38 (58.5)	
Sepsis focus, *n* (%)			0.46
Respiratory	42 (62.7)	34 (52.3)	
Abdominal	16 (23.8)	16 (24.6)	
Urinary	3 (4.5)	4 (6.2)	
Others	6 (9.0)	11 (16.9)	
Dialysis, *n* (%)	11 (16.4)	0 (0)	0.002
CKD, *n* (%)	57 (85.1)	7 (10.8)	<0.001
MV, *n* (%)	60 (89.6)	55 (84.6)	0.56
Length of ICU stay (days)	7.0 (5.0–15.0)	9.0 (4.0–16.5)	0.63
ICU mortality, *n* (%)	52.0 (77.6)	35.0 (53.8)	0.007

Data are expressed as the mean ± SD, median (including the lower and upper quartiles) or percentage

APACHE II Acute Physiology and Chronic Health Evaluation, *SOFA* Sequential Organ Failure Assessment, *RBC* red blood cells, *CKD* chronic kidney disease, *MV* mechanical ventilation, *ICU* intensive care unit

Table 2 Laboratory data of 132 patients with septic shock

Variable	Acute kidney injury		*p* value
	Yes (*n* = 67)	No (*n* = 65)	
Lactate (mmol/L)	2.2 (1.4–3.5)	2.1 (1.1–3.4)	0.78
Hemoglobin (g/dL)	11.0 (9.1–12.0)	11.6 (10.0–12.7)	0.025
Hematocrit (%)	32.0 ± 6.4	34.1 ± 5.7	0.06
Leukocytes ($10^3/mm^3$)	16.6 (12.2–21.6)	16.3 (12.2–24.0)	0.89
Sodium (mmol/L)	145 (140–149)	141 (137–148)	0.21
Potassium (mmol/L)	4.5 ± 0.9	4.1 ± 0.7	0.013
Phosphorus (mg/dL)	4.7 (3.4–6.6)	3.9 (2.7–4.9)	0.004
Glycemia (mg/dL)	145 (118–186)	146 (115–184)	0.87
CRP (mg/dL)	36.0 (28.0–44.1)	32.0 (8.5–41.5)	0.07
MDA (μmol/L)	1.65 (1.02–2.52)	1.25 (0.60–2.01)	0.009
Albumin (g/dL)	2.3 (2.0–2.5)	2.1 (1.8–2.8)	0.61
Urea (mg/dL)	95 (67–159)	53 (32–86)	<0.001
Creatinine (mg/dL)	2.1 (1.6–2.6)	0.7 (0.5–1.1)	<0.001

Data are expressed as median (including the lower and upper quartiles)

CRP C-reactive protein

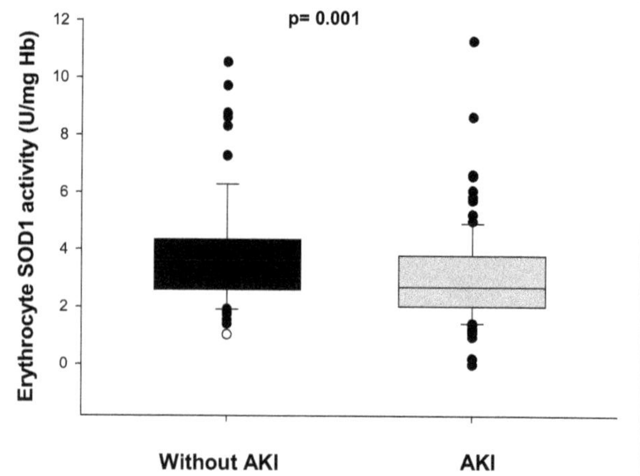

Fig. 2 Erythrocyte SOD1 activity in patients with septic shock

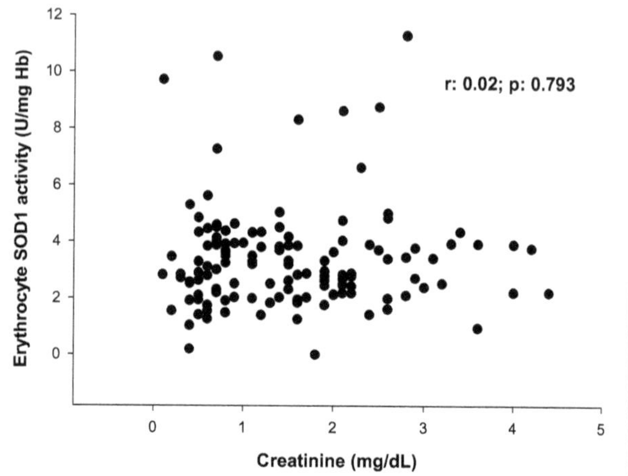

Fig. 3 Correlation of serum creatinine at ICU admission with erythrocyte SOD1 activity

Table 3 Cross-tabulation of erythrocyte SOD1 activity and acute kidney injury development

Erythrocyte SOD1 activity	Acute kidney injury		
	Yes	No	Total
<3.32 U/mg Hb (positive)	46	29	75
≥3.32 U/mg Hb (negative)	21	36	57
Total	67	65	132

Oxidative stress is characterized as an imbalance between ROS and antioxidant pathways, leading to oxidative damage to proteins, lipids and DNA. At the

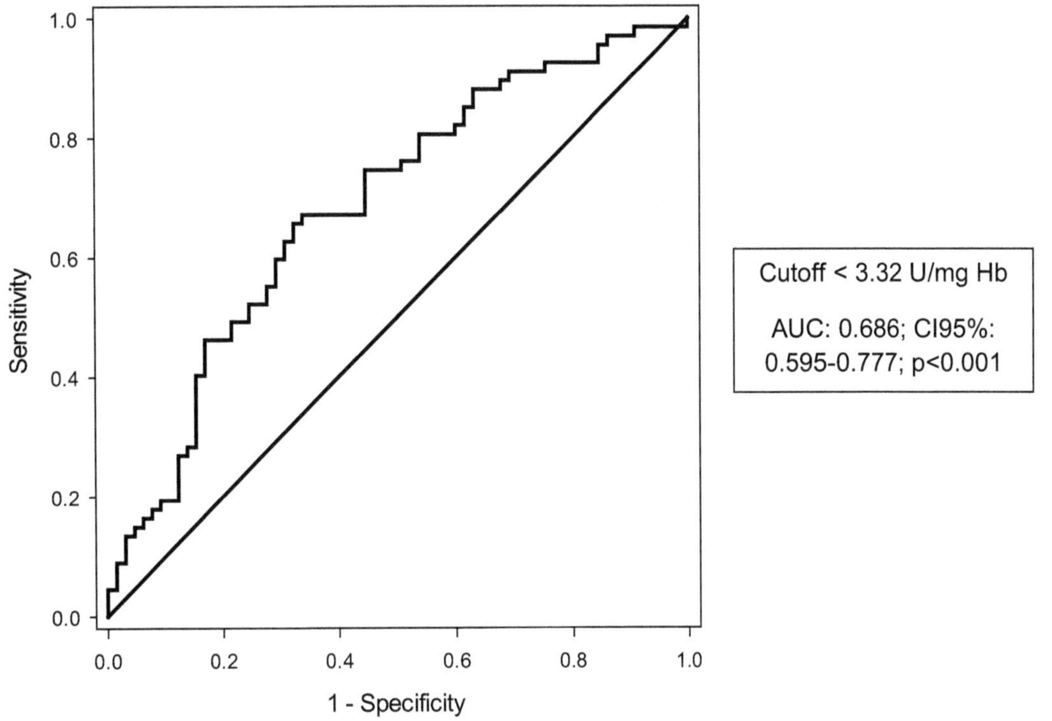

Fig. 4 ROC curve for the association between erythrocyte SOD1 activity and AKI development

Table 4 Logistic regression model for the prediction of acute kidney injury in 132 patients with septic shock

Variable	OR	IC 5–95 %	*p* value
SOD1 >3.32 U/mg Hb[a]	0.326	0.158–0.671	0.002
SOD1 >3.32 U/mg Hb[b]	0.129	0.033–0.508	0.003
SOD1 >3.32 U/mg Hb[c]	0.309	0.137–0.695	0.005

[a] Unadjusted

[b] Adjusted by gender, age, chronic kidney disease, admission category and APACHE II score

[c] Adjusted by APACHE II, phosphorus and hemoglobin

nanomolar scale, ROS play an important role in physiological processes by functioning as a second messenger in signal transduction pathways [32]. However, at the micromolar scale, ROS is associated with oxidative injury [32]. SOD is considered the first line of defense against ROS, consisting of three isoenzymes: copper/zinc SOD (SOD1), which is localized in the cytosol, nucleus and intermembrane space of mitochondria; manganese SOD (SOD2), which occurs in the mitochondrial matrix; and extracellular SOD (SOD3) [33]. SOD1 is the most abundant member of the family of antioxidant enzymes, representing approximately 90 % of SODs [34].

Experimental studies showed that SOD concentration and activity are reduced in chronic kidney injury [17, 19–21]. Vaziri et al. showed that SOD concentration was reduced and nicotinamide adenine dinucleotide phosphate (NADPH) oxidase expression was increased in the kidneys of rats submitted to nephrectomy [17]. Additionally, in studies with recombinant SOD molecules and SOD gene transfer, the animals submitted to these interventions presented reduced inflammation and oxidative stress in experimental models of ischemia–reperfusion and contrast-induced AKI [19–21].

In a clinical study with 134 individuals, Magalhães et al. compared hemodialyzed patients with healthy controls and showed that the activity of SOD is reduced in patients with chronic renal failure undergoing hemodialysis [16]. In our study, the activity of erythrocyte SOD1 was also lower in patients who developed AKI. This association remains statistically significant, even after adjustments for confounding variables in multivariate regression analysis. It is also important to note that erythrocyte SOD1 activity was lower and serum MDA concentration was higher in septic shock patients compared to control subjects. Thus, our results suggest that patients with septic shock had an impaired SOD1 response and increased oxidative stress, and this behavior was more pronounced in patients who developed AKI. In addition, this lower SOD1 activity occurred in the first 24 h of ICU admission.

The AUC of erythrocyte SOD1 activity was only 0.686; however, comparisons of AUCs of several biomarkers for AKI prediction showed also a poor performance with a huge variation in its values [35, 36]. Thus, our data suggest that erythrocyte SOD1 activity could be used as an early predictive marker of AKI.

It is important to remember that patients with chronic kidney disease have an increased risk to develop AKI. This could explain why our patients who developed AKI had higher levels of creatinine at ICU admission. Despite that, there was no correlation between creatinine at ICU admission and erythrocyte SOD1 activity. Thus, our results were not influenced by the initial difference in kidney function.

Considering that the development of AKI in patients with sepsis is related to increased mortality, the identification of early biomarkers of renal injury is extremely important. Erythrocyte SOD1 activity was associated with AKI detection 2.3 days before the KDIGO criteria. Our results have important clinical implications because we were able to identify patients at risk of developing AKI earlier. Thus, patients at risk of AKI could be treated more aggressively, improving septic shock outcomes.

We should consider some limitations of this study. We only included patients from a single medical center. Regarding AKI definition, we only have baseline serum creatinine of 55 % of patients who developed AKI, for the others we used the lowest value achieved during hospitalization in the absence of dialysis. Moreover, AKI was defined based upon the serum creatinine levels and not urine output. In addition, due to the relatively small number of patients, analysis of SOD1 according to the stage of AKI was not performed. Timing of antibiotic dosing was also not recorded, and blood was taken within the first 24 h, which is a relatively large window. Finally, the AUC of erythrocyte SOD1 activity was only 0.686, and our study is a preliminary data with a limited internal and external validity. Despite these limitations, we strongly believe that our data contribute relevant knowledge regarding the roles of SOD as early predictor of AKI in patients with septic shock.

Conclusions

In conclusion, our data suggest that erythrocyte SOD1 activity could play a role as an early marker of septic AKI and could be seen as a new research avenue in the field of biomarker in AKI. However, our study did not show a strong correlation between SOD activity and AKI. Nevertheless, these original data do warrant further research in order to confirm or not this hypothesis.

Abbreviations

AKI: acute kidney injury; AKIN criteria: acute kidney injury network criteria; APACHE II score: Acute Physiology and Chronic Health Evaluation II score; CI 95 %: confidence interval 95 %; CKD: chronic kidney disease; CRP: C-reactive protein; GFR: glomerular filtration rate; HPLC: high-performance liquid chromatography; ICU: intensive care unit; MDA: malondialdehyde; NGAL: neutrophil gelatinase-associated lipocalin; OR: odds ratio; ROS: reactive oxygen species; Scr: serum creatinine; SOFA score: Sequential Organ Failure Assessment score; SOD1: superoxide dismutase 1.

Authors' contributions

PSA, NBC, ESM and BFB were involved in acquisition of subjects and data, analysis and interpretation of data, revising the article critically; SET, GBS and ALB were involved in laboratorial analysis, statistical analysis, interpretation of data, revising the article critically; NAC, SARP, MFM, LAMZ, ALG and DP were involved in study design, analysis and interpretation of data, and drafting the manuscript. All authors revised the article critically for important intellectual content and approved the final version of the manuscript. All authors read and approved the final manuscript.

Author details

[1] Department of Internal Medicine, Botucatu Medical School, UNESP – Univ Estadual Paulista, Rubião Júnior s/n, Botucatu, SP CEP: 18618-970, Brazil.
[2] Department of Food and Experimental Nutrition, Faculty of Pharmaceutical Science, University of São Paulo, São Paulo, SP, Brazil.

Competing interests

The authors declare that they have no competing interests.

Funding

This study was funded by the State of São Paulo Research Foundation (FAPESP—2014/17262-0) and by CAPES ("Coordenação de Aperfeiçoamento de Pessoal de Nível Superior").

References

1. Lafrance JP, Miller DR. Acute kidney injury associates with increased long-term mortality. J Am Soc Nephrol. 2010;21:345–52.
2. Murugan R, Karajala-Subramanyam V, Lee M, Yende S, Kong L, Carter M, et al. Acute kidney injury in non-severe pneumonia is associated with an increased immune response and lower survival. Kidney Int. 2010;77:527–35.
3. Singbartl K, Kellum JA. AKI in the ICU: definition, epidemiology, risk stratification, and outcomes. Kidney Int. 2012;81:819–25.
4. Mehta RL, Chertow GM. Acute renal failure definitions and classification: time for change? J Am Soc Nephrol. 2003;14:2178–87.
5. Bjornsson TD. Use of serum creatinine concentrations to determine renal function. Clin Pharmacokinet. 1979;4:200–22.
6. American society of nephrology. American society of nephrology renal research report. J Am Soc Nephrol. 2005;16:1886–903.
7. Herget-Rosenthal S, Marggraf G, Husing J, Göring F, Pietruck F, Janssen O, et al. Early detection of acute renal failure by serum cystatin C. Kidney Int. 2004;66:1115–22.
8. Mishra J, Dent C, Tarabishi R, Mitsnefes MM, Ma Q, Kelly C, et al. Neutrophil gelatinase-associated lipocalin (NGAL) as a biomarker for acute renal injury after cardiac surgery. Lancet. 2005;365:1231–8.
9. Nga HS, Medeiros P, Menezes P, Bridi R, Balbi A, Ponce D. Sepsis and AKI in clinical emergency room patients: the role of urinary NGAL. Biomed Res Int. 2015;2015:413751.
10. Geus HRH, Betjes MG, Bakker J. Biomarkers for prediction of acute kidney injury: a narrative review on current status and future challenges. Clin Kidney J. 2012;5:102–8.

11. Vijayan A, Faubel S, Askenazi DJ, Cerda J, Fissell WH, Heung M, et al. Clinical use of the urine biomarker [TIMP-2] × [IGFBP7] for acute kidney injury risk assessment. Am J Kidney Dis. 2016. doi:10.1053/j.ajkd.2015.12.033.
12. Gomez H, Ince C, De Backer D, Pickkers P, Payen D, Hotchkiss J, et al. A unified theory of sepsis-induced acute kidney injury: inflammation, microcirculatory dysfunction, bioenergetics and the tubular cell adaptation to injury. Shock. 2014;41:3–11.
13. Himmelfarb J, Mcmonagle E, Freedman S, Klenzak J, McMenamin E, Le P, et al. Oxidative stress is increased in critically ill patients with acute renal failure. J Am Soc Nephrol. 2004;15:2449–56.
14. Noda Y, Ota K, Shirasawa T, Shimizu T. Copper/zinc superoxide dismutase insufficiency impairs progesterone secretion and fertility in female mice. Biol Reprod. 2012;86:1–8.
15. Rodrigo R, Libuy M, Feliú F, Hasson D. Oxidative stress-related biomarkers in essential hypertension and ischemia-reperfusion myocardial damage. Dis Markers. 2013;35:773–90.
16. Noleto Magalhães RC, Guedes Borges de Araujo C, Batista de Sousa Lima V, Machado Moita Neto J, do Nascimento Nogueira N, do Nascimento Marreiro D. Nutritional status of zinc and activity superoxide dismutase in chronic renal patients undergoing hemodialysis. Nutr Hosp. 2011;26:1456–61.
17. Vaziri ND, Dicus M, Ho ND, Boroujerdi-Rad L, Sindhu RK. Oxidative stress and dysregulation of superoxide dismutase and NADPH oxidase in renal insufficiency. Kidney Int. 2003;63:179–85.
18. Scholze A, Krueger K, Diedrich M, Räth C, Torges A, Jankowski V, et al. Superoxide dismutase type 1 in monocytes of chronic kidney disease patients. Amino Acids. 2011;41:427–38.
19. Yin M, Wheeler MD, Connor HD, Zhong Z, Bunzendahl H, Dikalova A, et al. Cu/Zn-superoxide dismutase gene attenuates ischemia-reperfusion injury in the rat kidney. J Am Soc Nephrol. 2001;12:2691–700.
20. Mortensen J, Shames B, Johnson CP, Nilakantan V. MnTMPyP, a superoxide dismutase/catalase mimetic, decreases inflammatory indices in ischemic acute kidney injury. Inflamm Res. 2011;60:299–307.
21. Pisani A, Sabbatini M, Riccio E, Rossano R, Andreucci M, Capasso C, et al. Effect of a recombinant manganese superoxide dismutase on prevention of contrast-induced acute kidney injury. Clin Exp Nephrol. 2014;18:424–31.
22. Fonseca I, Reguengo H, Almeida M, Dias L, Martins LS, Pedroso S, et al. Oxidative stress in kidney transplantation: malondialdehyde is an early predictive marker of graft dysfunction. Transplantation. 2014;97:1058–65.
23. Fonseca I, Reguengo H, Oliveira JC, Martins LS, Malheiro J, Almeida M, et al. A triple-biomarker approach for the detection of delayed graft function after kidney transplantation using serum creatinine, cystatin C, and malondialdehyde. Clin Biochem. 2015;48:1033–8.
24. Dellinger RP, Levy MM, Rhodes A, Annane D, Gerlach H, Opal SM, et al. Surviving Sepsis Campaign: international guidelines for management of severe sepsis and septic shock: 2012. Crit Care Med. 2013;41:580–637.
25. Clinical Practice Guidelines for Acute Kidney Injury; 2012. http://www.kdigo.org/clinical_practice_guidelines/AKI.php.
26. Gammelager H, Christiansen CF, Johansen MB, Tønnesen E, Jespersen B, Sørensen HT. Five-year risk of end-stage renal disease among intensive care patients surviving dialysis-requiring acute kidney injury: a nationwide cohort study. Crit Care. 2013;17:R145.
27. Siew ED, Matheny ME, Ikizler TA, Lewis JB, Miller RA, Waitman LR, et al. Commonly used surrogates for baseline renal function affect the classification and prognosis of acute kidney injury. Kidney Int. 2010;77:536–42.
28. Levey AS, Stevens LA, Schmid CH, Zhang YL, Castro AF 3rd, Feldman HI, et al. A new equation to estimate glomerular filtration rate. Ann Intern Med. 2009;150:604–12.
29. Nielsen F, Mikkelsen BB, Nielsen JB, Andersen HR, Grandjean P. Plasma malondialdehyde as biomarker for oxidative stress: reference interval and effects of life-style factors. Clin Chem. 1997;43:1209–14.
30. Ferro FE, de Sousa Lima VB, Soares NR, de Sousa Almondes KG, Pires LV, Cozzolino SM, et al. Parameters of metabolic syndrome and its relationship with zincemia and activities of superoxide dismutase and glutathione peroxidase in obese women. Biol Trace Elem Res. 2011;143:787–93.
31. Costa NA, Gut AL, Pimentel JAC, Cozzolino SM, Azevedo PS, Fernandes AA, et al. Erythrocyte selenium concentration predicts intensive care unit and hospital mortality in patients with septic shock: a prospective observational study. Crit Care. 2014;18:R92.
32. Droge W. Free radicals in the physiological control of cell function. Physiol Rev. 2002;82:47–95.
33. Okado-Matsumoto A, Fridovich I. Subcellular distribution of superoxide dismutases (SOD) in rat liver: Cu, Zn-SOD in mitochondria. J Biol Chem. 2001;276:38388–93.
34. Noor R, Mittal S, Iqbal J. Superoxide dismutase—applications and relevance to human diseases. Med Sci Monit. 2002;8:RA210–5.
35. Lameire NH, Vanholder RC, Van Biesen WA. How to use biomarkers efficiently in acute kidney injury. Kidney Int. 2011;79:1047–50.
36. Metzger J, Kirsch T, Schiffer E, Ulger P, Mentes E, Brand K, et al. Urinary excretion of twenty peptides forms an early and accurate diagnostic pattern of acute kidney injury. Kidney Int. 2010;78:1252–62.

3

Impact of a high loading dose of amikacin in patients with severe sepsis or septic shock

Nicolas Allou[1*], Astrid Bouteau[2], Jérôme Allyn[1], Aurélie Snauwaert[2], Dorothée Valance[1], Julien Jabot[1], Bruno Bouchet[1], Richard Galliot[1], Laure Corradi[1], Philippe Montravers[2] and Pascal Augustin[2]

Abstract

Background: The therapeutic effect of aminoglycosides is highest and optimal when the peak plasma concentration (C_{max})/minimal inhibitory concentration (MIC) ratio is between 8 and 10. The French guidelines recommend to use high doses of aminoglycosides for empiric antibiotic therapy in patients suffering from severe sepsis or septic shock. In clinical practice, the recommended target is an amikacin C_{max} between 60 and 80 mg/L, which corresponds to approximately 8 times the MIC breakpoint, as defined by the European Committee on Antimicrobial Susceptibility Testing. The aim of this study was to assess the incidence and impact on mortality of an amikacin concentration between 60 and 80 mg/L in patients suffering from severe sepsis or septic shock.

Methods: This was a prospective observational cohort study conducted in two intensive care units (ICU). Patients receiving amikacin at a loading dose of 30 mg/kg for severe sepsis or septic shock were enrolled in the cohort. The target C_{max} for amikacin was between 60 and 80 mg/L, as recommended by French guidelines (i.e. C_{max}/MIC breakpoint = 8–10).

Results: Over the study period, the amikacin C_{max} was <60 mg/L, between 60 and 80 mg/L, and >80 mg/L in 20 (18.2%), 46 (41.8%) and 44 (40%) of the 110 selected patients, respectively. Mortality rate was 40, 28.3 and 56.8% in the groups of patients with $C_{max} < 60$ mg/L, 60 mg/L $< C_{max} <$ 80 mg/L and $C_{max} > 80$ mg/L, respectively. Following multivariate analysis, mortality rate was significantly lower in the group of patients with amikacin C_{max} between 60 and 80 mg/L than in the group of patients with amikacin $C_{max} > 80$ mg/L ($P = 0.004$). The multivariate analysis also revealed that the factors independently associated with a higher in-ICU mortality rate were age ($P = 0.02$) and norepinephrine dose ($P = 0.0001$).

Conclusions: With a loading dose of 30 mg/kg of amikacin, concentration was potentially suboptimal ($C_{max} < 60$ mg/L) in only 18.2% of patients. The pharmacodynamic target (60 mg/L $< C_{max} <$ 80 mg/L) recommended by French guidelines was reached in 41.8% of patients and was associated with reduced in-ICU mortality. But amikacin overexposure (i.e. $C_{max} > 80$ mg/L) was frequent and potentially associated with increased mortality.

Keywords: Amikacin, Pharmacokinetics/pharmacodynamics, Severe sepsis/septic shock

Background

The usefulness of antimicrobial combination therapy, such as the use of aminoglycosides in patients with severe sepsis or septic shock, remains controversial [1, 2]. Nevertheless, early and appropriate antimicrobial therapy in septic shock patients has been reported to reduce in-hospital mortality [2]. In view of this, aminoglycosides are often combined with another antibiotic in patients with severe sepsis or septic shock in order to broaden the treatment's spectrum of activity and obtain bactericidal synergy. The therapeutic effect of aminoglycosides

*Correspondence: nicolas.allou@hotmail.fr
[1] Réanimation polyvalente, Hôpital Felix Guyon, Centre Hospitalier Universitaire Felix Guyon, Allée des Topazes, Bellepierre, 97405 Saint Denis, France
Full list of author information is available at the end of the article

is highest and optimal when the peak plasma concentration (C_{max})/minimal inhibitory concentration (MIC) ratio is between 8 and 10 [3]. However, in patients with severe sepsis or septic shock, aminoglycosides are frequently used in empiric antimicrobial treatment without the causal micro-organisms and their MICs being identified. The French guidelines recommend to use high doses of aminoglycosides for empiric antibiotic therapy in patients suffering from severe sepsis or septic shock, and, specifically, doses of 25–30 mg/kg in the case of amikacin [4, 5]. In clinical practice, the recommended target is an amikacin C_{max} between 60 and 80 mg/L [4], which corresponds to approximately 8–10 times the MIC breakpoint, as defined by the European Committee on Antimicrobial Susceptibility Testing (EUCAST) of *Pseudomonas aeruginosa* and Enterobacteriaceae [5]. Previous studies have shown that a loading dose of 25 mg/kg frequently leads to a suboptimal amikacin C_{max} (>30% of patients with C_{max} < 60 mg/L) [6, 7], prompting an increase in the loading dose to 30 mg/kg without improving outcomes [8, 9]. Yet the dose of 30 mg/kg has been evaluated in a limited number of patients (n < 50) [8, 9]. The aim of this study was to assess the incidence and impact on mortality of an amikacin concentration between 60 and 80 mg/L in patients suffering from severe sepsis or septic shock.

Methods

The present observational study was approved by the Ethics Committee of Félix Guyon University Hospital (R15003). The requirement to obtain written informed consent from patients was waived, as the study was non-interventional and followed our usual protocol. However, all patients or their legally authorised representative was verbally informed about the process of data collection and could refuse to participate.

The reporting of this study complies with the Strengthening the Reporting of Observational studies in Epidemiology recommendations statement [10].

Selection of the study sample

This prospective observational cohort study was conducted from April 2015 to December 2015 in one mixed medical/surgical ICU and in one surgical ICU at two French university hospitals.

All patients were over 18 years old and treated for severe sepsis or septic shock with a combination therapy of amikacin at a loading dose of 30 mg/kg (±2.5 mg/kg) on the day of enrolment.

The first dose of amikacin was calculated using the total body weight of the day for patients with a body mass index <30 kg/m^2. For patients with a body mass index ≥30 kg/m^2, the dose was calculated using the adjusted body weight, which was calculated as follows: ideal body weight (height (cm) − 100 − [height (cm) − 150]/4 for male gender and height (cm) − 100 − [height (cm) − 150]/2 for female gender) + 0.4 [total body weight at admission-ideal body weight].

Severe sepsis and septic shock were defined following the Surviving Sepsis Campaign guidelines [11].

Only the first day of amikacin administration was studied.

The prescribed duration of the continuous infusion was 30 min. Measurements of C_{max} and trough concentration were taken 30 min and 24 h after the end of infusion. All samples were analysed immediately. Amikacin dosages were measured using a fluorescence polarisation immunoassay [12].

Trough concentration was considered elevated if >2.5 mg/L and was assessed only if treatment length was >5 days or in cases of renal insufficiency, as recommended by French guidelines [4, 6].

The exclusion criteria were: treatment with amikacin within 7 days prior to inclusion; inappropriate dose of amikacin (<27.5 or >32.5 mg/kg); inappropriate duration of amikacin infusion (<25 or >35 min); and inappropriate delays in measuring the amikacin C_{max} (<20 or >40 min after the end of infusion).

Data collected and study endpoint

Patient comorbidities at ICU admission were recorded on inclusion.

After administering the loading dose of 30 mg/kg of amikacin, the main endpoint was to evaluate the impact of the amikacin C_{max} on the in-ICU mortality of patients with severe sepsis or septic shock.

Statistical analysis

Results were expressed as total number (percentage) for categorical variables and as median [25th–75th percentiles] for continuous variables. Continuous variables were compared using the Mann–Whitney test or the Kruskal–Wallis test, as appropriate. Categorical variables were compared using the Chi-square test or the Fisher's exact test, as appropriate. Risk factors for in-ICU mortality in bivariate analysis with P < 0.1 were entered into a multivariate logistic regression analysis using backward selection with P < 0.05.

We considered that 50 patients were needed in the non-survivors group to perform a multivariate analysis with ten variables [13]. Based on an in-ICU mortality rate of 50% in patients with severe sepsis or septic shock [6], we calculated that 100 patients had to be included in the study cohort for there to be a minimum of 50 patients in the non-survivors group. Collinearity between independent factors was investigated. When identified, the most clinically relevant factor was chosen for use in the multivariate model. A P value <0.05 was considered significant. Analyses were performed using SAS statistical software (8.2, Cary, NC, USA).

Results

Study population

Over the study period, 921 patients were hospitalised, of which 150 (16.3%) received amikacin for severe sepsis or septic shock. Among the latter, 40 were excluded: 15 had received aminoglycosides in the previous seven days; 15 had received an inappropriate dose of amikacin; and 10 had an incorrect C_{max} measurement taken. The remaining 110 patients formed the cohort.

Patient characteristics on ICU admission and study inclusion are shown in Tables 1, 2 and 3.

The median age was 61 [51–70], the median Simplified Acute Physiology Score 2 at admission was 54 [41–68], and the median SOFA score on the day of amikacin administration was 10 [8–11]. The sources of infection were respiratory in 57 cases (51.8%), intra-abdominal in 16 cases (14.5%) and catheter related in 9 cases (8.2%). Bacteraemia was present in 32 cases (29.1%) (Table 3).

The most frequently isolated bacteria were *P. aeruginosa* (19.1%), *Enterobacter* spp. (16.7%) and *Escherichia coli* (13.9%) (Table 3).

Amikacin dosages

The median dose of amikacin was 30 [29.2–30.6] mg/kg. Pharmacodynamic amikacin targets (60 mg/L < C_{max} < 80 mg/L) were achieved in 46 of the 110 patients (41.8%). Forty-four of the 110 patients (40%) had a C_{max} > 80 mg/L, and 20 of the 110 patients (18.2%) had a C_{max} < 60 mg/L. No patient had a C_{max} < 30 mg/L (Table 4).

Trough concentration was measured for 65 patients (68.2%). Among these, 51 (78.5%) had a trough concentration >2.5 mg/L.

Prognosis

The in-ICU mortality rate was 41.8%. A univariate analysis revealed that the amikacin C_{max} was not associated with a reduction in the in-ICU mortality rate (C_{max} was 73.6 [65.9–83.6] mg/L in survivors and 81.9 [66.5–89.7] mg/L in non-survivors, $P = 0.12$).

The univariate analysis also showed that the in-ICU mortality rate was lower in the group of patients with a C_{max} between 60 and 80 mg/L (28.3%) than in patients with a C_{max} > 80 mg/L (56.8%, $P = 0.006$).

Moreover, there was no statistically significant difference of mortality between the group of patients with a C_{max} between 60 and 80 mg/L and the group of patients with a C_{max} < 60 mg/L (40%, $P = 0.18$).

The univariate analysis of trough concentration measurements in 75 of the 110 patients (68.2%) revealed that a higher amikacin trough concentration was not associated with a higher in-ICU mortality rate (5.2 [2.3–10.4] mg/L in survivors versus 8.6 [4.2–14.3] mg/L in non-survivors, $P = 0.058$).

The proportion of micro-organisms with a greater than usual amikacin MIC (i.e. non-fermenting Gram-negative bacilli) in non-survivors was similar to that in survivors (16 of 64 in survivors group versus 6 out of 46 in non-survivors group, $P = 0.12$).

The other risk factors found to be predictive of in-ICU mortality (based on a bivariate analysis with $P < 0.1$) are exposed in Table 2.

Following multivariate analysis, compared to a C_{max} between 60 and 80 mg/L, C_{max} > 80 mg/L was associated with a higher probability of mortality (OR 95% CI 3.96 [1.54–10.2], $P = 0.004$), and C_{max} < 60 mg/L was not associated with a higher probability of mortality (OR 95% CI 1.92 [0.46–8.24], $P = 0.4$). The multivariate analysis also revealed that the factors independently associated with a higher mortality rate were a higher age ($P = 0.02$) and a higher norepinephrine dose ($P = 0.0001$) (Table 5).

In survivors, acute kidney injury was not associated with a C_{max} > 80 mg/L (15.8% of patients who developed acute kidney injury had a C_{max} > 80 mg/L, while 14.2% who did not had a C_{max} > 80 mg/L, $P = 0.88$).

An amikacin trough concentration >2.5 mg/L was not significantly associated with acute kidney injury ($P = 0.26$).

Discussion

To our knowledge, this is the largest study evaluating the incidence and impact on in-ICU mortality of an amikacin C_{max} achieved with a high loading dose of 30 mg/kg. Roger et al. and Galvez et al. evaluated the effects of a dose of 30 mg/kg of amikacin in 47 and 33 patients, respectively, but did not assess the impact of amikacin concentration on mortality [8, 9]. In these studies, the median C_{max} obtained with a loading dose of 30 mg/kg of amikacin was 75 mg/L. This is consistent with previous studies that reported values ranging from 72.1 to 75.8 mg/L [8, 9]. We found that, with a loading dose of 30 mg/kg of amikacin, the pharmacodynamic C_{max} target (i.e. >60 mg/L for the less susceptible bacteria) was frequently achieved (81.2% cases), a rate that is consistent with previous studies [8, 9].

Studies by Taccone et al. [7] and de Montmollin et al. [6], in which amikacin concentration following a loading dose of 25 mg/kg was evaluated, found a high frequency of underdosing (>30%). These results prompted an increase in the loading dose of amikacin with the aim

Table 1 Baseline patient characteristics at intensive care unit admission and at inclusion

Characteristics	Total ($n = 110$)	Amikacin C_{max} (mg/L)			P
		<60 ($n = 20$)	60–80 ($n = 46$)	>80 ($n = 44$)	
At ICU admission					
Age (years old)	61 [51–70]	57. 5 [50.5–69]	63 [45–69]	62 [55.5–70]	0.521
Male sex	78 (70.9)	14 (70)	33 (71.7)	31 (70.5)	0.986
Weight (kg)	70 [58.2–80]	60 [52.5–73.5]	70 [58.2–80]	72.5 [65–82]	0.029
Body mass index (kg/m^2)	24.6 [20.7–28]	21.1 [18.5–25.7]	23.7 [20.8–27.3]	26.6 [21.9–29]	0.023
APACHE II	23 [18–28]	25 [21–28]	23 [17–28]	22 [18–26]	0.309
Simplified Acute Physiology Score 2	54 [41–68]	62 [47–70]	54 [44–63]	52 [40–67]	0.361
History of congestive heart failure	12 (10.9)	1 (5)	8 (17.4)	3 (6.9)	0.177
Liver cirrhosis	4 (3.6)	0	2 (4.3)	2 (4.5)	0.63
Chronic obstructive pulmonary disease	26 (23.6)	5 (25)	10 (21.7)	11 (25)	0.924
Chronic kidney disease requiring dialysis	9 (8.2)	1 (5)	2 (4.3)	6 (13.6)	0.233
Cancer (<3 months)	16 (14.5)	4 (20)	10 (21.7)	2 (4.5)	0.051
Diabetes mellitus	39 (35.5)	7 (35)	12 (26.1)	20 (45.5)	0.158
Immunodepression	24 (21.8)	6 (30)	9 (19.6)	9 (20.5)	0.616
At the day of aminoglycoside administration					
Day since admission	1 [0–5]	1 [0–6]	0.5 [0–5]	1.5 [0–6.5]	0.834
Emergent surgery	25 (22.7)	9 (45)	12 (26.1)	4 (9.1)	0.005
Sequential Organ Failure Assessment score	10 [8–11]	10 [9–11]	10 [7–12]	10 [8–12]	0.950
Weight (kg)	70 [60–80]	66 [55.5–79]	71 [58.2–80]	72 [65.5–82]	0.104
Weight gain since ICU admission (kg)	0 [0–3]	0 [0–3]	0 [0–2]	0 [0–2]	0.847
Extracorporeal membrane oxygenation	15 (13.6)	4 (20)	5 (10.9)	6 (13.6)	0.611
Catecholamines	89 (80.9)	16 (80)	36 (78.3)	37 (84.1)	0.776
Norepinephrine (µg/kg/min)	0.44 [0.1–0.93]	0.88 [0.11–1.64]	0.46 [0.09–0.83]	0.41 [0.11–0.81]	0.343
PaO_2/FiO_2 ratio	177 [122–264]	155 [90–230]	203 [140–289]	159 [118–258]	0.234
Renal replacement therapy	40 (36.4)	12 (60)	15 (32.6)	13 (29.5)	0.05
Glomerular filtration rate (mL/min)	45 [18.6–86.2]	22.1 [0–90.4]	43.6 [24.6–86]	49.7 [22.5–83.9]	0.583
Lactate level (mmol/L)	2.3 [1.2–4]	2.7 [1.5–4]	2.3 [1.2–6.5]	1.7 [1.2–3.2]	0.315
Platelet count (G/L)	204 [97–307]	170 [84–218]	204 [90–340]	230 [141–325]	0.113
Hematocrit level (%)	29.3 [26–31.6]	30.3 [26.8–32.7]	29.7 [27.3–31.6]	27.7 [25.3–31.1]	0.284
Leucocyte count (G/L)	13.9 [8.9–21]	14.1 [7.1–17.7]	15.6 [8.9–23.2]	13 [9.2–20.3]	0.373
Glasgow Coma Scale score	15 [13–15]	15 [13–15]	15 [13–15]	15 [13–15]	0.661
Bilirubin level (mg/dL)	12 [8–20]	12.5 [9–20]	12 [9–29]	12 [7–19]	0.657
Prothrombin time (%)	66 [52–78]	66 [57–78]	64 [47–81]	67 [57–78]	0.606
Proteinemia (g/L)	56 [47–63]	46.5 [40.5–60.5]	55.5 [49–64]	59 [51–64.5]	0.007

Results are expressed as the median [25th–75th percentiles] or *n* (%) as appropriate

APACHE Acute Physiology and Chronic Health Evaluation, C_{max} peak plasma concentration, PaO_2/FiO_2 partial pressure of oxygen in arterial blood/fraction of inspired oxygen

of achieving a C_{max} > 60 mg/L in the highest number of patients [8, 9].

In our study, the amikacin C_{max} between 60 and 80 mg/L recommended by French guidelines [4] was associated with a reduction in the in-ICU mortality rate. In theory, a C_{max} of amikacin between 60 and 80 mg/L would be optimal for treating sepsis caused by less susceptible Enterobacteriaceae and non-fermenting Gram-negative bacterial infections (such as *P. aeruginosa*) with a MIC of 8 mg/L. This is highlighted in a study by Dubois et al. [14], in which 61% of the isolated *P. aeruginosa* strains had a MIC of 8 mg/L. However, in patients with severe sepsis or septic shock, aminoglycosides are frequently used in empiric antimicrobial treatment without the causal micro-organisms and their MICs being identified. One of the major potential advantages of using aminoglycoside combination therapy is to broaden antibiotic treatment in cases of resistant bacteria, which may be found in ICUs [15, 16]. Combination therapy can increase the success of empiric therapy in up to 20% of

Table 2 Baseline patient characteristics at intensive care unit admission and at inclusion (survivors/non-survivors)

Characteristics	Survivors ($n = 64$)	Non-survivors ($n = 46$)	P
At ICU admission			
Age (years old)	60 [45–69]	63 [57–73]	0.03
Male sex	49 (76.6)	29 (63)	0.12
Weight (kg)	70 [60–80]	70 [58–79]	0.84
Body mass index (kg/m^2)	24.6 [20.7–27.8]	24.4 [20.7–28]	0.58
APACHE II	21 [17–25]	26 [22–29]	0.0007
Simplified Acute Physiology Score 2	52 [41–60]	57 [45–73]	0.05
History of congestive heart failure	6 (9.4)	6 (13)	0.54
Liver cirrhosis	0	4 (8.7)	0.03
Chronic obstructive pulmonary disease	15 (23.4)	11 (23.9)	0.96
Chronic kidney disease requiring dialysis	4 (6.3)	5 (10.9)	0.38
Cancer (<3 months)	11 (17.2)	5 (10.9)	0.35
Diabetes mellitus	15 (23.4)	24 (52.2)	0.002
Immunodepression	16 (25)	8 (17.4)	0.34
At the day of aminoglycoside administration			
Day since admission	1 [0–5]	2 [0–7]	0.32
Emergent surgery	17 (26.6)	8 (17.4)	0.26
Sequential Organ Failure Assessment score	9 [7–10]	10 [9–13]	0.004
Weight (kg)	70 [60–81]	70.5 [60–80]	0.92
Weight gain since ICU admission (kg)	0 [0–2]	0 [0–3]	0.62
Extracorporeal membrane oxygenation	7 (10.9)	8 (17.4)	0.33
Catecholamines	49 (76.6)	40 (87)	0.17
Norepinephrine (µg/kg/min)	0.26 [0.04–0.61]	0.83 [0.41–1.65]	0.0002
PaO_2/FiO_2 ratio	200 [140–280]	147 [103–259]	0.06
Renal replacement therapy	19 (29.7)	21 (45.7)	0.09
Glomerular filtration rate (mL/min)	53.5 [29.7–90.4]	29.8 [0–65.9]	0.008
Lactate level (mmol/L)	1.7 [1.2–3.1]	3.2 [1.4–7]	0.01
Platelet count (G/L)	205 [105–339]	201 [86–270]	0.47
Hematocrit level (%)	29.2 [26–31.3]	29.7 [26–32.4]	0.54
Leucocyte count (G/L)	15.6 [9.4–22.3]	13.4 [7.8–18.7]	0.22
Glasgow Coma Scale score	15 [14, 15]	15 [12–15]	0.23
Bilirubin level (mg/dL)	12 [8–17]	145 [9–26]	0.22
Prothrombin time (%)	72 [57–81]	60 [47–75]	0.01
Proteinemia (g/L)	58 [49–64]	52 [46–62]	0.1
Amikacin C_{max} between 60 and 80 mg/L	34 (53.1)	13 (28.3)	0.009

Results are expressed as the median [25th–75th percentiles] or n (%) as appropriate

APACHE Acute Physiology and Chronic Health Evaluation, C_{max} peak plasma concentration, PaO_2/FiO_2 partial pressure of oxygen in arterial blood/fraction of inspired oxygen

patients [17, 18]. A high C_{max} is therefore likely necessary given that *P. aeruginosa* is one of the most frequently isolated micro-organisms, even in cases of early-onset sepsis [19, 20].

We agree with Roger et al. [8] that a lower amikacin C_{max} may be enough to treat sepsis. In their study, all isolated strains had an amikacin MIC $\leq$ 4 mg/L, meaning that a C_{max} between 32 and 64 mg/L would be sufficient to meet pharmacokinetic/pharmacodynamic parameters in all patients (i.e. C_{max}/MIC > 8) [8]. In the present study, we found that with a high dose of 30 mg/kg of amikacin, C_{max} > 80 mg/L was frequently observed and was associated with higher mortality rates. We did not identify a clear hypothesis to explain the relationship between amikacin concentration >80 mg/L and mortality. Similar mortality results were found in a small randomised study of 99 patients by Galvez et al. [9] compared three dosing regimens (15, 25 and 30 mg/kg) of amikacin in patients with severe sepsis or septic shock. In the 15, 25 and 30 mg/kg amikacin-treated groups, the study found that a

Table 3 Sites of infection and isolated micro-organisms

	N
Sites of infection	110
Pulmonary	57
Catheter	9
Intra-abdominal	13
Skin and soft tissue	6
Urinary tract	6
Other	3
Unknown	16
Bacteraemia	32
Isolated micro-organisms	108
Cocci	24
Staphylococcus aureus	13
Other staphylococci	3
Enterococcus spp.	5
Streptococcus spp.	3
Bacilli	84
Enterobacteriaceae	56
Escherichia coli	15
Enterobacter spp.	18
Serratia marcescens	3
Klebsiella spp.	14
Other Enterobacteriaceae	6
Pseudomonas aeruginosa	21
Acinetobacter baumannii	2
Other bacilli	5
None	36

Table 4 Amikacin pharmacokinetic/pharmacodynamic parameters

Variable	$n = 110$
Dose (mg)	2100 [1800–2400]
Dose (mg/kg)	30 [29.2–30.6]
Peak plasma concentration (mg/L)	75 [66.1–86.1]
Patients with a peak concentration >80 mg/L	44 (40)
Patients with a peak concentration between 60 and 80 mg/L	46 (41.8)
Patients with a peak concentration <60 mg/L	20 (18.2)
Patients with a peak concentration <30 mg/L	0
Trough concentration >2.5 mg/L[a]	51 (78.5)

Results are expressed as the median [25th–75th percentiles] or *n* (%)

[a] Trough concentration was not measured for 45 patients

C_{max} > 60 mg/L was reached in 0, 39 and 76% of patients, respectively, but the mortality rate was 0, 9.1 and 22.2%, respectively. This study was not, however, designed to statistically analyse mortality. We found that patients with amikacin overexposures tended to have greater amikacin trough concentrations ($P = 0.08$). It is well established that aminoglycosides are associated with nephrotoxicity [21, 22], and that a high amikacin C_{max} in ICU is associated with higher trough-level concentrations [6]. Nevertheless, it is difficult to consider these high C_{max} as "overexposure" and further studies are needed. Moreover, recent in vitro and in vivo studies suggest that higher aminoglycosides exposure should be targeted for difficult to treat pathogens [23, 24]. To date, there is a lack of data on aminoglycoside-related toxicity in once-daily dose and short-duration aminoglycoside therapy. The present study was not designed to analyse and evaluate the association between acute kidney injury and trough concentration or aminoglycoside C_{max}, in that trough concentrations were not measured in all patients, as suggested by French guidelines [4]. Furthermore, previous studies suggest that aminoglycoside-associated acute kidney injury cannot be solely attributed to aminoglycosides, because other factors are frequently associated with acute kidney injury in the ICU, including sepsis, septic shock or nephrotoxic drugs [25, 26].

Table 5 Multivariate analysis of risk factors for in-intensive care unit mortality

Variables	Adjusted odds ratio (CI 95%)	*P* value
Age (per year increment)	1.044 (1.01–1.08)	0.02
Norepinephrine (per μg/kg/min increment)	3.94 (1.9–8.15)	0.0001
Amikacin C_{max}		
Between 60 and 80 mg/L	Reference	Reference
<60 mg/L	1.92 (0.46–8.24)	0.4
>80 mg/L	3.96 (1.54–10.2)	0.004
Prothrombin time	0.98 (0.96–1.01)	0.118
PaO_2/FiO_2 ratio	0.99 (0.99–1)	0.28
Diabetes mellitus	1.6 (0.59–4.38)	0.32
Glomerular filtration rate (mL/min)	0.99 (0.98–1.01)	0.43
Lactate level	1.01 (0.89–1.14)	0.53
SOFA	1.03 (0.81–1.3)	0.18

The Hosmer–Lemeshow goodness-of-fit test *P* value was 0.248. The Nagelkerke and Cox/Snell R^2 were, respectively, 0.347 and 0.258

CI confidence intervals, C_{max} peak plasma concentration, PaO_2/FiO_2 partial O_2 pressure in arterial blood/fraction of the inspired oxygen ratio, *SOFA* Sequential Organ Failure Assessment

Despite the current trend to increase doses of antibiotics in ICUs for pharmacokinetic/pharmacodynamic purposes, no beneficial effect on outcome has been clearly demonstrated [6–8]. In clinical practice, in Europe physicians are still using low doses of aminoglycosides, as shown by a recent survey of antimicrobial prescribing practices in ICUs, where aminoglycosides were administered at "low" doses (5 mg/kg for gentamicin and 15 mg/kg for amikacin) [27].

This study has severe limitations. Given that it was not a randomised controlled trial comparing different loading regimens, we cannot conclude a direct causal relationship between the amikacin C_{max} and the mortality rate. We did not evaluate the subsequent amikacin C_{max} after the first injection of the study, and MIC of isolated bacteria was not determined for amikacin. Although the study population may be considered small, to our knowledge this is the largest cohort to have been selected for evaluating the impact of high doses of 30 mg/kg of amikacin in patients with severe sepsis or septic shock [8, 9]; moreover, other studies confined their analysis to pharmacokinetics/pharmacodynamics parameters [8, 9]. We agree that analysing pharmacokinetics/pharmacodynamics parameters of medications is one of the first steps before launching an impact study [28]. Nevertheless, aminoglycosides are associated with well-known and severe side effects and analysing outcomes when increasing usual doses is indispensable. Previous studies reported that when high doses of aminoglycosides are administered, sampling within 90 min of the infusion provides information that leads to the overestimation of the peak serum concentration/minimum inhibitory concentration ratio and to the inaccurate calculation of pharmacokinetic parameters [29, 30]. Nevertheless, these studies were confined to gentamicin concentrations in a limited number of healthy volunteers (<13) [29, 30]. By contrast, recent studies [6–10] have reported measurements of amikacin C_{max} performed 30 min after infusion, as suggested by French guidelines [4].

Conclusion

This study suggests that with a high loading dose of 30 mg/kg the amikacin C_{max} between 60 and 80 mg/L recommended by French guidelines is associated with reduced in-hospital mortality, but that it is difficult to achieve in ICU patients (<50%). Amikacin overexposure (i.e. C_{max} > 80 mg/L) was frequent and potentially associated with increased mortality.

Abbreviations

APACHE: Acute Physiology and Chronic Health Evaluation; C_{max}: peak plasma concentration; ICU: intensive care unit; EUCAST: European Committee on Antimicrobial Susceptibility Testing; MIC: minimal inhibiting concentration; SAPS: Simplified Acute Physiology Score; SOFA: Sequential Organ Failure Assessment.

Authors' contributions

Drs. NA, AB, PA and JA had full access to all of the data in the study and take responsibility for the integrity of the data and the accuracy of the data analysis. NA, JA, PA and PM contributed to study concept and design. NA, PA, AB, AS, DV, JJ, BB, RG and LC helped in acquisition of data. NA, JA, PA and PM analysed and interpreted the data. NA, JA, AB, AS, DV, JJ, PM and PA drafted the manuscript. NA, AB, JA, AS, DV, JJ, BB, RG, LC, PM and PA critically revised the manuscript for important intellectual content. JA, NA, RG and PA contributed to statistical analysis. AB, NA, AS, RG and DV helped in administrative, technical or material support. JA, NA, PM, PA and AB helped in study supervision. All authors read and approved the final manuscript.

Author details

[1] Réanimation polyvalente, Hôpital Felix Guyon, Centre Hospitalier Universitaire Felix Guyon, Allée des Topazes, Bellepierre, 97405 Saint Denis, France. [2] Département d'Anesthésie Réanimation, AP-HP, Centre Hospitalier Universitaire Bichat-Claude-Bernard, 46, rue Henri-Huchard, 75018 Paris, France.

Acknowledgements

This work was internally funded. Obtained funding support was provided solely from institutional and/or departmental sources.

Presented in part at the International Congress of the French Society of Anaesthesia and Intensive Care, Paris, France, September 17–19, 2015.

Competing interests

The authors declare that they have no competing interests.

References

1. Kumar A, Safdar N, Kethireddy S, Chateau D. A survival benefit of combination antibiotic therapy for serious infections associated with sepsis and septic shock is contingent only on the risk of death: a meta-analytic/meta-regression study. Crit Care Med. 2010;38:1651–4.
2. Kumar A, Zarychanski R, Light B, et al. Early combination antibiotic therapy yields improved survival compared with monotherapy in septic shock: a propensity-matched analysis. Crit Care Med. 2010;38:1773–85.
3. Moore RD, Lietman PS, Smith CR. Clinical response to aminoglycoside therapy: importance of the ratio of peak concentration to minimal inhibitory concentration. J Infect Dis. 1987;155:93–9.
4. Update on good use of injectable aminoglycosides, gentamycin, tobramycin, netilmycin, amikacin. Pharmacological properties, indications, dosage, and mode of administration, treatment monitoring. Med et Mal Infect 2012; 42:301–308.
5. EUCAST. European Committee on Antimicrobial Susceptibility Testing 2015. www.eucast.org/.
6. de Montmollin E, Bouadma L, Gault N, et al. Predictors of insufficient amikacin peak concentration in critically ill patients receiving a 25 mg/kg total body weight regimen. Intensive Care Med. 2014;40:998–1005.
7. Taccone FS, Laterre PF, Spapen H, et al. Revisiting the loading dose of amikacin for patients with severe sepsis and septic shock. Crit Care. 2010;14:R53.
8. Roger C, Nucci B, Louart B, et al. Impact of 30 mg/kg amikacin and 8 mg/kg gentamicin on serum concentrations in critically ill patients with severe sepsis. J Antimicrob Chemother. 2016;71:208–12.
9. Galvez R, Luengo C, Cornejo R, et al. Higher than recommended amikacin loading doses achieve pharmacokinetic targets without associated toxicity. Int J Antimicrob Agents. 2011;38:146–51.
10. von Elm E, Altman DG, Egger M, et al. The Strengthening the Reporting of Observational Studies in Epidemiology (STROBE) statement: guidelines for reporting observational studies. Lancet. 2007;370:1453–7.
11. Dellinger RP, Levy MM, Rhodes A, et al. Surviving sepsis campaign: international guidelines for management of severe sepsis and septic shock, 2012. Intensive Care Med. 2013;39:165–228.
12. Blaser J, Konig C, Fatio R, et al. Multicenter quality control study of amikacin assay for monitoring once-daily dosing regimens. International Antimicrobial Therapy Cooperative Group of the European Organization for Research and Treatment of Cancer. Ther Drug Monit. 1995;17:133–6.
13. Vittinghoff E, McCulloch CE. Relaxing the rule of ten events per variable in logistic and Cox regression. Am J Epidemiol. 2007;165:710–8.
14. Dubois V, Arpin C, Dupart V, et al. Beta-lactam and aminoglycoside resistance rates and mechanisms among *Pseudomonas aeruginosa* in French general practice (community and private healthcare centres). J Antimicrob Chemother. 2008;62:316–23.

15. Durante-Mangoni E, Grammatikos A, Utili R, et al. Do we still need the aminoglycosides? Int J Antimicrob Agents. 2009;33:201–5.
16. Leibovici L, Vidal L, Paul M. Aminoglycoside drugs in clinical practice: an evidence-based approach. J Antimicrob Chemother. 2009;63:246–51.
17. Bhat S, Fujitani S, Potoski BA, et al. *Pseudomonas aeruginosa* infections in the intensive care unit: can the adequacy of empirical beta-lactam antibiotic therapy be improved? Int J Antimicrob Agents. 2007;30:458–62.
18. Beardsley JR, Williamson JC, Johnson JW, et al. Using local microbiologic data to develop institution-specific guidelines for the treatment of hospital-acquired pneumonia. Chest. 2006;130:787–93.
19. Verhamme KM, De Coster W, De Roo L, De Beenhouwer H, Nollet G, Verbeke J, Demeyer I, Jordens P. Pathogens in early-onset and late-onset intensive care unit–acquired pneumonia. Infect Control Hosp Epidemiol. 2007;28:389–97.
20. Allou N, Allyn J, Snauwaert A, Welsch C, Lucet JC, Kortbaoui R, Desmard M, Augustin P, Montravers P. Postoperative pneumonia following cardiac surgery acquired in non-ventilated patients versus acquired in mechanically ventilated patients: is there any difference? Crit Care. 2015;11(19):116. doi:10.1186/s13054-015-0845-5.
21. Paul M, Lador A, Grozinsky-Glasberg S, et al. Beta lactam antibiotic monotherapy versus beta lactam-aminoglycoside antibiotic combination therapy for sepsis. Cochrane Database Syst Rev. 2014;1:CD003344.
22. Buchholtz K, Larsen CT, Hassager C, et al. Severity of gentamicin's nephrotoxic effect on patients with infective endocarditis: a prospective observational cohort study of 373 patients. Clin Infect Dis. 2009;48:65–71.
23. Rees VE, Bulitta JB, Oliver A et al. Resistance suppression by high-intensity, short-duration aminoglycoside exposure against hypermutable and non-hypermutable *Pseudomonas aeruginosa*. J Antimicrob Chemother. 2016 Aug 11. pii: dkw297.
24. Pajot O, Burdet C, Couffignal C, et al. Impact of imipenem and amikacin pharmacokinetic/pharmacodynamic parameters on microbiological outcome of Gram-negative bacilli ventilator-associated pneumonia. J Antimicrob Chemother. 2015;70:1487–94.
25. Boyer A, Gruson D, Bouchet S, et al. Aminoglycosides in septic shock: an overview, with specific consideration given to their nephrotoxic risk. Drug Saf. 2013;36:217–30.
26. Taber SS, Mueller BA. Drug-associated renal dysfunction. Crit Care Clin. 2006;22:357–74.
27. Tabah A, De Waele J, Lipman J et al; Working Group for Antimicrobial Use in the ICU within the Infection Section of the European Society of Intensive Care Medicine (ESICM). The ADMIN-ICU survey: a survey on antimicrobial dosing and monitoring in ICUs. J Antimicrob Chemother 2015; 70:2671–2677.
28. Reilly BM, Evans AT. Translating clinical research into clinical practice: impact of using prediction rules to make decisions. Ann Intern Med. 2006;144:201–9.
29. McNamara DR, Nafziger AN, Menhinick AM, et al. A dose-ranging study of gentamicin pharmacokinetics: implications for extended interval aminoglycoside therapy. J Clin Pharmacol. 2001;41:374–7.
30. Demczar DJ, Nafziger AN, Bertino JS Jr. Pharmacokinetics of gentamicin at traditional versus high doses: implications for once-daily aminoglycoside dosing. Antimicrob Agents Chemother. 1997;41:1115–9.

4

Early risk factors and the role of fluid administration in developing acute respiratory distress syndrome in septic patients

Raghu R. Seethala[1,2*], Peter C. Hou[1,2], Imoigele P. Aisiku[1], Gyorgy Frendl[2,3], Pauline K. Park[4], Mark E. Mikkelsen[5], Steven Y. Chang[6], Ognjen Gajic[7] and Jonathan Sevransky[8]

Abstract

Background: Sepsis is a major risk factor for acute respiratory distress syndrome (ARDS). However, there remains a paucity of literature examining risk factors for ARDS in septic patients early in their course. This study examined the role of early fluid administration and identified other risk factors within the first 6 h of hospital presentation associated with developing ARDS in septic patients.

Methods: This was a secondary analysis of septic adult patients presenting to the Emergency Department or being admitted for high-risk elective surgery from the multicenter observational cohort study, US Critical Injury and Illness trial Group-Lung Injury Prevention Study 1 (USCIITG-LIPS 1, NCT00889772). Multivariable logistic regression was performed to identify potential early risk factors for ARDS. Stratified analysis by shock status was performed to examine the association between early fluid administration and ARDS.

Results: Of the 5584 patients in the original study cohort, 2534 (45.4%) met our criteria for sepsis. One hundred and fifty-six (6.2%) of these patients developed ARDS during the hospital stay. In multivariable analyses, Acute Physiology and Chronic Health Evaluation (APACHE) II score (OR 1.10, 95% CI 1.07–1.13), age (OR 0.97, 95% CI 0.96–0.98), total fluid infused in the first 6 h (in liters) (OR 1.15, 95% CI 1.03–1.29), shock (OR 2.57, 95% CI 1.62–4.08), pneumonia as a site of infection (OR 2.31, 95% CI 1.59–3.36), pancreatitis (OR 3.86, 95% CI 1.33–11.24), and acute abdomen (OR 3.77, 95% CI 1.37–10.41) were associated with developing ARDS. In the stratified analysis, total fluid infused in the first 6 h (in liters) (OR 1.05, 95% CI 0.87–1.28) was not associated with the development of ARDS in the shock group, while there was an association in the non-shock group (OR 1.21, 95% CI 1.05–1.38).

Conclusions: In septic patients, the following risk factors identified within the first 6 h of hospital presentation were associated with ARDS: APACHE II score, presence of shock, pulmonary source of infection, pancreatitis, and presence of an acute abdomen. In septic patients without shock, the amount of fluid infused during the first 6 h of hospital presentation was associated with developing ARDS.

Keywords: Sepsis, Acute respiratory distress syndrome, Fluid resuscitation, Pneumonia, Acute lung injury

Background

Acute respiratory distress syndrome (ARDS) is a common condition encountered in the intensive care unit (ICU), with close to 10% of all patients admitted to the ICU developing ARDS [1]. Sepsis has long been recognized as a major risk factor for the development of ARDS. Prior investigations have reported approximately up to 40% of ARDS patients also having a diagnosis of sepsis [2, 3]. Previous work has described risk factors in septic shock patients that are predictive of ARDS, but this work has largely focused on patients admitted to the ICU [4]. Recent international sepsis guidelines have highlighted the importance of early recognition and treatment and

*Correspondence: rseethala@bwh.harvard.edu
[1] Division of Emergency Critical Care Medicine, Department of Emergency Medicine, Brigham and Women's Hospital, 75 Francis St., Neville House, Boston, MA 02115, USA
Full list of author information is available at the end of the article

have specifically focused on the first 3 and 6 h of care [5]. Multiple studies have demonstrated improved mortality and outcomes with increased adherence to these guidelines [6, 7]. It is likely that during this critical 6-h period of initial presentation there are readily identifiable risk factors in the sepsis population that predispose them to developing ARDS. Despite these observations, literature examining risk factors for ARDS in septic patients early in their course like in the emergency department remains sparse. There have been preliminary data on the epidemiology of ARDS in septic patients in the emergency department, but these studies have been limited by their retrospective nature, only including a single center, and small sample size [8, 9].

Early fluid administration may be an important modifiable risk factor for the development of ARDS in sepsis patients. There has been recent debate regarding the optimal fluid strategy in septic patients. One of the most important components of sepsis resuscitation bundles is fluid resuscitation. Three recently published sepsis trials found that protocolized resuscitation did not perform any better than usual or standard care by physicians [10–12]. The mortality rates in these studies were much lower than prior studies, and this has led to speculation that the early aggressive volume resuscitation instituted in these studies partially explains this observed lower mortality. On the other hand, there have been several studies demonstrating worse outcomes with larger fluid resuscitation and positive fluid balance during ICU stay in septic patients [13–16]. Sepsis is a highly inflamed state, with increased capillary permeability. Excessive volume administration could lead to increased pulmonary edema and subsequent ARDS. In spite of this, the role of volume resuscitation and developing ARDS during the early period of sepsis has not been extensively studied.

In a large multicenter cohort of septic patients, we sought to identify risk factors readily detectable during the first 6 h of hospital presentation that were associated with the development of ARDS and examine the association of fluid administration during the first 6 h and ARDS.

Methods

Study design and setting

This was a secondary analysis of a multicenter observational cohort study, US Critical Injury and Illness trial Group-Lung Injury Prevention Study 1 (USCIITG-LIPS 1, NCT00889772) [17]; patients were enrolled prospectively in 19 hospitals and retrospectively (after hospital discharge) in three hospitals over a 6-month period, beginning in March 2009. The hospitals included both community and academic medical centers with 20 of the hospitals located in the USA and two hospitals located in Turkey. The study was approved by the institutional review board at each participating institution. Approval was also granted for ancillary studies such as the present investigation.

Study patients

The original study included consecutive adult patients with one or more study-defined ARDS risk factors admitted to the hospital through the Emergency Department or admitted for high-risk elective surgery. This was a subgroup analysis that included patients with sepsis as an ARDS risk factor. These patients were followed during their initial hospital stay to assess for the development of ARDS. We defined sepsis as those with the presence of known or suspected infection with 2 or more systemic inflammatory response syndrome (SIRS) criteria or the diagnosis of pneumonia at the time of enrollment. Patients with the diagnosis of ARDS at the time of initial presentation were excluded.

Data collection

As detailed in the original lung injury prediction score (LIPS) study [17], demographics, comorbidities, and clinical variables were collected during the first 6 h of initial evaluation. Data were entered into a secure electronic database (REDCap).

Outcome

The primary outcome was development of ARDS during the hospital stay. ARDS was defined according to the Berlin definition [18]. The Berlin definition was retrospectively applied to the data, as this definition was not yet published at the time of the data collection.

Statistical analysis

Continuous data were reported as means and standard deviations. Categorical data were reported as counts and percentages. As appropriate, Student's t tests and Chi-square tests were used to compare characteristics between the ARDS and non-ARDS groups. Logistic regression was performed to examine the association of potential risk factors and development of ARDS in this sepsis cohort. We a priori hypothesized the following risk factors would be associated with ARDS in septic patients: Acute Physiology and Chronic Health Evaluation (APACHE) II score, age, total fluid infused during first 6 h, presence of shock, race, gender, pneumonia as site of infection, and blood product transfusion. Shock was defined as presence of hypotension (systolic blood pressure <90 mmHg, or decrease of 40 mmHg from baseline, or mean arterial pressure <65 mmHg) with evidence of inadequate tissue perfusion on physical examination (altered mental status not explained by other causes other than the hemodynamic status and urine output less than 0.5 ml/Kg/min). The definitions of all clinical variables are available in the online data supplement of the original study [17]. Total fluid infused during first 6 h was calculated by adding the total amount of crystalloid, colloid, and other infusions received during that time period. We additionally examined the risk factors identified in the original LIPS study that were associated with ARDS [17].

We performed univariable analysis of the risk factors identified in the original LIPS study. Risk factors with a p value <0.2 were then entered into a multivariable model. Additionally, using a forced entry strategy, the a priori hypothesized risk factors were also entered into the multivariable model. We then used stepwise backward elimination, retaining variables with a p value <0.2, to select the optimal model. Variables in which less than 1% of the study population had the variable present, or in which >30% of the values were missing were excluded from analysis. We additionally hypothesized that the association between total amount of fluid infused during the first 6 h and development of ARDS would differ between the shock and non-shock groups and thus performed a stratified analysis by shock status.

Odds ratio (OR) and 95% CI were reported. Imputation with mean value was used to analyze continuous variables with missing data. Missing indicator method was used to analyze categorical variables with missing data. The following variables had >5% missing data: total fluid infused during first 6 h (28%), alcohol use (10%), blood product transfusion (23%), obesity (20%), tobacco use (7%), and FIO_2 >0.35 (8%). Sensitivity analysis was performed using complete case analysis. All analyses were performed using SAS version 9.4 (SAS Institute, Cary, NC). In the final model, a p value <0.05 was considered significant.

Results

A total of 5584 patients were included in the original LIPS study cohort (309 of these patients were enrolled retrospectively). Out of 5584, 2534 patients (45.4%) in the original study cohort met our predefined criteria for sepsis and were analyzed (Fig. 1). One hundred and fifty-six (6.2%) of these patients developed ARDS during the hospital stay. Mean time to development of ARDS was 4.5 ± 5.3 days, with approximately 50% of the cases occurring in the first 2 days of hospitalization, and 80% occurring within 5 days. 1209 (47.7%) of the sepsis cohort were admitted to the ICU, and 170 (6.7%) died during their in-hospital stay. Of the patients that developed ARDS, 54 (34.6%) died, while 116 (4.9%) of the patients that did not develop ARDS died. The mean

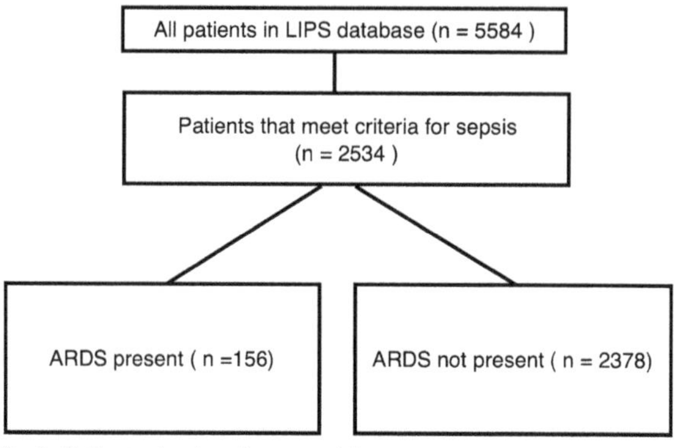

Fig. 1 Patient selection diagram with outcomes

hospital length of stay for septic patients with ARDS was 19.1 ± 16.2 days and for those without ARDS was 7.6 ± 8.1 days (p < 0.001). Patient characteristics are listed in Table 1.

In univariable analysis, APACHE II score, age, total fluid infused during first 6 h, shock, race, gender, pneumonia, blood product transfusion, aspiration, pancreatitis, acute abdomen, tachypnea, hypoxemia, and FIO_2 >0.35 were all associated with the increased odds of development of ARDS, while the diagnosis of diabetes mellitus was found to be protective against ARDS (Table 2).

The final multivariable model is demonstrated in Table 3. APACHE II score (OR 1.10, 95% CI 1.07–1.13), age (OR 0.97, 95% CI 0.96–0.98), total fluid infused in the first 6 h (in liters) (OR 1.15, 95% CI 1.03–1.29), shock (OR 2.57, 95% CI 1.62–4.08), pneumonia as a site of infection (OR 2.31, 95% CI 1.59–3.36), pancreatitis (OR 3.86, 95% CI 1.33–11.24), and acute abdomen (OR 3.77, 95% CI 1.37–10.41) were all associated with the development of ARDS. We performed a sensitivity analysis with complete case analysis that yielded similar results (Additional file 1: Table S1).

We also observed that during the first 6 h of hospital presentation the incidence of ARDS increased with increasing fluid administration (Fig. 2). The stratified analysis according to the presence of shock revealed that the relationship between amount of fluid infused in first 6 h and the development of ARDS was not present within the subgroup of patients with shock (OR 1.05, 95% CI 0.87–1.28) (Table 4). This association was still present in the non-shock group (OR 1.21, 95% CI 1.05–1.38).

Discussion

In this large cohort of patients with sepsis and pneumonia, we found that the rate of developing ARDS was low. Although only 6% of at-risk patients developed ARDS,

Table 1 Characteristics of patients in the sepsis cohort

	Total ($n = 2534$)	ARDS ($n = 156$)	No ARDS ($n = 2378$)	p value
APACHE II	11.7 ± 6.4	16.3 ± 7.4	11.4 ± 6.2	<0.001
Age (years)	58.5 ± 18.8	54.9 ± 17.3	58.8 ± 18.9	0.01
Total fluid infused during first 6 h (L)	1.49 ± 1.51	2.54 ± 2.31	1.41 ± 1.42	<0.001
Race				0.04
White	1448 (59.2)	97 (63.8)	1351 (58.9)	
Black	724 (29.6)	31 (20.4)	693 (30.2)	
Asian	35 (1.4)	3 (2.0)	32 (1.4)	
Other	240 (9.8)	21 (13.8)	219 (9.5)	
Shock	234 (9.23)	44 (28.2)	190 (8.0)	<0.001
Male	1298 (51.2)	94 (60.3)	1204 (50.6)	0.02
Pneumonia as site of infection	1234 (48.7)	91 (58.33)	1143 (48.1)	0.01
Alcohol use	596 (26.0)	41 (29.3)	555 (25.8)	0.36
Blood product transfusion	51 (2.6)	10 (8.6)	41 (2.2)	<0.001
Aspiration	103 (4.1)	15 (9.6)	88 (3.7)	<0.001
Pancreatitis	24 (1.0)	5 (3.2)	19 (0.8)	0.003
Thoracic surgery	6 (0.2)	0 (0.0)	6 (0.3)	0.53
Spine surgery	3 (0.1)	2 (1.3)	1 (0.0)	<0.001
Acute abdomen	42 (1.7)	6 (3.9)	36 (1.5)	0.03
Cardiac surgery	3 (0.1)	0 (0.0)	3 (0.1)	0.66
Aortic surgery	3 (0.1)	0 (0.0)	3 (0.1)	0.66
Lung contusion	2 (0.1)	0 (0.0)	2 (0.1)	0.72
Near drowning	0 (0)	0	0	NA
Brain injury	11 (0.4)	3 (1.9)	8 (0.34)	0.004
Smoke inhalation	4 (0.2)	1 (0.6)	3 (0.1)	0.12
Long-bone fractures	5 (0.2)	3 (1.9)	2 (0.1)	<0.001
Obesity (BMI > 30)	598 (23.6)	44 (28.2)	554 (23.3)	0.16
Chemotherapy	131 (5.2)	10 (6.4)	121 (5.1)	0.47
Diabetes mellitus	733 (28.9)	33 (21.1)	700 (29.4)	0.03
Tobacco use				0.83
Never	1177 (49.7)	73 (51.4)	1104 (49.6)	
Former	652 (27.6)	36 (25.4)	616 (27.7)	
Current	538 (22.7)	33 (23.3)	505 (22.7)	
Emergency surgery	41 (1.6)	5 (3.2)	36 (1.5)	0.10
Tachypnea (RR > 30)	239 (9.7)	30 (20.0)	209 (9.0)	<0.001
Hypoxemia (SpO_2 < 95%)	861 (34.6)	68 (44.2)	793 (34.0)	0.01
FIO_2 >0.35	395 (17.0)	61 (41.2)	334 (15.4)	<0.001
Hypoalbuminemia	695 (54.9)	64 (74.4)	631 (53.4)	<0.001
Acidosis (pH < 7.35)	231 (42.5)	50 (55.6)	181 (40.0)	0.006

Data are presented as mean ± SD or n (%) unless otherwise indicated

APACHE Acute Physiology and Chronic Health Evaluation, *BMI* body mass index, *RR* respiratory rate

mortality was significantly higher in those who developed ARDS. We found that APACHE II score, age, higher volume of early fluid administration, pulmonary source of sepsis, shock, pancreatitis, and acute abdomen were all associated with the development of ARDS. Of these exposures, fluid administration appears to be the only potentially modifiable exposure.

Our results highlight the role of the amount of fluid administered to septic patients during the first 6 h of care and the development of ARDS. Other studies support our findings that increased fluid administration may be associated with the development of ARDS. Jia et al. [19] demonstrated that a positive fluid balance during the first 48 h of mechanically ventilated patients is associated with the development of ARDS. In addition, after initial resuscitation, conservative fluid-management strategies compared to liberal strategies have increased days alive and off the ventilator in patients

Table 2 Univariable logistic regression of early risk factors for ARDS in sepsis cohort

	Odds ratio (95% CI)	*p* value
APACHE II	1.11 (1.08–1.13)	<0.001
Age (years)	0.99 (0.98–1.0)	0.01
Total fluid infused during first 6 h (L)	1.40 (1.28–1.54)	<0.001
Race		
White	Reference	Reference
Black	0.62 (0.41–0.94)	0.02
Asian	1.31 (0.39–4.34)	0.59
Other	1.34 (0.82–2.19)	0.25
Shock	4.52 (3.10–6.61)	<0.001
Gender (male)	1.48 (1.06–2.06)	0.02
Pneumonia as site of infection	1.51 (1.09–2.10)	0.01
Alcohol use	1.19 (0.82–1.74)	0.36
Blood product transfusion	4.10 (2.00–8.41)	<0.001
Aspiration	2.77 (1.56–4.91)	<0.001
Pancreatitis	4.11 (1.51–11.16)	0.003
Acute abdomen	2.60 (1.08–6.27)	0.03
Obesity (BMI > 30)	1.29 (0.90–1.86)	0.16
Chemotherapy	1.28 (0.66–2.49)	0.47
Diabetes mellitus	0.64 (0.43–0.95)	0.03
Tobacco use		
Never	Reference	Reference
Former	0.88 (0.59–1.33)	0.56
Current	0.99 (0.65–1.51)	0.81
Emergency surgery	2.16 (0.83–5.57)	0.11
Tachypnea (RR > 30)	2.52 (1.65–3.86)	<0.001
Hypoxemia (SpO_2 < 95%)	1.54 (1.11–2.14)	0.01
FIO_2 >0.35	3.86 (2.72–5.46)	<0.001

For continuous variables, the odds ratio indicates the increased odds of ARDS for a 1-unit increase of the variable

APACHE Acute Physiology and Chronic Health Evaluation, *BMI* body mass index, *RR* respiratory rate

with established ARDS, many of whom had sepsis as a risk factor [20]. Multiple studies have demonstrated that increasing extravascular lung water is associated with mortality in ARDS patients [21–23]. A positive fluid balance has also been associated with increased mortality in septic shock patients [13].

Conversely, early resuscitation in sepsis has been shown to decrease inflammatory markers [24]. Therefore, fluid resuscitation during this early phase of sepsis may actually be beneficial and decrease the risk of ARDS by limiting the inflammatory cascade. One study demonstrated in septic patients with the diagnosis of ARDS aggressive fluid resuscitation in the first 6 h followed by conservative fluid management in the next 7 days was the optimal fluid therapy in terms of mortality [25]. A prior investigation demonstrated that inadequate resuscitation for patients in septic shock was an independent risk

Table 3 Multivariable logistic regression of early risk factors for ARDS in sepsis cohort

	Odds ratio (95% CI)	*p* value
APACHE II	1.10 (1.07–1.13)	<0.001
Age (years)	0.97 (0.96–0.98)	<0.001
Total fluid infused during first 6 h (L)	1.15 (1.03–1.29)	0.01
Shock	2.57 (1.62–4.08)	<0.001
Gender (male)	1.30 (0.92–1.85)	0.14
Race		
White	Reference	Reference
Black	0.56 (0.36–0.87)	0.08
Asian	1.14 (0.32–4.11)	0.58
Other	1.14 (0.66–1.96)	0.29
Pneumonia as site of infection	2.31 (1.59–3.36)	<0.001
Pancreatitis	3.86 (1.33–11.24)	0.01
Acute abdomen	3.77 (1.37–10.41)	0.01
Diabetes mellitus	0.74 (0.48–1.12)	0.16
Tachypnea (RR > 30)	1.41 (1.00–1.97)	0.05

For continuous variables, the odds ratio indicates the increased odds of ARDS for a 1-unit increase in the variable

APACHE Acute Physiology and Chronic Health Evaluation, *RR* respiratory rate

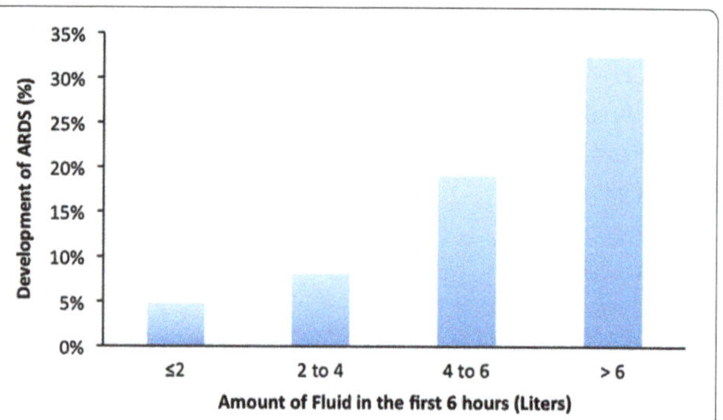

Fig. 2 Frequency of acute respiratory distress syndrome (ARDS) development according to amount of fluid administered during the first 6 h of hospital presentation

Table 4 Shock subgroup analysis: multivariable analysis of total volume in first 6 h and the development of ARDS

	Odds ratio (95% CI)	*p* value
Shock	1.05 (0.87–1.28)	0.60
No shock	1.21 (1.05–1.38)	0.01

The odds ratio indicates the increased odds of ARDS for a 1-l increase in volume of fluids administered

factor for ARDS [4]. Another study demonstrated that total volume of fluid infused during the first 24 h of care of severe sepsis and septic shock patients did not increase risk of ARDS [26].

Our stratified analysis showed that fluid administration during the first 6 h was not significantly associated with ARDS in the subgroup of patients with shock. However, we did demonstrate that the association between amount of fluid infused in the first 6 h and the development of ARDS was present in patients without shock. This may suggest that septic patients without shock are at the highest risk of ARDS with early excessive fluid administration. It is important to note that only 9% of our patients had shock. Larger size studies with sufficient power are necessary to examine this issue. Interestingly, this phenomenon has also been observed in patients with severe blunt trauma. A multicenter prospective study demonstrated that blunt trauma patients with prehospital hypotension and higher crystalloid infusion did not have an increased incidence of ARDS, while blunt trauma patients without prehospital hypotension and higher crystalloid infusion did have a higher incidence of ARDS [27].

Despite multiple randomized control trials comparing different early resuscitation protocols for septic patients, this relationship between early fluid resuscitation in septic patients and ARDS has not been well studied. Unfortunately, none of these trials specifically looked at ARDS as an outcome. The original early goal-directed therapy (EGDT) trial did not measure the incidence of ARDS directly, but did report the need for mechanical ventilation [28]. The patients randomized to the EGDT group received more fluids in the first 6 h and had a significantly decreased requirement of mechanical ventilation. This suggests in that patient population early aggressive fluid administration was not associated with respiratory impairment and in fact was associated with improved respiratory outcomes. Our results do not contradict those findings. The patients in the EGDT study were considerably sicker than our cohort. They had an initial APACHE score of 21 and an overall mortality of 37%. As we have demonstrated in our study, it is in the less sick patients without shock in which we observed the association of increased early fluids and ARDS. The subsequent three sepsis trials comparing standard care to EGDT did not demonstrate a significant association between EGDT and respiratory outcomes [10–12]. This may be due to the fact that there was not a large difference in amount of fluid received between the control and interventional arms. In the PROMISE and ARISE trials, the difference in the amount of fluids given in the first 6 h between the control and intervention groups was between 200 and 250 cc. However, in the PROCESS trial there were three arms: EGDT, another protocolized resuscitation, and standard care. The standard care group had a significantly lower volume infused in the first 6 h: 2.3L (standard care) versus 2.8L (EGDT) and 3.3L (other protocolized resuscitation) ($p < 0.001$) and had a trend toward less respiratory failure. At this point, it is unclear what the optimal fluid strategy is during the early phase of sepsis to prevent ARDS. It likely depends on several factors including severity of illness and hemodynamic status.

Our findings are also consistent with prior investigations that demonstrated severity of illness, pneumonia as a source of infection, and shock at presentation as risk factors for ARDS in septic patients [8]. We additionally found that pancreatitis and acute abdomen were risk factors for ARDS in this cohort. This is not surprising, given that lung and abdomen have been identified as the most frequent sources of infection in patients with ARDS [29]. The contribution of pulmonary sepsis to ARDS is likely multifactorial. Septic patients with pneumonia have a direct lung injury from the pneumonia itself and then indirect lung injury from the sepsis inflammatory cascade, which can both lead to ARDS. It has also long been known that ARDS is a major complication of severe pancreatitis. ARDS has been reported to be the major cause of death of acute pancreatitis patients that die within one week of presentation [30, 31].

Blood product administration is a known risk factor for lung injury and progression to ARDS in critically ill patients [19, 32–34]. Our study found an association with ARDS in univariable analysis, but our multivariable analysis did not. We were likely underpowered to demonstrate such an association, since only 2.6% of our patients received blood products. In contrast to our results, Iscimen et al. [4] found that blood product transfusion in the septic shock population independently predicted ARDS. Their study differed from ours in that it only evaluated patients in septic shock, and over 50% of the patients received some blood product transfusion.

Our study has several strengths. This was a large multicenter study, and the majority of data were prospectively collected. Additionally, our study is generalizable to patients with the entire spectrum of sepsis, since our study included sepsis and septic shock. Our study also has some limitations. First, we did not collect data on some important risk factors that have been associated with ARDS in sepsis including time to antibiotics and lactate level. Second, we have incomplete data on some of the covariates. We dealt with the missing data using established epidemiologic methods. We also performed a sensitivity analysis with complete case analysis and found that our results were similar. Third, there is risk for misclassification from medical chart review. This risk was reduced since the vast majority of these patients were enrolled prospectively with close follow-up. Fourth, there is the limitation that most ARDS investigations share regarding the reproducibility of diagnosis of ARDS. In order to mitigate this limitation, mandatory structured training in ARDS assessment was instituted and site-principal investigators were responsible for ensuring quality. Finally, we are able to demonstrate association, but not demonstrate causality. Future studies, including advanced adjustment techniques, are warranted to confirm the relationship between initial fluid administration and ARDS development. However, because the application of propensity score methods for continuous exposures is less well developed than their use for binary exposures, we adjusted for potential confounders using multivariable logistic regression models [35].

Conclusions

In septic patients, we demonstrated that the following variables present upon initial hospital presentation: Severity of illness, age, pulmonary source of sepsis, presence of shock, pancreatitis, and acute abdomen were associated with developing ARDS. In septic patients without shock, we also identified another important association between a potentially modifiable risk factor, the amount of fluid infused in the first 6 h, and the development of ARDS. Future investigations should focus on determining the optimal early resuscitation strategies for septic patients based on severity of sepsis and examine the outcome of ARDS.

Abbreviations

ARDS: acute respiratory distress syndrome; APACHE: Acute Physiology and Chronic Health Evaluation; ICU: intensive care unit; LIPS: lung injury prediction score; OR: odds ratio; SIRS: systemic inflammatory response syndrome.

Authors' contributions

RS, PH, and JS contributed to the study design and concept. RS, MM, and JS contributed to analysis and interpretation of data. RS, PH, IA, GF, PP, MM, SC, OG, and JS contributed to the writing and review. All authors read and approved the final manuscript.

Author details

[1] Division of Emergency Critical Care Medicine, Department of Emergency Medicine, Brigham and Women's Hospital, 75 Francis St., Neville House, Boston, MA 02115, USA. [2] Surgical ICU Translational Research (STAR) Center, Brigham and Women's Hospital, Boston, MA, USA. [3] Department of Anesthesiology, Perioperative and Pain Medicine, Brigham and Women's Hospital, Boston, MA, USA. [4] Division of Acute Care Surgery, Department of Surgery, University of Michigan Health System, Ann Arbor, MI, USA. [5] Division of Pulmonary, Allergy, and Critical Care Medicine, Department of Medicine, Perelman School of Medicine, University of Pennsylvania, Philadelphia, PA, USA. [6] Division of Pulmonary and Critical Care, Department of Medicine, UCLA, Los Angeles, CA, USA. [7] Division of Pulmonary and Critical Care Medicine, Department of Medicine, Mayo Clinic, Rochester, MN, USA. [8] Division of Pulmonary, Allergy and Critical Care, Department of Medicine, Emory University, Atlanta, GA, USA.

Acknowledgements

We thank the US Critical Illness and Injury Trials Group: Lung Injury Prevention Study for collaborating with us on this investigation (see "Appendix" for a listing of collaborating investigators and clinical centers).

Competing interests

The authors declare that they have no competing interests.

Appendix: US Critical Illness and Injury Trials Group: Lung Injury Prevention Study Participating Centers and Investigators

Mayo Clinic, Rochester, Minnesota: Adil Ahmed, M.D.; Ognjen Gajic, M.D.; Michael Malinchoc, M.S.; Daryl J. Kor, M.D.; Bekele Afessa, M.D.; Rodrigo Cartin-Ceba, M.D.; Rickey E. Carter, Ph.D.; Departments of Internal Medicine, Health Sciences Research and Anesthesiology

University of Missouri, Missouri, Columbia: University of Missouri-Columbia: Ousama Dabbagh, M.D., M.S.P.H., Associate Professor of Clinical Medicine; Nivedita Nagam, M.D.; Shilpa Patel, M.D.; Ammar Kar; and Brian Hess

University of Michigan, Ann Arbor, Michigan: Pauline K. Park, M.D., F.A.C.S., F.C.C.S., Co-Director, Surgical Intensive Care Unit, Associate Professor, Surgery; Julie Harris, Clinical Research Coordinator; Lena Napolitano, M.D.; Krishnan Raghavendran, M.B.B.S.; Robert C. Hyzy, M.D.; James Blum, M.D.; Christy Dean

University of Texas Southwestern Medical Center in Dallas, Dallas, Texas: Adebola Adesanya, M.D.; Srikanth Hosur, M.D.; Victor Enoh, M.D.; Department of Anesthesiology, Division of Critical Care Medicine

University of Medicine and Dentistry of New Jersey, New Jersey: Steven Y. Chang, Ph.D., M.D., Assistant Professor, MICU Director, Pulmonary and Critical Care Medicine; Amee Patrawalla, M.D., M.P.H.; Marie Elie, M.D.

Brigham and Women's Hospital, Boston, Massachusetts: Peter C. Hou, M.D.; Jonathan M. Barry, B.A.; Ian Shempp, B.S.; Atul Malhotra, M.D.; Gyorgy Frendl, M.D., Ph.D.; Departments of Emergency Medicine, Surgery, Internal Medicine and Anesthesiology,

Perioperative and Pain Medicine, Division of Burn, Trauma, and Surgical Critical Care

Wright State University Boonshoft School of Medicine and Miami Valley Hospital, Dayton, Ohio: Harry Anderson III, M.D., Professor of Surgery; Kathryn Tchorz, M.D., Associate Professor of Surgery; Mary C. McCarthy, M.D., Professor of Surgery; David Uddin, Ph.D., D.A.B.C.C., C.I.P., Director of Research

Wake Forest University Health Sciences, Winston-Salem, North Carolina: J. Jason Hoth, M.D., Assistant Professor of Surgery; Barbara Yoza, Ph.D., Study Coordinator

University of Pennsylvania, Philadelphia, Pennsylvania: Mark Mikkelsen, M.D., M.S.C.E., Assistant Professor of Medicine, Pulmonary, Allergy, and Critical Care Division; Jason D. Christie, M.D.; David F. Gaieski, M.D.; Paul Lanken, M.D.; Nuala Meyer, M.D.; Chirag Shah, M.D.

Temple University School of Medicine, Philadelphia, Pennsylvania: Nina T. Gentile, M.D., Associate Professor and Director, Clinical Research, Department of Emergency Medicine, Temple University School of Medicine; Karen Stevenson, M.D., Resident, Department of Emergency Medicine; Brent Freeman, B.S., Research Coordinator; Sujatha Srinivasan, M.D., Resident, Department of Emergency Medicine

Mount Sinai School of Medicine, New York, New York: Michelle Ng Gong, M.D., M.S., Assistant Professor, Pulmonary, Critical Care, and Sleep Medicine, Department of Medicine

Beth Israel Deaconess Medical Center, Boston, Massachusetts: Daniel Talmor, M.D., Director of Anesthesia and Critical Care, Associate Professor of Anaesthesia, Harvard Medical School, Boston, Massachusetts; S. Patrick Bender, M.D.; Mauricio Garcia, M.D.

Massachusetts General Hospital Harvard Medical School, Boston, Massachusetts: Ednan Bajwa, M.D., M.P.H., Instructor in Medicine; Atul Malhotra, M.D., Assistant Professor; B. Taylor Thompson, Associate Professor; David C. Christiani, M.D., M.P.H., Professor

University of Washington, Harborview, Seattle, Washington: Timothy R. Watkins, M.D., Acting Instructor, Department of Medicine, Division of Pulmonary and Critical Care Medicine; Steven Deem, M.D.; Miriam Treggiari, M.D., M.P.H.

Mayo Clinic Jacksonville: Emir Festic, M.D.; Augustine Lee, M.D.; John Daniels, M.D.

Akdeniz University, Antalyia, Turkey: Melike Cengiz, M.D., Ph.D.; Murat Yilmaz, M.D.

Uludag University, Bursa, Turkey: Remzi Iscimen, M.D.

Bridgeport Hospital, Yale New Haven Health, New Haven, Connecticut: David Kaufman, M.D., Section Chief, Pulmonary, Critical Care, and Sleep Medicine, Medical Director, Respiratory Therapy

Emory University, Atlanta, Georgia: Annette Esper, M.D.; Greg Martin, M.D.

University of Illinois at Chicago, Chicago, Illinois: Rux ana Sadikot, M.D., M.R.C.P.

University of Colorado, Boulder, Colorado: Ivor Douglas, M.D.

Johns Hopkins University: Jonathan Sevransky, M.D., M.H.S., Assistant Professor of Medicine, Medical Director, JHBMC MICU.

References

1. Brun-Buisson C, Minelli C, Bertolini G, Brazzi L, Pimentel J, Lewandowski K, et al. Epidemiology and outcome of acute lung injury in European intensive care units. Results from the ALIVE study. Intensive Care Med. 2004;30(1):51–61. doi:10.1007/s00134-003-2022-6.
2. Hudson LD, Milberg JA, Anardi D, Maunder RJ. Clinical risks for development of the acute respiratory distress syndrome. Am J Respir Crit Care Med. 1995;151(2 Pt 1):293–301. doi:10.1164/ajrccm.151.2.7842182.
3. Rubenfeld GD, Caldwell E, Peabody E, Weaver J, Martin DP, Neff M, et al. Incidence and outcomes of acute lung injury. N Engl J Med. 2005;353(16):1685–93. doi:10.1056/NEJMoa050333.
4. Iscimen R, Cartin-Ceba R, Yilmaz M, Khan H, Hubmayr RD, Afessa B, et al. Risk factors for the development of acute lung injury in patients with septic shock: an observational cohort study. Crit Care Med. 2008;36(5):1518–22. doi:10.1097/CCM.0b013e31816fc2c0.
5. Dellinger RP, Levy MM, Rhodes A, Annane D, Gerlach H, Opal SM, et al. Surviving sepsis campaign: international guidelines for management of severe sepsis and septic shock: 2012. Crit Care Med. 2013;41(2):580–637. doi:10.1097/CCM.0b013e31827e83af.
6. Levy MM, Rhodes A, Phillips GS, Townsend SR, Schorr CA, Beale R, et al. Surviving Sepsis Campaign: association between performance metrics and outcomes in a 7.5-year study. Crit Care Med. 2015;43(1):3–12. doi:10.1097/CCM.0000000000000723.
7. Damiani E, Donati A, Serafini G, Rinaldi L, Adrario E, Pelaia P, et al. Effect of performance improvement programs on compliance with sepsis bundles and mortality: a systematic review and meta-analysis of observational studies. PLoS ONE. 2015;10(5):e0125827. doi:10.1371/journal.pone.0125827.
8. Mikkelsen ME, Shah CV, Meyer NJ, Gaieski DF, Lyon S, Miltiades AN, et al. The epidemiology of acute respiratory distress syndrome in patients presenting to the emergency department with severe sepsis. Shock. 2013;40(5):375–81. doi:10.1097/SHK.0b013e3182a64682.
9. Fuller BM, Mohr NM, Dettmer M, Kennedy S, Cullison K, Bavolek R, et al. Mechanical ventilation and acute lung injury in emergency department patients with severe sepsis and septic shock: an observational study. Acad Emerg Med. 2013;20(7):659–69. doi:10.1111/acem.12167.
10. Pro CI, Yealy DM, Kellum JA, Huang DT, Barnato AE, Weissfeld LA, et al. A randomized trial of protocol-based care for early septic shock. N Engl J Med. 2014;370(18):1683–93. doi:10.1056/NEJMoa1401602.
11. Investigators A, Group ACT, Peake SL, Delaney A, Bailey M, Bellomo R, et al. Goal-directed resuscitation for patients with early septic shock. N Engl J Med. 2014;371(16):1496–506. doi:10.1056/NEJMoa1404380.
12. Mouncey PR, Osborn TM, Power GS, Harrison DA, Sadique MZ, Grieve RD, et al. Trial of early, goal-directed resuscitation for septic shock. N Engl J Med. 2015;372(14):1301–11. doi:10.1056/NEJMoa1500896.
13. Boyd JH, Forbes J, Nakada TA, Walley KR, Russell JA. Fluid resuscitation in septic shock: a positive fluid balance and elevated central venous pressure are associated with increased mortality. Crit Care Med. 2011;39(2):259–65. doi:10.1097/CCM.0b013e3181feeb15.
14. Micek ST, McEvoy C, McKenzie M, Hampton N, Doherty JA, Kollef MH. Fluid balance and cardiac function in septic shock as predictors of hospital mortality. Crit Care. 2013;17(5):R246. doi:10.1186/cc13072.
15. de Oliveira FS, Freitas FG, Ferreira EM, de Castro I, Bafi AT, de Azevedo LC, et al. Positive fluid balance as a prognostic factor for mortality and acute kidney injury in severe sepsis and septic shock. J Crit Care. 2015;30(1):97–101. doi:10.1016/j.jcrc.2014.09.002.
16. Sirvent JM, Ferri C, Baro A, Murcia C, Lorencio C. Fluid balance in sepsis and septic shock as a determining factor of mortality. Am J Emerg Med. 2015;33(2):186–9. doi:10.1016/j.ajem.2014.11.016.
17. Gajic O, Dabbagh O, Park PK, Adesanya A, Chang SY, Hou P, et al. Early identification of patients at risk of acute lung injury: evaluation of lung injury prediction score in a multicenter cohort study. Am J Respir Crit Care Med. 2011;183(4):462–70. doi:10.1164/rccm.201004-0549OC.
18. Force ADT, Ranieri VM, Rubenfeld GD, Thompson BT, Ferguson ND, Caldwell E, et al. Acute respiratory distress syndrome: the Berlin definition. JAMA. 2012;307(23):2526–33. doi:10.1001/jama.2012.5669.
19. Jia X, Malhotra A, Saeed M, Mark RG, Talmor D. Risk factors for ARDS in patients receiving mechanical ventilation for >48 h. Chest. 2008;133(4):853–61. doi:10.1378/chest.07-1121.
20. National Heart L, Blood Institute Acute Respiratory Distress Syndrome Clinical Trials N, Wiedemann HP, Wheeler AP, Bernard GR, Thompson BT, et al. Comparison of two fluid-management strategies in acute lung injury. N Engl J Med. 2006;354(24):2564–75. doi:10.1056/NEJMoa062200.

21. Phillips CR, Chesnutt MS, Smith SM. Extravascular lung water in sepsis-associated acute respiratory distress syndrome: indexing with predicted body weight improves correlation with severity of illness and survival. Crit Care Med. 2008;36(1):69–73. doi:10.1097/01.CCM.0000295314.01232.BE.
22. Craig TR, Duffy MJ, Shyamsundar M, McDowell C, McLaughlin B, Elborn JS, et al. Extravascular lung water indexed to predicted body weight is a novel predictor of intensive care unit mortality in patients with acute lung injury. Crit Care Med. 2010;38(1):114–20. doi:10.1097/CCM.0b013e3181b43050.
23. Jozwiak M, Silva S, Persichini R, Anguel N, Osman D, Richard C, et al. Extravascular lung water is an independent prognostic factor in patients with acute respiratory distress syndrome. Crit Care Med. 2013;41(2):472–80. doi:10.1097/CCM.0b013e31826ab377.
24. Rivers EP, Kruse JA, Jacobsen G, Shah K, Loomba M, Otero R, et al. The influence of early hemodynamic optimization on biomarker patterns of severe sepsis and septic shock. Crit Care Med. 2007;35(9):2016–24.
25. Murphy CV, Schramm GE, Doherty JA, Reichley RM, Gajic O, Afessa B, et al. The importance of fluid management in acute lung injury secondary to septic shock. Chest. 2009;136(1):102–9. doi:10.1378/chest.08-2706.
26. Chang DW, Huynh R, Sandoval E, Han N, Coil CJ, Spellberg BJ. Volume of fluids administered during resuscitation for severe sepsis and septic shock and the development of the acute respiratory distress syndrome. J Crit Care. 2014;29(6):1011–5. doi:10.1016/j.jcrc.2014.06.005.
27. Brown JB, Cohen MJ, Minei JP, Maier RV, West MA, Billiar TR, et al. Goal-directed resuscitation in the prehospital setting: a propensity-adjusted analysis. J Trauma Acute Care Surg. 2013;74(5):1207–12. doi:10.1097/TA.0b013e31828c44fd **(discussion 12-4)**.
28. Rivers E, Nguyen B, Havstad S, Ressler J, Muzzin A, Knoblich B, et al. Early goal-directed therapy in the treatment of severe sepsis and septic shock. N Engl J Med. 2001;345(19):1368–77. doi:10.1056/NEJMoa010307.
29. Sheu CC, Gong MN, Zhai R, Bajwa EK, Chen F, Thompson BT, et al. The influence of infection sites on development and mortality of ARDS. Intensive Care Med. 2010;36(6):963–70. doi:10.1007/s00134-010-1851-3.
30. Jacobs ML, Daggett WM, Civette JM, Vasu MA, Lawson DW, Warshaw AL, et al. Acute pancreatitis: analysis of factors influencing survival. Ann Surg. 1977;185(1):43–51.
31. Raghu MG, Wig JD, Kochhar R, Gupta D, Gupta R, Yadav TD, et al. Lung complications in acute pancreatitis. JOP. 2007;8(2):177–85.
32. Khan H, Belsher J, Yilmaz M, Afessa B, Winters JL, Moore SB, et al. Fresh-frozen plasma and platelet transfusions are associated with development of acute lung injury in critically ill medical patients. Chest. 2007;131(5):1308–14. doi:10.1378/chest.06-3048.
33. Gong MN, Thompson BT, Williams P, Pothier L, Boyce PD, Christiani DC. Clinical predictors of and mortality in acute respiratory distress syndrome: potential role of red cell transfusion. Crit Care Med. 2005;33(6):1191–8.
34. Gajic O, Rana R, Winters JL, Yilmaz M, Mendez JL, Rickman OB, et al. Transfusion-related acute lung injury in the critically ill: prospective nested case–control study. Am J Respir Crit Care Med. 2007;176(9):886–91. doi:10.1164/rccm.200702-271OC.
35. Elliot MR, Zhang N, Small DS. Application of propensity scores to a continuous exposure: effect of lead exposure in early childhood on reading and mathematics scores. Obs Stud. 2015;1:30–55.

5

Superior accuracy of mid-regional proadrenomedullin for mortality prediction in sepsis with varying levels of illness severity

David Andaluz-Ojeda[1,2], H. Bryant Nguyen[3], Nicolas Meunier-Beillard[4], Ramón Cicuéndez[1,2], Jean-Pierre Quenot[4], Dolores Calvo[5], Auguste Dargent[4], Esther Zarca[5], Cristina Andrés[5], Leonor Nogales[1,2], Jose María Eiros[6], Eduardo Tamayo[2,7], Francisco Gandía[1,2], Jesús F. Bermejo-Martín[2*] and Pierre Emmanuel Charles[4]

Abstract

Background: The use of novel sepsis biomarkers has increased in recent years. However, their prognostic value with respect to illness severity has not been explored. In this work, we examined the ability of mid-regional proadrenomedullin (MR-proADM) in predicting mortality in sepsis patients with different degrees of organ failure, compared to that of procalcitonin, C-reactive protein and lactate.

Methods: This was a two-centre prospective observational cohort, enrolling severe sepsis or septic shock patients admitted to the ICU. Plasma biomarkers were measured during the first 12 h of admission. The association between biomarkers and 28-day mortality was assessed by Cox regression analysis and Kaplan–Meier curves. Patients were divided into three groups as evaluated by the Sequential Organ Failure Assessment (SOFA) score. The accuracy of the biomarkers for mortality was determined by area under the receiver operating characteristic curve (AUROC) analysis.

Results: A total of 326 patients with severe sepsis (21.7%) or septic shock (79.3%) were enrolled with a 28-day mortality rate of 31.0%. Only MR-proADM and lactate were associated with mortality in the multivariate analysis: hazard ratio 8.5 versus 3.4 ($p < 0.001$). MR-proADM showed the best AUROC for mortality prediction at 28 days in the analysis over the entire cohort (AUROC [95% CI] 0.79 [0.74–0.84]) ($p < 0.001$). When patients were stratified by the degree of organ failure, MR-proADM was the only biomarker to predict mortality in all severity groups (SOFA ≤ 6, SOFA $= 7$–12, and SOFA ≥ 13), AUROC [95% CI] of 0.75 [0.61–0.88], 0.74 [0.66–0.83] and 0.73 [0.59–0.86], respectively ($p < 0.05$). All patients with MR-proADM concentrations ≤ 0.88 nmol/L survived up to 28 days. In patients with SOFA ≤ 6, the addition of MR-proADM to the SOFA score increased the ability of SOFA to identify non-survivors, AUROC [95% CI] 0.70 [0.58–0.82] and 0.77 [0.66–0.88], respectively ($p < 0.05$ for both).

Conclusions: The performance of prognostic biomarkers in sepsis is highly influenced by disease severity. MR-proADM accuracy to predict mortality is not affected by the degree of organ failure. Thus, it is a good candidate in the early identification of sepsis patients with moderate disease severity but at risk of mortality.

Keywords: MR-proADM, Biomarkers, Sepsis, Mortality, SOFA

Background

Sepsis remains the primary cause of death in intensive care unit (ICU) patients despite improvements in antibiotic and early hemodynamic management. In Europe, sepsis occurrence in acutely ill patients results in an ICU mortality rate ranging between 27 and 54% depending on the severity [1]. In the USA, the Centre for Disease Control estimates that 500,000 people develop sepsis and 200,000 die each year [2, 3]. The prompt diagnosis and assessment of high risk sepsis patients is

*Correspondence: jfbermejo@saludcastillayleon.es
[2] Group for Biomedical Research in Sepsis (Bio·Sepsis), Hospital Clínico Universitario, Avda Ramón y Cajal 3, 47005 Valladolid, Spain
Full list of author information is available at the end of the article

therefore highly desirable, increasing the possibility of initiating early and specific treatments. Thus, clinical severity scores such as Sequential Organ Failure Assessment (SOFA) score can play a critical role [4]. However, the isolated use of these scoring systems to guide decision-making in sepsis has been heavily criticized [5]. A standardized assessment tool for the early identification of sepsis patients upon admission with a range of severity levels would be of dramatic value in aiding clinical decision-making and optimizing the use of health care resources. Accordingly, a number of prognostic biomarkers have been proposed in the field of sepsis over the last decades—many more than in other diseases. Most of these molecules are hormones, cytokines or circulating proteins related to inflammation or the coagulation system and may require considerable time, effort and costs to be measured [6].

Adrenomedullin (ADM) is a peptide which can act as a hormone and is produced by multiple tissues during physiologic and infectious stress with varying physiological functions, including vasodilatory, anti-inflammatory and antimicrobial activity, which is further enhanced by its regulation and modulation of complement activity [7]. Thus, ADM is considered a "hormokine", characterized by a hormone-like behaviour in non-inflammatory conditions when it is only produced by endocrine cells, and by a cytokine-like behaviour in sepsis when it is ubiquitously hyper-expressed. Moreover, exogenous ADM has been shown to reduce acute lung injury, vascular permeability and death in animal models of sepsis, whilst endogenous over-expression similarly ameliorates the sepsis insult [8, 9]. Measurement of circulating ADM is complicated by a rapid degradation and clearance from the circulation, and is further masked by a binding protein (complement factor H), preventing its detection by standard immunoassay. The mid-regional fragment of proadrenomedullin (MR-proADM), comprising of amino acids 45–92, is more stable and directly reflects levels of the rapidly degraded active ADM peptide [10]. Increased MR-proADM concentrations have been identified in the plasma of patients with community acquired pneumonia (CAP) and are widely used in the risk and severity assessment of this condition [11–13]. However, very few are available for severe sepsis and septic shock patients. Additionally, the influence of disease severity on the performance of prognostic biomarkers in sepsis has not been appropriately studied yet.

In this study, we aimed to evaluate the ability of MR-proADM levels to predict 28-day mortality in sepsis patients, compared to other standard biomarkers (procalcitonin (PCT), C-reactive protein (CRP), and lactate), in three different levels of disease severity as measured by the SOFA score.

Methods

Patient selection, inclusion and exclusion criteria

This study was a prospective observational cohort of patients recruited consecutively from two intensive care units (ICU) in Spain and France. Adult patients with age ≥18 years and admitted to the ICU from April 2013 to January 2016 were enrolled within 12 h after meeting criteria for severe sepsis or septic shock, based on the SEPSIS-2 definition by the American College of Chest Physicians/Society of Critical Care Medicine Consensus Conference [14]. Enrolled patients also had SOFA score ≥2 and therefore met criteria for the new SEPSIS-3 definition for sepsis [15]. Patients with human immunodeficiency virus (HIV) infection and those undergoing radiotherapy or receiving immunosuppressive drugs, including chemotherapy or systemic steroids, in the 3 months prior to admission to the ICU were considered to be immunosuppressed. Exclusion criteria were age <18 years, the presence of pregnancy, the absence of a blood sample available for biomarker profiling within the first 12 h following ICU admission, or lack of informed consent. Clinical data recorded from the medical records included demographics, comorbidities, laboratories, microbiology, and biomarker levels. The severity of illness was assessed on admission by calculating the Sequential Organ Failure Assessment (SOFA) score.

Biomarker evaluation

Plasma samples for biomarker profiling were collected as close as possible to the moment of ICU admission, and always within the first 12 h. Plasma MR-proADM measurement was performed by TRACE technology (Time Resolved Amplified Cryptate Emission) using a new sandwich immunoassay (Kryptor Compact Plus Analyser, BRAHMS, Hennigsdorf, Germany); limit of detection 0.05 nmol/L. PCT measurement was performed by electrochemiluminescence immunoassay (ECLIA) on a chemistry analyser (Cobas 6000, Roche Diagnostics, Meylan, France); limit of detection 0.02 ng/ml. Serum CRP and lactate were measured by particle-enhanced immunoturbidimetric and colorimetric assay, respectively (e501 Module Analyser, Roche Diagnostics, Meylan, France); limit of detection 0.15 mg/dL and 0.2 mmol/L, respectively.

Statistical analysis

Differences in demographic and clinical characteristics between survivors and non-survivors were assessed using the Chi-square test for categorical variables. Student's t test or Mann–Whitney U test were, respectively, used to compare continuous variables based upon the presence or absence of normal distribution. The association between biomarkers and the risk of mortality was assessed by Cox regression analysis, adjusted by confounding variables. Time was censored at 28 days following admission to the ICU. The first 24 h of ICU admission was considered as day 1 in the analysis. Variables yielding a $p < 0.05$ in the univariate regression analysis were further included in the multivariate analysis. Biomarkers were log transformed in order to reach a normal distribution. The impact of biomarkers on mean survival time was assessed by using Kaplan–Meier curves and the Mantel–Haenszel log-rank test. Similar to the Cox regression analysis, time was censored at 28 days following admission to the ICU. Accuracy and predictive values of the biomarkers for mortality were evaluated by calculating the area under the receiver operating characteristic (AUROC) curve. Patients were distributed into three groups depending on disease severity as assessed by the SOFA score using two predefined cut-offs, one with a sensitivity close to 90% and the other showing a specificity close to 90% for detecting non-survivors at 28 days (Additional file 1: Figure S1). Data were analysed by using the IBM SPSS 20.0 software (SPSS, Chicago, Ill).

Results

Patient characteristics and biomarker concentrations

Three hundred and twenty-six patients (326) with severe sepsis (21.7%) or septic shock (79.3%) were enrolled with a 28-day mortality rate of 25.5 and 34.9% in Valladolid and Dijon, respectively, and an overall mortality rate of 31.0% across both sites (Table 1). The median age was 65 years and 54.3% of patients were male. Compared to survivors, non-survivors were older and presented with higher SOFA scores, and an increased incidence of septic shock, mechanical ventilation, renal replacement therapy, neoplasia, cardiovascular disease, chronic renal failure, immunosuppression, and respiratory disease (all $p < 0.05$). The most common source of infection was of respiratory and urologic origin, regardless of outcome.

Table 1 Clinical characteristics of the patients: data are presented as mean (S.D.) or median (IQR) where appropriate

	Survivors $n = 225$	Non-survivors $n = 101$	Total $n = 326$	p
Patients from Valladolid (n, %)	102 (45.3%)	35 (34.7%)	137	0.071
Patients from Dijon (n, %)	123 (54.7%)	66 (65.3%)	189	
Male (n, %)	133 (59.1%)	68 (67.3%)	201 (61.4%)	0.098
Age (years) (mean, SD)	63 (14)	69 (12)	65.4 (14)	<0.001
SOFA (mean, SD)	8 (3.4)	11 (3.5)	9 (3.7)	<0.001
Septic shock (n, %)	152 (67.5%)	87 (86.1%)	239 (73.3%)	0.020
Mechanical ventilation (n, %)	150 (66.7%)	89 (88.1%)	239 (73.3%)	<0.001
RRT (n, %)	40 (17.7%)	45 (44.6%)	85 (26.2%)	<0.001
ICU stay (days) (mean, SD)	12.9 (18)	7.7 (6.7)	11.2 (15.6)	0.012
Neoplasia (n, %)	47 (21%)	35 (34.7%)	82 (25.2%)	0.007
Diabetes (n, %)	58 (25.8%)	29 (28.7%)	87 (26.7%)	0.330
COPD (n, %)	33 (14.7%)	16 (15.8%)	49 (15%)	0.450
Cardiovascular disease (n, %)	56 (25%)	41 (40.6%)	97 (29.8%)	0.030
Chronic renal failure (n, %)	16 (7.1%)	16 (15.8%)	32 (9.8%)	0.014
Immunosuppression (n, %)	21 (9.3%)	25 (24.8%)	46 (14.1%)	<0.001
Respiratory infection (n, %)	98 (43.6%)	58 (57.4%)	156 (48%)	0.014
Urologic infection (n, %)	75 (33.3%)	36 (35.6%)	111 (34%)	0.380
Abdominal infection (n, %)	25 (11.1%)	10 (9.9%)	35 (10.7%)	0.450
Other infection (n, %)	32 (14%)	11 (10.9%)	43 (13%)	0.40
Primary or secondary bacteremia (n, %)	69 (30.7%)	38 (37.6%)	107 (32.8%)	0.130
Gram − bacteria (n, %)	62 (27.6%)	28 (27.7%)	90 (27.6%)	0.975
Gram + bacteria (n, %)	47 (20.9%)	22 (21.8%)	69 (21.2%)	0.855
Fungi (n, %)	3 (1.3%)	5 (5%)	8 (2.5%)	0.050
Virus (n, %)	15 (6.7%)	5 (5%)	20 (6.1%)	0.550
MR-proADM (nmol/L) (median, IQR)	2.68 (3.56)	7.44 (6.84)	3.62 (5.6)	<0.001
Lactate (mmol/L) (median, IQR)	2.00 (1.54)	3.60 (5.53)	2.12 (2.28)	<0.001
CRP (mg/dl) (median, IQR)	147.8 (193.6)	163.0 (181.9)	155.0 (189)	0.200
PCT (ng/ml) (median, IQR)	2.9 (17.5)	5.8 (36.7)	3.54 (27.5)	0.001

Values expressed in percentages (%) indicate the proportion of survivors and non-survivors at 28 days for specific variables

Mortality rates depending on the source of infection were as follows: 37.2% in patients suffering from a respiratory infection, 32.4% in those with an urological infection, 28.6% in patients with an abdominal infection, 35.5% in those showing a primary or secondary bacteremia and 25.6% in those patients with an infection of other origin. Regarding microbiological identification, both survivors and non-survivors showed a similar presence of Gram−, Gram+ and virus pathogens. Fungal infections were more frequent in non-survivors. The most common cause of death was multi-organ dysfunction syndrome (n = 58; 57.4%), followed by refractory shock (n = 9; 8.9%) and refractory hypoxemia (n = 8; 7.9%). A limitation of therapeutic effort was applied to 21 patients. MR-proADM, PCT and lactate concentrations were all significantly elevated in non-surviving patients compared to survivors (all $p < 0.01$), whereas CRP levels remained similar in both groups. Levels of MR-proADM depending on the source of infection were as follows [median (interquartile range)] respiratory infection [3.6 nmol/L (5.6)], urological infection [4.6 nmol/L (5.4)], abdominal infection [4.9 nmol/L (6.5)], bacteremia [3.8 nmol/L (5.1)], and [3.5 nmol/L (5.8)] in infections of other origin. Levels of MR-proADM depending on the infecting microbe were [median (interquartile range)]: fungal infection [6.1 nmol/L (5.6)], Gram − bacteria [4.9 nmol/L (5.9)], Gram + bacteria [4.1 nmol/L (6.2)] or viruses [1.2 nmol/L (3.4)].

Survival analysis

MR-proADM, PCT and lactate showed a significant association with mortality in the univariate Cox regression analysis (Table 2). After adjusting for confounders and compared to PCT, CRP, and lactate, MR-proADM showed the strongest independent association with the risk of mortality (hazard ratio 8.5; 95% confidence interval 4.2–17.4; $p < 0.001$; Table 2). In addition, Kaplan–Meier analysis showed that no patients with a MR-proADM value ≤0.88 nmol/L died in the first 28 days following ICU admission (Fig. 1). This cut-off was selected since it provided a sensitivity of 100% in identifying non-survivors in the AUROC (Fig. 2).

Adjusting variables were: age, septic shock, cardiovascular disease, immunosuppression, chronic renal failure, neoplasia, respiratory source of infection, renal replacement therapy, hospital (Valladolid/Dijon), presence of fungal infection, limitation of therapeutic effort.

The influence of disease severity on biomarker performance

MR-proADM showed the best AUROC for mortality prediction at 28 days in the analysis over the entire cohort, even better than that of SOFA score (Fig. 2). When patients were stratified by the degree of organ failure, MR-proADM was the only biomarker able to discriminate non-survivors from survivors at 28 days in those patients with the lowest degree of disease severity (SOFA score ≤ 6), (AUROC [95% confidence interval (95% CI)] 0.75 [0.61–0.88]), (p = 0.006) (Fig. 3). In the moderately severe patients (SOFA score 7–12), MR-proADM showed a higher AUROC than that observed with lactate (0.74 [0.66–0.83] vs. 0.61 [0.52–0.71], respectively, Fig. 3). In the most severe patients (SOFA score ≥13), MR-proADM and lactate had a similar AUROC (0.73 [0.59–0.86] vs. 0.72 [0.59–0.86], respectively, Fig. 3). Neither CRP nor PCT was predictive of 28-day mortality in any severity group based on the SOFA score, with AUROCs ranging from 0.43 to 0.60.

The threshold values (cut-off) of MR-proADM were determined by having the highest specificity with a pre-fixed sensitivity of at least 0.80 for identifying non-survivors. For patients with SOFA scores ≤6, 7–12, and ≥13, the MR-proADM cut-offs were 1.79, 3.25, and 5.58 nmol/L, respectively (Table 3).

Table 2 Uni- and multivariate Cox regression analysis for mortality prediction at 28 days following ICU admission

	Univariate		Multivariate	
	HR (95% CI)	p	HR (95% CI)	p
MR-proADM	11.2 (6.3–19.8)	<0.001	8.5 (4.2–17.4)	<0.001
Lactate	3.8 (2.6–5.5)	<0.001	3.4 (2.0–5.8)	<0.001
CRP	1.3 (0.8–1.9)	0.266	–	–
PCT	1.4 (1.2–1.8)	0.001	1.1 (0.9–1.4)	0.326
SOFA	1.2 (1.2–1.3)	<0.001	1.2 (1.1–1.3)	<0.001

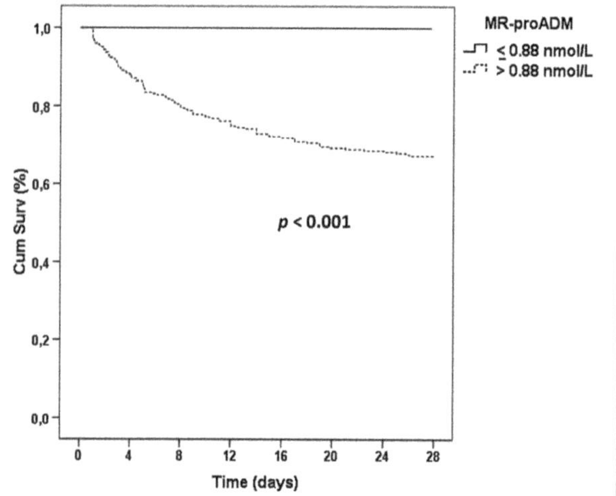

Fig. 1 Kaplan–Meier analysis for mortality prediction at 28 days

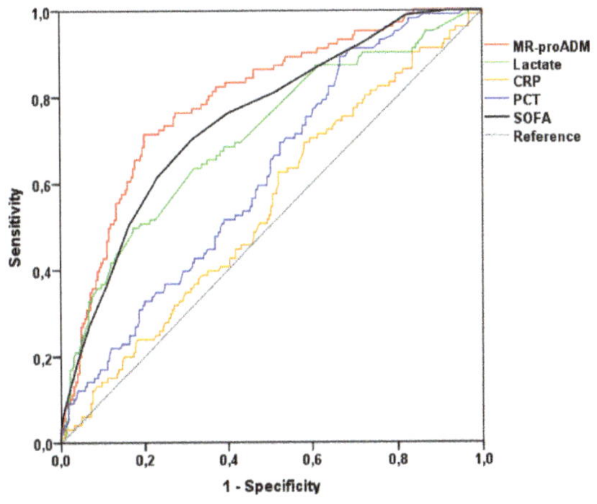

	AUROC [95 %CI]	p
MR-proADM	0.79 [0.74 - 0.84]	< 0.001
Lactate	0.71 [0.64 - 0.77]	< 0.001
CRP	0.54 [0.47 - 0.61]	0.248
PCT	0.61 [0.55 - 0.68]	< 0.001
SOFA	0.75 [0.69 - 0.80]	< 0.001

Fig. 2 AUROC analysis for identifying non-survivors at 28 days (entire cohort)

The length of ICU stay in each severity group was [mean, (SD)]: SOFA ≤ 6: 11.0 days (18.3); SOFA 7–12: 12.4 days (16.0) and SOFA ≥ 13: 8.4 days (7.6). The mortality rates for each severity group were 12.8, 30.6 and 59.7%, respectively.

MR-proADM improves mortality prediction in the less severely ill patients

We evaluated the combination of MR-proADM and SOFA score in predicting mortality, such that patients with MR-proADM concentrations >1.79 nmol/L were considered to have a 1 point increase in the SOFA score. In patients with SOFA ≤ 6, the MR-proADM modified SOFA score (ADM-SOFA) showed an increased ability to identify non-survivors compared to SOFA alone, AUROC [95% CI] SOFA 0.70 [0.58–0.82] and ADM-SOFA 0.77 [0.66–0.88].

Discussion

Severity in sepsis depends on the extent of organ failure as evaluated by the SOFA score, which in turn is directly associated with the risk of mortality [15]. Nonetheless,

SOFA ≤ 6 N= 94 patients	SOFA 7-12 N= 170 patients	SOFA ≥ 13 N= 62 patients

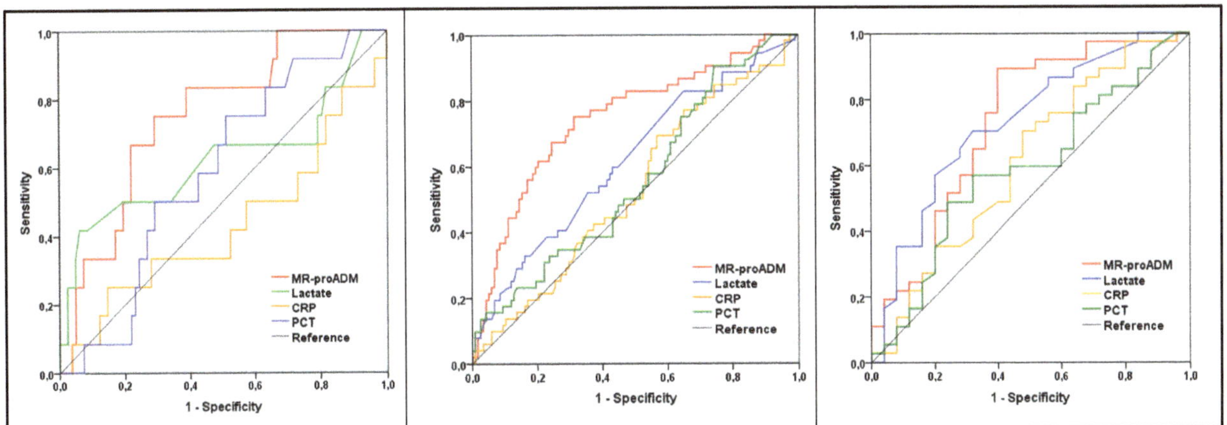

SOFA ≤ 6

	AUROC [95%CI]	p
MR-proADM	0.75 [0.61 - 0.88]	0.006
Lactate	0.62 [0.41 - 0.83]	0.165
CRP	0.43 [0.23 - 0.62]	0.428
PCT	0.58 [0.44 - 0.73]	0.341

SOFA 7-12

	AUROC [95%CI]	p
MR-proADM	0.74 [0.66 - 0.83]	0.000
Lactate	0.61 [0.52 - 0.71]	0.018
CRP	0.53 [0.44 - 0.62]	0.549
PCT	0.56 [0.46 - 0.65]	0.250

SOFA ≥ 13

	AUROC [95%CI]	p
MR-proADM	0.73 [0.59 - 0.86]	0.003
Lactate	0.72 [0.59 - 0.86]	0.003
CRP	0.6 0 [0.46 - 0.75]	0.168
PCT	0.58 [0.44 - 0.73]	0.279

Fig. 3 AUROC analysis for identifying non-survivors at 28 days depending on biomarker levels in the three severity groups

Table 3 MR-proADM cut-off (nmol/L) with the highest accuracy for predicting 28-day mortality based on SOFA score

	Cut-off	Sensitivity	Specificity	PPV	NPV	+LR	−LR
SOFA ≤ 6	1.79	83.0	61.0	23.8	96.2	2.14	0.27
SOFA 7–12	3.25	83.0	52.0	43.4	87.0	1.74	0.33
SOFA ≥ 13	5.58	83.8	60.0	75.6	71.4	2.09	0.27

PPV positive predictive value, *NPV* negative predictive value, *+LR* positive likelihood ratio, *−LR* negative likelihood ratio

the emergence of an increasing number of biomarkers may provide a new avenue with which to improve prognostic accuracy in a simple and rapid manner. In this regard, our study suggests that MR-proADM may be a promising biomarker. However, previous studies evaluating the prognostic role of MR-proADM in sepsis have provided conflicting results. Christ-Crain et al. [16] found that MR-proADM yielded an AUROC of 0.81 for detecting ICU mortality in a group of 53 patients with sepsis. In contrast, Suberviola et al. [17] found limited value of MR-proADM for predicting hospital mortality in 137 sepsis patients, with an AUROC of 0.62. Yet Marino et al. [18] showed that in 101 patients with sepsis, severe sepsis or septic shock, plasma adrenomedullin was strongly associated with the severity of disease, vasopressor requirement and 28-day mortality. These divergent results on the prognostic role of MR-proADM may be explained by differences in patient characteristics, disease severity, infectious source, surgical versus medical and small sample sizes across the various studies.

In the present study, we demonstrated for the first time that the performance of biomarkers to predict mortality in sepsis strongly depends on the degree of organ failure upon ICU admission. Stratifying patients based on their SOFA score allowed us to demonstrate that MR-proADM was the only biomarker able to identify non-survivors in all the severity groups. This is particularly important for the less severely ill patients (SOFA score ≤ 6), since this group represents either the earliest presentation in the clinical course of sepsis and/or the less severe form of this disease.

Thus, MR-proADM may be a good candidate, after validation in further studies, to be incorporated in an early sepsis management protocol, since it can provide rapid prognostic value and help to guide diagnostic interventions and treatment decisions, consequently resembling the role of troponin in myocardial infarction or d-dimer in pulmonary embolism. The cut-off value of MR-proADM identified for this group of patients (1.79 nmol/L) could be very useful in this regard. This cut-off is able to detect mortality with a good sensitivity and a high negative predictive value. Thus, MR-proADM may potentially help stratify patients in clinical trials examining novel therapies for sepsis.

MR-proADM showed greater predictive value for the risk of mortality than other more commonly used biomarkers, including lactate, in patients with an intermediate degree of organ failure (SOFA score 7–12). In contrast, both MR-proADM and lactate performed similarly in the most severe patients (SOFA ≥ 13). Therefore, our results support the importance of considering the degree of organ failure when designing studies for the discovery of prognostic biomarkers in sepsis.

The assessment of organ failure by using the SOFA score was recently proposed by the SEPSIS-3 consensus to identify high risk patients with suspected infection [15]. Our results show that a "positive" MR-proADM value may improve the ability of SOFA to predict mortality in sepsis. Interestingly, a combination of MR-proADM with clinical scores such as PSI or CURB-65 also performed better than the clinical scores alone in patients with Community Acquired Pneumonia (CAP) or lower respiratory tract infections (LRTI) [12, 19–21]. As a result, MR-proADM could be used as a reliable risk-stratification tool with the ability to predict mortality or adverse events and to guide clinical decisions. Further clinical studies evaluating strategies combining MR-proADM with other classical severity scores and/or biomarkers for improving the recognition and prognostication of sepsis are therefore warranted [22, 23].

Finally, we observed that an MR-proADM value lower than 0.88 nmol/L may allow to "rule out" mortality in the 28 days following admission to the ICU. This cut-off may be especially useful for guiding early clinical decisions, when the clinical signs of overt organ failure are not yet apparent.

Indeed, our results are similar to those of previous studies. Albrich et al. found that patients with LRTI and MR-proADM concentrations <0.75 nmol/L had an overall mortality of less than 0.5% (11). Furthermore, Krüger et al. showed that patients with CAP and an MR-proADM concentration of <0.9 nmol/L had a survival probability of 99.3% (12). Bello et al. [24] also found an optimal MR-proADM cut-off for predicting 30-day mortality in patients with CAP of 1.06 nmol/L.

Our study is limited in that we evaluated MR-proADM and other biomarker levels only on the day of ICU admission. As a result, we cannot extrapolate our findings to the emergency department or general ward. MR-proADM monitoring over time may further illustrate a temporal trend, which can indicate the success of specific therapies and consequently increase its outcome predictive value [25]. Finally, in our cohort, MR-proADM levels slightly differed depending on the source of infection. Fungal infections induced the highest levels of MR-proADM, while viral infection induced the lowest. This was likely related to the fact that fungal infections resulted in a higher disease severity (median SOFA score of 12 vs. 9 points in patients with no fungal infection), while viral infections resulted in a milder disease severity (median SOFA score of 6.5 vs. 9 points in patients with no viral infection). The potential influence of the source of infection and the type of microbe on MR-proADM's ability to predict mortality in sepsis merits further investigation.

Conclusions

Our results demonstrate that the performance of biomarkers in determining the risk of mortality in sepsis is influenced by disease severity. In patients with moderate severity, MR-proADM outperformed other standard biomarkers. As a consequence, MR-proADM may aid the early identification of sepsis patients requiring urgent ICU admission as well as facilitating the subsequent clinical management of these patients.

Abbreviations

ADM: adrenomedullin; MR-proADM: mid-regional proadrenomedullin; CRP: C-reactive protein; PCT: procalcitonin; SOFA: Sequential Organ Failure Assessment Score; CI: confidence interval; AUROC: area under receiver operating characteristics; PPV: positive predictive value; NPV: negative predictive value; LR: likelihood ratio; HR: hazard ratio; PSI: Pneumonia Severity Index; RRT: renal replacement therapy.

Authors' contributions

RC, J-PQ, AD, LN, NM-B, FG recruited the patients and collected the clinical information. They critically reviewed the manuscript draft. DC, EZ, CA performed the laboratory works and critically reviewed the manuscript draft. JME, ET critically reviewed the manuscript draft. DA-O, JFB -M, PEC participated in the design of study, statistical analysis and interpretation of the data and drafted the manuscript. HBN participated in the statistical analysis and interpretation of the data and drafted the manuscript. All authors read and approved the final manuscript.

Author details

[1] Servicio de Medicina Intensiva, Hospital Clínico Universitario, Avda Ramón y Cajal 3, 47005 Valladolid, Spain. [2] Group for Biomedical Research in Sepsis (Bio·Sepsis), Hospital Clínico Universitario, Avda Ramón y Cajal 3, 47005 Valladolid, Spain. [3] Division of Pulmonary and Critical Care Medicine, Department of Medicine, Loma Linda University, Loma Linda, CA, USA. [4] Service de Réanimation Médicale, Hôpital Bocage Central, C.H.U. DIJON, 14 rue Gaffarel, B.P. 77908-21079, Dijon Cedex, France. [5] Servicio de Análisis Clínicos, Hospital Clínico Universitario, Avda Ramón y Cajal 3, 47005 Valladolid, Spain. [6] Departmento de Microbiología, Facultad de Medicina, Universidad de Valladolid, Avda/Ramón y Cajal 7, 47005 Valladolid, Spain. [7] Servicio de Anestesiología y Reanimación, Hospital Clínico Universitario, Avda/Ramón y Cajal 3, 47005 Valladolid, Spain.

Acknowledgements

The authors thank the ICU nursery team for its contribution to this study in collecting the biological samples. The authors also thank Darius Wilson for kindly providing technical support.

Competing interests

D. Andaluz-Ojeda, B. Nguyen and P.E. Charles have participated in Advisory Board and Speaker Bureau for Thermo Fisher; J.F. Bermejo-Martin has participated in Advisory Board for Thermo Fisher. The remainder authors that they have no competing interests.

Funding

Thermo Fisher provided reagents for the biomarker evaluation. This study was supported by 'Fondo de Investigaciones Sanitarias, Instituto de Salud Carlos III', Spain, Grant (Nos. PI15/01959 and PI13/02110) and Programa de Intensificación de la Actividad Investigadora de la Gerencia Regional de Salud de la Consejería de Sanidad de Castilla y León (INT/M/06/16).

References

1. Vincent J-L. Clinical sepsis and septic shock—definition, diagnosis and management principles. Langenbecks Arch Surg Dtsch Ges Für Chir. 2008;393:817–24.
2. Jean-Baptiste E. Cellular mechanisms in sepsis. J Intensive Care Med. 2007;22:63–72.
3. Hoyert DL, Xu J. Deaths: preliminary data for 2011. Natl Vital Stat Rep Cent Dis Control Prev Natl Cent Health Stat Natl Vital Stat Syst. 2012;61:1–51.
4. Vincent JL, Moreno R, Takala J, Willatts S, De Mendonça A, Bruining H, et al. The SOFA (sepsis-related organ failure assessment) score to describe organ dysfunction/failure. On behalf of the working group on sepsis-related problems of the European society of intensive care medicine. Intensive Care Med. 1996;22:707–10.
5. Vincent J-L, Opal SM, Marshall JC. Ten reasons why we should NOT use severity scores as entry criteria for clinical trials or in our treatment decisions. Crit Care Med. 2010;38:283–7.
6. Pierrakos C, Vincent J-L. Sepsis biomarkers: a review. Crit Care Lond Engl. 2010;14:R15.
7. Hirata Y, Mitaka C, Sato K, Nagura T, Tsunoda Y, Amaha K, et al. Increased circulating adrenomedullin, a novel vasodilatory peptide, in sepsis. J Clin Endocrinol Metab. 1996;81:1449–53.
8. Müller-Redetzky HC, Will D, Hellwig K, Kummer W, Tschernig T, Pfeil U, et al. Mechanical ventilation drives pneumococcal pneumonia into lung injury and sepsis in mice: protection by adrenomedullin. Crit Care Lond Engl. 2014;18:R73.
9. Pugin J. Adrenomedullin: a vasodilator to treat sepsis? Crit Care Lond Engl. 2014;18:152.
10. Struck J, Tao C, Morgenthaler NG, Bergmann A. Identification of an adrenomedullin precursor fragment in plasma of sepsis patients. Peptides. 2004;25:1369–72.
11. Huang DT, Angus DC, Kellum JA, Pugh NA, Weissfeld LA, Struck J, et al. Midregional proadrenomedullin as a prognostic tool in community-acquired pneumonia. Chest. 2009;136:823–31.
12. Albrich WC, Dusemund F, Rüegger K, Christ-Crain M, Zimmerli W, Bregenzer T, et al. Enhancement of CURB65 score with proadrenomedullin (CURB65-A) for outcome prediction in lower respiratory tract infections: derivation of a clinical algorithm. BMC Infect Dis. 2011;11:112.

13. Krüger S, Ewig S, Giersdorf S, Hartmann O, Suttorp N, Welte T, et al. Cardiovascular and inflammatory biomarkers to predict short- and long-term survival in community-acquired pneumonia: results from the German Competence Network, CAPNETZ. Am J Respir Crit Care Med. 2010;182:1426–34.
14. Bone RC, Balk RA, Cerra FB, Dellinger RP, Fein AM, Knaus WA, et al. Definitions for sepsis and organ failure and guidelines for the use of innovative therapies in sepsis. The ACCP/SCCM consensus conference committee. American College of Chest Physicians/Society of Critical Care Medicine. 1992. Chest. 2009;136:e28.
15. Singer M, Deutschman CS, Seymour CW, Shankar-Hari M, Annane D, Bauer M, et al. The third international consensus definitions for sepsis and septic shock (sepsis-3). JAMA. 2016;315:801–10.
16. Christ-Crain M, Morgenthaler NG, Struck J, Harbarth S, Bergmann A, Müller B. Mid-regional pro-adrenomedullin as a prognostic marker in sepsis: an observational study. Crit Care Lond Engl. 2005;9:R816–24.
17. Suberviola B, Castellanos-Ortega A, Ruiz Ruiz A, Lopez-Hoyos M, Santibañez M. Hospital mortality prognostication in sepsis using the new biomarkers suPAR and proADM in a single determination on ICU admission. Intensive Care Med. 2013;39:1945–52.
18. Marino R, Struck J, Maisel AS, Magrini L, Bergmann A, Di Somma S. Plasma adrenomedullin is associated with short-term mortality and vasopressor requirement in patients admitted with sepsis. Crit Care Lond Engl. 2014;18:R34.
19. Christ-Crain M, Morgenthaler NG, Stolz D, Müller C, Bingisser R, Harbarth S, et al. Pro-adrenomedullin to predict severity and outcome in community-acquired pneumonia [ISRCTN04176397]. Crit Care Lond Engl. 2006;10:R96.
20. Courtais C, Kuster N, Dupuy A-M, Folschveiller M, Jreige R, Bargnoux A-S, et al. Proadrenomedullin, a useful tool for risk stratification in high Pneumonia Severity Index score community acquired pneumonia. Am J Emerg Med. 2013;31:215–21.
21. Renaud B, Schuetz P, Claessens Y-E, Labarère J, Albrich W, Mueller B. Proadrenomedullin improves risk of early admission to ICU score for predicting early severe community-acquired pneumonia. Chest. 2012;142:1447–54.
22. Guignant C, Voirin N, Venet F, Poitevin F, Malcus C, Bohé J, et al. Assessment of pro-vasopressin and pro-adrenomedullin as predictors of 28-day mortality in septic shock patients. Intensive Care Med. 2009;35:1859–67.
23. Travaglino F, De Berardinis B, Magrini L, Bongiovanni C, Candelli M, Silveri NG, et al. Utility of procalcitonin (PCT) and mid regional pro-adrenomedullin (MR-proADM) in risk stratification of critically ill febrile patients in Emergency Department (ED). A comparison with APACHE II score. BMC Infect Dis. 2012;12:184.
24. Bello S, Lasierra AB, Mincholé E, Fandos S, Ruiz MA, Vera E, et al. Prognostic power of proadrenomedullin in community-acquired pneumonia is independent of aetiology. Eur Respir J. 2012;39:1144–55.
25. Andaluz-Ojeda D, Cicuéndez R, Calvo D, Largo E, Nogales L, Muñoz MF, et al. Sustained value of proadrenomedullin as mortality predictor in severe sepsis. J Infect. 2015;71:136–9.

Epidemiology of sepsis in Catalonia: analysis of incidence and outcomes in a European setting

Juan Carlos Yébenes[1,2,3,16*], Juan Carlos Ruiz-Rodriguez[4,5], Ricard Ferrer[4,5,6], Montserrat Clèries[7], Anna Bosch[7], Carol Lorencio[8], Alejandro Rodriguez[2,9,10], Xavier Nuvials[11,12], Ignacio Martin-Loeches[13], Antoni Artigas[6,14,15] and SOCMIC (Catalonian Critical Care Society) Sepsis Working Group

Abstract

Background: Up-to-date identification of local trends in sepsis incidence and outcomes is of considerable public health importance. The aim of our study was to estimate annual incidence rates and in-hospital mortality trends for hospitalized patients with sepsis in a European setting, while avoiding selection bias in relation to different complexity hospitals.

Methods: A large retrospective analysis of a 5-year period (2008–2012) was conducted of hospital discharge records obtained from the Catalan Health System (CatSalut) Minimum Basic Data Set for Acute-Care Hospitals (a mandatory population-based register of admissions to all public and private acute-care hospitals in Catalonia). Patients hospitalized with sepsis were detected on the basis of ICD-9-CM codes used to identify acute organ dysfunction and infectious processes.

Results: Of 4,761,726 discharges from all acute-care hospitals in Catalonia, 82,300 cases (1.72%) had sepsis diagnoses. Annual incidence was 212.7 per 100,000 inhabitants/year, rising from 167.2 in 2008 to 261.8 in 2012. Length of hospital stay fell from 18.4 to 15.3 days ($p < .00001$), representing a relative reduction of 17%. Hospital mortality fell from 23.7 to 19.7% ($p < .0001$), representing a relative reduction of 16.9%. These differences were confirmed in the multivariate analysis (adjusted for age group, sex, comorbidities, ICU admission, emergency admission, organ dysfunction, number of organ failures, sepsis source and bacteraemia).

Conclusions: Sepsis incidence has risen in recent years, whereas mortality has fallen. Our findings confirm reports for other parts of the world, in the context of scarce administrative data on sepsis in Europe.

Keywords: Sepsis, Septic shock, Mortality, Epidemiology

Background

Sepsis has been recently redefined as an infection that leads to organ dysfunction [1]. Although a hospitalized patient with sepsis is more likely to die than a patient with heart attack or stroke [2], sepsis is still not evaluated with the same urgency as other critical conditions. Sepsis mortality can be reduced considerably by adopting early recognition protocols and using standardized emergency treatment, but fewer than 1 in 7 patients are actively intervened in this way [3]. Treatment ineffectiveness is often due to late sepsis diagnosis—mainly a failure by caregivers or healthcare professionals to suspect sepsis. The clinical symptoms and laboratory signs currently used for diagnostic purposes are not specific for sepsis, and there is a lack of reliable systems for timely detection of septic patients.

Proper detection of sepsis and its progression are essential to patient management. Epidemiology case studies using administrative hospital data have reported both

*Correspondence: jyebenes@csdm.cat
[16] Servei de Medicina Intensiva, Hospital de Mataró, Carretera de Cirera s/n, 08304 Mataró, Spain
Full list of author information is available at the end of the article

growing incidence and declining mortality rates associated with severe sepsis in several different countries but mainly in the USA, Australia and New Zealand [4–11]. However, administrative data may be affected by changes in coding practices that distort incidence and mortality estimates. Recently, Stevenson et al. [12] compared incidence and mortality trends in trial data with those observed in administrative data, observing that, since 1991, risk-standardized 28-day severe sepsis mortality has tended to decline in parallel for both methods; this which would indicate that trends in severe sepsis mortality as calculated from administrative data and International Classification of Diseases, 9th revision, Clinical Modification (ICD-9-CM) algorithms are likely to be accurate.

Catalonia, an autonomous region in Spain, has actively begun to advocate more vigorous efforts to decrease the sepsis burden through the development of an Inter-hospital Sepsis Emergency Code, operational between the Catalan Health Service (CatSalut) and seven local medical societies [13]. Since the identification of trends in sepsis outcomes is of considerable public health importance, the aim of our study was to estimate population and annual in-hospital incidence rates and in-hospital mortality trends for patients with sepsis between 2008 and 2012 in Catalonia, before implementation of the Inter-hospital Sepsis Emergency Code designed to coordinate and optimize care of patients with sepsis.

Methods

Data sources

A retrospective analysis was conducted of hospital discharge records from the Minimum Basic Data Set for the Catalan Health System (CatSalut) Acute-Care Hospitals (a mandatory population-based register of admissions to all public and private acute-care hospitals in Catalonia) enables evaluation and optimization of resource use, provides support to and improves healthcare planning and facilitates procurement management and payments. To ensure data quality, the CMBD-HA input data are systematically validated internally and periodically validated externally. The data set contains demographic and clinical data for patient care episodes, including age, sex, length of stay (days), one primary diagnosis, up to nine secondary diagnoses, one primary procedure, up to seven secondary procedures and status on discharge (alive or dead). Official data from the register of insured persons maintained by CatSalut were used to estimate crude and specific hospitalization rates (universal coverage for 7,601,813 inhabitants in 2012).

Patients

Sepsis, formerly severe sepsis [1] was defined by the presence of infection and at least one organ dysfunction. Patients hospitalized with sepsis were detected, according ICD-9-CM codes used to identify acute organ dysfunction and infectious processes following the Angus methodology [5], over a 5-year period (2008–2012). To avoid overlaps, we excluded patients who were transferred from one acute-care hospital to another during the same severe sepsis episode.

Coding

Diagnoses and procedures were coded using the ICD-9-CM, whose codes to identify patients with sepsis were updated in 2000 to the following: 995.91 (sepsis), 995.92 (severe sepsis) and 785.52 (septic shock) (Supplementary Appendix: Additional file 1). Although information was not available regarding the unit or department where patients were treated (intensive care unit (ICU), internal medicine unit, etc.), we indirectly deduced ICU admission from procedures typically used in intensive care management (Supplementary Appendix: Additional file 1). The Charlson comorbidity index with its 17 comorbid disease categories [13] was used to assess the presence of underlying comorbidities. The ICD-9-CM codes used to identify acute organ dysfunction and infectious processes are listed in Supplementary Appendix: Additional file 1.

Statistical analysis

The hospitalization rate was defined as the yearly number of admissions per 100,000 population (excluded were 1590 admissions from non-residents in Catalonia). Crude overall and specific hospitalization rates by age and sex were calculated. Continuous variables and discrete variables were compared using analysis of variance and the Chi-square test, respectively. Multivariate logistic regression, adjusted for other significant variables, was used to analyse hospital mortality risk by year of admission for the study population and for the ICU and non-ICU patient groups; variables were entered one by one and retained when their significance was <.10 and were clinically plausible. For the regression analysis, each of the clinical attributes included (comorbidities, acute organ failure and infection) were treated as binary (dummy) variables indicating the presence or absence of these conditions; a single patient could therefore account for more than one attribute. The area under the receiver operating characteristic curve (AUROC) was used to evaluate how well the multivariate logistic regression model discriminated between patients with severe sepsis who were discharged alive versus those who died in-hospital [14]. Data analysis was performed using SPSS 18.0 software (SPSS Inc, Chicago, IL, USA).

Results

Incidence and main features of severe sepsis

Of 4,761,726 discharges from all acute-care hospitals during the study period, 82,300 (1.72%) had sepsis. Demographic characteristics and comorbidities for patients with sepsis are shown in Table 1.

Annual incidence in the population was 212.7 per 100,000 inhabitants/year, increasing from 167.2 in 2008 to 261.8 per 100,000 inhabitants/year in 2012 (Fig. 1). Sepsis was significantly associated with age (more frequent in older patients) and sex (208.3 cases for men versus 156.0 cases for women per 100,000 inhabitants/year) (Fig. 2).

The most frequent origins of sepsis were urinary and respiratory tract infections, accounting for 37.2 and 32.5% of cases, respectively, followed by the abdomen (11%). Almost a quarter (24.7%) of cases presented bacteraemia. Acute kidney injury was the most frequent organ failure (58.4%), followed by respiratory failure (20.5%) and central nervous system failure (19.7%). Cardiovascular dysfunction was reported in 4.9% of cases. Two or more acute organ failures were documented in 14% of cases (Table 1).

Hospital outcomes

In-hospital mortality over the study period was 21.6% (95% confidence interval (CI); 18.6–24.9). Hospital mortality was higher in older patients with higher Charlson comorbidity score, in patients with bacteraemia (39.3% in patients with positive versus 15.8% in patients with negative blood cultures), and was also higher in patients with more organ failures (three or more, 63.4%). Respiratory and abdominal origins were associated with higher mortality (24 and 28%, respectively). Mean (SD) length of stay was 16.7 (19.5) days, with no clinically relevant differences for patients who died in-hospital versus who were discharged alive (despite a value of $p < .001$) (Table 1 and Table 2).

Incidence and in-hospital outcome trends

Incidence of sepsis increased in the five-year study period from 12,809 cases to 20,228 cases (mean 16,460 cases per year over the period), representing 1.3 and 2.1% ($p < .0001$) of hospital admissions, respectively (Fig. 2). Observed in the same period were an increase in mean age, from 69.1 to 72.8 years ($p < .0001$), and an increase in mean Charlson comorbidities score, from 4.9 to 5.3 ($p < .001$) (Fig. 3).

Length of hospital stay decreased from 18.4 to 15.3 days ($p < .0001$), representing a relative reduction of 17% (Fig. 3). Univariate analysis showed that hospital mortality also decreased—from 23.7 to 19.7% ($p < .0001$)—for a relative reduction of 18.6% (Fig. 2). These differences were confirmed in the multivariate analysis adjusted for all significant variables (age group, sex, comorbidities, ICU admission, emergency admission, organ dysfunction, number of organ failures, infection source and presence of bacteraemia) (Tables 1, 2). Differences between 2008 and all the ensuing years except 2009 were statistically significant. The logistic regression (reference year 2008) indicated a mortality odds ratio (OR) for patients with sepsis in 2012 of 0.772 (95% CI 0.727–0.820) (Table 3). The falling trend in the mortality OR was linear throughout the study period for all patients with sepsis, whether or not treated in the ICU. Values for the AUROC were calculated to evaluate how well the multivariate logistic regression model discriminated between patients discharged alive and discharged dead: 0.782 (95% CI 0.779–0.786) for all patients, 0.746 (0.741–0.752) for non-ICU patients and 0.749 (0.743–0.756) for ICU patients.

Discussion

Most epidemiological data on sepsis refers to the first decade of twenty-first century and almost exclusively refer to the USA. This is a large observational study of patients discharged from all national health system acute-care hospitals conducted in a European setting. We estimated the mean sepsis incidence to be 212.7 cases per 100,000 inhabitants/year and in-hospital mortality to be 21.6%. Incidence and mortality varied over time, with a yearly increase in incidence of 7.3%, a yearly relative reduction of 3.3% in length of stay and a yearly reduction in in-hospital mortality of 3.4%. After adjustments for relevant clinical and epidemiological variables, the reduction in mortality remained statistically significant.

The estimated incidence of sepsis in our study was lower than reported in the USA and slightly higher than reported in smaller European studies [2, 6, 7]. Previous studies conducted in Spain reported incidences of between 110 and 230 cases per 100,000 inhabitants/year [15, 16], versus the 212.7 cases observed in our study. Differences in calculated incidences may be related to structural or functional organization [17] or may be due to discharge diagnosis coding. Nonetheless, we would like to emphasize the importance of using local data to monitor trends in activity and results over time. Moreover, the number of sepsis cases in our study increased yearly, a finding which is consistent with findings reported in other epidemiological studies [10–12].

Estimates of sepsis incidence and trends are also essential to estimate the resources needed to care for these patients. Sepsis incidence is increasing compared to incidence for other leading causes of mortality such as acute myocardial infarction or ischaemic stroke. The CatSalut data on hospital admissions/year for severe sepsis (five-year mean, 16,460 cases) are close to the combined numbers for acute coronary syndrome and ischaemic stroke admissions together, at 11,000 and 8000, respectively [18, 19]. However, incidence rates for acute coronary syndrome and ischaemic stroke, unlike for sepsis, are stable

[19–21]. In the USA, the percentage of septic patients with a fatal outcome increased from 14% in 2000 to 16% in 2010; in contrast, mortality for respiratory failure decreased from 25 to 17%, for heart attack from 10 to 8%, for cancer from 8 to 4% and for stroke from 6 to 5% [22].

Prospective versus retrospective analysis observed differences in incidence and source of sepsis. Prospective monitoring is laborious, costly and complex and can also be affected by issues such as inclusion criteria or data sources [23, 24]. Although retrospective analyses from hospital discharges—as in our study—can also be affected by definitions, codes and analytical methods, they serve an important function in analysing local trends and outcomes. Gaieski [24] observed a 3.5-fold difference in estimates of absolute incidence using different database abstraction methods. Nonetheless, trends were similar irrespective of the methodology. Stevenson et al. [12] recently found that severe sepsis mortality was 10% higher for patients included in the control group of clinical trials compared to administrative data (collected according to Angus' criteria) [5]; nonetheless, mortality trends were similar, irrespective of the data source—and were also similar to the 3% yearly reduction found in our study. Stevenson et al. consequently concluded that administrative data are useful in monitoring mortality trends in patients with severe sepsis.

Table 1 Profile of patients with severe sepsis in Catalonia 2008–2012

	Total *N* = 82,300	Alive on discharge *N* = 64,511	Dead on discharge *N* = 17,789	*p*
	Mean (SD)	Mean (SD)	Mean (SD)	
Age (years)	71.2 (19.7)	70.6 (20.4)	73.3 (16.6)	<.0001
Length of hospital stay (days)	16.7 (19.5)	16.8 (19.3)	16.3 (20.3)	<.001
Charlson comorbidity index	5.1 (2.6)	5.0 (2.6)	5.6 (2.7)	<.0001
	%	%	%	*p*
Age (years)				
<15	3.2	3.7	1.4	<.0001
15–44	6.1	6.6	4.2	
45–64	16.4	16.2	17.3	
65–74	17.5	17.3	18.4	
75–84	32.9	32.8	33.6	
>84	23.8	23.5	25.0	
Sex				
Males	56.7	56.1	59.0	<.0001
Comorbidities				
Chronic kidney disease	23.8	24.5	20.9	<.0001
COPD	22.4	22.9	20.6	<.0001
Cancer	14.5	12.5	21.5	<.0001
Metastasis	4.8	5.8	8.3	<.0001
Peripheral vascular disease	4.4	4.2	4.9	<.0001
Complicated diabetes	4.0	4.3	3.0	<.0001
Liver disease: mild	9.7	8.7	13.1	<.0001
Liver disease: moderate–severe	3.0	2.4	4.9	<.0001
Myocardial infarction	3.8	3.6	4.7	<.0001
Congestive heart failure	20.1	19.1	23.8	<.0001
Cerebrovascular disease	6.7	6.5	7.6	<.0001
AIDS/HIV infection	1.0	0.9	1.3	<.0001
Emergency stay (%)	89.4	89.8	87.8	<.0001
ICU admissions	28.2	22.3	49.8	<.0001
Admission year				
2008	15.6	15.1	17.1	<.0001
2009	17.9	17.4	19.6	
2010	19.7	19.6	20.0	
2011	22.3	22.6	21.0	

Table 1 continued

	%	%	%	*p*
2012	24.6	25.2	22.3	
Sepsis origins				
Urinary	37.2	41.1	23.0	<.0001
Respiratory	32.5	31.4	36.4	<.0001
Abdominal	11.0	10.1	14.3	<.0001
Skin and soft tissues	4.1	4.2	3.9	.06
Endocarditis	1.6	1.5	2.0	<.0001
Device-related	1.1	1.2	0.6	<.0001
CNS	0.9	0.9	1.2	<.0001
Others	37.9	41.0	26.5	<.0001
Bacteraemia	24.7	19.1	44.9	<.0001
Organ dysfunction				
Kidney	58.4	56.9	63.7	<.0001
Lung	20.5	15.7	37.9	<.0001
CNS	19.7	21.6	12.7	<.0001
Haematologic	11.1	11.0	11.5	.054
Cardiovascular	4.9	5.2	3.6	<.0001
Liver	1.3	0.7	3.3	<.0001
Number of organ failures				
1	86.3	89.7	72.9	<.0001
2	12.0	9.4	21.8	
3	1.6	0.8	4.7	
4 or more	0.2	0.1	0.6	

Data are presented as mean and standard deviation or %

AIDS acquired immune deficiency syndrome, *CNS* central nervous system, *COPD* chronic obstructive pulmonary disease, *HIV* human immunodeficiency virus, *ICU* intensive care unit

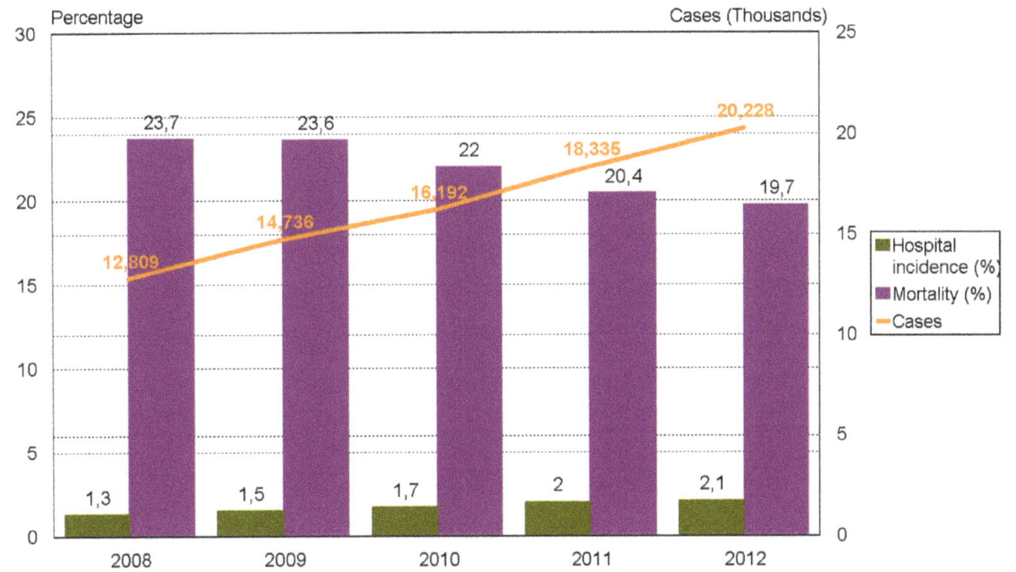

Fig. 1 Number of cases, mortality rates and hospital incidence rates for sepsis in Catalonia (2008–2012). Incidence of sepsis increased from 12,809 cases to 20,228 cases in the 5-year study period (mean 16,460 cases per year), representing 1.3 and 2.1% ($p < .0001$) of hospital admissions and an average yearly increase of 6%. However, hospital mortality decreased from 23.7 to 19.7% ($p < .0001$) for a yearly relative reduction of 3.4%

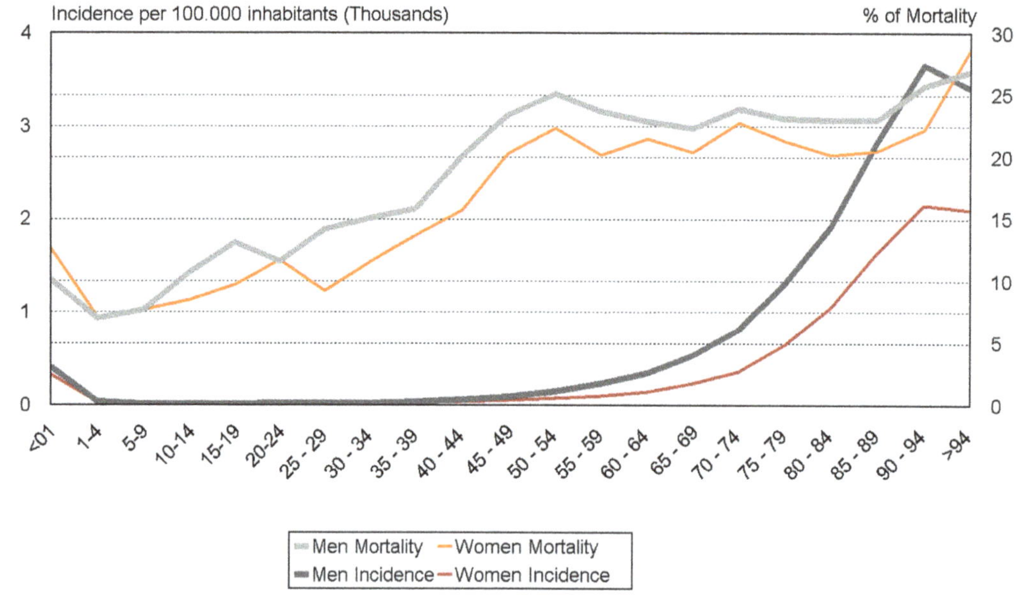

Fig. 2 Age-specific incidence and mortality rates for all cases of severe sepsis by sex in Catalonia (2008–2012). The *dark line* represents incidence (*thicker* for men and *thinner* for women) expressed as a thousand cases per 100,000 inhabitants. Age-adjusted mortality is expressed as the number of deaths with respect to the number of cases grouped according to 5-year age brackets

Table 2 Overall mortality by patient characteristics, sepsis origins, presence of bacteraemia and organ dysfunction by year of admission in Catalonia (2008–2012)

Condition	*N*	Presence of condition (%)						In-hospital mortality (%)
		2008	2009	2010	2011	2012	*p*	
Mortality		23.7	23.6	22.0	20.4	19.7	<.0001	
Source of sepsis								
Urinary tract	30,600	33.6	35.0	37.1	39.8	38.8	<.0001	13.9
Respiratory tract	26,748	34.2	34.0	31.2	30.9	32.7	<.0001	24.2
Abdomen	9065	10.7	11.2	11.3	11.0	10.9	NS	28.0
Skin and soft tissues	3394	3.9	4.0	4.0	4.4	4.2	NS	20.3
Endocarditis	1326	1.8	1.8	1.9	1.4	1.4	<.0001	27.3
Device-related	869	1.1	1.1	1.2	1.1	0.9	.016	11.6
CNS	775	1.2	1.1	1.1	0.7	0.7	<.0001	27.5
Other	31,149	37.4	37.5	39.2	38.1	37.1	.001	15.1
Bacteraemia	20,285	25.5	25.5	24.5	24.8	23.5	<.0001	39.3
Organ dysfunction								
Kidney	48,072	50.8	53.5	57.1	61.9	64.7	<.0001	23.6
Respiratory	16,876	26.1	24.1	20.9	17.9	16.3	<.0001	40.0
CNS	16,177	20.5	19.6	19.1	18.9	20.3	<.0001	13.9
Haematologic	9158	11.6	12.3	12.2	11.2	9.1	<.0001	22.4
Cardiovascular	3988	5.3	5.4	4.7	4.6	4.4	<.0001	16.1
Liver	1058	1.0	1.3	1.3	1.3	1.4	.029	55.9
Number of organ failures								
1	70,874	86.6	85.9	86.5	86.0	85.8	NS	18.5
2	9964	11.7	12.2	11.8	12.4	12.3		39.0
3 or more	1462	1.7	1.9	1.9	1.7	1.8		63.4

Data are presented as number of cases or %

CNS central nervous system, *NS* non-significant

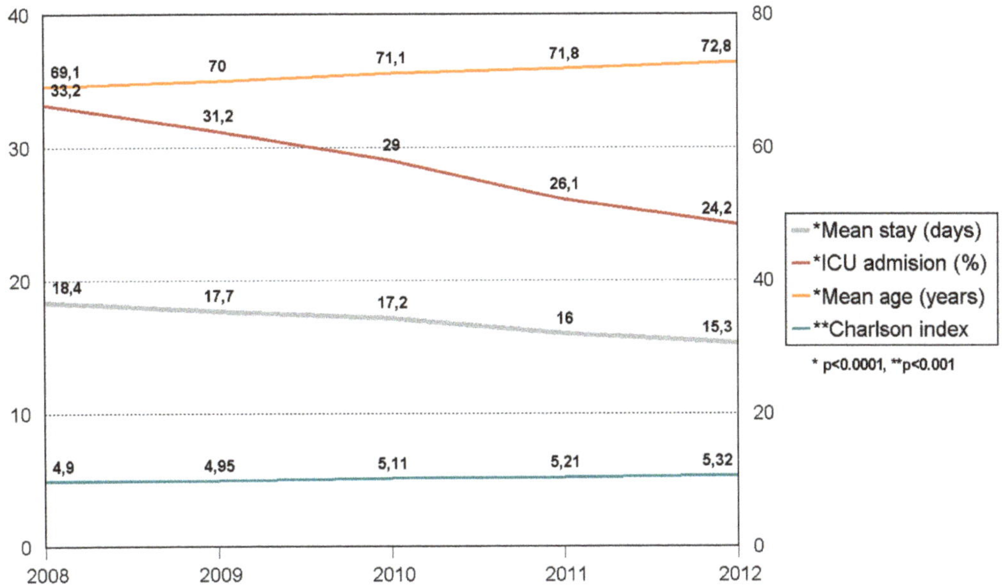

Fig. 3 Trends for main characteristics and hospital stay for patients with sepsis in Catalonia (2008–2012)

Table 3 Univariate and multivariate analyses of in-hospital mortality by year of admission in Catalonia (2008–2012)

	Univariate analysis			Multivariate analysis		
	N	% mortality	*p*	OR	95% CI for OR	*p*
All patients *N* = 82,300						
2008	12,809	23.7	<.0001	1	–	–
2009	14,736	23.6		0.988	0.928–1.052	NS
2010	16,192	22.0		0.911	0.856–0.969	.003
2011	18,335	20.4		0.818	0.770–0.870	<.0001
2012	20,228	19.7		0.772	0.727–0.820	<.0001
Non-ICU patients *N* = 59,064						
2008	8551	15.8	<.0001	1	–	–
2009	10,137	16.3		1.028	0.945–1.117	NS
2010	11,497	15.4		0.941	0.867–1.022	NS
2011	13,545	14.8		0.859	0.793–0.931	<.0001
2012	15,334	13.9		0.769	0.711–0.832	<.0001
ICU patients *N* = 23,236						
2008	4258	39.5	.002	1	–	–
2009	4599	39.6		0.938	0.854–1.031	NS
2010	4695	38.2		0.868	0.790–0.953	.003
2011	4790	36.0		0.757	0.686–0.832	<.0001
2012	4894	37.6		0.778	0.702–0.855	<.0001

Data are presented as number of death or %. The multivariate analysis is adjusted by sex, age group, comorbidities, ICU admission, emergency admission, organ dysfunction, number of organ failures, septic origins and bacteraemia

CI confidence interval, *ICU* intensive care unit, *OR* odds ratio, *NS* non-significant

Length of stay and mortality both decrease yearly during the study period—to a statistically significant degree according to the multivariate analysis adjusted for demographic data, comorbidities, infection source and number of organ failures. The external validity of our findings is supported by the fact that mortality in 2008 was the same as that reports by the PROWESS-SHOCK study placebo group [25]. Other recent large randomized clinical trials

(RCTs) have reported mortality rates of 18–30% [26, 27], further confirming the likely validity of 2008 as our baseline year. Kaukonen et al. [11], who recently reported similar results for Australia and New Zealand, observed an annual absolute decrease of 1.3% in risk, from 24% in 2008 to 19% in 2012. In our study, multivariate analysis revealed a robust association between mortality and year of detection, as adjusted for confounding factors including sex, age group, comorbidities, ICU admission, emergency admission, organ dysfunction, number of organ failures, septic focus and the presence of bacteraemia. Although our study was not designed to address this issue, a potential improvement in the management of sepsis could be suggested, explained in part as a consequence of training and increased clinical awareness [3, 28–30].

Our results suggest also that sepsis outcomes should be interpreted according to the year of data collection and the presence of comorbidities. Moreover, underpowered RCTs would be avoided if these effects were taken into account in estimating statistical power and sample size. Yearly reduction in crude mortality rates should be expected, bearing in mind that overestimated mortality rates may lead to underpowered studies which might, in turn, lead to potentially useful treatments being downgraded due to lack of evidence. Furthermore, excluding elderly patients and patients with comorbidities from RCTs represents a form of selection bias; Kaukonen et al. [11], for instance, reported a 4.6% mortality rate for comorbidity-free patients and young patients (versus our rate of 21.6%). Another issue is that sepsis outcomes are too often viewed as binary: The patient dies (failure) or survives (success). Studies also tend to focus on in-hospital mortality and length of stay as an outcome measure for ICU patients, overlooking the fact that many patients admitted for sepsis die after discharge. There is an unmet need to improve knowledge regarding long-term effects in patients with sepsis [1–8], so other outcome indicators such as long-term morbidity and quality of life are likely to be included in future trials.

Just under a quarter (24.7%) of our patients presented with bacteraemia, associated with higher mortality. Patients with bacteraemia could represent a suitable population to monitor prospectively in clinical practice, as bacteraemia, unlike sepsis, is easily identified retrospectively, is easily distinguished from other non-infectious diseases that cause organ dysfunction and is also easily stratified using the sepsis-related organ failure assessment (SOFA) instrument [31].

The main strengths of our study are the large cohort of patients included in a European setting, the fact of including 100% of admissions to both public and private hospitals of Catalonia Health System, the long period of data collection and the use of a previously validated strategy. Our study has several limitations. The fact that cases of sepsis were identified indirectly using ICD-9-CM codes implies less accuracy in identifying cases and a poor clinical analysis compared to prospective methods. Urinary infections appear as the main focus of sepsis in our study. The relevance of each focus can be affected by population characteristics or methodology. It also can affect incidence or severity results. Case recruitment may also have been affected by coding, as reflected in our results for cardiovascular dysfunction. Hypotension was poorly documented on discharge. Incidence, as reported in our study, probably does not reflect clinical incidence. Cardiovascular dysfunction incidence rates of 7.2–42% have been reported for epidemiological or retrospective studies, in contrast to rates of up 90% for prospective studies [4, 5, 9, 13, 15, 32, 33]. Our study cannot account for reasons for reduced mortality and shorter stays. Inclusion of a specific severity scores, such as SOFA, in the multivariate analysis would allow insights into whether mortality reduction is related to the inclusion of less severe patients. Unfortunately, our study design does not admit this conclusion. Given that the CMBD-HA does not specifically collect data about ICU admission, the category 'ICU stay' was deduced from procedures typically used in ICUs. We think that since this definition is highly specific but not sensitive, we cannot rule out the possibility that some septic patients with less severity were excluded from ICU admission.

Conclusions

Sepsis incidence has risen continuously in recent years in Catalonia. While mortality and length of stay have fallen, despite increases in age and in comorbidities, our findings corroborate results reported for other parts of the world, in the context of scarce administrative data on sepsis in Europe.

Abbreviations

AIDS: acquired immune deficiency syndrome; CI: confidence interval; CMBD-HA: Minimum Basic Data Set—Acute-Care Hospitals; COPD: chronic obstructive pulmonary disease; ICD-9-CM: International Classification of Diseases, 9th revision, Clinical Modification; ICU: intensive care unit; NS: non-significant; OR: odds ratio; RCT: randomized clinical trials; SD: standard deviation; SOFA: sepsis-related organ failure assessment.

Authors' contributions

JCY, JCR, RF, MC, AB and AA conceived and designed the work. Data acquisition and statistical analysis were performed by MC and AB; interpretation of the data for the work was carried out by JCY, JCR, RF, MC, AB and AA; all authors were involved in draft redaction and/or revision for important intellectual content; all authors read and approved the final manuscript.

Author details
[1] Critical Care Department, Hospital de Mataró, Mataró, Spain. [2] Grup de Recerca en Sepsis, Imflamació i Seguretat (AGAUR 2014-SGR926), Barcelona, Spain. [3] Escola Superior de Ciencies de la Salut, Universitat Pompeu Fabra, Mataró, Spain. [4] Critical Care Department, Vall d'Hebron University Hospital, Barcelona, Spain. [5] Shock, Organ Dysfunction and Resuscitation (SODIR) Research Group, Vall d' Hebron Research Institut, Universitat Autònoma de Barcelona, Barcelona, Spain. [6] CIBER Enfermedades Respiratorias, Madrid, Spain. [7] Divisió d'Anàlisi de la Demanda i l'Activitat, Servei Català de la Salut (CatSalut), Barcelona, Spain. [8] Critical Care Department, Hospital Universitari Dr. Josep Trueta, Girona, Spain. [9] Critical Care Department, Hospital Universitari Joan XXIII, Tarragona, Spain. [10] IISPV/URV, Tarragona, Spain. [11] Critical Care Department, Hospital Universitari Arnau de Vilanova, Lleida, Spain. [12] Institut de Recerca Biomèdica (IRB), Lleida, Spain. [13] Multidisciplinary Intensive Care Research Organization (MICRO), St James's University Hospital, Trinity Centre for Health Sciences, Dublin, Ireland. [14] Critical Care Center, Sabadell Hospital, Corporació Sanitaria Universitaria Parc Tauli, Sabadell, Spain. [15] Universitat Autonoma de Barcelona, Sabadell, Spain. [16] Servei de Medicina Intensiva, Hospital de Mataró, Carretera de Cirera s/n, 08304 Mataró, Spain.

Acknowledgements
Group Authorship: SOCMIC (Catalan Critical Care Society) Sepsis Working Group Members: Abdo Taché, Servei de Medicina Intensiva, Hospital Universitari Dr Josep Trueta de Girona; Antoni Margarit, Servei de Medicina Intensiva, Hospital Nostra Senyora Meritxell d'Andorra; Assumpta Ricart, Servei de Urgències, Hospital Universitari Vall d' Hebron; Adolf Ruiz-Sanmartin, Servei de Medicina Intensiva, Hospital Universitari Vall d' Hebron; Begoña Balsera, Servei de Medicina Intensiva, Hospital Universitari Arnau de Vilanova de Lleida; Berta Cisteró, Servei de Urgències, Hospital Parc Taulí de Sabadell; Candelària de Haro, Servei de Medicina Intensiva, Hospital Parc Taulí de Sabadell; Concepció Rovira, Servei de Medicina Intensiva, Hospital Sant Joan de Reus; Eva Torrents, Hospital Parc Taulí de Sabadell; Francisco Álvarez-Lerma, Servei de Medicina Intensiva, Hospital del Mar de Barcelona; Herbert Baquerizo, Servei de Urgències, Hospital Sant Joan de Déu de Manresa; Joan Balcells, Servei de Pediatria, Hospital Universitari Vall d'Hebrón de Barcelona; José L. Echarte, Servei de Urgències, Hospital del Mar de Barcelona; José Luna, Servei de Medicina Intensiva, Hospital de Tortosa Verge de la Cinta; Josep M. Sirvent, Servei de Medicina Intensiva, Hospital Universitari Dr Josep Trueta de Girona; Juan Méndez, Servei de Medicina Intensiva, Hospital de Mataró; Lluís Zapata, Servei de Medicina Intensiva, Hospital de Sant Pau i Santa Creu de Barcelona; Lluïsa Bordejé, Servei de Medicina Intensiva, Hospital Universitari Germans Trias i Pujol de Badalona; Lourdes Jiménez, Servei de Medicina Intensiva, Hospital Universitari Arnau de Vilanova de Lleida; Maite Martínez-Izquierdo, Servei de Urgències, Hospital del Mar de Barcelona; María L. Martínez, Hospital Parc Taulí de Sabadell; María P. Gracia-Arnillas, Servei de Medicina Intensiva, Hospital del Mar de Barcelona; Mercedes Palomar, Servei de Medicina Intensiva Hospital Universitari Arnau de Vilanova de Lleida; Miguel Sánchez, Servei de Urgències, Hospital Clínic de Barcelona; Pablo Pujol, Servei de Medicina Intensiva, Hospital Universitari Dr Josep Trueta de Girona; Pau Garro, Servei de Medicina Intensiva, Hospital General de Granollers; Pau Torrabadella, Servei de Medicina Intensiva, Hospital Universitari Germans Trias i Pujol de Badalona; Paula Vera, Servei de Medicina Intensiva, Hospital de Sant Pau i Santa Creu de Barcelona; Roger Bisbal, Servei de Medicina Intensiva, Hospital de Mataró; Ruth Hernández, Servei de Urgències, Hospital de Sant Joan Despí Moisès Broggi; Teresa M. Tomasa, Servei de Medicina Intensiva, Hospital Universitari Germans Trias i Pujol de Badalona; Víctor Pérez-Claveria, Servei de Urgències, Hospital de Mataró.

Competing interests
The authors declare that they have no competing interests.

Funding
The study was partially funded by the Mataró Sepsis Challenge (www.sepsis-challenge.cat) through the Fundació Salut del Consorci Sanitari del Maresme.

Prior presentation
This study was reported in part as a communication at the 43rd Annual Congress of the Society of Critical Care Medicine (SCCM, January, 2014, San Francisco, California, USA), the 27th Annual Congress of the European Society of Intensive Care Medicine (ESICM, September 2014, Barcelona, Spain) and the 36th Annual Congress of the Catalan Society of Critical Care Medicine (SOCMIC, March, 2015, Barcelona, Spain).

References

1. Singer M, Deutschman C, Seymour C, Shankar-Hari M, Annane D, Bauer M, Bellomo R, et al. The third international consensus definitions for sepsis and septic shock (sepsis-3). JAMA. 2016;315:801–10.
2. Hall MJ, Levant S, DeFrances CJ. Trends in inpatient hospital deaths: National Hospital Discharge Survey, 2000–2010. NCHS data brief, no 118. Hyattsville: National Center for Health Statistics; 2013.
3. Ferrer R, Artigas A, Levy MM, Edusepsis Study Group et al. Improvement in process of care and outcome after a multicenter severe sepsis educational program in Spain. JAMA. 2008;299:2294–303.
4. Martin G, Mannino D, Eaton S, et al. The epidemiology of sepsis in the United States from 1979 through 2000. N Engl J Med. 2003;348:1546–54.
5. Angus DC, Linde-Swirble T, Lidicker J, et al. Epidemiology of severe sepsis in the United States: analysis of incidence, outcome, and associated costs of care. Crit Care Med. 2001;29:1303–10.
6. Padkin A, Goldfrad C, Brady AR, et al. Epidemiology of severe sepsis occurring in the first 24 hrs in intensive care units in England, Wales, and Northern Ireland. Crit Care Med. 2003;31:2332–8.
7. Brun-Buisson C, Meshaka P, Pinton P, EPISEPSIS Study Group et al. EPISEPSIS: a reappraisal of the epidemiology and outcome of severe sepsis in French intensive care units. Intensive Care Med. 2004;30(4):580–8.
8. Finfer S, Bellomo R, Lipman J, et al. Adult-population incidence of severe sepsis in Australian and New Zealand intensive care units. Intensive Care Med. 2004;30(4):589–96.
9. Dombrovskiy VY, Martin AA, Sunderram J, et al. Rapid increase in hospitalization and mortality rates for severe sepsis in the United States: a trend analysis from 1993 to 2003. Crit Care Med. 2007;35(5):1244–50.
10. Lagu T, Rothberg MB, Shieh MS, et al. Hospitalizations, costs, and outcomes of severe sepsis in the United States 2003–2007. Crit Care Med. 2012;40(3):754–61.
11. Kaukonen KM, Bailey M, Suzuki S, et al. Mortality related to severe sepsis and septic shock among critically ill patients in Australia and New Zealand, 2000–2012. JAMA. 2014;311(13):1308–16.
12. Stevenson EK, Rubenstein AR, Radin GT, et al. Two decades of mortality trends among patients with severe sepsis: a comparative meta-analysis. Crit Care Med. 2014;42:625–31.
13. Quan H, Sundararajan V, Halfon P, et al. Coding algorithms for defining comorbidities in ICD-9-CM and ICD-10 administrative data. Med Care. 2005;43:1130–9.
14. Hanley JA, McNeil BJ. The meaning and use of the area under a receiver operating characteristic (ROC) curve. Radiology. 1982;143:29–36.
15. Iñigo J, Sendra JM, Díaz R, Bouza C, Sarría-Santamera A. Epidemiology and costs of severe sepsis in Madrid. A hospital discharge study. Med Intensiva. 2006;30:197–203.
16. Andreu Ballester JC, Ballester F, González Sánchez A, et al. Epidemiology of sepsis in the Valencian Community (Spain), 1995–2004. Infect Control Hosp Epidemiol. 2008;29:630–4.
17. Levy MM, Artigas A, Phillips GS, et al. Outcomes of the Surviving Sepsis Campaign in intensive care units in the USA and Europe: a prospective cohort study. Lancet Infect Dis. 2012;12:919–24.
18. Dégano I, Elosua R, Marrugat J. Epidemiology of acute coronary syndromes in Spain: estimation of the number of cases and trends from 2005 to 2049. Rev Esp Cardiol. 2013;66(6):472–81.
19. Colls C, Abillera S, Garcia ALtes A, Gallofre M. Beneficis de l'organització de l'atenció sanitària a les persones amb ictus: mortalitat evitada i impacte econòmic. Edita:AQuAS, 1st ed. Barcelona. Observatori del Sistema de Salut de Catalunya; 2013.

20. Sans S, Puigdefabregas A, Paluzie G, Monterde D, et al. Increasing trends of acute myocardial infarction in Spain: the MONICA-Catalonia Study. Eur Heart J. 2005;26:505–15.
21. Gil M, Martı H, Elosua R, et al. Análisis de la tendencia en la letalidad, incidencia y mortalidad por infarto de miocardio en Girona entre 1990 y 1999. Rev Esp Cardiol. 2007;60:349–56.
22. Hall MJ, Williams SN, DeFrances CJ et al. Inpatient care for septicemia or sepsis: a challenge for patients and hospitals. NCHS data brief 2011;62:1–8. CDC National Hospital Discharge Survey. http://www.cdc.gov/nchs/nhds.htm. Accessed 17 Oct 2014.
23. Klein Klouwenberg PM, Ong DS, Bonten MJ, et al. Classification of sepsis, severe sepsis and septic shock: the impact of minor variations in data capture and definition of SIRS criteria. Intensive Care Med. 2012;38:811–9.
24. Gaieski DF, Edwards JM, Kallan MJ, et al. Benchmarking the incidence and mortality of severe sepsis in the United States. Crit Care Med. 2013;41:1167–74.
25. Ranieri M, Thompson T, Barie P, et al. Drotrecogin alfa (activated) in adults with septic shock. N Engl J Med. 2012;366:2055–64.
26. Caironi P, Tognoni G, Masson S, et al. Albumin replacement in patients with severe sepsis or septic shock. N Engl J Med. 2014;370:1412–21.
27. The ProCESS Investigators. A randomized trial of protocol-based care for early septic shock. N Engl J Med. 2014;370:1683–93.
28. Iwashyna TJ, Angus DC. Declining case fatality rates for severe sepsis: good data bring good news with ambiguous implications. JAMA. 2014;311(13):1295–7.
29. Levy MM, Dellinger RP, Townsend SR, Campaign SS, et al. The Surviving Sepsis Campaign: results of an international guideline-based performance improvement program targeting severe sepsis. Crit Care Med. 2010;38:367–74.
30. Suarez D, Ferrer R, Artigas A, Edusepsis Study Group et al. Cost-effectiveness of the Surviving Sepsis Campaign protocol for severe sepsis: a prospective nation-wide study in Spain. Intensive Care Med. 2011;37:444–52.
31. Routsi C, Pratikaki M, Sotiropoulou C, et al. Application of the sequential organ failure assessment (SOFA) score to bacteremic ICU patients. Infection. 2007;35(4):240–4.
32. Bouza C, Lopez-Cuadrado T, Amate-Blanco JM. Use of explicit ICD9-CM codes to identify adult severe sepsis: impacts on epidemiological estimates. Crit Care. 2016;20:313. doi:10.1186/s13054-016-1497-9.
33. Esteban A, Frutos-Vivar F, Ferguson ND, et al. Sepsis incidence and outcome: contrasting the intensive care unit with the hospital ward. Crit Care Med. 2007;35(5):1284–9.

7

A hypoperfusion context may aid to interpret hyperlactatemia in sepsis-3 septic shock patients: a proof-of-concept study

Leyla Alegría[1], Magdalena Vera[1], Jorge Dreyse[1], Ricardo Castro[1], David Carpio[1], Carolina Henriquez[1], Daniela Gajardo[1], Sebastian Bravo[1], Felipe Araneda[1], Eduardo Kattan[1], Pedro Torres[2], Gustavo Ospina-Tascón[3], Jean-Louis Teboul[4], Jan Bakker[1,5] and Glenn Hernández[1*]

Abstract

Background: Persistent hyperlactatemia is particularly difficult to interpret in septic shock. Besides hypoperfusion, adrenergic-driven lactate production and impaired lactate clearance are important contributors. However, clinical recognition of different sources of hyperlactatemia is unfortunately not a common practice and patients are treated with the same strategy despite the risk of over-resuscitation in some. Indeed, pursuing additional resuscitation in non-hypoperfusion-related cases might lead to the toxicity of fluid overload and vasoactive drugs. We hypothesized that two different clinical patterns can be recognized in septic shock patients through a multimodal perfusion monitoring. Hyperlactatemic patients with a hypoperfusion context probably represent a more severe acute circulatory dysfunction, and the absence of a hypoperfusion context is eventually associated with a good outcome. We performed a retrospective analysis of a database of septic shock patients with persistent hyperlactatemia after initial resuscitation.

Results: We defined hypoperfusion context by the presence of a $ScvO_2 < 70\%$, or a $P(cv\text{-}a)CO_2 \geq 6$ mmHg, or a CRT ≥ 4 s together with hyperlactatemia. Ninety patients were included, of whom seventy exhibited a hypoperfusion-related pattern and 20 did not. Although lactate values were comparable at baseline (4.8 ± 2.8 vs. 4.7 ± 3.7 mmol/L), patients with a hypoperfusion context exhibited a more severe circulatory dysfunction with higher vasopressor requirements, and a trend to longer mechanical ventilation days, ICU stay, and more rescue therapies. Only one of the 20 hyperlactatemic patients without a hypoperfusion context died (5%) compared to 11 of the 70 with hypoperfusion-related hyperlactatemia (16%).

Conclusions: Two different clinical patterns among hyperlactatemic septic shock patients may be identified according to hypoperfusion context. Patients with hyperlactatemia plus low $ScvO_2$, or high $P(cv\text{-}a)CO_2$, or high CRT values exhibited a more severe circulatory dysfunction. This provides a starting point to launch further prospective studies to confirm if this approach can lead to a more selective resuscitation strategy.

Keywords: Septic shock, Hyperlactatemia, Resuscitation, Hypoperfusion, Central venous oxygen saturation, Central venous-arterial PCO_2 gradient, Capillary refill time

Background

Sepsis-3 consensus defined septic shock as vasopressor requirement to maintain mean arterial pressure (MAP) >65 mmHg and a serum lactate level >2 mmol/L despite fluid resuscitation [1], and claimed that these criteria will identify patients with a homogeneous high risk of death, allegedly in excess of 40% [1]. Unfortunately, neither this new definition [1], or the Surviving Sepsis Campaign (SSC) [2] recognizes the heterogeneous sources of lactate in septic shock or the existence of different clinical patterns among hyperlactatemic patients. Therefore,

*Correspondence: glenn@med.puc.cl; glennguru@gmail.com
[1] Departamento de Medicina Intensiva, Facultad de Medicina, Pontificia Universidad Católica de Chile, Marcoleta 367, Santiago 8320000, Chile
Full list of author information is available at the end of the article

normalization of lactate is recommended as a goal for septic shock resuscitation under the assumption that tissue hypoxia is the main source of lactate generation [2].

However, persistent hyperlactatemia is particularly difficult to interpret in the clinical setting. Besides hypoperfusion, adrenergic-driven aerobic lactate production and impaired hepatic lactate clearance have been suggested as important contributors [3–5]. Recognizing a clinical pattern of hypoperfusion-related hyperlactatemia appears as highly relevant since optimizing systemic blood flow in this setting could revert ongoing hypoperfusion and improve prognosis [6, 7]. In contrast, pursuing additional resuscitation in non-hypoperfusion-related cases might lead to the toxicity of fluid overload and excessive vasoactive drugs, eventually increasing morbidity or mortality [4].

Recognition of clinical patterns among septic shock patients with persistent hyperlactatemia is unfortunately not a common practice around the world, and hyperlactatemic patients are treated with the same strategy despite the risk of over-resuscitation in some. Nevertheless, a multimodal perfusion monitoring could aid in identifying a hypoperfusion context [4]. Indeed, the combination of hyperlactatemia with pCO_2-related markers of tissue hypoxia provides a stronger prognostic signal than either one alone [8]. In a lactate-driven resuscitation protocol, Jansen et al. [7] recommended systemic flow optimization exclusively in hyperlactatemic patients with concomitant low central venous oxygen saturation ($ScvO_2$). Hernandez et al. [9] demonstrated that variables such as $ScvO_2$, central venous-arterial PCO_2 gradient ($P(cv\text{-}a)CO_2$) and peripheral perfusion as assessed by the capillary refill time (CRT) exhibit a very fast normalization rate in relation to systemic flow optimization, whereas lactate shows a biphasic response with an initial rapid improvement in parallel with the above-mentioned variables, followed by a much slower trend thereafter. Thus, a concomitant low $ScvO_2$, or high $P(cv\text{-}a)CO_2$, or an abnormal peripheral perfusion defines a hypoperfusion context on which increasing systemic flow may contribute to serum lactate decrease.

Is the opposite true? Can resuscitation be safely stopped in hyperlactatemic septic shock patients without a hypoperfusion context? A recent pilot study by van Genderen et al. [10] indeed suggests that stopping fluid resuscitation when peripheral perfusion is normalized is not only safe, but also associated with less positive fluid balances and organ dysfunctions in septic shock patients with hyperlactatemia. However, this aspect is currently being addressed by ongoing studies.

We hypothesized that two different clinical patterns can be recognized in septic shock patients as defined by sepsis-3 consensus, according to the presence of a hypoperfusion context. Hyperlactatemic patients with a hypoperfusion context probably represent a more severe acute circulatory dysfunction, and the absence of a hypoperfusion context is eventually associated with a good outcome. We designed this retrospective proof-of-concept study to test our primary hypothesis. If this proves to be true, then it could be safe to launch a prospective study testing a restrictive resuscitation strategy in the latter, while concentrating resuscitation efforts in the former.

Methods

We evaluated all septic shock patients admitted to our intensive care unit (ICU) at the University Hospital of the Pontificia Universidad Católica de Chile during the 18-month period from July 2013 to December 2014. These patients were managed according to a local algorithm [9] and entered into a prospective dataset. The Institutional Review Board of our Institution approved this study and waived the need of an informed consent because of the retrospective observational nature of the study (CEC-MEDUC; 16-182, 2016).

Study population

Patients ≥18 years old were included if they presented: (a) septic shock according to sepsis-3 Definitions (requirement of vasopressors to sustain MAP ≥65 mmHg and hyperlactatemia >2 mmol/l after initial fluid resuscitation) [1]; (b) concomitant values for $ScvO_2$, $P(cv\text{-}a)CO_2$ and CRT; (c) full commitment for resuscitation; and (d) complete follow-up in the dataset and medical charts until hospital discharge.

Study protocol

Hypoperfusion context was defined by the presence of a $ScvO_2$ <70%, or a P(cv-a) CO_2 ≥6 mmHg, or a CRT ≥4 s together with hyperlactatemia after initial fluid resuscitation in the ICU. Patients without any abnormality were classified as with a non-hypoperfusion context. Both subgroups were compared in clinical-demographic data and severity scores at baseline; and macrohemodynamic and perfusion parameters, hemodynamic interventions and main outcomes.

All patients were managed according to our local algorithm aimed at macrohemodynamic stabilization and improvement of hypoperfusion [9]. A central venous catheter and an arterial line were inserted in all. A pulmonary artery catheter was recommended for those with a concomitant acute respiratory distress syndrome and/or past medical history of heart failure. Perfusion targets were normalization of $ScvO_2$, $P(cv\text{-}a)CO_2$, CRT and mottling, and a clear tendency to a decrease in arterial lactate levels. The algorithm was described elsewhere [9], but briefly preload optimization guided by dynamic predictors of fluid responsiveness was the first step to improve systemic blood flow. Pulse pressure variation was the preferred dynamic parameter when feasible. Echocardiography was not routinely performed during the study period except as an aid to assess preload status through inferior vena cava distensibility when necessary. Fluid challenges were repeated until the perfusion targets mentioned above were normalized, or the selected dynamic predictor of fluid responsiveness turned negative, or a safety limit of an increase in central venous pressure ≥5 mmHg after a fluid bolus was reached. Norepinephrine (NE) was the vasopressor of choice and adjusted to a MAP ≥65 mmHg. Low-dose dobutamine or milrinone was restricted to patients with persistent or worsening hypoperfusion after preload optimization. Hemoglobin concentrations were maintained at 8 g/dL or higher to optimize arterial O_2 content. Mechanical ventilation settings were adjusted according to current recommendations. High-volume hemofiltration (HVHF) was used as rescue therapy in patients evolving with refractory septic shock.

Statistical analysis

Categorical data were analyzed with Chi-square, *t* test for paired samples and Wilcoxon test when appropriate. We tested the discriminating value of each perfusion variable alone or in combination.

All data are presented as mean ± standard deviation (SD). All reported p values are two-sided, with a significant alpha level at 5%. STATA 13 (STATA Corp, Tx, USA) statistical package was used for analysis.

Results

A total of 116 septic shock patients were admitted during the study period. Of these, ninety patients (57% female, mean age 66 ± 16 years) fulfilling the inclusion criteria were analyzed. Twenty-six patients were excluded from further analysis because of normal lactate levels at ICU admission (7), absence of data on one of the three parameters that define hypoperfusion context (10), no full commitment for full resuscitation (4), or early transfer to other hospitals (5).

The main sepsis sources were abdominal ($n = 46$), pulmonary ($n = 21$), urinary ($n = 15$), and others ($n = 8$). Seventy patients exhibited a hypoperfusion context after initial resuscitation in the ICU, and 20 did not. The main clinical, demographic and physiological characteristics according to subgroups at baseline are presented in Table 1.

Although lactate values at baseline (4.8 ± 2.8 vs. 4.7 ± 3.7 mmol/L) were comparable, the hypoperfusion-context subgroup presented a more severe circulatory dysfunction as expressed by higher NE requirements and a trend to a worse SOFA score (Table 1). As expected according to our local algorithm, patients categorized as with a hypoperfusion context received more dobutamine (31 vs. 5%; $p < 0.01$), and tended to receive more fluids (6732 ± 2524 vs. 5940 ± 2756 ml; $p = 0.2$).

Table 1 Clinical, demographic, severity scores, perfusion and hemodynamic variables at baseline according to hypoperfusion context

	Hypoperfusion context (70)	Non-hypoperfusion context (20)	p value
Age (years)	66 ± 17	65 ± 13	0.9
Charlson index	1.9 ± 2.2	1.6 ± 0.3	0.7
APACHE II score	22 ± 7	20 ± 5	0.2
SOFA score	9.5 ± 3.8	8.4 ± 2.6	0.1
Heart rate (beats/s)	104 ± 23	115 ± 24	0.07
MAP (mmHg)	75 ± 19	77 ± 21	0.6
SAP (mmHg)	108 ± 27	111 ± 27	0.6
DAP (mmHg)	59 ± 14	57 ± 12	0.6
Arterial lactate (mmol/L)	4.8 ± 2.8	4.7 ± 3.7	0.9
ScvO2 (%)	71.3 ± 9.5	74.8 ± 7	<0.05
P(cv-a) CO_2	7.6 ± 2.5	5.5 ± 2.2	<0.001
CRT (s)	5.4 ± 2.3	4.2 ± 2.6	<0.001
NE (mcg/kg/min)	0.19 ± 0.24	0.09 ± 0.11	<0.05

A $p < 0.05$ was considered as significant

Values are expressed as mean ± SD

APACHE Acute Physiology and Chronic Health Evaluation, *SOFA* Sequential Organ Failure Assessment, *MAP* mean arterial pressure, *SAP* systolic arterial pressure, *DAP* diastolic arterial pressure, *P*(cv-a)CO_2 central venous-arterial pCO_2 gradient, *CRT* capillary refill time, *NE* norepinephrine

Lactate decreased at the same rate in both groups (6 h lactate: 4 ± 2.7 vs. 3.9 ± 2.7 mmol/l, $p = 0.9$; 24 h lactate: 3.2 ± 3.0 vs. 2.7 ± 2.1 mmol/l, $p = 0.4$; 6 h lactate clearance: 13 ± 39 vs. 7 ± 48%, $p = 0.58$; 24 h lactate clearance: 27 ± 61 vs. 32 ± 39%, $p = 0.7$). However, within the hypoperfusion-context subgroup, 24-h lactate levels significantly decreased only in survivors with no change in non-survivors (Additional file 1: Figure S1). In addition, P(cv-a)CO_2 (7.6 ± 2.6 to 4.4 ± 2.3 mmHg; $p < 0.001$) and CRT (5.4 ± 2.2 to 3.1 ± 2.9 s; $p < 0.001$) decreased only in survivors.

Regarding main outcomes, patients with a hypoperfusion context exhibited a more severe circulatory dysfunction requiring higher NE doses at 6 h, and tended to have longer duration of mechanical ventilation, and higher use of HVHF as rescue therapy, in addition to longer ICU and hospital stays (Fig. 1). Eleven of 70 patients (16%) with a hypoperfusion context died as compared to only one of twenty in those without, although this difference was not significant.

The effect of using the criterion of "at least one abnormal perfusion parameter" among the three considered for

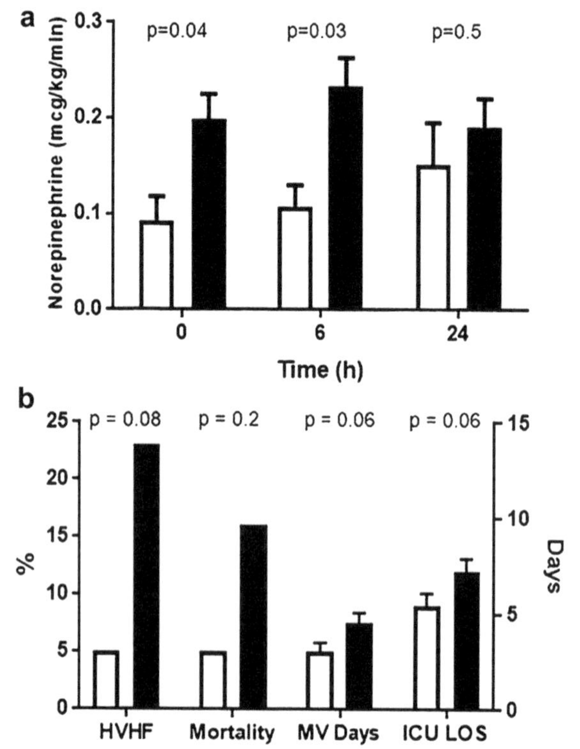

Fig. 1 Severity criteria to compare hyperlactatemic patients without versus with a hypoperfusion context. **a** Mean norepinephrine doses for both subgroups at baseline, 6 and 24 h. *Black boxes* describe hypoperfusion-context subgroup; *white boxes* represent non-hypoperfusion context subgroup. **b** Comparison of the use of rescue therapy and several outcome parameters between subgroups. *HVHF* high-volume hemofiltration, *Mortality* hospital mortality, *MV* mechanical ventilation, *ICU* intensive care unit, *LOS* length of stay

defining a hypoperfusion context, as compared to each one individually to discriminate survivors versus non-survivors is shown in the distributional Fig. 2. Although the purpose of this figure is only to show visually the impact of using different criteria, it appears that the best discriminating capacity is for "at least one abnormal perfusion parameter." In addition, the effect of testing different combinations of these three perfusion parameters ($ScvO_2$, $P(cv\text{-}a)CO_2$, and CRT) to define hypoperfusion context and the effect on outcomes variables is shown in Additional file 2: Table S1.

Discussion

Our main finding is that a multimodal perfusion monitoring in sepsis-3 septic shock patients may aid to differentiate two clinical patterns according to the presence of a hypoperfusion context. Patients with hyperlactatemia associated with either low $ScvO_2$, or high $P(cv\text{-}a)CO_2$, or high CRT values exhibit a more severe circulatory dysfunction. The absence of a hypoperfusion context among septic shock patients with hyperlactatemia is associated with a good outcome. These findings do not support sepsis-3 statement that the new septic shock definition identifies a group of patients with a homogenous high mortality risk [1]. On the other hand, they provide the basis for the development of a prospective study aimed at testing a safe restrictive fluid resuscitation strategy in septic shock patients without a hypoperfusion context, while concentrating resuscitation efforts in those with hypoperfusion criteria. The presence of a low $ScvO_2$ in the setting of persistent hyperlactatemia clearly indicates an imbalance in the oxygen transport/oxygen consumption relationship [7, 11]. A high $Pcv\text{–}aCO_2$ might identify patients who remain inadequately resuscitated and constitutes a marker of global perfusion that could aid in identifying a hypoperfusion-related hyperlactatemia [12, 13]. Assessment of peripheral perfusion may provide additional physiological information. An abnormal peripheral perfusion may be caused by adrenergic-induced skin vasoconstriction secondary to a low systemic blood flow and should prompt a reassessment of the hemodynamic state, in particular the volume status [10, 14]. Under the best of our knowledge, this is the first study that uses the three variables together to define a hypoperfusion context, an aspect that has to be highlighted because of the individual limitations of every isolated parameter. As a matter of fact, $ScvO_2$ can be normal in the setting of severe microcirculatory abnormalities [4, 12], $Pcv\text{-}aCO_2$ might be normal in hyperdynamic states even in the presence of tissue hypoxia [13], and peripheral perfusion may be difficult to assess under some circumstances. However, our results show that when the three are normal in hyperlactatemic patients, mortality as well as morbidity is very low, and thus the presence of tissue hypoxia as the cause of hyperlactatemia appear as unlikely in this setting, although of course it cannot be ruled out completely.

Remarkably, lactate values were comparable between subgroups at baseline (mean of 4.7–4.8 mmol/l) at a level where patients would not only have been diagnosed as septic shock according to sepsis-3 criteria [1], but also considered for inclusion in the EDGT trial [11]. However, adding hypoperfusion-context criteria to clinical assessment might aid in differentiating two clinical patterns with marked different risks as demonstrated by our study. Of course our design does not allow us to establish sensitivity or specificity or predictive value of these criteria to track real hypoxia-related hyperlactatemia, but at least our findings are hypothesis-generating, and might build up the foundations for future trials on septic shock patients that focus resuscitation efforts on selected populations. Anyway, hypoxia is a cellular event that is hardly diagnosed by clinical means. In the past, lactate/pyruvate ratio or more recently, the venous-arterial CO_2

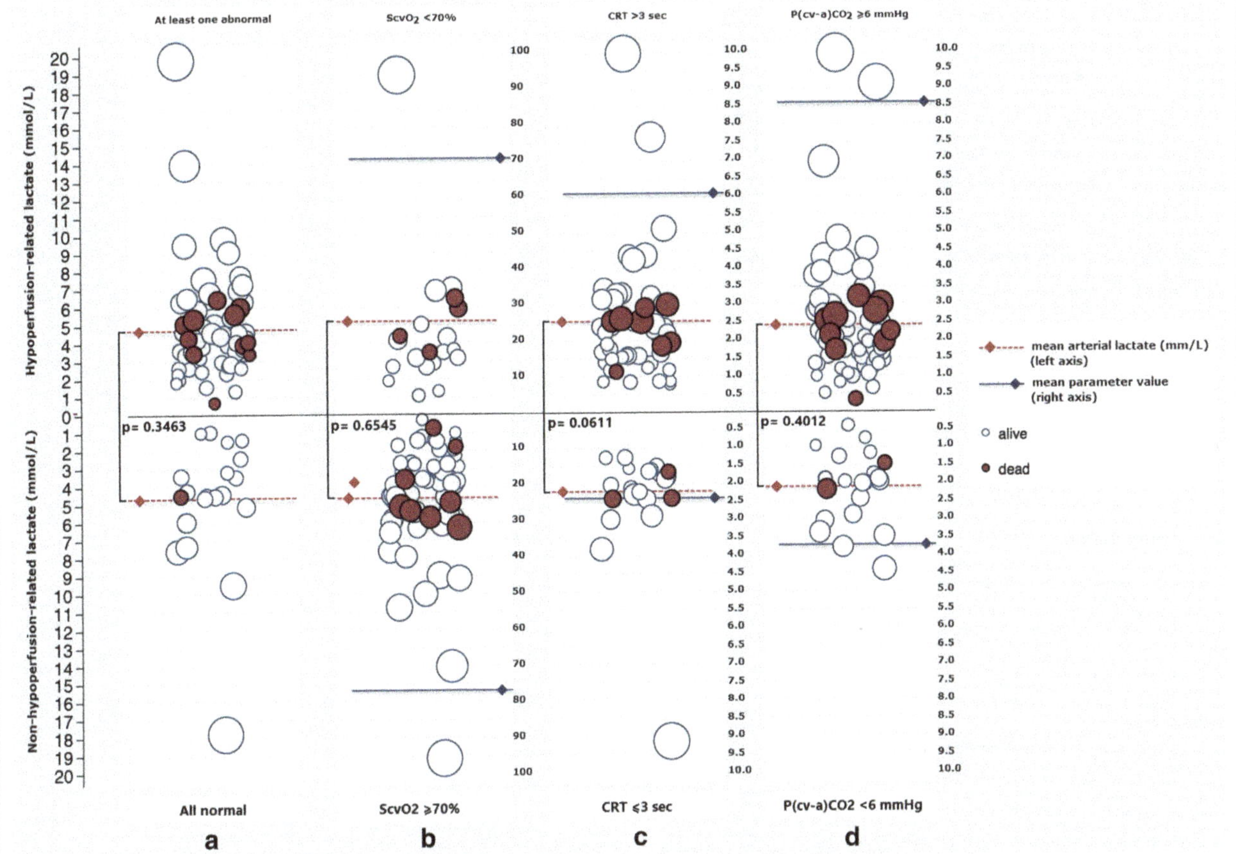

Fig. 2 Distributional figure: the figure displays different plausible allocation of patients under *four* distinctive hypoperfusion-context descriptors and their relationship with outcome in hyperlactatemic septic shock patients. The figure shows the distribution of patients according to the presence of abnormal $ScvO_2$, CRT, and $P(cv-a)CO_2$, and its relationship with hospital mortality where *white* and *black circles* represent survivors and non-survivors, respectively. **a** Comparing patients with normal perfusion criteria (*bottom*) versus those with at least one abnormal criterion (*top*). **b** Comparing patients with normal (*bottom*) versus abnormal $ScvO_2$ (*top*). **c** Comparing patients with normal (*bottom*) versus abnormal CRT (*top*). **d** Comparing patients with normal (*bottom*) versus abnormal $P(cv-a)CO_2$ (*top*). The *p* values represent the difference in mean lactate values among patients fulfilling or not the descriptors tested. No difference in lactate values was observed when using any of these descriptors although there are trends for difference in survival, especially when using the "at least one abnormal perfusion parameter" criterion as shown in the *first column*. *$ScvO_2$* central venous oxygen saturation, *CRT* capillary refill time, *$P(cv-a)CO_2$* central venous-to-arterial carbon dioxide difference

to arterial-venous O_2 content difference ratio have been proposed for this purpose, although both ratios have important theoretical and practical drawbacks [3, 8]. Our study has several drawbacks related to its retrospective nature and inclusion of a relatively small number of patients. Several variables exhibited a trend to be worse in the hypoperfusion-related subgroup but were short of significance, thus weakening our conclusions. Additionally, each variable proposed to define a hypoperfusion context has its own limitations. We also did not calculate the lactate/pyruvate or venous-arterial CO_2 to arterial-venous O_2 content difference ratios, closers indicators of tissue hypoxia according to several physiological studies. The parallel decrease in lactate levels in subgroups with versus without a hypoperfusion context could be viewed as contradictory, but when addressing this aspect more profoundly, the rate of decrease in lactate values in presumably hypoperfused patients was slowed by the performance of non-survivors who tended to increase lactate over time as compared to survivors (Additional file 1: Figure S1). This highlights the difficulties in interpreting lactate dynamics in septic shock patients subjected to a nonselective resuscitation strategy, as was also observed in another previous study [7]. However, despite these limitations, we could effectively differentiate two clinical patterns among hyperlactatemic septic shock patients when applying a monitoring model that includes three easily assessable perfusion-related parameters.

Conclusion

A mutimodal perfusion monitoring can identify two clinical patterns among hyperlactatemic septic shock patients according to widely used hypoperfusion-related criteria. Patients with hyperlactatemia plus low ScvO2, or high P(cv-a)CO_2, or high CRT values exhibit a more severe circulatory dysfunction with increased morbidity. This provides a starting point to launch further prospective studies to confirm if this approach can lead to a more rational and selective resuscitation strategy.

Abbreviations

MAP: mean arterial pressure; ScvO2: central venous oxygen saturation; P(cv-a)CO_2: central venous-arterial PCO_2 gradient; SSC: Surviving Sepsis Campaign; CRT: capillary refill time; ICU: intensive care unit.

Authors' contributions

LA and GH are guarantors of the entire manuscript; LA, GH, RC, GOT, JLT, and JB designed the study; MV, JD, CH, DG, PT, EK, and SB collected and analyzed all of the data. All of the authors helped in the data interpretation and the manuscript draft. All authors read and approved the final manuscript.

Author details

[1] Departamento de Medicina Intensiva, Facultad de Medicina, Pontificia Universidad Católica de Chile, Marcoleta 367, Santiago 8320000, Chile. [2] Hospital San Francisco, Quito, Ecuador. [3] Intensive Care Medicine Department, Fundación Valle del Lili - Universidad ICESI, Cali, Colombia. [4] Assistance Publique-Hôpitaux de Paris, Hôpitaux universitaires Paris-Sud, Hôpital de Bicêtre, Service de Réanimation Médicale, Le Kremlin-Bicêtre, France. [5] Department of Intensive Care Adults, Erasmus University Medical Center, Rotterdam, The Netherlands.

Competing interests

The authors declare that they have no competing interests.

Financial support

The study was financed by an internal grant from the Departamento de Medicina Intensiva, Facultad de Medicina, Pontificia Universidad Católica de Chile.

References

1. Singer M, Deutschman CS, Seymour CW, Shankar-Hari M, Annane D, Bauer M, et al. The third international consensus definitions for sepsis and septic shock (Sepsis-3). JAMA. 2016;315:801–10.
2. Dellinger RP, Levy MM, Rhodes A, Annane D, Gerlach H, Opal SM, et al. Surviving Sepsis Campaign: international guidelines for management of severe sepsis and septic shock, 2012. Crit Care Med. 2013;41:580–637.
3. Garcia-Alvarez M, Marik P, Bellomo R. Sepsis-associated hyperlactatemia. Crit Care. 2014;18:503.
4. Hernandez G, Bruhn A, Castro R, Regueira T. The holistic view on perfusion monitoring in septic shock. Curr Opinion Crit Care. 2012;18:280–6.
5. Tapia P, Soto D, Bruhn A, Alegria L, Jarufe N, Luengo C, et al. Impairment of exogenous lactate clearance in experimental hyperdynamic septic shock is not related to total liver hypoperfusion. Crit Care. 2015;19:188.
6. Cecconi M, De Backer D, Antonelli M, Beale R, Bakker J, Hofer C, et al. Consensus on circulatory shock and hemodynamic monitoring. Task force of the European Society of Intensive Care Medicine. Intensive Care Med. 2014;40:1795–815.
7. Jansen TC, van Bommel J, Schoonderbeek FJ, Sleeswijk Visser SJ, van der Klooster JM, et al. Early lactate-guided therapy in intensive care unit patients: a multicenter, open-label, randomized controlled trial. Am J Respir Crit Care Med. 2010;182:752–61.
8. Ospina-Tascon GA, Umana M, Bermudez W, Bautista-Rincon DF, Hernandez G, Bruhn A, et al. Combination of arterial lactate levels and venous-arterial CO_2 to arterial-venous O_2 content difference ratio as markers of resuscitation in patients with septic shock. Intensive Care Med. 2015;41:796–805.
9. Hernandez G, Luengo C, Bruhn A, Kattan E, Friedman G, Ospina-Tascon GA, et al. When to stop septic shock resuscitation: clues from a dynamic perfusion monitoring. Ann Intensive Care. 2014;4:30.
10. van Genderen ME, Engels N, van der Valk RJP, Lima A, Klijn E, Bakker J, et al. Early peripheral perfusion-guided fluid therapy in patients with septic shock. Am J Respir Crit Care Med. 2015;191:477–80.
11. Rivers E, Nguyen B, Havstad S, Ressler J, Muzzin A, Knoblich B, et al. Early goal-directed therapy in the treatment of severe sepsis and septic shock. N Engl J Med. 2001;345:1368–77.
12. Vallée F, Vallet B, Mathe O, Parraguette J, Mari A, Silva S, et al. Central venous-to-arterial carbon dioxide difference: An additional target for goal-directed therapy in septic shock? Intensive Care Med. 2008;34:2218–25.
13. Ospina-Tascón GA, Bautista-Rincón DF, Umaña M, Tafur JD, Gutiérrez A, García AF, et al. Persistently high venous-to-arterial carbon dioxide differences during early resuscitation are associated with poor outcomes in septic shock. Crit Care. 2013;17:R294.
14. Hernandez G, Pedreros C, Veas E, Bruhn A, Romero C, Rovegno M, et al. Evolution of peripheral vs metabolic perfusion parameters during septic shock resuscitation: a clinical-physiologic study. J Crit Care. 2012;27:283–8.

The impact of a multifaceted intervention including sepsis electronic alert system and sepsis response team on the outcomes of patients with sepsis and septic shock

Yaseen M. Arabi[1*], Hasan M. Al-Dorzi[2], Ahmed Alamry[2], Ra'ed Hijazi[2], Sami Alsolamy[2], Majid Al Salamah[2], Hani M. Tamim[2,3], Saad Al-Qahtani[2], Abdulaziz Al-Dawood[2], Abdellatif M. Marini[2], Fatimah H. Al Ehnidi[2], Shihab Mundekkadan[2], Amal Matroud[2], Mohamed S. Mohamed[2] and Saadi Taher[2]

Abstract

Background: Compliance with the clinical practice guidelines of sepsis management has been low. The objective of our study was to describe the results of implementing a multifaceted intervention including an electronic alert (e-alert) with a sepsis response team (SRT) on the outcome of patients with sepsis and septic shock presenting to the emergency department.

Methods: This was a pre–post two-phased implementation study that consisted of a pre-intervention phase (January 01, 2011–September 24, 2012), intervention phase I (multifaceted intervention including e-alert, from September 25, 2012–March 03, 2013) and intervention phase II when SRT was added (March 04, 2013–October 30, 2013) in a 900-bed tertiary-care academic hospital. We recorded baseline characteristics and processes of care in adult patients presenting with sepsis or septic shock. The primary outcome measures were hospital mortality. Secondary outcomes were the need for mechanical ventilation and length of stay in the intensive unit and in the hospital.

Results: After implementing the multifaceted intervention including e-alert and SRT, cases were identified with less severe clinical and laboratory abnormalities and the processes of care improved. When adjusted to propensity score, the interventions were associated with reduction in hospital mortality [for intervention phase II compared to pre-intervention: adjusted odds ratio (aOR) 0.71, 95% CI 0.58–0.85, $p = 0.003$], reduction in the need for mechanical ventilation (aOR 0.45, 95% CI 0.37–0.55, $p < 0.0001$) and reduction in ICU LOS and hospital LOS for all patients as well as ICU LOS for survivors.

Conclusions: Implementing a multifaceted intervention including sepsis e-alert with SRT was associated with earlier identification of sepsis, increase in compliance with sepsis resuscitation bundle and reduction in the need for mechanical ventilation and reduction in hospital mortality and LOS.

Keywords: Sepsis, Shock, Intensive care unit, Hospital mortality, Quality improvement, Patient safety, Health service administration, Emergency department, Sepsis resuscitation bundle

*Correspondence: arabi@ngha.med.sa; yaseenarabi@yahoo.com
[1] Intensive Care Department, MC-1425, Respiratory Services, College of Medicine, King Abdullah International Medical Research Center, King Saud bin Abdulaziz University for Health Sciences, P.O. Box 22490, Riyadh 11426, Kingdom of Saudi Arabia
Full list of author information is available at the end of the article

Background

Despite the major burden of sepsis as a leading cause of human death, studies have repeatedly demonstrated that the compliance with the clinical practice guidelines for sepsis management, grouped in the sepsis resuscitation bundle, is low and that this low compliance is associated with increased mortality [1–9]. As a result, the Surviving Sepsis Campaign (SSC) has recommended performance improvement efforts be undertaken [10, 11] and the National Quality Forum has endorsed the bundle implementation [12]. Thus, several institutional, national and international improvement projects have been launched [13–16].

However, transitioning evidence into sustainable clinical improvement in sepsis management has been a complex task [17–19]. Implementation barriers include delayed identification of septic patients, unawareness of or disagreement with guidelines, guideline complexity, lack of resources [17–19], staff shortage and unavailability of specialized setting required to put therapy into routine practice [9]. In the face of this complexity, different implementation strategies have been utilized, including education, posters, reminders, audit and feedback, paper-based and electronic sepsis screening tools, clinical pathways, rapid response teams and sepsis response teams (SRTs) [20–28]. The differential or the synergistic effect of these strategies on changing sepsis management practice has not been studied. However, it has been shown in other settings that these interventions vary in effectiveness. Two systematic reviews showed that educational activities and audits had low leverage on changing physician practices and reminders had a slightly larger effect [29, 30]. Automation and forcing function have higher leverage [31], and a multifaceted approach may be the most effective [29, 30]. Yet, many sepsis improvement projects invested in potentially low-leverage interventions leading to modest change in sepsis bundle compliance and mortality. The use of automation and forced function in sepsis management may be achieved by combining an electronic sepsis alert (e-alert) system for timely sepsis identification with a sepsis response team for timely management. Although there are a few reports on implementing these two interventions individually [32–34], the inclusion of the two as components of a multifaceted intervention, which may have a synergistic effect [26], has not been studied.

The objective of this study was to examine the impact of an improvement project utilizing a multifaceted intervention that includes an e-alert system and SRT on the compliance with the sepsis resuscitation bundle and outcome of adult patients with sepsis and septic shock presenting to the emergency department (ED).

Methods

Setting

The study was conducted in a 900-bed tertiary-care academic hospital accredited by Joint Commission International. The ED receives >200,000 patients per year is staffed by board-certified emergency medicine physicians and has 15 resuscitation beds for high-acuity patients and 49 beds for moderate-acuity patients. The Intensive Care Department staffs 5 ICUs on a 24-h/7-day in-house basis [35], has a rapid response team [36] and provides coverage for boarding patients in the ED who meet ICU admission criteria.

Study design

This was a pre–post implementation study that consisted of a pre-intervention phase and a 2-step implementation (intervention phases I and II). During the study period, there were no major changes in the hospital admission criteria, nursing or medical care plans, or staffing structure. The study was approved by the Institutional Review Board of Ministry of National Guard-Health affairs, and informed consent requirement was waived.

Pre-intervention phase

In this phase (January 01, 2011–September 24, 2012), patients presenting to the ED were triaged based on illness severity according to the Canadian Triage and Acuity Scale [37], evaluated first by the ED nurses and physicians, and then referred to a primary admitting service. Critically ill septic patients were subsequently referred to the intensive care team. Identifying patient as having sepsis and initial resuscitation were based on clinical assessment by the ED physicians, the primary admitting service, the intensive care team or a combination of these services. During this phase, the sepsis bundle had not been implemented.

Intervention phase I

In this phase (September 25, 2012–March 03, 2013), sepsis e-alert and computerized physician order entry (CPOE) sepsis management order-set (based on the SCC sepsis bundle) were implemented and were accompanied by an educational campaign targeting the ED healthcare providers. A clinical pathway was also generated after multidisciplinary discussions (Additional file 1: Figure S1, Figure S2, Table S1). Additionally, weekly text messages were sent to the phones of the ED and ICU physicians about the bundle compliance rates highlighting the element of the bundle that had the lowest compliance.

This phase required considerable planning, which started in October 2011 as a multidisciplinary quality improvement project aimed at improving sepsis management through the implementation of the SSC bundle. Root-cause analysis was conducted to search for the probable causes of low bundle compliance. In addition, the flow of septic patients from the ED to the ICU was mapped to understand related processes and bottlenecks. After analysis, the low compliance was attributed to multiple factors including delays in sepsis recognition, insufficient awareness of sepsis resuscitation bundle and the complexity of the care processes. For the intervention phase I, the project focused on improving early sepsis recognition through building an electronic sepsis screening tool (e-alert) in the hospital electronic health record (EHR) system (QuadraMed® Computerized Patient Record System, Reston, VA, USA) and on simplifying the care process by building a CPOE order-set that incorporated the required orders in groups on one platform. The e-alert was based on identifying abnormal vital signs and certain laboratory tests, all captured from the EHR. We used in designing our e-alert the formal definition of sepsis (previously called severe sepsis) with includes a combination of the Systemic Inflammatory Response Syndrome (SIRS) criteria and one organ dysfunction, because this quality improvement project was performed the new definition for sepsis (Sepsis-3) became available [38.] When a patient demonstrated any two SIRS criteria (temperature >38 °C OR <36 °C; heart rate >90 beats/min; respiratory rate >20 breaths/min; WBC count >12,000/mm^3 OR <4000/mm^3) AND at least one of the following organ dysfunctions (systolic blood pressure 86–90 mmHg with intravenous fluids or <86 mmHg regardless of fluids; blood oxygen saturation of 85–90% with supplemental oxygen or <85% without oxygen; lactate >2 mmol/L) OR two of the above organ dysfunctions, an e-alert was sent to the nursing work-list prompting her/him to contact the treating medical team. The treating physician would then evaluate the patient, confirm the presence or absence of these conditions and use the CPOE order-set if indicated. The development and testing of both the e-alert and the CPOE order-set went through multiple PDSA (plan, do, study, act) cycles with small-scale testing, documentation and learning in the EHR system development (in-production) domain until the activation date. During these PDSA cycles, certain triggers were added to the e-alert (systolic blood pressure 86–90 mmHg with intravenous fluids or <86 mmHg regardless of fluids; blood oxygen saturation of 85–90% with supplemental oxygen or <85% without oxygen) to improve specificity. We could not use reduced level of consciousness in building the e-alert, because it was recorded as a text and not as a numeric value in our EHR.

Intervention phase II

On March 04, 2013, and through October 30, 2013, a dedicated 24/7 SRT was launched in addition to the interventions already in place from intervention phase I. The SRT consisted of an intensive care registrar physician and a nurse who were trained on sepsis management using didactic lectures and simulation-based learning. The bedside nurse activated the SRT after being prompted by the e-alert or when sepsis was clinically suspected. The SRT assessed the patient for the presence of sepsis, followed the same clinical pathway used in intervention phase I and provided sepsis management as needed in collaboration with the treating team.

Data collection and outcome measures

Starting October 2011, we collected patient-level data prospectively by a dedicated data collector using the 2008 SSC data collection tool [39]. Additional data were collected retrospectively for the period January 2011–September 2011, to expand the baseline data of pre-intervention phase. Sepsis (originally severe sepsis) was defined as SIRS with acute organ dysfunction secondary to documented or suspected infection. The organ dysfunctions that were used to build the e-alert were hypotension, hypoxia and increased lactate as defined above. Septic shock was defined as sepsis (originally severe sepsis) with persistent hypotension after fluid resuscitation with at least 20 mL/kg of crystalloid (or equivalent). We recorded the compliance with the following individual elements of the 2008 SSC resuscitation bundle and the time to intervention: [1] serum lactate obtained within 6 h of presentation, [2] blood cultures taken before the administration of broad-spectrum antibiotics, [3] broad-spectrum antibiotics administered within 3 h of ED admission, [4] 20 mL/kg of crystalloid (or equivalent) administered in patients who were hypotensive or had lactate >4 mmol/L; and in patients who remained hypotensive or had lactate >4 mmol/L, [6] achievement of central venous pressure (CVP) ≥8 mmHg and central venous oxygen saturation ($ScvO_2$) ≥70% and initiation of vasopressors. Based on recent evidence arising from the recent clinical trials on early goal-directed therapy [40–42], we evaluated bundle compliance with the first 4 elements only and we did not include CVP and $ScvO_2$. The primary outcome measure was hospital mortality. Secondary outcome measures were the need for mechanical ventilation during this episode of sepsis, ICU and hospital length of stay (LOS) for all patients for survivors.

Statistical analysis

All statistical analyses were performed using SAS software (version 9.1; SAS Institute, Cary, NC). Continuous variables were presented as means with standard deviations, and categorical variables as absolute and relative frequencies. Mann–Whitney and Chi-square tests were used to compare differences between the phases as appropriate. To account for the differences in baseline characteristics among the three phases, we generated propensity scores using the following variables that were clinically relevant and statistically associated with the different phases (Table 1): pneumonia, hypothermia, acutely altered mental status, hypoxia, leukopenia, increased creatinine, thrombocytopenia, hyperbilirubinemia, coagulopathy and lactate levels. To check the balancing effect of propensity scores, we used the propensity scores as covariates in an analysis of covariance for continuous baseline variables and in multinomial logistic regression for categorical baseline variables. We used multivariate logistic and linear regression analysis to examine the association of implementation phase with mortality and LOS after adjustment to propensity scores. A p value <0.05 was considered to be statistically significant. We constructed control charts with upper and lower control limits for the 4-element bundle compliance and for hospital mortality using CHARTrunner, version 3.6.88 (PQ Systems, Dayton OH, USA).

Results

Patients baseline characteristics

At the time of identification, patients in the intervention phases I and II were less likely to have hypothermia, altered mental status, hypotension, hypoxemia,

Table 1 Baseline characteristics of patients with sepsis and septic shock on presentation in the three study phases: pre-intervention (A), intervention phase I (B) and intervention phase II (C)

All patients	Pre-intervention A	Intervention phase I B	Intervention phase II C	Crude p value			p value after propensity score adjustment		
	$N=436$	$N=195$	$N=699$	B vs. A	C vs. B	C vs. A	B vs. A	C vs. B	C vs. A
Source of sepsis, no. (%)									
Pneumonia	228 (52.3)	93 (47.7)	281 (40.2)	0.29	0.06	<0.0001	0.99	0.98	0.96
Urinary tract infection	70 (16.1)	28 (14.4)	107 (15.3)	0.59	0.74	0.74	0.78	0.90	0.38
Acute abdominal infection	40 (9.2)	8 (3.6)	47 (6.7)	0.03	0.18	0.13	0.05	0.37	0.17
Soft tissue infection	8 (1.8)	8 (4.1)	32 (4.6)	0.10	0.78	0.01	0.42	0.84	0.56
Other infections	138 (31.7)	68 (34.9)	254 (36.3)	0.43	0.71	0.11	0.92	0.60	0.48
Signs and symptoms, no. (%)									
Hyperthermia[a]	114 (26.2)	52 (26.7)	172 (24.6)	0.89	0.56	0.56	0.81	0.15	0.47
Hypothermia[a]	34 (7.8)	6 (3.1)	7 (1.0)	0.02	0.04	<0.0001	0.99	0.86	0.81
Acutely altered mental status	157 (36.0)	48 (24.6)	59 (8.4)	0.005	<0.0001	<0.0001	0.98	0.67	0.71
Chills and rigors	11 (2.5)	7 (3.6)	2 (0.3)	0.46	0.001	0.0006	0.55	0.0007	0.02
Tachycardia[a]	354 (81.2)	168 (86.2)	624 (89.3)	0.13	0.23	0.0001	0.76	0.44	0.49
Tachypnea[a]	368 (84.4)	174 (89.2)	583 (83.4)	0.11	0.05	0.66	0.44	0.34	0.92
Hypotension[a]	368 (84.4)	111 (56.9)	265 (37.9)	<0.0001	<0.0001	<0.0001	0.004	0.42	<0.0001
Hypoxia[a]	101 (23.2)	79 (40.5)	227 (32.5)	<0.0001	0.04	0.0008	0.94	0.96	0.99
Laboratory findings, no. (%)									
Leukocytosis[a]	237 (54.4)	85 (43.6)	229 (32.8)	0.01	0.005	<0.0001	0.14	0.003	<0.0001
Leukopenia[a]	36 (8.3)	6 (3.1)	21 (3.0)	0.02	0.96	<0.0001	0.99	0.99	0.92
Increased creatinine[a]	107 (24.5)	4 (2.1)	1 (0.1)	<0.0001	0.009	<0.0001	0.97	0.99	0.68
Thrombocytopenia[a]	40 (9.2)	0 (0.0)	1 (0.1)	<0.0001	1.0	<0.0001	0.43	0.99	0.70
Hyperbilirubinemia[a]	44 (10.1)	1 (0.5)	1 (0.1)	<0.0001	0.39	<0.0001	0.82	0.94	0.68
Hyperlactatemia[a]	168 (38.5)	70 (35.9)	320 (45.8)	0.53	0.01	0.02	0.99	0.99	0.98
Coagulopathy[a]	67 (15.4)	2 (1.0)	1 (0.1)	<0.0001	0.12	<0.0001	0.87	0.86	0.67
Classification, no. (%)									
Sepsis	108 (24.8)	99 (50.8)	584 (83.6)	<0.0001	<0.0001	<0.0001	0.93	0.78	0.68
Septic shock	328 (75.2)	96 (49.2)	115 (16.5)						

[a] Hyperthermia: temperature >38 °C, hypothermia: temperature <36 °C, tachycardia: heart rate >90/min, tachypnea: respiratory rate >20/min, hypotension: systolic blood pressure <90, mean arterial pressure <65 or systolic blood pressure decrease >40 mmHg from baseline, hypoxia: oxygen requirement to maintain oxygen saturation >90%, leukocytosis: WBC count >12 × 10^9/L, leucopenia: white blood cell count <4 × 10^9/L, increased creatinine: creatinine increase >176.8 mmol/L, thrombocytopenia: platelet count <100 × 10^9/L, hyperbilirubinemia: bilirubin >34.2 mmol/L, hyperlactatemia: lactate >2 mmol/L, coagulopathy: international normalized ratio (INR) >1

leukopenia, elevated creatinine, thrombocytopenia, hyperbilirubinemia and coagulopathy compared to patients in the pre-intervention phase (Table 1). These differences in symptoms and signs, and key laboratory findings between the three phases suggest that the implementation of multifaceted interventions including sepsis e-alert and SRT was associated with earlier identification of sepsis.

Propensity scores

The balancing effect of the generated propensity scores is shown in Table 1. When adjusted to propensity scores, all baseline characteristics were balanced.

Interventions during the course of treatment

Intervention phases I and II were associated with improvement in most measured processes of sepsis care. The frequency of measuring lactate (at any time and within 6 h) and the time to obtaining lactate all improved. Similarly the frequency of obtaining blood cultures (at any time and before antibiotics) and the time to blood cultures improved. Antibiotics administration within 3 h and the time to antibiotics followed a similar pattern. In patients with persistent hypotension or lactate >4 mmol/L, CVP $\geq$8 mmHg and $ScvO_2$ of $\geq$70% were achieved more often (Table 2). As a result, the overall compliance with 4-element bundle increased from 19.3 to 44.6 to 69.4% (p values <0.0001 after adjustment to propensity scores) (Table 2; Fig. 1).

Outcomes

Intervention phase II was associated with reduction in crude hospital mortality and ICU LOS (Fig. 1; Table 3). When adjusted to propensity score, intervention phase II was associated with a significant reduction in hospital mortality [adjusted odds ratio (aOR) 0.71, 95% CI 0.58–0.85, $p = 0.003$] and in the need for mechanical ventilation (aOR 0.45, 95% CI 0.37–0.55, $p < 0.0001$). In addition, intervention phase II was associated with reduction in ICU LOS and hospital LOS for all patients as well as ICU LOS for survivors (Table 3).

Discussion

Our study demonstrates that the implementation of a multifaceted intervention including a sepsis e-alert with an SRT was associated with improvement in the care process of sepsis management; improvement in the timeliness of lactate measurement, obtaining of blood cultures, antibiotic administration and achievement of CVP and $ScvO_2$ targets and reduction in the need for mechanical ventilation and reduction in hospital mortality and LOS.

Quality improvement projects that implemented sepsis resuscitation bundle [43] have been shown to reduce mortality in several settings [20, 22, 26]. However, the effect varied considerably and was often modest, particularly when instruction-based interventions were used [22]. Our study showed a substantial improvement when a multifaceted approach was used that included an e-alert with SRT. The use of e-alert with SRT exemplifies the use of automation and forcing function in improving adherence to the best practice.

Timely recognition of sepsis is key to improving its management. A sepsis e-alert that is activated as soon as abnormal values are entered in the EHR may serve as a decision support system that bypasses the shortcomings of human processes. In addition, electronic screening for sepsis is more reliable and sustainable than paper-based screening tools as demonstrated in other settings [44]. Our data show that the e-alert identified patients with sepsis cases at earlier stage, which is a major aim of the project. However, early recognition may raise concerns about workload increase and overtreatment. However, in our project, physicians reviewed all cases before initiating treatment; thus reducing the risk of overtreatment. Additionally, it is our belief that the implications of overtreatment, if exists, are small compared to the substantial advantage of timely sepsis management.

Improving compliance with evidence-based time-sensitive therapies may be achieved by using condition-specific teams, as shown with acute myocardial infarction [45], stroke [46] and trauma teams [47]. Such teams are more focused, knowledgeable and experienced thus reducing care variation and increasing reliability. Only few studies have examined SRT implementation. A prospective cohort study examined the impact of 'team' vs. 'non-team' models on implementing sepsis bundle in multiple Asian countries [21]. In the non-team model, ED physicians completed the bundle in the ED as a standard care [21]. In the team model, the implementation was championed by intensivists with the bundle completed in the ICU and was associated with a greater improvement in the compliance [21]. Another study examined the impact of daily auditing with weekly feedback and SRT activation in patients admitted to the medical ICU with sepsis or septic shock [26]. The compliance rate with the sepsis resuscitation bundle increased from 12.7% at baseline to 37.7 and 53.7% during the weekly feedback and SRT activation periods, respectively ($p < 0.001$) [26]. The overall hospital mortality rates were 30.3, 28.3 and 22.0% during baseline, weekly feedback and SRT team periods, respectively ($p = 0.03$) [26]. In this study, the SRT was involved only in managing patients admitted to the medical ICU and required restructuring the existing ICU service, without adding new manpower [26].

There have been a heated debate about using CVP and $ScvO_2$ as treatment goals in patients with sepsis; a debate

Table 2 Sepsis-related interventions during the treatment period for patients with sepsis or septic shock in the three study phases: pre-intervention (A), intervention phase I (B) and intervention phase II (C)

Variable	Pre-intervention A	Intervention phase I B	Intervention phase II C	*p* value			*p* value after propensity scores adjustments		
All patients	***N*** **= 436**	***N*** **= 195**	***N*** **= 699**	**B vs. A**	**C vs. B**	**C vs. A**	**B vs. A**	**C vs. B**	**C vs. A**
Lactate measured at any time, no. (%)	406 (93.1)	191 (97.9)	682 (97.6)	0.01	1.0	0.0003	0.02	0.72	0.009
Time to lactate (h), mean ± SD	9.3 ± 22.1	2.5 ± 5.3	1.1 ± 3.7	<0.0001	0.0008	<0.0001	0.002	0.0002	<0.0001
Lactate (mmol/L), mean ± SD	3.9 ± 3.6	3.3 ± 2.3	3.4 ± 5.5	0.01	0.93	0.03	0.76	0.28	0.26
Measure lactate within 6 h, no. (%)	270 (61.9)	168 (86.2)	663 (94.9)	<0.0001	<0.0001	<0.0001	<0.0001	<0.0001	<0.0001
Blood culture obtained at any time, no. (%)[a]	238 (54.6)	119/194 (61.3)	592/679 (87.2)	0.11	<0.0001	<0.0001	0.16	<0.0001	<0.0001
Time to blood culture (h), mean ± SD	2.4 ± 6.7	0.9 ± 1.4	0.9 ± 2.5	0.001	0.94	0.0008	0.02	0.84	0.0001
Blood culture before antibiotics, no. (%)	219 (50.2)	116 (59.5)	565 (80.8)	0.02	<0.0001	<0.0001	0.10	<0.0001	<0.0001
Antibiotics administered at any time, no. (%)[a]	266/269 (98.9)	136/137 (99.3)	439/448 (98.0)	1.0	0.47	0.55	0.97	0.45	0.87
Time to antibiotic administration (h), mean ± SD	4.8 ± 6.7	3.0 ± 3.6	1.9 ± 3.3	0.0004	0.002	<0.0001	0.002	0.002	0.01
Antibiotics within 3 h, no. (%)	295 (67.7)	149 (76.4)	625 (89.4)	<0.0001	<0.0001	<0.0001	0.01	0.0001	<0.0001
Patients with hypotension/lactate >4 mmol/L	***N*** **= 406**	***N*** **= 149**	***N*** **= 361**						
Fluids delivered at any time, no. (%)[a]	399 (98.3)	148 (99.3)	344 (95.3)	0.69	0.02	0.02	0.51	0.15	0.51
MAP raised and remained >65 mmHg, no. (%)	88/399 (22.1)	53/148 (35.8)	229/344 (67.8)	0.001	<0.0001	<0.0001	0.02	0.50	0.09
Vasopressors administered, no. (%)	299/311 (96.1)	91/95 (95.8)	101/115 (87.8)	1.0	0.04	0.002	0.72	0.07	0.05
Fluids (≥20 mL/kg) and vasopressors in the first 6 h, no. (%)	364/412 (88.4)	144/153 (94.1)	324/370 (87.6)	0.04	0.03	0.74	0.04	0.08	0.85
Compliance with the 4 elements bundle	84 (19.3)	87 (44.6)	485 (69.4)	<0.0001	<0.0001	<0.0001	<0.0001	<0.0001	<0.0001
Patients with persistent hypotension/lactate >4 mmol/L	***N*** **= 333**	***N*** **= 115**	***N*** **= 209**						
CVP ≥ 8 mmHg achieved, no. (%)									
Within 6 h	71/358 (19.8)	24/121 (19.8)	64/245 (26.1)	0.99	0.18	0.07	0.47	0.0002	<0.0001
Within 24 h	190 (57.2)	51 (44.4)	98 (46.9)	0.002	0.69	<0.0001	0.06	0.004	0.66
After 24 h	42 (12.7)	6 (5.2)	7 (3.4)						
Time to CVP (h), mean ± SD	16.3 ± 21.8	11.3 ± 10.4	8.1 ± 9.5	0.01	0.05	<0.0001	0.25	0.02	0.005
$ScvO_2$ ≥ 70% achieved, no. (%)									
Within 6 h	65/358 (18.2)	19/121 (15.7)	56/245 (22.9)	0.53	0.11	0.16	0.69	<0.0001	0.0006
Within 24 h	106 (31.9)	26 (22.6)	78 (37.3)	0.03	0.57	0.006	0.003	<0.0001	0.31
After 24 h	37 (11.1)	5 (4.4)	7 (3.6)						
Time to $ScvO_2$ (h) mean ± SD	20.8 ± 52.1	9.8 ± 13.7	8.2 ± 12.7	<0.0001	<0.0001	<0.0001	0.41	0.40	0.09

[a] Patients who had cultures or received antibiotics prior to meeting sepsis and septic shock criteria were not included

[a] 20 mL/kg of crystalloid fluids *CVP* central venous pressure, *MAP* mean arterial pressure, *$ScvO_2$* central venous oxygen saturation. Denominators are equal to '*N*' in all three phases unless otherwise specified

that manifested intensely among our staff during the course of our project. Three recent trials of early goal-directed therapy demonstrated that routine use of central hemodynamic and oxygen-saturation monitoring compared to their use at-physician discretion did not result in better outcomes [40–42] resulted in removal of these elements from the sepsis resuscitation bundle [48]. Our data show significant improvement in outcomes even with modest increase in the compliance with the CVP and $ScvO_2$ elements, supporting the notion that the key to improving sepsis outcome lies mainly in the early recognition, early fluid administration and early antibiotic therapy [48]. Why bundle compliance fell short of 100% even in the SRT phase?. An important reason is that the 2008 SCC bundle accounts for compliance achievement rather than attempting-to-achieve therapeutic

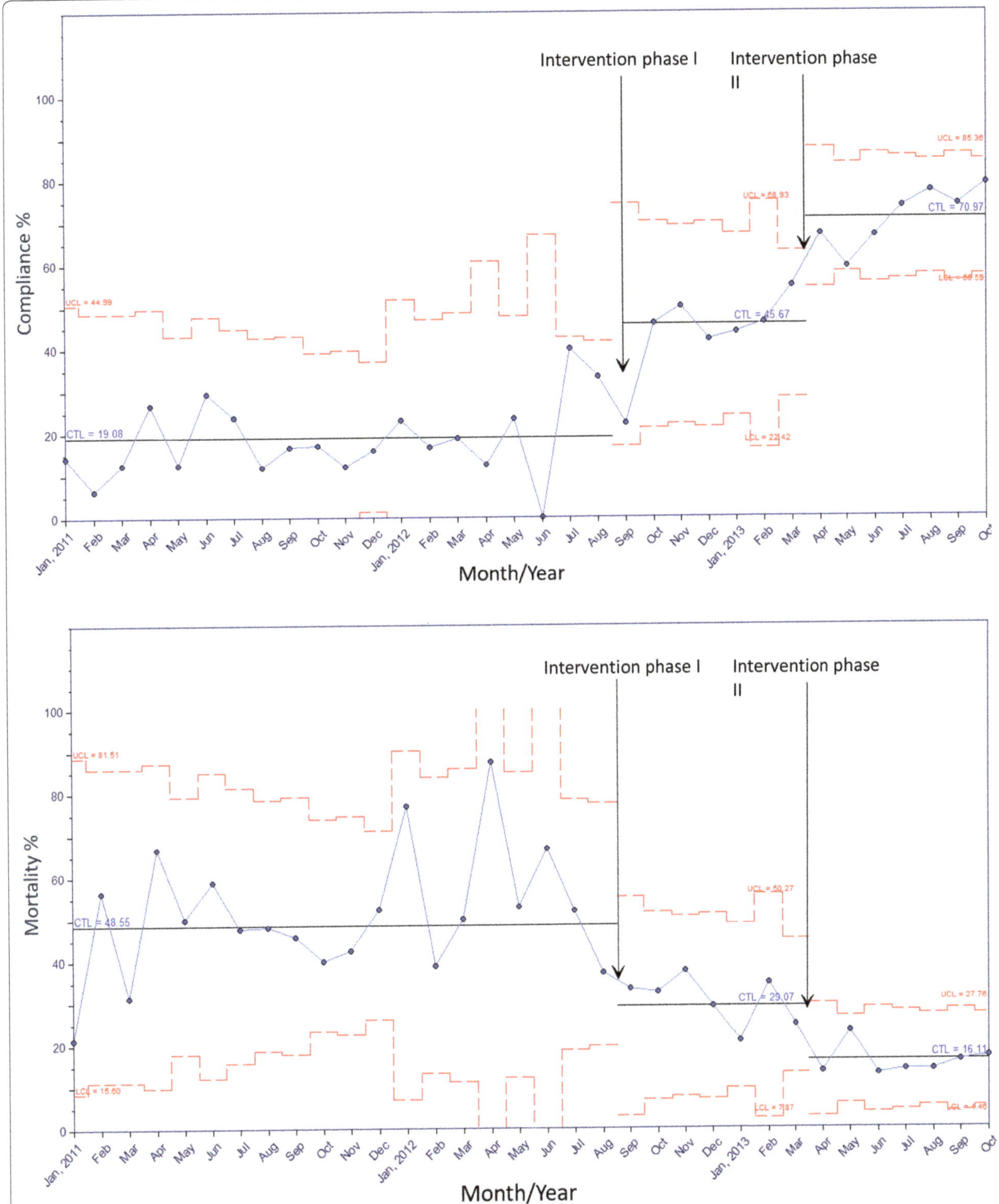

Fig. 1 Control chart with *upper* and *lower* control limits of the overall compliance with the resuscitation bundle and the mortality in the three phases. The two arrows on the chart show the time of initiation of the intervention phases I and II

Table 3 Outcomes among patients with sepsis or septic shock in the three study phases: pre-intervention (A), intervention phase I (B) and intervention phase II (C) with adjustment to propensity scores

Variable	Pre-intervention A	Intervention phase I B	Intervention phase II C	Propensity scores adjusted OR or correlation coefficient* (95% CI, *p* value)		
All patients	$N = 436$	$N = 195$	$N = 699$	**B vs. A**	**C vs. B**	**C vs. A**
Hospital mortality, no. (%)	208 (47.7)	60 (30.8)	118 (16.9)	0.73 (0.48–1.09, 0.13)	0.78 (0.51–1.17, 0.23)	0.71 (0.58–0.85, 0.003)
ICU LOS (days), mean ± SD	13.3 ± 17.4	8.6 ± 8.3	5.1 ± 11.4	−4.49 (−7.39 to −1.59, 0.002)*	−1.54 (−3.38 to 0.29, 0.09)*	−2.72 (−3.92 to −1.52, <0.0001)*
Mechanical ventilation, no. (%)	265 (60.8)	54 (27.7)	78 (11.2)	0.33 (0.22–0.49, <0.0001)	0.64 (0.41–0.99, 0.05)	0.45 (0.37–0.55, <0.0001)
ICU LOS among survivors (days), mean ± SD	15.9 ± 19.5	11.9 ± 10.4	8.2 ± 13.8	−5.88 (−11.44 to −0.22, 0.04)*	−1.05 (−5.22 to 3.10, 0.61)*	−3.55 (−6.13 to −0.98, 0.007)*
Hospital LOS (days), mean ± SD	29.3 ± 33.9	25.7 ± 40.9	15.3 ± 23.5	−1.37 (−8.28 to 5.53, 0.70)*	−8.42 (−13.29 to −3.54, 0.0007)*	−5.35 (−7.76 to −2.94, <0.0001)*
Hospital LOS among survivors (days), mean ± SD	28.1 ± 30.8	24.7 ± 37.7	20.6 ± 28.6	−1.76 (−12.09 to 8.57, 0.73)*	−6.22 (−16.9 to 4.48, 0.25)*	−3.45 (−7.83 to 0.92, 0.12)*

LOS length of stay, * correlation coefficient (95% CI, *p* value)

goals within the recommended time [49], which has been revised in the 2012 version. Other reasons may include the complexity and high number of interventions, involvement of multiple players, resistance to change and the long waiting time to access care in our ED.

Our study has demonstrated that early identification and management of sepsis was associated with a reduction the need for mechanical ventilation and vasopressor therapy illustrating the notion that organ dysfunction in sepsis is preventable by early treatment. Some physicians prefer a slower pace of fluid resuscitation than what has been recommended in the SSC guidelines with the perception that a faster approach may precipitate pulmonary edema. While this concern may be valid in selected patients with very poor cardiovascular status, our study shows that early fluid resuscitation is generally associated with reduction in the need for mechanical ventilation.

SRT implementation, which is complex and intensive, should take into account factors that facilitate its sustainability, such as senior and clinical leadership engagement, evidence credibility, staff involvement and training, infrastructure and alignment with the organization strategic aim and culture [50]. SRT implementation, monitoring of compliance and comparing of outcomes require considerable infrastructure, resources and costs, which should be considered before adopting such an intervention. Nevertheless, we believe that the SRT may be a cost-effective intervention given the significant reduction in LOS, although a proper cost-effectiveness analysis is needed.

Our results should be interpreted in light of the study strengths and limitations. Strengths include the prospective design and the use of data to drive improvement. Limitations include being a single-center study and the pre–post nature. The study was limited to the ED intervention and did not include septic patients who were referred from the wards or were already in the ICUs. Because baseline compliance was low, the room for improvement was large. Therefore, it is possible that impact of this intervention could be less in centers with better performance at baseline. In addition, the e-alert system was built internally using the existing EHR and based on the available data and has not been validated externally. However, this will be likely the case for most similar projects, and our data can be used to support the concept of e-alert rather that a particular system. It remains to be studied whether designing an e-alert for sepsis screening using the new Sepsis-3 criteria would be superior to e-alerts based on the SIRS criteria like ours. Due to the nature of the database, we evaluated the timing of antibiotic therapy, but not antibiotic adequacy or adherence to local guidelines. Our data show learning effect, as reflected by improvement in compliance preceding the actual date of each phase on the control chart. Preparation to any intervention, whether the e-alert or the SRT was discussed among the staff who were invited to provide their input into the project; therefore, it is not surprising to see this learning effect. Such phenomenon is not unusual in quality improvement projects. We think that having this learning effect or 'contamination' is acceptable as improving the care was the final goal; however, this may have underestimated the difference between the phases. Nevertheless, the intervention phases I and II are distinct phases; with the second phase has manpower implications; therefore, we analyzed them as separate phases. Due to the nature of the SSC database, certain data elements were not available such as age, gender, comorbidities and severity of illness. Although our analysis suggests that the propensity scores were able to balance the baseline differences, the availability of such data elements may have further improved their performance. The possibility of ascertainment bias (detection of milder cases) is inherent in studies that implement screening systems. However, the differences remained significant after adjustment to propensity scores.

In conclusion, the implementation of a multifaceted intervention including a sepsis e-alert system with SRT was associated with improvement in care processes of sepsis and septic shock and reduced need for mechanical ventilation as well as reduced mortality and LOS.

Abbreviations

CI: confidence interval; CPOE: computerized physician order entry; CVP: central venous pressure; e-alert: electronic alert; ED: emergency department; EHR: electronic health record; ICU: intensive care department; LOS: length of stay; PDSA: plan, do, study and act; SAS: statistical analysis software; $ScvO_2$: central venous oxygen saturation; SRT: sepsis response team; SSC: surviving sepsis campaign.

Authors' contributions

YMA, HA, MS, SS, AM, ST contributed to study conception and design; YMA, HA, SQ, AA, SS, AM, FH, SM, AM, MM, ST helped in acquisition of data; YMA, AA, HA, RH, MS, HT, FH, SM, AM, MM analyzed and interpreted the data; YMA, AA, HA, MS, SA, AM, SM drafted the manuscript; YMA, AA, HA, RH, MS, HT, SQ, AA, SA, AM, FH, SM, AM, MM, ST critically revised the manuscript for important intellectual content; YMA, HMT statistically analyzed the study; YMA, AA, HA, RH, MS, HT, SQ, AA, SA, AM, FH, SM, AM, MM, ST finally approved the version; YMA, HD, RH supervised the study. All authors read and approved the final manuscript.

Author details

[1] Intensive Care Department, MC-1425, Respiratory Services, College of Medicine, King Abdullah International Medical Research Center, King Saud bin Abdulaziz University for Health Sciences, P.O. Box 22490, Riyadh 11426, Kingdom of Saudi Arabia. [2] King Abdullah International Medical Research Center, King Saud bin Abdulaziz University for Health Sciences, Riyadh, Kingdom of Saudi Arabia. [3] Department of Internal Medicine, American University of Beirut- Medical Center, Beirut, Lebanon.

Acknowledgements

Other Sepsis Improvement Team Members

John Alchin, CCRN[5], Syed Kamran Asad, MBBS[1], Aslam Patta, MBBS[1], Saeed Obbed, MBBS[1], Mohammed Almadani, MD[1], Tahir Khan, MBBS[1], Ijaz Tasawar, MBBS[1], Vusala Razayeva, MBBS[1], Magdi Ibrahim, MBBS[1], Erick Elvena, RN[1], Grace Teo, RN[1], Komathi Govindan, RN[1], Emily Carmona, RN[1], Norhaiza Kassim, RN[1], Musharaf Sadat, MBBS[1], Tarek Dabbagh, MD[1,4], Souzan M. Al Owais, RPh, CPHQ[2], Basit Baig, MD, MBBS, MSc[2], Majed Al Thagafi, MD, FRCPC[3,4], Khaled Rajhi, MD[3,4], Khalid Al Johani, MD[3,4]

[1]Intensive Care Department, King Abdulaziz Medical City

[2]Department of Quality Management, King Abdulaziz Medical City

[3]Emergency Medicine Department, King Abdulaziz Medical City

[4]King Saud bin Abdulaziz University for Health Sciences (KSAU-HS)

[5]Clinical Nursing, King Abdulaziz Medical City

All from Ministry of National Guard-Health Affairs, Riyadh, Saudi Arabia.

Competing interests

The authors declare that they have no competing interests.

Funding

This study was funded by King Abdullah International Medical Research Center (KAIMRC), Riyadh, Saudi Arabia.

References

1. Levy MM, Artigas A, Phillips GS, Rhodes A, Beale R, Osborn T, et al. Outcomes of the Surviving Sepsis Campaign in intensive care units in the USA and Europe: a prospective cohort study. Lancet Infect Dis. 2012;12(12):919–24.
2. Phua J, Koh Y, Du B, Tang YQ, Divatia JV, Tan CC, et al. Management of severe sepsis in patients admitted to Asian intensive care units: prospective cohort study. BMJ. 2011;342:d3245.
3. Jones AE, Focht A, Horton JM, Kline JA. Prospective external validation of the clinical effectiveness of an emergency department-based early goal-directed therapy protocol for severe sepsis and septic shock. Chest. 2007;132(2):425–32.
4. Kortgen A, Niederprum P, Bauer M. Implementation of an evidence-based "standard operating procedure" and outcome in septic shock. Crit Care Med. 2006;34(4):943–9.
5. Lin SM, Huang CD, Lin HC, Liu CY, Wang CH, Kuo HP. A modified goal-directed protocol improves clinical outcomes in intensive care unit patients with septic shock: a randomized controlled trial. Shock. 2006;26(6):551–7.
6. Nguyen HB, Corbett SW, Steele R, Banta J, Clark RT, Hayes SR, et al. Implementation of a bundle of quality indicators for the early management of severe sepsis and septic shock is associated with decreased mortality. Crit Care Med. 2007;35(4):1105–12.
7. Micek ST, Roubinian N, Heuring T, Bode M, Williams J, Harrison C, et al. Before-after study of a standardized hospital order set for the management of septic shock. Crit Care Med. 2006;34(11):2707–13.
8. Sebat F, Musthafa AA, Johnson D, Kramer AA, Shoffner D, Eliason M, et al. Effect of a rapid response system for patients in shock on time to treatment and mortality during 5 years. Crit Care Med. 2007;35(11):2568–75.
9. Shapiro NI, Howell MD, Talmor D, Lahey D, Ngo L, Buras J, et al. Implementation and outcomes of the Multiple Urgent Sepsis Therapies (MUST) protocol. Crit Care Med. 2006;34(4):1025–32.
10. Dellinger RP, Levy MM, Rhodes A, Annane D, Gerlach H, Opal SM, et al. Surviving sepsis campaign: international guidelines for management of severe sepsis and septic shock: 2012. Crit Care Med. 2013;41(2):580–637.
11. Rhodes A, Evans LE, Alhazzani W, Levy MM, Antonelli M, Ferrer R, et al. Surviving Sepsis Campaign: international guidelines for management of sepsis and septic shock: 2016. Intensive Care Med. 2017;43:304–77.
12. National Quality Forum: severe sepsis and septic shock: management bundle. http://www.qualityforum.org/Home.aspx.
13. World Sepsis Day. http://www.world-sepsis-day.org.
14. Sepsis UK Core Team. http://sepsistrust.org/meet-the-team/sepsis-uk-core-team/.
15. NSW Health System: Clinical Excellence Commission. http://www.cec.health.nsw.gov.au/programs/sepsis.
16. College of Emergency Medicine: standards for severe sepsis and septic shock in adults. http://www.collemergencymed.ac.uk/code/document.asp?id=4717.
17. Jones AE. Evidence-based therapies for sepsis care in the emergency department: striking a balance between feasibility and necessity. Acad Emerg Med. 2006;13(1):82–3.
18. Carlbom DJ, Rubenfeld GD. Barriers to implementing protocol-based sepsis resuscitation in the emergency department–results of a national survey. Crit Care Med. 2007;35(11):2525–32.
19. Jones AE, Shapiro NI, Roshon M. Implementing early goal-directed therapy in the emergency setting: the challenges and experiences of translating research innovations into clinical reality in academic and community settings. Acad Emerg Med. 2007;14(11):1072–8.
20. Wang Z, Xiong Y, Schorr C, Dellinger RP. Impact of sepsis bundle strategy on outcomes of patients suffering from severe sepsis and septic shock in china. J Emerg Med. 2013;44(4):735–41.
21. Na S, Kuan WS, Mahadevan M, Li CH, Shrikhande P, Ray S, et al. Implementation of early goal-directed therapy and the surviving sepsis campaign resuscitation bundle in Asia. Int J Qual Health Care. 2012;24(5):452–62.
22. Ferrer R, Artigas A, Levy MM, Blanco J, Gonzalez-Diaz G, Garnacho-Montero J, et al. Improvement in process of care and outcome after a multicenter severe sepsis educational program in Spain. JAMA. 2008;299(19):2294–303.

23. Castellanos-Ortega A, Suberviola B, Garcia-Astudillo LA, Holanda MS, Ortiz F, Llorca J, et al. Impact of the Surviving Sepsis Campaign protocols on hospital length of stay and mortality in septic shock patients: results of a three-year follow-up quasi-experimental study. Crit Care Med. 2010;38(4):1036–43.
24. Levy MM, Dellinger RP, Townsend SR, Linde-Zwirble WT, Marshall JC, Bion J, et al. The Surviving Sepsis Campaign: results of an international guideline-based performance improvement program targeting severe sepsis. Intensive Care Med. 2010;36(2):222–31.
25. Giuliano KK, Lecardo M, Staul L. Impact of protocol watch on compliance with the surviving sepsis campaign. Am J Crit Care. 2011;20(4):313–21.
26. Schramm GE, Kashyap R, Mullon JJ, Gajic O, Afessa B. Septic shock: a multidisciplinary response team and weekly feedback to clinicians improve the process of care and mortality. Crit Care Med. 2011;39(2):252–8.
27. Laguna-Perez A, Chilet-Rosell E, Delgado Lacosta M, Alvarez-Dardet C, Uris Selles J, Munoz-Mendoza CL. Clinical pathway intervention compliance and effectiveness when used in the treatment of patients with severe sepsis and septic shock at an Intensive Care Unit in Spain. Rev Lat Am Enfermagem. 2012;20(4):635–43.
28. Shiramizo SC, Marra AR, Durao MS, Paes AT, Edmond MB, Pavao dos Santos OF. Decreasing mortality in severe sepsis and septic shock patients by implementing a sepsis bundle in a hospital setting. PLoS ONE. 2011;6(11):e26790.
29. Grimshaw JM, Thomas RE, MacLennan G, Fraser C, Ramsay CR, Vale L, et al. Effectiveness and efficiency of guideline dissemination and implementation strategies. Health Technol Assess. 2004;8(6):iii–iv, 1–72.
30. Cheung A, Weir M, Mayhew A, Kozloff N, Brown K, Grimshaw J. Overview of systematic reviews of the effectiveness of reminders in improving healthcare professional behavior. Syst Rev. 2012;1:36.
31. Davis DA, Taylor-Vaisey A. Translating guidelines into practice. A systematic review of theoretic concepts, practical experience and research evidence in the adoption of clinical practice guidelines. CMAJ. 1997;157(4):408–16.
32. Sawyer AM, Deal EN, Labelle AJ, Witt C, Thiel SW, Heard K, et al. Implementation of a real-time computerized sepsis alert in nonintensive care unit patients. Crit Care Med. 2011;39(3):469–73.
33. Meurer WJ, Smith BL, Losman ED, Sherman D, Yaksich JD, Jared JD, et al. Real-time identification of serious infection in geriatric patients using clinical information system surveillance. J Am Geriatr Soc. 2009;57(1):40–5.
34. Nelson JL, Smith BL, Jared JD, Younger JG. Prospective trial of real-time electronic surveillance to expedite early care of severe sepsis. Ann Emerg Med. 2011;57(5):500–4.
35. Arabi Y, Alshimemeri A, Taher S. Weekend and weeknight admissions have the same outcome of weekday admissions to an intensive care unit with onsite intensivist coverage. Crit Care Med. 2006;34(3):605–11.
36. Al-Qahtani S, Al-Dorzi HM, Tamim HM, Hussain S, Fong L, Taher S, et al. Impact of an intensivist-led multidisciplinary extended rapid response team on hospital-wide cardiopulmonary arrests and mortality. Crit Care Med. 2013;41(2):506–17.
37. Bullard MJ, Unger B, Spence J, Grafstein E. Revisions to the Canadian Emergency Department Triage and Acuity Scale (CTAS) adult guidelines. CJEM. 2008;10(2):136–51.
38. Singer M, Deutschman CS, Seymour CW, Shankar-Hari M, Annane D, Bauer M, et al. The third international consensus definitions for sepsis and septic shock (sepsis-3). JAMA. 2016;315(8):801–10.
39. Dellinger RP, Levy MM, Carlet JM, Bion J, Parker MM, Jaeschke R, et al. Sepsis Campaign: international guidelines for management of severe sepsis and septic shock: 2008. Crit Care Med. 2008;36(1):296–327.
40. Mouncey PR, Osborn TM, Power GS, Harrison DA, Sadique MZ, Grieve RD, et al. Trial of early, goal-directed resuscitation for septic shock. N Engl J Med. 2015;372(14):1301–11.
41. ARISE Investigators; ANZICS Clinical Trials Group, Peake SL, Delaney A, Bailey M, Bellomo R, et al. Goal-directed resuscitation for patients with early septic shock. N Engl J Med. 2014;371(16):1496–506.
42. Pro CI, Yealy DM, Kellum JA, Huang DT, Barnato AE, Weissfeld LA, et al. A randomized trial of protocol-based care for early septic shock. N Engl J Med. 2014;370(18):1683–93.
43. Dellinger RP, Carlet JM, Masur H, Gerlach H, Calandra T, Cohen J, et al. Surviving Sepsis Campaign guidelines for management of severe sepsis and septic shock. Crit Care Med. 2004;32(3):858–73.
44. Lecumberri R, Marques M, Diaz-Navarlaz MT, Panizo E, Toledo J, Garcia-Mouriz A, et al. Maintained effectiveness of an electronic alert system to prevent venous thromboembolism among hospitalized patients. Thromb Haemost. 2008;100(4):699–704.
45. Bradley EH, Curry LA, Webster TR, Mattera JA, Roumanis SA, Radford MJ, et al. Achieving rapid door-to-balloon times: how top hospitals improve complex clinical systems. Circulation. 2006;113(8):1079–85.
46. Hamidon BB, Dewey HM. Impact of acute stroke team emergency calls on in-hospital delays in acute stroke care. J Clin Neurosci. 2007;14(9):831–4.
47. Vernon DD, Furnival RA, Hansen KW, Diller EM, Bolte RG, Johnson DG, et al. Effect of a pediatric trauma response team on emergency department treatment time and mortality of pediatric trauma victims. Pediatrics. 1999;103(1):20–4.
48. Lilly CM. The ProCESS trial—a new era of sepsis management. N Engl J Med. 2014;370:1750-1.
49. Berg GM, Vasquez DG, Hale LS, Nyberg SM, Moran DA. Evaluation of process variations in noncompliance in the implementation of evidence-based sepsis care. J Healthc Qual. 2013;35(1):60–9.
50. Maher L, Gustafson D, Evans A. NHS sustainability model and guide. NHS Institute for Innovation and Improvement. 2005.

9

Red blood cell transfusion in the resuscitation of septic patients with hematological malignancies

Adrien Mirouse[1], Matthieu Resche-Rigon[2], Virginie Lemiale[3], Djamel Mokart[4], Achille Kouatchet[5], Julien Mayaux[6], François Vincent[7], Martine Nyunga[8], Fabrice Bruneel[9], Antoine Rabbat[10], Christine Lebert[11], Pierre Perez[12], Anne Renault[13], Anne-Pascale Meert[14], Dominique Benoit[15], Rebecca Hamidfar[16], Mercé Jourdain[17], Michaël Darmon[18], Elie Azoulay[3], Frédéric Pène[1*] and on behalf of the Groupe de Recherche sur la Réanimation Respiratoire en Onco-Hématologie (Grrr-OH)

Abstract

Background: Indications for red blood cell (RBC) transfusion in septic acute circulatory failure remain unclear. We addressed the practices and the prognostic impact of RBC transfusion in the early resuscitation of severe sepsis and septic shock in patients with hematological malignancies.

Methods: We performed a retrospective analysis of a prospectively collected database of patients with hematological malignancies who required intensive care unit (ICU) admission in 2010–2011. Patients with a main admission diagnosis of severe sepsis or septic shock were included in the present study. We assessed RBC transfusion during the first two days as part of initial resuscitation.

Results: Among the 1011 patients of the primary cohort, 631 (62.4%) were admitted to the ICU for severe sepsis (55%) or septic shock (45%). Among them, 210 (33.3%) patients received a median of 2 [interquartile 1–3] packed red cells during the first 48 h. Hemoglobin levels were lower in transfused patients at days 1 and 2 and became similar to those of non-transfused patients at day 3. Early RBC transfusion was more likely in patients with myeloid neoplasms and neutropenia. Transfused patients displayed more severe presentations as assessed by higher admission SOFA scores and blood lactate levels and the further requirements for organ failure supports. RBC transfusion within the first two days was associated with higher day 7 (20.5 vs. 13.3%, $p = 0.02$), in-ICU (39 vs. 25.2%, $p < 0.001$) and in-hospital (51 vs. 36.6%, $p < 0.001$) mortality rates. RBC transfusion remained independently associated with increased in-hospital mortality in multivariate logistic regression (OR 1.52 [1.03–2.26], $p = 0.03$) and propensity score-adjusted (OR 1.64 [1.05–2.57], $p = 0.03$) analysis.

Conclusions: RBC transfusion is commonly used in the early resuscitation of septic patients with hematological malignancies. Although it was preferentially provided to the most severe patients, we found it possibly associated with an increased risk of death.

Keywords: Hematological malignancy, Severe sepsis, Septic shock, Anemia, Red blood cell transfusion

*Correspondence: frederic.pene@aphp.fr
[1] Réanimation médicale, hôpital Cochin, Assistance Publique-Hôpitaux de Paris (AP-HP) and Université Paris Descartes, 27 rue du Faubourg Saint-Jacques, 75014 Paris, France
Full list of author information is available at the end of the article

Background

Septic shock is a frequent and dreaded complication in patients with malignancies. Following the overall improvement in the management of the disease, the last two decades have witnessed dramatic improvements in the prognosis of cancer patients presenting with severe sepsis and septic shock [1–4]. A major advance in the general management of sepsis was the implementation of aggressive resuscitation strategies, primarily inspired from the pivotal study by Rivers and colleagues, which promoted a protocol-guided hemodynamic resuscitation based on circulatory and tissue oxygenation objectives, the so-called early goal-directed therapy (EGDT) [5]. The genuine EGDT algorithm included a hematocrit target of 30% in case of persistent tissue hypoxia. Two-thirds of EGDT-treated patients therefore received red blood cell (RBC) transfusion within the early 72 h of resuscitation. However, the own prognostic value of RBC transfusion was not specifically assessed. Moreover, the study was performed in the late 1990s at the time when liberal fluid filling accounted for a high incidence of dilution anemia. All three recent replication studies of early goal-directed therapy retrieved lower requirements in RBC transfusion along with a more restrictive fluid filling policy [6–8]. Indications of RBC transfusion in the resuscitation of severe sepsis remain unclear [9], and it is noteworthy that the 2012 Surviving Sepsis Campaign guidelines were not able to provide any firm recommendation about the optimal transfusion threshold during hemodynamic instability [10]. Owing to the remaining controversy about optimal hemoglobin thresholds for transfusion in sepsis resuscitation, additional data are needed to optimize practices at the bedside.

Cancer patients with septic shock are at high risk of untractable multiple organ failure within the first days of ICU admission [11]. Early and aggressive resuscitation through restoration of both hemodynamics and tissue oxygenation is a major therapeutic goal in this setting. The optimal threshold for RBC transfusion and the eventual benefit in septic acute circulatory failure are debated. This issue appears particularly relevant to patients with hematological malignancies since the high prevalence of anemia imposed by malignant bone marrow infiltration or by cytotoxic treatments makes them particularly liable to urgent RBC transfusion in this setting in contrast to patients with delayed ICU-acquired anemia. This question was not specifically addressed by the leading trials about transfusion strategies in critically ill patients, since patients with chronic anemia were excluded from the pivotal TRICC trial and cancer patients were underrepresented in the TRISS trial [12–14]. We herein addressed the practices and the prognostic value of RBC transfusion as part of early sepsis resuscitation in a large cohort of patients with hematological malignancies who were admitted to the intensive care unit (ICU) for the main diagnosis of severe sepsis and septic shock.

Patients and methods

Study design

We conducted a substudy of a prospective, multicenter observational study that included 1011 consecutive adult patients with hematological malignancies who required ICU admission in 2010–2011. The study was approved by the appropriate ethics committees in France and Belgium. The methods and primary results of the study have been already published elsewhere [15]. The study involved 17 centers in France and Belgium, which may display different transfusion practices toward patients with hemodynamic instability. Blood banks followed similar national procedures for the collection, pre-storage leucoreduction, storage duration and delivery of RBC concentrates.

Patients

We focused on patients with a primary diagnosis of severe sepsis or septic shock according to the common definitions of the Surviving Sepsis Campaign [10]. Briefly, severe sepsis was defined by a clinically or microbiologically documented infection associated with organ failure. Septic shock was defined as an acute circulatory failure requiring vasopressor support. We collected the requirements for RBC transfusion during the first 48 h as part of initial resuscitation, thereby identifying transfused and non-transfused patients.

The following data were prospectively collected: demographic features (age and gender), performance status prior to the acute complication, comorbidities using the Charlson comorbidity index, features of the underlying hematological malignancy (type of disease, time from diagnosis, status, hematopoietic stem cell transplantation). Newly diagnosed malignancies were defined as diagnosed within the past 4 weeks. The sepsis-related organ failure assessment (SOFA) score was computed on admission then daily throughout the stay in the ICU [16]. The features and management features of sepsis included the primary source of infection and the pathogen involved, as well as requirements for life-supporting interventions including vasopressor support, noninvasive/invasive mechanical ventilation and renal replacement therapy during the ICU stay.

Statistical analysis

Quantitative variables were described as median [interquartile range] and categorical variables as number (percentage). The primary endpoint was vital status at hospital discharge. Multivariate logistic regression was used to assess the impact of day 1–2 transfusion on hospital mortality. The covariates identified as determinants of death in the primary analyses were entered into the model. Log-linearity was checked for continuous variables. Non-log-linear variables were dichotomised. Hosmer–Lemeshow goodness-of-fit tests were performed on multivariate regression models.

In order to limit bias in between-group comparisons, a propensity score-based approach was used to assess the impact of transfusion on hospital mortality, ICU mortality and 7-day mortality. The propensity score was defined as the probability that a patient with specific baseline characteristics receives transfusion. Then, two patients with identical propensity score values can be considered as comparable, and matching on the propensity score has been shown as one of the most efficient method for treatment effect assessment. We computed the propensity score using logistic regression to predict transfusion based on baseline characteristics known to be linked to the mortality and/or possibly to transfusion. Each subject treated by transfusion was randomly selected and then matched (without replacement) to the nearest untreated subject based on calipers of width of 0.2 of the standard deviation of the logit of the propensity score [17]. An inverse probability weighting approach for propensity score was also considered as sensitivity analysis. Missing data were handled using multiple imputation by chained equation. Fifty complete dataset were created using 10 iterations of the chained equation process. Rubin's rules were applied after the evaluation of the treatment effect on each complete dataset.

All tests were two-sided and p values <0.05 were considered as indicating significant association. Analyses were performed using the R statistical software version 2.15.0 (http://www.Rproject.org).

Results

Among the 1011 patients of the primary cohort, 347 (34.3%) were admitted to the ICU for severe sepsis and 284 (28%) for septic shock. Of those 631 patients, 210 (33%) received transfusions of 2 [1–3] packed red cells as part of the initial resuscitation strategy during the first two days in the ICU (148 (23.5%) and 89 (14.5%) at days 1 and 2, respectively). Among transfused patients, 6 (3%) presented concurrent bleeding at the time of admission. Hemoglobin levels were lower in transfused patients at day 1 (7.8 [7.1–8.8] vs. 9.7 [8.7–11] g/dL, $p < 0.001$) and day 2 (8.9 [7.9–9.9] vs. 9.3 [8.4–10.2] g/dL, $p = 0.001$) and became similar to those of non-transfused patients at day 3 (8.9 [8.2–9.8] vs. 8.9 [8–10]) (Fig. 1).

The other characteristics of non-transfused and transfused patients are shown and compared in Table 1. Early RBC transfusion was more likely in patients with acute myeloid leukemia and neutropenia. Transfused patients appeared with more severe presentations and tissue dysoxia as assessed by higher admission SOFA scores (8 [5–11] vs. 6 [4–9], $p < 0.001$), higher blood lactate levels (2.3 [1.5–4.9] vs. 2.0 [1.2–3.7] mmol/L, $p = 0.02$) (Additional file 1: Fig. S1) and the further requirements for organ failure supports including vasopressive drugs (70 vs. 57.7%, $p = 0.004$), invasive mechanical ventilation (55.2 vs. 48.7%, $p = 0.01$) and renal replacement therapy (30.5 vs. 22.2%, $p = 0.03$).

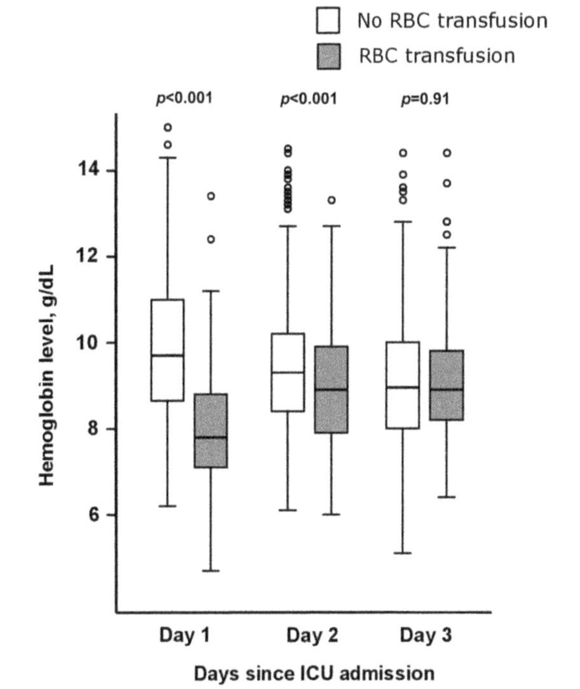

Fig. 1 Hemoglobin levels in non-transfused ($n = 421$) and transfused ($n = 210$) patients. *ICU* intensive care unit, *RBC* red blood cell

The overall in-ICU and in-hospital mortality rates were 28.9 and 41.4%, respectively. In univariate analysis, RBC transfusion within the first 48 h was associated with increased mortality at day 7 (20.5 vs. 13.3%, $p = 0.02$), in the ICU (39 vs. 25.2%, $p < 0.001$) and in the hospital (51 vs. 36.6%, $p < 0.001$) (Table 2; Fig. 2a). After adjustment with other relevant variables including the hemoglobin level on ICU admission and septic shock, RBC transfusion was no longer associated with 7-day mortality (OR 1.11 [0.66–1.87], $p = 0.7$), but tended to be associated with higher in-ICU and in-hospital mortality rate (OR 1.44 [0.94–2.21], $p = 0.09$ and OR 1.52 [1.03–2.26], $p = 0.03$, respectively). Other variables associated with in-hospital mortality were poor performance status, severity on admission as assessed by SOFA score, allogeneic hematopoietic stem cell transplantation, increased time to ICU admission and invasive aspergillosis. Partial

Table 1 Characteristics of patients without and with red blood cell transfusions at day 1/2

Characteristics	No RBC transfusion ($n = 421$)	RBC transfusion ($n = 210$)	*p*
Demographics			
Age (years)	60 [49–71]	60 [49–69]	0.68
Male gender	268 (63.7%)	138 (65.7%)	0.30
Comorbid illnesses			
Performance status 3–4	87 (20.7%)	51 (24.3%)	0.35
Charlson comorbidity index	4 [3–6]	4 [2–5]	0.77
Cardiovascular comorbidity	155 (36.8%)	77 (36.7%)	1
Coronary disease	31 (7.3%)	19 (9.0%)	0.53
Chronic heart failure	20 (4.8%)	14 (6.7%)	0.35
Peripheral arterial disease	19 (4.5%)	6 (2.8%)	0.39
Underlying malignancy			0.01
Non-Hodgkin lymphoma	149 (35.4%)	53 (25.2%)	
Hodgkin lymphoma	13 (3.1%)	2 (1.0%)	
Chronic lymphocytic leukemia	37 (8.8%)	13 (6.2%)	
Acute lymphocytic leukemia	23 (5.5%)	20 (9.5%)	
Acute myeloid leukemia	88 (20.9%)	69 (32.3%)	
Chronic myeloid leukemia	8 (1.9%)	4 (1.9%)	
Myeloma	56 (13.3%)	26 (12.4%)	
Myelodysplastic syndrome	23 (5.5%)	12 (5.7%)	
Others	24 (5.7%)	11 (5.2%)	
Time between diagnosis and ICU admission (days)	294 [38–1309]	199 [29–817]	0.06
Hematopoietic stem cell transplantation			
Autologous	50 (11.9%)	26 (12.4%)	0.72
Allogeneic	77 (18.3%)	33 (15.7%)	0.49
Malignancy status			
Newly diagnosed	120 (28.6%)	70 (33.3%)	0.95
Partial/complete remission	115 (27.5%)	54 (25.7%)	0.54
Time between hospital and ICU admissions (days)	6 [1–21]	8 [1–19]	0.38
ICU admission characteristics			
SOFA	6 [4–9]	8 [5–11]	<0.001
Hemoglobin (g/dL)	9.7 [8.7–11]	7.8 [7.1–8.8]	<0.001
Hemoglobin ranges [*n* (%)]			0.001
>9 g/dL	259 (66.1%)	44 (21.9%)	
7–9 g/dL	126 (32.1%)	117 (58.2%)	
<7 g/dL	7 (1.8%)	40 (19.9%)	
Platelet count (G/L)	77 [32–170]	31 [16–63]	<0.001
Neutropenia	122 (29.0%)	107 (51.0%)	<0.001
Lactate level (mmol/L)	2.0 [1.2–3.7]	2.3 [1.5–4.9]	0.02
Source of infection			
Pneumonia	252 (59.9%)	106 (50.5%)	0.03
Abdominal	15.7%	17.6%	0.61
Urinary tract	26 (6.2%)	10 (4.8%)	0.59
Catheter-related	5.0%	3.3%	0.46
Pathogens			
Gram-negative bacteria	108 (25.7%)	67 (31.9%)	0.12
Gram-positive bacteria	60 (14.3%)	21 (10.0%)	0.69
Aspergillus	46 (10.9%)	23 (11.0%)	1.00
Pneumocystis	20 (4.8%)	2 (1.0%)	0.02

Table 1 continued

Characteristics	No RBC transfusion ($n = 421$)	RBC transfusion ($n = 210$)	p
Life-supporting interventions			
Vasopressive drugs	243 (57.7%)	147 (70%)	0.004
Invasive ventilation	205 (48.7%)	116 (55.2%)	0.01
Renal replacement therapy	92 (22.2%)	62 (30.5%)	0.03
Platelet transfusions			
Day 1	70 (16.6%)	96 (45.7%)	<0.001
Day 2	58 (13.7%)	82 (39.0%)	<0.001
Mortality			
ICU mortality	106 (25.2%)	82 (39.0%)	<0.001
Hospital mortality	154 (36.6%)	107 (51.0%)	<0.001

ICU intensive care unit, *RBC* red blood cell, *SOFA* sequential organ failure assessment

or complete remission was associated with improved survival (Table 3).

In order to refine the statistical adjustment between non-transfused and transfused patients, we built a propensity score of being transfused during the first two days following ICU admission. The propensity score was based on hemoglobin level at the time of ICU admission and on the following characteristics: age, gender, performance status, days since hospital admission, allogeneic hematopoietic stem cell transplantation, hematological malignancy type and status, time between its diagnosis and ICU admission, time between hospital and ICU admissions, neutropenia, aspergillosis, chemotherapy, admission SOFA score and septic shock. This score allowed matching 142 patients who did receive RBC transfusion as part of the initial resuscitation to 142 counterparts who did not. As shown in Fig. 2b, propensity score-matched transfused and non-transfused patients displayed similar survival trends (OR for in-hospital death 1.25 [0.75–2.05], $p = 0.39$). When including all 631 patients in a weighting analysis, day 1/2 RBC transfusion was still associated with increased hospital mortality (OR 1.64 [1.05–2.57], $p = 0.03$).

Discussion

There is no doubt that the prognosis of critically ill patients with hematological malignancies has dramatically improved, and admission to the ICU is now viewed as a bridge to cure rather than a terminal process. The reasons for this trend are multiple, including general improvements in the prognosis of cancer, better and early identification of patients likely to benefit from intensive care and advances in the management of acute life-threatening disorders [18]. However, severe infections resulting in shock and/or acute respiratory failure represent dreaded complications in cancer patients and still account for a large number of deaths regardless of the stage of malignancy. It is clear that cancer patients already benefited from advances in the field of sepsis, but it remains a major area for improvement for this vulnerable population. Nevertheless, such immunocompromised patients were either underrepresented or even excluded from the leading clinical trials in severe sepsis and septic shock. Whether they are entitled to strictly similar management as non-immunocompromised patients is questionable.

The poor prognosis of hematological patients with severe sepsis is commonly attributed to the underlying immune defects resulting in impaired and delayed pathogen clearance, but additional mechanisms related to the disease itself or to its treatment may also worsen organ failures. For instance, endothelial or cardiac toxicity by chemotherapy and radiotherapy may contribute to the pathophysiology of acute circulatory failure [19], while lactic acidosis may not only reflect systemic tissue hypoperfusion but might also result from altered metabolism of tumor cells. However, intensity and duration or vasopressor support appear quite similar in cancer patients, either untreated or treated with chemotherapy, and in patients free of cancer but harboring alternative comorbidities [20]. Furthermore, microvascular derangements have been reported in non-septic patients with chemotherapy-induced neutropenia, albeit microcirculatory alterations induced by septic shock appeared quite similar in neutropenic and non-neutropenic patients [21]. Most importantly, cancer patients commonly display chronic anemia likely to contribute to the impaired oxygen delivery encountered in severe sepsis and septic shock and appear then liable to RBC transfusion early in the course of hemodynamic resuscitation.

The general practice of RBC transfusion in the ICU is guided by the apparently opposite objectives of preserving an appropriate tissue oxygenation while minimizing the number of packed red cells transfused.

Table 2 Characteristics of in-hospital survivors and deceased

Characteristics	In-hospital survivors ($n = 370$)	In-hospital deceased ($n = 261$)	p
Demographics			
Age (years)	58.5 [47–67.75]	63 [52–71]	0.01
Male gender	240 (64.9%)	166 (63.6%)	0.81
Comorbid illnesses			
Performance status 3–4	61 (16.5%)	77 (29.5%)	0.0001
Charlson comorbidity index	4 [2–5]	4 [3–6]	0.008
Underlying malignancy			0.90
Lymphoid disease	179 (48.4%)	131 (50.2%)	
Myeloid disease	121 (32.7%)	83 (31.8%)	
Time between diagnosis and ICU admission (days)	91 [14; 444]	90 [11; 396]	0.58
Hematopoietic stem cell transplantation			0.04
Autologous	52 (14.1%)	24 (9.2%)	
Allogeneic	55 (14.9%)	55 (21.1%)	
Malignancy status			0.019
Newly diagnosed	106 (28.7%)	84 (32.2%)	
Partial/complete remission	116 (31.4%)	53 (21.4%)	
Time between hospital and ICU admissions (days)	4 [0–16]	9 [1–25]	<0.0001
ICU admission characteristics			
SOFA score	6 [4–8]	8 [5–11.75]	<0.0001
Neutropenia	125 (33.8%)	104 (39.9%)	0.14
Lactate (mmol/L)	1.9 (1.125–3.575)	2.4 [1.6–5.6]	0.0001
Hemoglobin level (g/dL)			
Day 1	9.2 [8–10.7]	8.9 [7.8–10.2]	0.02
Day 2	9.2 [8.3–10.2]	9.1 [8.3–10]	0.33
Day 3	9 [8.1–10]	8.9 [8.2–9.975]	0.88
Day 7	8.8 [8.1–9.8]	8.8 [8.3–9.95]	0.53
RBC transfusion			
Day 1 and/or 2	103 (27.8%)	107 (41%)	0.0008
Day 3	42 (12.4%)	39 (17.3%)	0.13
Day 7	16 (10.6%)	21 (16.7%)	0.19
Source of infection			
Pneumonia	190 (51.4%)	68 (64.3%)	0.002
Abdominal	69 (18.7%)	34 (13.0%)	0.076
Urinary tract	21 (5.7%)	15 (5.8%)	1.00
Catheter-related	21 (5.7%)	7 (2.7%)	0.11
Pathogens			
Gram-negative bacteria	101 (27.3%)	74 (28.4%)	0.84
Gram-positive bacteria	56 (15.1%)	25 (9.6%)	0.053
Aspergillus	27 (7.3%)	42 (16.1%)	0.0008
Pneumocystis	17 (4.6%)	5 (1.9%)	0.11
Life-supporting interventions			
Vasopressive drugs	184 (49.7%)	206 (78.9%)	<0.0001
Invasive ventilation	124 (33.5%)	197 (75.5)	<0.0001
Renal replacement therapy	56 (15.4%)	98 (38.7%)	<0.0001

ICU intensive care unit, *RBC* red blood cell, *SOFA* sequential organ failure assessment

Studies investigating RBC transfusion in the ICU have so far been performed in general populations in which anemia is mostly acquired during the ICU stay as a result of dilution and blood loss, associated with an impaired erythropoietic response. In 1999, the pivotal TRICC study by Hebert and colleagues showed that a restrictive

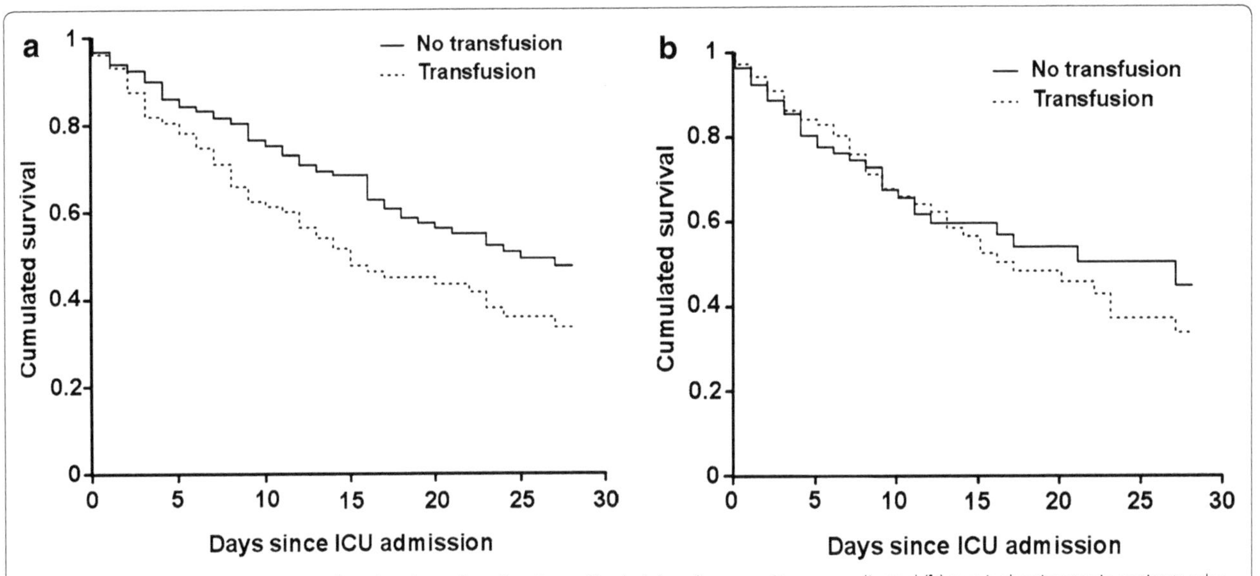

Fig. 2 Survival estimates in non-transfused and transfused patients. Crude (**a**) and propensity score-adjusted (**b**) survival estimates in patients who did or did not receive red blood cell transfusion during the first two days of resuscitation. **a** Encompasses the whole cohort (631 patients distributed into 421 non-transfused and 210 transfused). **b** Includes 142 transfused patients with 142 propensity score-matched non-transfused counterparts. *ICU* intensive care unit

Table 3 Determinants of hospital mortality: multivariate analysis

Characteristics	Odds ratio (95% CI)	*p*
RBC transfusion at day 1/2	1.52 (1.03–2.26)	0.03
Hemoglobin level at ICU admission	1.0 (0.95–1.06)	0.87
Performance status 3–4	1.97 (1.29–3.02)	0.002
Lactate level at ICU admission	1.01 (0.96–1.05)	0.79
SOFA score at ICU admission	1.14 (1.1–1.21)	<0.001
Septic shock	1.30 (0.86–1.96)	0.21
Allogeneic HSCT recipient	2.14 (1.28–3.57)	0.004
Remission	0.53 (0.34–0.84)	0.007
Time between hospital and ICU admissions >1 day	1.69 (1.14–2.51)	0.009
Invasive aspergillosis	1.91 (1.08–3.4)	0.02

All variables entered into the model appear in the table. Hosmer–Lemeshow goodness of fit of the multivariate model was tested on each imputed dataset, with p values ranging from 0.22 to 0.96

CI confidence interval, *HSCT* hematopoietic stem cell transplantation, *ICU* intensive care unit, *RBC* red blood cell, *OR* odds ratio, *SOFA* sequential organ failure assessment

strategy of non-leucodepleted RBC transfusion to maintain hemoglobin above 7 g/dL was at least as effective as a liberal transfusion strategy aimed to maintain hemoglobin >10 g/dL in critically ill patients [12]. As of today, the recommendations for RBC transfusion in the ICU remain largely based on this study. Of note, this study excluded patients with a previous history of chronic anemia.

However, some studies challenged the general implementation of this restrictive strategy and suggested that a higher transfusion threshold might be beneficial in septic patients for whom oxygen delivery is of paramount importance. This was first derived from the study by Rivers and colleagues, in which most EGDT-treated patients had received RBC transfusion to maintain a hematocrit level above 30% [5]. Since then, three studies using propensity-adjusted analysis also reported that RBC transfusion was associated with improved survival in septic shock [22–24]. Furthermore, a Brazilian monocenter randomized study reported that a liberal RBC transfusion strategy (hemoglobin >9 g/dL) versus a restrictive strategy (hemoglobin >7 g/dL) improved survival in critically ill patients admitted to the ICU following major cancer surgery [25]. The reasons for this finding remain intriguing, but possibly related to a lower incidence of both cardiovascular complications and superinfections. The same team reported a benefit from a liberal transfusion strategy applied throughout the ICU stay in solid cancer patients with septic shock [26]. A multicenter randomized Scandinavian study addressed the transfusion policy in septic shock patients, of whom 7.5% had hematological malignancies and 9.5% had metastatic cancer. Patients were randomized to either a restrictive or a liberal transfusion policy to maintain hemoglobin levels higher than 7 or 9 g/dL, respectively [13]. Similar survival rates were reported in the restrictive and liberal randomization arms. Subgroup analysis in patients with hematological malignancies or metastatic cancer also retrieved similar survival rates in both randomization arms [27]. However, it should be emphasized that most patients had already been efficiently resuscitated and restored tissue oxygenation at the time of randomization. Although this study suggests that a restrictive transfusion policy can be safely implemented in most patients with septic shock, we do think that it does not provide a definite answer for patients with persistent and/or marked circulatory failure.

The trend in increased mortality in transfused patients is the most intriguing result of our study. Although this is in line with several case–control studies which suggested that RBC transfusion was associated with higher mortality and increased incidence of ICU-acquired complications in critically ill patients, the interpretation of this finding deserves caution. On one hand, this could suggest that requirements of RBC transfusion, presumably imposed by persistent tissue dysoxia, could represent a very potent prognostic factor even when adjusted to the classical determinants of death in this setting. On the other hand, there are considerable interindividual variations in the microcirculatory and tissue oxygenation responses to RBC transfusion [28, 29]. Increase in blood viscosity by RBC transfusion and storage lesions can result in paradoxical impairment on microcirculation and tissue oxygenation. While not being immediately fully efficient for oxygen delivery to tissue, red cells may then sludge within capillaries, interact with endothelial cells and promote inflammatory processes [30, 31]. However, recent studies using leucodepleted packed red cells did not retrieve any impact of storage duration on restoration of tissue oxygenation or survival status in critically ill patients with anemia [32, 33]. Finally, RBC transfusion may represent a risk factor for hospital-acquired infection as a result of transfusion-induced immunomodulation [34, 35]. Although we could not reliably collect the incidence of ICU-acquired complications, it is noteworthy that the non-adjusted survival curves of transfused and non-transfused patients forked as early as three days after ICU admission, suggesting that the poor impact of RBC transfusion was related to early events rather than secondary ICU-acquired complications.

One strength of this study is the prospective collection of data, although it was a secondary analysis of a database that was not designed to this specific aim. In general, data from the first three days were complete and accurate, but data collected later on were less detailed. Thus, the estimation of packed red cells transfused within the first three days was accurate, whereas daily transfusions thereafter were not collected. Nonetheless, neither the volume of fluid loading nor the fluid balance was accurately recorded in the database. In the same way, the incidence of delayed ICU-acquired infectious and non-infectious complications and the definite causes of death could not be reliably estimated. In the absence of guidelines, indications of RBC transfusion in this setting were probably quite inconsistent across centers. Hemoglobin levels in the RBC transfusion group were often higher than the recommended 7 g/dl threshold. However, this was an observational study reflecting routine practice. With respect to the lower hemoglobin levels and the severity of circulatory dysfunctions in transfused patients, it is likely that physicians followed a common pragmatic decision-making process at the bedside, based not only on a sole hemoglobin level but also on markers of tissue dysoxia. However, such an observational study can only provide exploratory data and statistical link, but is no substitute to prospective interventional studies.

Conclusion

RBC transfusions are frequently used as part of the initial resuscitation of severe sepsis or septic shock in patients with hematological malignancies. Although RBC transfusion was preferentially administrated to the most severe patients, we found it possibly associated with an increased risk of death. Since the definite indications of RBC transfusions in resuscitation of severe sepsis remain of underlying anemia represent a relevant subgroup to questionable, cancer patients with a high prevalence address this question in a prospective manner.

Abbreviations

EGDT: early goal-directed therapy; HSCT: hematopoietic stem cell transplantation; ICU: intensive care unit; RBC: red blood cell; SOFA: sepsis-related organ failure assessment.

Authors' contributions

AM, MRR, EA and FP made substantial contributions to the conception of the work, the acquisition, analysis and interpretation of data for the work. They drafted the work and revised it critically for important intellectual content. They gave final approval of the version to be published. They agree to be accountable for all aspects of the work in ensuring that questions related to the accuracy or integrity of any part of the work are appropriately investigated and resolved. VL, DM, AK, JM, FV, MN, FB, AR, CL, PP, AR, APM, DB, RH, MJ, MD made substantial contributions to the acquisition of data for the work. They revised the work critically for important intellectual content. They gave final approval of the version to be published. They agree to be accountable for all aspects of the work in ensuring that questions related to the accuracy or integrity of any part of the work are appropriately investigated and resolved. All authors read and approved the final manuscript.

Presented at the congress "Réanimation 2016" of the French Intensive Care Society, 13–15 January 2016, Paris, France.

Author details
[1] Réanimation médicale, hôpital Cochin, Assistance Publique-Hôpitaux de Paris (AP-HP) and Université Paris Descartes, 27 rue du Faubourg Saint-Jacques, 75014 Paris, France. [2] Département de biostatistiques, Hôpital Saint-Louis, AP-HP and Université Paris Diderot, Paris, France. [3] Réanimation médicale, Hôpital Saint-Louis, AP-HP and Université Paris Diderot, Paris, France. [4] Département d'anesthésie-réanimation, Institut Paoli-Calmettes, Marseille, France. [5] Réanimation médicale et médecine hyperbare, CHU d'Angers, Angers, France. [6] Réanimation médicale, Hôpital de la Pitié-Salpêtrière, AP-HP and Université Pierre et Marie Curie, Paris, France. [7] Réanimation polyvalente, Centre Hospitalier Intercommunal, Montfermeil, France. [8] Centre Hospitalier de Roubaix, Roubaix, France. [9] Réanimation polyvalente, Hôpital André Mignot, Le Chesnay, France. [10] Unité de soins intensifs respiratoires, Hôpital Cochin, AP-HP and Université Paris Descartes, Paris, France. [11] Réanimation polyvalente, Centre Hospitalier Départemental, La Roche-sur-Yon, France. [12] Réanimation médicale, Hôpital Brabois, Nancy, France. [13] Réanimation médicale, Centre Hospitalier de Brest, Brest, France. [14] Service des soins intensifs et urgences oncologiques, Institut Jules Bordet, Brussels, Belgium. [15] Ghent University Hospital, Ghent, Belgium. [16] Réanimation médicale, CHU Grenoble-Alpes, Grenoble, France. [17] Université de Lille and Réanimation Polyvalente, CHU de Lille, Lille, France. [18] Réanimation médicale, Centre Hospitalier de Saint-Etienne, Saint-Etienne, France.

Competing interests
The authors declare that they have no competing interests.

Funding
French Ministry of Health No. PHRC AOM 08235 and French Intensive Care Society.

References

1. Larché J, Azoulay E, Fieux F, Mesnard L, Moreau D, Thiery G, et al. Improved survival of critically ill cancer patients with septic shock. Intensive Care Med. 2003;29(10):1688–95.
2. Pène F, Percheron S, Lemiale V, Viallon V, Claessens Y-E, Marqué S, et al. Temporal changes in management and outcome of septic shock in patients with malignancies in the intensive care unit. Crit Care Med. 2008;36(3):690–6.
3. Zuber B, Tran T-C, Aegerter P, Grimaldi D, Charpentier J, Guidet B, et al. Impact of case volume on survival of septic shock in patients with malignancies. Crit Care Med. 2012;40(1):55–62.
4. Legrand M, Max A, Peigne V, Mariotte E, Canet E, Debrumetz A, et al. Survival in neutropenic patients with severe sepsis or septic shock. Crit Care Med. 2012;40(1):43–9.
5. Rivers E, Nguyen B, Havstad S, Ressler J, Muzzin A, Knoblich B, et al. Early goal-directed therapy in the treatment of severe sepsis and septic shock. N Engl J Med. 2001;345(19):1368–77.
6. Investigators ProCESS, Yealy DM, Kellum JA, Huang DT, Barnato AE, Weissfeld LA, et al. A randomized trial of protocol-based care for early septic shock. N Engl J Med. 2014;370(18):1683–93.
7. ARISE Investigators, ANZICS Clinical Trials Group, Peake SL, Delaney A, Bailey M, Bellomo R, et al. Goal-directed resuscitation for patients with early septic shock. N Engl J Med. 2014;371(16):1496–506.
8. Mouncey PR, Osborn TM, Power GS, Harrison DA, Sadique MZ, Grieve RD, et al. Trial of early, goal-directed resuscitation for septic shock. N Engl J Med. 2015;372(14):1301–11.
9. Dupuis C, Sonneville R, Adrie C, Gros A, Darmon M, Bouadma L, et al. Impact of transfusion on patients with sepsis admitted in intensive care unit: a systematic review and meta-analysis. Ann Intensive Care. 2017;7(1):5.
10. Dellinger RP, Levy MM, Rhodes A, Annane D, Gerlach H, Opal SM, et al. Surviving Sepsis Campaign: international guidelines for management of severe sepsis and septic shock, 2012. Intensive Care Med. 2013;39(2):165–228.
11. Daviaud F, Grimaldi D, Dechartres A, Charpentier J, Geri G, Marin N, et al. Timing and causes of death in septic shock. Ann Intensive Care. 2015;5(1):16.
12. Hébert PC, Wells G, Blajchman MA, Marshall J, Martin C, Pagliarello G, et al. A multicenter, randomized, controlled clinical trial of transfusion requirements in critical care. Transfusion Requirements in Critical Care Investigators, Canadian Critical Care Trials Group. N Engl J Med. 1999;340(6):409–17.
13. Holst LB, Haase N, Wetterslev J, Wernerman J, Guttormsen AB, Karlsson S, et al. Lower versus higher hemoglobin threshold for transfusion in septic shock. N Engl J Med. 2014;371(15):1381–91.
14. Carson JL, Stanworth SJ, Roubinian N, Fergusson DA, Triulzi D, Doree C, et al. Transfusion thresholds and other strategies for guiding allogeneic red blood cell transfusion. In: Cochrane database of systematic reviews [Internet]. Wiley; 2016 [cited 2017 Mar 16]. http://onlinelibrary.wiley.com/doi/10.1002/14651858.CD002042.pub4/abstract.
15. Azoulay E, Mokart D, Pène F, Lambert J, Kouatchet A, Mayaux J, et al. Outcomes of critically ill patients with hematologic malignancies: prospective multicenter data from France and Belgium—a groupe de recherche respiratoire en réanimation onco-hématologique study. J Clin Oncol. 2013;31(22):2810–8.
16. Vincent JL, Moreno R, Takala J, Willatts S, De Mendonça A, Bruining H, et al. The SOFA (Sepsis-related Organ Failure Assessment) score to describe organ dysfunction/failure. On behalf of the Working Group on Sepsis-Related Problems of the European Society of Intensive Care Medicine. Intensive Care Med. 1996;22(7):707–10.
17. Austin PC. Some methods of propensity-score matching had superior performance to others: results of an empirical investigation and Monte Carlo simulations. Biom J. 2009;51(1):171–84.
18. Azoulay E, Pène F, Darmon M, Lengliné E, Benoit D, Soares M, et al. Managing critically Ill hematology patients: time to think differently. Blood Rev. 2015;29(6):359–67.
19. Mokart D, Sannini A, Brun J-P, Faucher M, Blaise D, Blache J-L, et al. N-terminal pro-brain natriuretic peptide as an early prognostic factor in cancer patients developing septic shock. Crit Care. 2007;11(2):R37.
20. Schnell D, Besset S, Lengliné E, Maziers N, Zafrani L, Reuter D, et al. Impact of a recent chemotherapy on the duration and intensity of the norepinephrine support during septic shock. Shock. 2013;39(2):138–43.
21. Karvunidis T, Chvojka J, Lysak D, Sykora R, Krouzecky A, Radej J, et al. Septic shock and chemotherapy-induced cytopenia: effects on microcirculation. Intensive Care Med. 2012;38(8):1336–44.
22. Vincent J-L, Sakr Y, Sprung C, Harboe S, Damas P. Sepsis Occurrence in Acutely Ill Patients (SOAP) Investigators. Are blood transfusions associated with greater mortality rates? Results of the Sepsis Occurrence in Acutely Ill Patients study. Anesthesiology. 2008;108(1):31–9.
23. Park DW, Chun B-C, Kwon S-S, Yoon YK, Choi WS, Sohn JW, et al. Red blood cell transfusions are associated with lower mortality in patients with severe sepsis and septic shock: a propensity-matched analysis. Crit Care Med. 2012;40(12):3140–5.
24. Mark DG, Morehouse JW, Hung Y-Y, Kene MV, Elms AR, Liu V, et al. In-hospital mortality following treatment with red blood cell transfusion or inotropic therapy during early goal-directed therapy for septic shock: a retrospective propensity-adjusted analysis. Crit Care. 2014;18(5):496.
25. de Almeida JP, Vincent J-L, Galas FRBG, de Almeida EPM, Fukushima JT, Osawa EA, et al. Transfusion requirements in surgical oncology patients: a prospective, randomized controlled trial. Anesthesiology. 2015;122(1):29–38.
26. Bergamin FS, Almeida JP, Landoni G, Galas FRBG, Fukushima JT, Fominskiy E, et al. Liberal versus restrictive transfusion strategy in critically ill oncologic patients: the transfusion requirements in critically ill oncologic patients randomized controlled trial. Crit Care Med. 2017. doi:10.1097/CCM.0000000000002283.
27. Rygård SL, Holst LB, Wetterslev J, Johansson PI, Perner A, TRISS Trial Group, et al. Higher vs. lower haemoglobin threshold for transfusion in septic

shock: subgroup analyses of the TRISS trial. Acta Anaesthesiol Scand. 2017;61(2):166–75.
28. Sakr Y, Chierego M, Piagnerelli M, Verdant C, Dubois M-J, Koch M, et al. Microvascular response to red blood cell transfusion in patients with severe sepsis. Crit Care Med. 2007;35(7):1639–44.
29. Kopterides P, Theodorakopoulou M, Nikitas N, Ilias I, Vassiliadi DA, Orfanos SE, et al. Red blood cell transfusion affects microdialysis-assessed interstitial lactate/pyruvate ratio in critically ill patients with late sepsis. Intensive Care Med. 2012;38(11):1843–50.
30. Marik PE, Sibbald WJ. Effect of stored-blood transfusion on oxygen delivery in patients with sepsis. JAMA. 1993;269(23):3024–9.
31. Aubron C, Nichol A, Cooper DJ, Bellomo R. Age of red blood cells and transfusion in critically ill patients. Ann Intensive Care. 2013;3(1):2.
32. Lacroix J, Hébert PC, Fergusson DA, Tinmouth A, Cook DJ, Marshall JC, et al. Age of transfused blood in critically ill adults. N Engl J Med. 2015;372(15):1410–8.
33. Dhabangi A, Ainomugisha B, Cserti-Gazdewich C, Ddungu H, Kyeyune D, Musisi E, et al. Effect of transfusion of red blood cells with longer vs shorter storage duration on elevated blood lactate levels in children with severe anemia: the total randomized clinical trial. JAMA. 2015;314(23):2514–23.
34. Shorr AF, Jackson WL, Kelly KM, Fu M, Kollef MH. Transfusion practice and blood stream infections in critically ill patients. Chest. 2005;127(5):1722–8.
35. Rohde JM, Dimcheff DE, Blumberg N, Saint S, Langa KM, Kuhn L, et al. Health care-associated infection after red blood cell transfusion: a systematic review and meta-analysis. JAMA. 2014;311(13):1317–26.

Hemofiltration induces generation of leukocyte-derived CD31+/CD41−microvesicles in sepsis

Georg Franz Lehner[1], Ulrich Harler[1], Clemens Feistritzer[2], Viktoria Maria Haller[1], Julia Hasslacher[1], Romuald Bellmann[1] and Michael Joannidis[1*]

Abstract

Background: Microvesicles (MV) are extracellular vesicles known to be associated with cellular activation and inflammation. Hemofiltration is an effective blood purification technique for patients with renal failure and possibly also eliminates inflammatory mediators in the setting of sepsis. On the other hand, proinflammatory stimuli are induced by blood contacting the artificial membrane during extracorporeal blood purification. In chronic dialysis patients a systemic increase in MV has been described. The aim of the study was to investigate whether hemofilter passage of blood in continuous veno-venous hemofiltration (CVVH) alters MV composition and levels in critically ill patients with sepsis.

Methods: Pre- and postfilter bloods as well as ultrafiltrate samples from intensive care unit patients with severe sepsis were obtained during CVVH with regional citrate anticoagulation. MV subtypes in blood were analyzed by high-sensitivity flow cytometry. Additionally, tissue factor (TF) levels and MV-associated TF activities as well as MV activities were quantified. All parameters were corrected for hemoconcentration applied during CVVH.

Results: Twelve patients were analyzed. A significant increase in presumably mostly leukocyte-derived CD31+/CD41− MV (1.32 (1.09–1.93)-fold [median (25th–75th quartiles)], $p = 0.021$) was observed post- to prefilter, whereas platelet-derived MV as well as AnnexinV-binding MV were unaltered. Increments of AnnexinV+, CD42b+ and CD31+/CD41− MV post- to prefilter correlated with filtration fraction (FF) (all $p < 0.05$). Significant reductions in MV activity [0.72 (0.62–0.84)-fold, $p = 0.002$] and TF level [0.95 (0.87–0.99)-fold, $p = 0.0093$] were detected postfilter compared to prefilter. No MV activity was measurable in ultrafiltrate samples.

Conclusions: Despite clearing a fraction of small PS-exposing MV CVVH does not eliminate larger MV. Concurrently, CVVH induces the release of CD31+/CD4− MV that indicate leukocyte activation during hemofilter passage in septic patients. Increments of several MV subtypes within the hemofilter correlate with FF, which supports common recommendations to keep FF low. A fraction of TF is being cleared by CVVH via ultrafiltration.

Keywords: Sepsis, Microvesicles, Microparticles, Hemofiltration, Continuous veno-venous hemofiltration, Renal replacement therapy, Tissue factor, Leukocytes, Platelets

Background

Continuous veno-venous hemofiltration (CVVH) is a frequently used renal replacement therapy (RRT) modality in critically ill patients [1]. Although it is an effective and life-saving treatment in the presence of renal failure, its beneficial effect as sole supportive sepsis therapy is still controversial [2, 3]. It has been shown that hemofiltration is able to influence levels of circulating mediators such as inflammatory cytokines by adsorption or filtration [4]. However, these potentially favorable effects might be offset by proinflammatory stimuli that are induced by

*Correspondence: michael.joannidis@i-med.ac.at
[1] Division of Intensive Care and Emergency Medicine, Department of Internal Medicine, Medical University Innsbruck, Anichstrasse 35, 6020 Innsbruck, Austria
Full list of author information is available at the end of the article

blood contacting an artificial membrane during extracorporeal blood purification itself [5–7]. This effect may be enhanced when heparin is used for anticoagulation and attenuated during regional citrate anticoagulation [8]. Microvesicles (MV) are extracellular vesicles sized between approximately 100 nm and 1 µm that are released by several cell types upon stimulation or apoptosis [9, 10]. They mediate pleiotropic inflammatory signals during sepsis [11] and are associated with the occurrence of disseminated intravascular coagulation [12]. In patients with chronic renal failure increased systemic levels of platelet-derived as well as procoagulatory AnnexinV-binding MV were found in blood following RRT [13]. However, it is not known whether this increase reflects secondary systemic effects of RRT or a MV release within the hemofilter.

The aim of this study was to examine the influence of blood membrane contact during a single hemofilter passage in CVVH with citrate anticoagulation on MV levels and composition in patients with severe sepsis.

Methods

Patients

Patients from a tertiary intensive care unit (ICU) that required RRT and fulfilled at least two systemic inflammatory response syndrome (SIRS) criteria [14] in the presence of a suspected or proven sepsis focus were prospectively enrolled in the study from January 2012 to March 2013. Patients were excluded if they were younger than 18 years, moribund, pregnant or breast-feeding. The study was approved by the Ethics Committee from the Medical University Innsbruck (protocol UN 2705a 244/4.20). Subjects provided written informed consent either prior to enrollment or post hoc. Vital parameters were obtained, routine laboratory values measured, as well as acute physiology and chronic health evaluation (APACHE II) score [15], simplified acute physiology score (SAPS II) [16] and sequential organ failure assessment score (SOFA) [17] computed.

Hemofiltration and sample collection

RRT was conducted in CVVH mode by using a ST150 (Gambro Hospital Austria GmbH, Wiener Neudorf, Austria) hemofilter in a Prismaflex® machine (Gambro Hospital Austria GmbH) with postdilution. Phoxilium® was used as substitution fluid. Anticoagulation was performed as regional citrate anticoagulation with Prismocitrate® 18/0, aiming at a postfilter iCa^{2+} level of 0.35–0.45 mmol/l. Prefilter blood was obtained from a port located after citrate and prefilter substitution fluid influx, and postfilter blood from a port located directly after the hemofilter. Blood was drawn in 3-ml S-Monovette® tubes (Sarstedt, AG & Co., Nümbrecht, Germany) with 3.2% citrate. Ultrafiltrate and blood samples were immediately centrifuged at 20 °C in a Hettich Rotanta 46 RC centrifuge at 1550 g for 15 min with acceleration and deceleration set at 8. The supernatant plasma from blood samples was then further centrifuged at 13000 *g* for 2 min in a Hettich Micro R22 centrifuge set at maximum acceleration and deceleration, and platelet-free plasma (PFP) obtained. Samples were flash-frozen in liquid nitrogen and stored at −80 °C. Upon analysis samples were thawed at 37 °C in a water bath for 2 min and then kept on wet ice.

Quantification of microvesicles by high-sensitivity flow cytometry

PFP was labeled for 30 min at room temperature with AnnexinV–FITC (1.5 µg/ml [final concentration]) to label phosphatidylserine (PS) on MV, CD31-PE (PECAM; platelet endothelial cell adhesion molecule; 0.39 µg/ml) which is present on MV from endothelial cells, platelets as well as leukocytes and CD42b-APC (GPIbα; glycoprotein Ib alpha; 0.78 µg/ml; all from BD Pharmingen, San Jose, CA) as well as CD41-PC7 (GPIIb; glycoprotein IIb; 0.78 µg/ml; Beckman-Coulter, Miami, FL) to label platelet-derived MV. AnnexinV and antibodies were filtered with a 0.1-µm filter (Millipore, Darmstadt, Germany), and PBS and AnnexinV-binding buffer with a 0.2-µm syringe filter (Sarstedt, Nümbrecht, Germany). Following the addition of CytoCount™ beads (DakoCytomation, Glostrup, Denmark) and 500 µl of AnnexinV-binding buffer (BD Pharmigen) specimens were measured with a Gallios™ flow cytometer with the threshold set at forward scatter (FS) by using Gallios™ Cytometry List Mode Data Acquisition and Analysis Software 1.2 (both Beckman Coulter, Bra, CA). Isotype controls prepared analogously were run in parallel to assess background signals of samples that showed potential artifacts in flow cytometry. These controls were labeled with AnnexinV–FITC and matched irrelevant antibodies of the same isotype and diluted in calcium-free phosphate-buffered saline (PBS from PAA Laboratories, Pasching, Austria) instead of AnnexinV-binding buffer. Artifact-containing parameters were excluded in subsequent analyses (Additional file 1: Fig. S1). Flow cytometric data were analyzed with Kaluza®, version 1.2 (Beckman Coulter). The gating strategy defined MV in a size range between 0.3 and 1.0 µm polystyrene bead-equivalents (LB3 and 89904 from Sigma-Aldrich, Saint Louis, MO) that showed a positivity concerning the aforementioned markers. The number of MV per µl PFP was determined by referring to CytoCount™ beads.

Table 1 Patient characteristics

Age (years)	64 (11)
Gender (% male)	83
SOFA	14 (4)
SAPS II	67 (16)
APACHE II	29 (6)
Vasopressor requirement (%)	92
Leukocyte count (G/l)	15 (10)
Platelet count (G/l)	127 (145)
CRP (mg/dl)	19.3 (9.6)
PCT (ng/l)	39.9 (75.3)
ICU survival (%)	33
Hospital survival (%)	25

SOFA and laboratory parameters refer to the day of blood draw. Metric variables are presented as mean (standard deviation)

G/l Giga (10^9) cells per liter, *SOFA* sequential organ failure assessment score, *APACHE II* acute physiology and chronic health evaluation, *SAPS II* simplified acute physiology score, *CRP* C-reactive protein, *PCT* procalcitonin

Microvesicle activity and tissue factor measurements

PFP and ultrafiltrate samples were analyzed with three solid-phase-capturing assays as recommended by the manufacturers. The quantity of PS, here referred to as MV activity, which is also one aspect of the procoagulatory potential of MV, was measured with the Zymuphen MP activity assay (Hyphen BioMed, Neuville sur Oise, France). The amount of tissue factor was assessed by using the Imubind® tissue factor ELISA (Sekisu Diagnostics, Stamford, CT). The procoagulatory ability of TF in the presence of PS on MV, here referred to as TF activity, was analyzed with the Zymuphen MP-TF assay (Hyphen BioMed).

Calculation of hemofiltration flow rates and statistical analyses

Absolute amounts of microvesicles entering and leaving the hemofilter were calculated by multiplying the measured MV counts (MV/µl) with the plasma flow or ultrafiltrate flow at the distinct sampling site per minute:

$$\text{Amount}_{\text{prefilter}} = C_{\text{meas}} \times \left(\text{BF} \times \left(1 - \frac{\text{HCT}}{100}\right) + \frac{\text{CF}}{60}\right) \times 1000$$

$$\text{Amount}_{\text{postfilter}} = C_{\text{meas}} \times \left(BF \times \left(1 - \frac{\text{HCT}}{100}\right) + \frac{\text{CF}}{60} - \frac{\text{UF}}{60}\right) \times 1000$$

$$\text{Amount}_{\text{UF}} = C_{\text{meas}} \times \frac{\text{UF} \times 1000}{60}$$

$$\text{FF} = \frac{\text{UF}}{\text{BF} \times \left(1 - \frac{\text{HCT}}{100}\right) \times 60 + \text{CF}}$$

C_{meas}—concentration of MV measured at specific port (MV/µl); $\text{Amount}_{\text{prefilter}}$—amount of MV entering the hemofilter (MV/min); $\text{Amount}_{\text{postfilter}}$—amount of MV leaving the hemofilter via blood (MV/min); $\text{Amount}_{\text{UF}}$—amount of MV leaving the hemofilter via ultrafiltrate (MV/min); BF—blood flow (ml/min); CF—flow of citrate-containing solution (ml/h); UF—ultrafiltrate flow (ml/h), as determined by the Prismaflex® machine; HCT—hematocrit (%); and FF—filtration fraction.

Statistical analyses were performed with GraphPad Prism® version 5 (GraphPad Software Inc., La Jolla, CA) and SPSS® version 23 (IBM, Armonk, NY). Data were tested for normality by using the Shapiro–Wilk test. For comparison of amounts before and after the hemofilter the Wilcoxon signed-rank test was used. Correlations were analyzed in SPSS by using the Spearman rho test. Quantitative data are presented as median and 25th–75th quartiles, if not indicated otherwise. P values below 0.05 were considered statistically significant.

Results

Patients

Twelve eligible patients from a tertiary ICU with severe sepsis or septic shock requiring RRT due to renal failure were included in the study. Blood culture was positive in six patients. Primary sepsis focus was the lung in six patients, urinary tract in two patients and soft tissue in one patient. In three patients no distinct focus could be determined in addition to a positive blood culture. Additional patient characteristics are presented in Table 1.

Table 2 provides an overview of the hemofiltration settings.

Microvesicles and tissue factor in pre- and postfilter blood samples

To examine whether hemofiltration alters counts of several MV subtypes in blood the absolute amounts of MV subtypes entering and leaving the hemofilter per time were compared. Ratios of the amounts of distinct parameters in blood that enter and leave the hemofilter are shown in Table 3.

Table 2 Hemofiltration settings at the time of blood draw presented as mean (standard deviation)

Blood flow (ml/min)	126 (9)
Citrate flow (ml/h)	1240 (102)
Substitution fluid flow (ml/h)	921 (304)
Patient fluid withdrawal (ml/h)	83 (83)
Ultrafiltrate flow (ml/h)	2249 (298)
Filter runtime at the time of sampling (h)	7 (7.5)
Filter survival (h)	59.6 (17.5)

Table 3 Ratios of the amounts leaving the filter/entering the filter via blood presented as median (quartiles)

Parameter	Ratio amount postfilter/prefilter blood	p
AnnexinV+	0.94 (0.84–1.93)	1.0
CD41+	1.00 (0.93–1.80)	0.7334
CD42b+	1.02 (0.70–1.41)	0.8501
CD31+/CD41−	*1.32 (1.09–1.93)*	*0.0210*
CD31+/CD42b−	1.01 (0.91–1.91)	0.4697
MV activity	*0.72 (0.62–0.84)*	*0.0020*
TF activity	1.05 (0.85–1.36)	0.5186
TF level	*0.95 (0.87–0.99)*	*0.0093*

P values refer to the comparison of absolute amounts/minute leaving to the amounts/minute entering the hemofilter *via* blood

A significant increase in probably mostly leukocyte-derived CD31+/CD41− MV [8.45×10^6 ($3.37 \times 10^6 - 2.03 \times 10^7$) vs. 1.19×10^7 ($5.49 \times 10^6 - 2.53 \times 10^7$) MV/min; $p = 0.021$] (Fig. 1a) was detected after the hemofilter passage. However, no significant differences in counts of platelet-derived CD41+ and CD42b+ MV, AnnexinV+ MV or TF activity (all $p > 0.05$) were found (Fig. 1b–d, f). There were significant correlations between filtration fraction (FF) and the ratios of post- to prefilter MV (Fig. 2) of AnnexinV+, CD42b+ and CD31+/CD41− MV (Spearman's correlation coefficient (r_s) = 0.683, $p = 0.042$; $r_s = 0.664$, $p = 0.018$; $r_s = 0.720$, $p = 0.008$, respectively).

A measure of the total amount of PS-exposing MV, i.e., MV activity (Fig. 1e), revealed a statistically significant decrease during hemofilter [0.088 (0.027–0.243) vs. 0.067 (0.021–0.223) nmol/min; $p = 0.002$]. The comparison of TF levels (Fig. 1g) before and after the hemofilter showed a significant decrease after the hemofilter [27877 (22103–37793) vs. 25811 (18736–35164) pg/min, ($p = 0.0376$) pg/min; $p = 0.0093$)]. No significant correlation was detected between FF and alterations in MV activity, TF activity or TF level.

There were no correlations between platelet or leukocyte counts and the observed alterations of MV or TF during hemofilter passage. No associations between filter runtime and MV alterations were detected.

Three patients showing artifacts in AnnexinV+ MV counts and one patient with artifacts in measurements of MV activities were therefore excluded from analyses. However, this did not relevantly change statistics.

Microvesicles and tissue factor in ultrafiltrate

To investigate whether MV or fragments of them are ultrafiltrated during hemofilter passage solid-phase-capturing assays were used to examine the ultrafiltrate, such as the MV activity assay to detect MV. This assay captures PS and is therefore able to detect also MV that are sized below the detection limit of high-sensitivity flow cytometry which is approximately 0.3 μm. However, no relevant MV activity could be detected in ultrafiltrate samples (i.e., absolute activities ≤0.05 nM). A remarkable fraction of TF (in average approximately 4.6% of the TF amount that enters the hemofilter) was found in the ultrafiltrate [1229 (408–2218) pg/min, corresponding to an average sieving coefficient of 0.12 (Fig. 1g). However, there was no relevant TF activity measurable in ultrafiltrate (i.e., absolute activities ≤0.05 pg/ml) (Fig. 1f).

Discussion

This is the first study analyzing MV levels as well as TF in blood before and after the hemofilter in CVVH. The major findings of this study are that (1) CVVH clears small PS-exposing MV but not larger MV, (2) subsets of MV are generated within the hemofilter indicating leukocyte activation during hemofilter passage, (3) the extent of MV generation correlates with FF, and (4) a fraction of TF is being cleared via ultrafiltration.

Effects of hemofiltration on microvesicle counts and composition

We could show that CVVH has differential effects on distinct MV subtypes. On the one hand, we observed a reduction in MV activity during hemofilter passage, but no change in AnnexinV+ MV. Although both parameters are measures of PS-exposing MV, they reflect different fractions of PS + MV: MV activity comprises the overall amount of PS + MV, whereas AnnexinV+ MV, measured with hs-FC, exclusively PS + MV that are larger than approximately 0.3 μm. Thus, our data indicate that CVVH clears a fraction small PS-exposing MV. Since no MV activity was measurable in the ultrafiltrate, we assume mechanisms other than filtration such as adsorption being responsible for the clearance of small MV. The findings from our clinical study are compatible with a study from Abdelhafeez et al. [18] who analyzed the effects of CVVH on MV counts in an ex vivo model of CVVH and reported a reduction in MV over a period of 70 min, as shown for endothelium-derived MV. In line with our findings, they propose that mechanisms other than filtration seem to be responsible for the reduction in MV [18]. In conclusion, our data suggest that CVVH clears a fraction of small PS-exposing MV from blood of septic patients.

On the other hand, we found a significantly higher amount of CD31+/CD41− MV after the hemofilter. According to their surface epitope pattern this MV subtype can either be derived from leukocytes or endothelial cells. However, CD31+/CD41− MV that are generated within the hemofilter are probably predominantly leukocyte derived. There are two aspects corroborating this

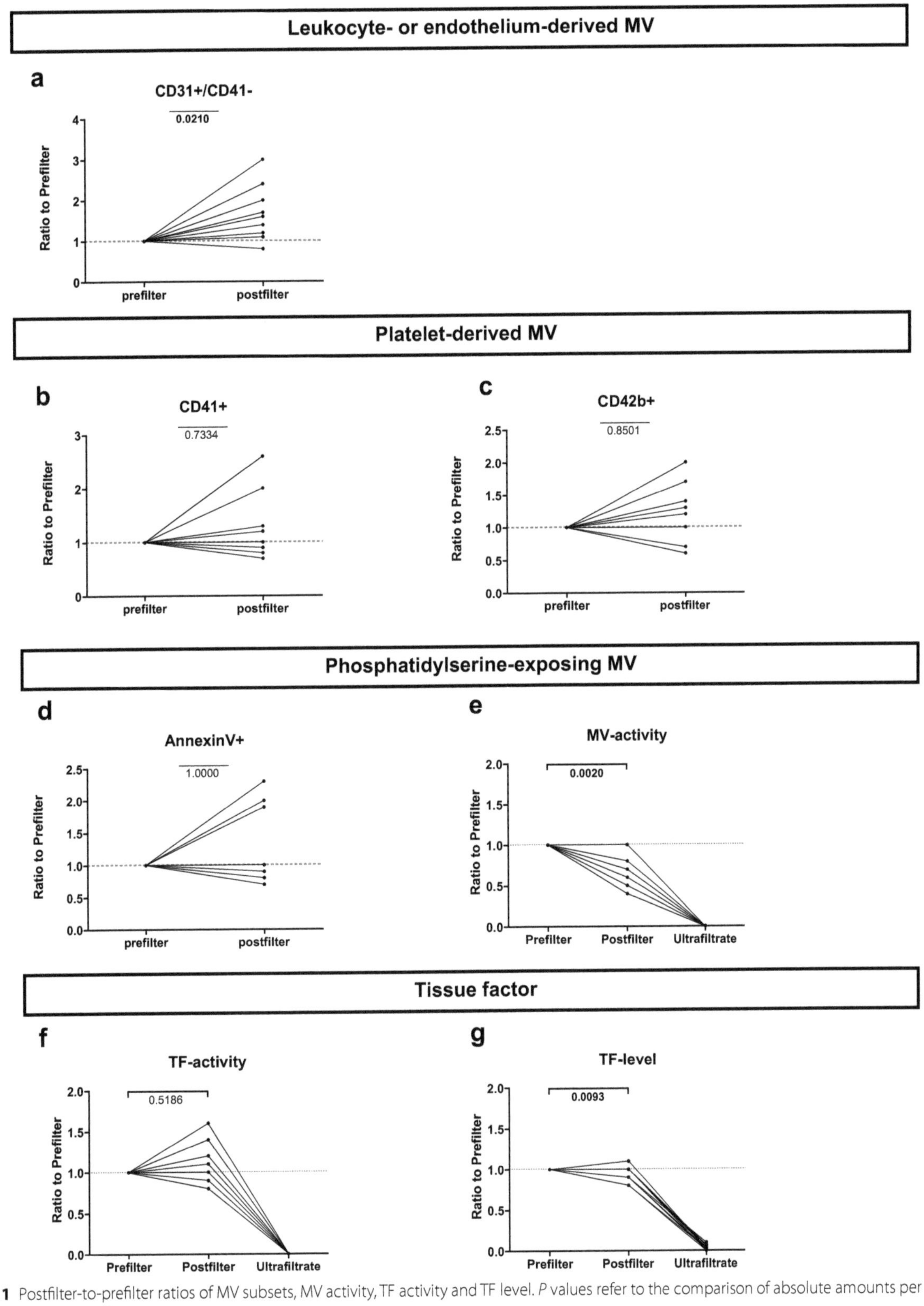

Fig. 1 Postfilter-to-prefilter ratios of MV subsets, MV activity, TF activity and TF level. *P* values refer to the comparison of absolute amounts per minute pre- to postfilter

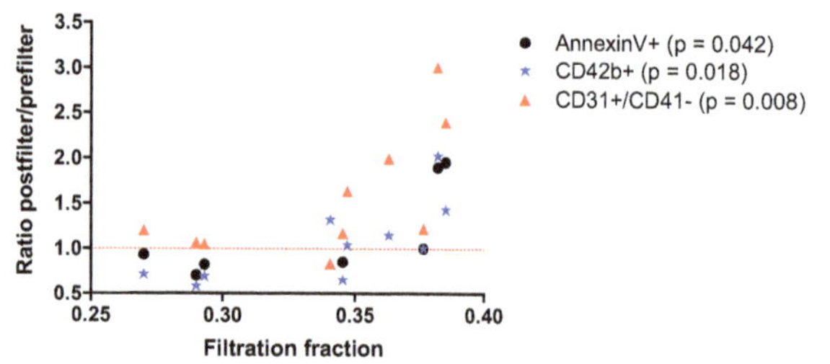

Fig. 2 Correlations of MV subtypes (post- to prefilter Ratios) with filtration fraction

assumption: Firstly, recent data suggest that the majority of MV exposing this not endothelium-specific CD31+/CD41− pattern are predominantly not derived from endothelial cells, but rather from leukocytes in patients with septic shock [19]. Secondly, it is evident that CD31+/CD41− MV that are released during a single hemofilter passage are originating from circulating cells. Despite low levels of circulating endothelial cells (CEC) present in patients with septic shock (approximately between 10 and 30 cells per ml) [20] it is likely that the observed significant increase in CD31+/CD41− MV is rather produced by leukocytes which are around half a million times more abundant than CEC. Our findings and conclusions are in accordance with a study from Kozek-Langenecker et al. [21] who directly assessed activation status of cells. Likewise, they report activation of leukocytes and also platelets within the hemofilter during CVVH with heparin anticoagulation [21]. In line with this, Faure et al. [13] found even higher systemic counts of leukocyte- and platelet-derived MV in patients with chronic renal failure that were dialyzed with heparin anticoagulation compared to patients without dialysis. Moreover, they observed a pronounced systemic increase in CD41+ platelet-derived MV and also in AnnexinV+ MV after the hemodialysis session [13]. We could not find increased levels of platelet-derived MV after hemofilter passage. This may be explained by the use of regional citrate anticoagulation in all patients, which has previously been demonstrated to result in significantly less platelet activation than heparin anticoagulation [6, 7].

Correlation of filtration fraction with MV generation

Interestingly, we found correlations between FF and increments of platelet- and presumably leukocyte-derived as well as procoagulant AnnexinV+ MV. The usually recommended FF is below 25% in postdilution mode [22], since higher FF frequently leads to hemofilter clotting [5]. As shown in Fig. 2, the induction of MV generation within the hemofilter seems to be more pronounced when FF is above 30%, probably due to increased shear stress at higher FF. This prominent effect at higher FF seems even to apply to platelet-derived and AnnexinV+ MV which did not significantly change in septic patients overall. We speculate that the generation of MV within the hemofilter might contribute to hemofilter clotting occurring when high FF is applied. However, this remains to be investigated in a larger study.

Mechanisms contributing to the presumed cellular activation and the subsequent MV generation within the hemofilter might include a high shear stress or contact with the hemofilter membrane [5–7, 23–25]. Such effects of CVVH might even be more pronounced in a septic state where cells are already preactivated or highly susceptible to activation. Accordingly, septic shock patients exhibit already threefold higher levels of presumably mostly leukocyte-derived CD31+/CD41− MV compared to healthy subjects, as recently reported [19]. As calcium is a key mediator for neutrophil degranulation that is induced by dialysis membranes [23] and as influx of extracellular calcium is required for vesiculation of platelets induced by shear stress [24] one might speculate that MV release might even be more pronounced in CVVH without citrate anticoagulation [6], but this needs to be tested.

Clearance of tissue factor by hemofiltration

Subsets of leukocytes, such as monocytes, are able to release MV and also associated TF upon activation [26, 27]. Based on the assumption that the above-mentioned increase in CD31+/CD41− predominantly reflects leukocyte activation we wanted to investigate whether we can find evidence for an accompanying TF generation during CVVH. Former studies reporting TF levels during hemofiltration analyzed exclusively systemic TF levels [28, 29]. Although Cardigan et al. [28] observed an increase in 50% of patients while on CVVH, no significant systemic increase could be detected in the most recent study from Bouman et al. [29]. So far, it was unclear whether potential alterations in systemic TF levels reflect secondary systemic inflammatory effects that are triggered by hemofiltration or if these alterations are due to TF generation or clearance within the hemofilter. Our study adds two new key answers to this matter: First, we provide evidence that hemofilter passage leads to a reduction in TF levels. Additionally, we demonstrate that a fraction of TF is being ultrafiltrated.

Strengths and limitations

A major strength of our study is that we assessed alterations in MV levels occurring directly and exclusively within the hemofilter. Limitations of the study are the relatively small number of patients as well as the lack of information concerning kinetics in the extracorporeal system or the systemic circulation because we did not take serial measurements due to the complexity of analysis. Since no conclusion can be drawn regarding whether the generation of CD31+/CD41− MV within the hemofilter may impact systemic levels or patient outcome, the clinical implications of MV generation within the hemofilter remain to be further elucidated.

Conclusions

In conclusion, CVVH clears a fraction of small PS-exposing MV by mechanisms other than filtration, but does not eliminate larger MV. CVVH induces the release of CD31+/CD41− MV that indicate leukocyte activation during hemofilter passage in septic patients. The generation of MV within the hemofilter seems to be particularly pronounced when FF is above 30%, which supports the clinical relevance of the usual recommendation to keep FF below 25%. A fraction of TF is being cleared by CVVH via ultrafiltration. Our findings show that MV analysis can be used to assess the effects caused by contact of blood with the hemofilter. Evaluation of MV patterns might be a promising instrument helping to refine extracorporeal therapeutic systems and biocompatibility of hemofilter membranes in future.

Abbreviations

CVVH: continuous veno-venous hemofiltration (CVVH); RRT: renal replacement therapy; MV: microvesicles; ICU: intensive care unit; SIRS: systemic inflammatory response syndrome; APCAHE II: acute physiology and chronic health evaluation score; SAPS II: simplified acute physiology score; SOFA: sequential organ failure assessment score; PFP: platelet-free plasma; PECAM: platelet endothelial cell adhesion molecule; GPIbα: glycoprotein Ib alpha; GPIIb: glycoprotein IIb; PBS: phosphate-buffered saline; CRP: C-reactive protein; PCT: procalcitonin; CEC: circulating endothelial cells; TAT: thrombin–antithrombin; FVII: factor VII; C_{meas}: concentration of MV measured at specific port (MV/μl); $Amount_{prefilter}$: amount of MV entering the hemofilter (MV/min); $Amount_{postfilter}$: amount of MV leaving the hemofilter via blood (MV/min); $Amount_{UF}$: amount of MV leaving the hemofilter via ultrafiltrate (MV/min); BF: blood flow (ml/min); CF: flow of citrate-containing solution (ml/h); UF: ultrafiltrate flow (ml/h); FF: filtration fraction.

Authors' contributions

GFL designed and coordinated the study, enrolled patients, carried out the analyses and wrote the manuscript. UH enrolled patients, participated in the coordination of the study and refinement of the manuscript. CF participated in the design of the study, the analysis and refinement of the manuscript. VMH took measurement of microvesicles and participated in the refinement of the manuscript. JH participated in the design of the study. RB participated in the enrollment of patients, calculation of hemofilter flow rates and refinement of the manuscript. MJ designed and coordinated the study, enrolled patients and refined the manuscript.

Author details

[1] Division of Intensive Care and Emergency Medicine, Department of Internal Medicine, Medical University Innsbruck, Anichstrasse 35, 6020 Innsbruck, Austria. [2] Department of Internal Medicine V - Haematology and Oncology, Medical University Innsbruck, Anichstrasse 35, 6020 Innsbruck, Austria.

Acknowledgements

None.

Competing interests

The authors declare that they have no competing interests.

Funding

Supported by funds of the Oesterreichische Nationalbank (Oesterreichische Nationalbank, Anniversary Fund, project numbers 13861 and 15708).

References

1. Jörres, A. Acute kidney injury: choice of the initial modality for renal replacement therapy. Med Klin Intensivmed Notfmed. 2015;110(4):251–5.
2. Payen D, Mateo J, Cavaillon JM, Fraisse F, Floriot C, Vicaut E, et al. Impact of continuous venovenous hemofiltration on organ failure during the early phase of severe sepsis: a randomized controlled trial. Crit Care Med. 2009;37(3):803–10.
3. Honore PM, Jamez J, Wauthier M, Lee PA, Dugernier T, Pirenne B, et al. Prospective evaluation of short-term, high-volume isovolemic hemofiltration on the hemodynamic course and outcome in patients with intractable circulatory failure resulting from septic shock. Crit Care Med. 2000;28(11):3581–7.
4. De Vriese AS, Colardyn FA, Philippe JJ, Vanholder RC, De Sutter JH, Lameire NH. Cytokine removal during continuous hemofiltration in septic patients. J Am Soc Nephrol. 1999;10(4):846–53.
5. Joannidis M, Oudemans-van Straaten HM. Clinical review: patency of the circuit in continuous renal replacement therapy. Crit Care. 2007;11(4):218.
6. Gritters M, Grooteman MP, Schoorl M, Schoorl M, Bartels PC, Scheffer PG, et al. Citrate anticoagulation abolishes degranulation of polymorphonuclear cells and platelets and reduces oxidative stress during haemodialysis. Nephrol Dial Transplant. 2006;21(1):153–9.
7. Oudemans-van Straaten HM, Kellum JA, Bellomo R. Clinical review: anticoagulation for continuous renal replacement therapy–heparin or citrate? Crit Care. 2011;15(1):202.
8. Oudemans-van Straaten HM. Hemostasis and thrombosis in continuous renal replacement treatment. Semin Thromb Hemost. 2015;41(1):91–8.
9. Thery C, Ostrowski M, Segura E. Membrane vesicles as conveyors of immune responses. Nat Rev Immunol. 2009;9(8):581–93.
10. Gyorgy B, Szabo TG, Pasztoi M, Pal Z, Misjak P, Aradi B, et al. Membrane vesicles, current state-of-the-art: emerging role of extracellular vesicles. Cell Mol Life Sci. 2011;68(16):2667–88.
11. Mastronardi ML, Mostefai HA, Meziani F, Martinez MC, Asfar P, Andriantsitohaina R. Circulating microparticles from septic shock patients exert differential tissue expression of enzymes related to inflammation and oxidative stress. Crit Care Med. 2011;39(7):1739–48.
12. Delabranche X, Boisrame-Helms J, Asfar P, Berger A, Mootien Y, Lavigne T, et al. Microparticles are new biomarkers of septic shock-induced disseminated intravascular coagulopathy. Intensive Care Med. 2013;39(10):1695–703.
13. Faure V, Dou L, Sabatier F, Cerini C, Sampol J, Berland Y, et al. Elevation of circulating endothelial microparticles in patients with chronic renal failure. J Thromb Haemost. 2006;4(3):566–73.
14. Bone RC, Balk RA, Cerra FB, Dellinger RP, Fein AM, Knaus WA, et al. Definitions for sepsis and organ failure and guidelines for the use of innovative therapies in sepsis. The ACCP/SCCM Consensus Conference Committee. American College of Chest Physicians/Society of Critical Care Medicine. Chest. 1992;101(6):1644–55.
15. Knaus WA, Draper EA, Wagner DP, Zimmerman JE. APACHE II: a severity of disease classification system. Crit Care Med. 1985;13(10):818–29.

16. Le Gall JR, Lemeshow S, Saulnier F. A new simplified acute physiology score (SAPS II) based on a European/North American multicenter study. JAMA. 1993;270(24):2957–63.
17. Vincent JL, Moreno R, Takala J, Willatts S, De Mendonca A, Bruining H, et al. The SOFA (Sepsis-related Organ Failure Assessment) score to describe organ dysfunction/failure. On behalf of the Working Group on sepsis-related problems of the European Society of Intensive Care Medicine. Intensive Care Med. 1996;22(7):707–10.
18. Abdelhafeez AH, Jeziorczak PM, Schaid TR, Hoefs SL, Kaul S, Nanchal R, et al. Clinical CVVH model removes endothelium-derived microparticles from circulation. J Extracell Vesicles. 2014;3(1):23498. doi:10.3402/jev.v3.23498.
19. Lehner GF, Harler U, Haller VM, Feistritzer C, Hasslacher J, Dunzendorfer S, et al. Characterization of microvesicles in septic shock using high-sensitivity flow cytometry. Shock. 2016;46(4):373–81.
20. Mutunga M, Fulton B, Bullock R, Batchelor A, Gascoigne A, Gillespie JI, et al. Circulating endothelial cells in patients with septic shock. Am J Respir Crit Care Med. 2001;163(1):195–200.
21. Kozek-Langenecker SA, Spiss CK, Michalek-Sauberer A, Felfernig M, Zimpfer M. Effect of prostacyclin on platelets, polymorphonuclear cells, and heterotypic cell aggregation during hemofiltration. Crit Care Med. 2003;31(3):864–8.
22. Klein SJ, Joannidis M. Renal replacement therapy in acute kidney injury. Med Klin Intensivmed Notfmed. 2017;112(5):437–443.
23. Bohler J, Donauer J, Birmelin M, Schollmeyer PJ, Horl WH. Mediators of complement-independent granulocyte activation during haemodialysis: role of calcium, prostaglandins and leukotrienes. Nephrol Dial Transplant. 1993;8(12):1359–65.
24. Miyazaki Y, Nomura S, Miyake T, Kagawa H, Kitada C, Taniguchi H, et al. High shear stress can initiate both platelet aggregation and shedding of procoagulant containing microparticles. Blood. 1996;88(9):3456–64.
25. Lehner GF, Schopf M, Harler U, Pechlaner C, Joannidis M. Repeated premature hemofilter clotting during regional citrate anticoagulation as indicator of heparin induced thrombocytopenia. Blood Purif. 2014;38(2):127–30.
26. Egorina EM, Sovershaev MA, Olsen JO, Osterud B. Granulocytes do not express but acquire monocyte-derived tissue factor in whole blood: evidence for a direct transfer. Blood. 2008;111(3):1208–16.
27. Key NS, Mackman N. Tissue factor and its measurement in whole blood, plasma, and microparticles. Semin Thromb Hemost. 2010;36(8):865–75.
28. Cardigan RA, McGloin H, Mackie IJ, Machin SJ, Singer M. Activation of the tissue factor pathway occurs during continuous venovenous hemofiltration. Kidney Int. 1999;55(4):1568–74.
29. Bouman CS, de Pont AC, Meijers JC, Bakhtiari K, Roem D, Zeerleder S, et al. The effects of continuous venovenous hemofiltration on coagulation activation. Crit Care. 2006;10(5):R150.

11

Comparison of diagnostic accuracy in sepsis between presepsin, procalcitonin, and C-reactive protein

Chin-Chieh Wu[1], Hao-Min Lan[2], Shih-Tsung Han[3], Chung-Hsien Chaou[3], Chun-Fu Yeh[4], Su-Hsun Liu[2,5], Chih-Huang Li[3], Gerald N. Blaney III[1], Zhen-Ying Liu[1] and Kuan-Fu Chen[1,3,6,7*]

Abstract

Background: The soluble cluster of differentiation 14 (or presepsin) is a free fragment of glycoprotein expressed on monocytes and macrophages. Although many studies have been conducted recently, the diagnostic performance of presepsin for sepsis remains debated. We performed a systematic review and meta-analysis of the available literature to assess the accuracy of presepsin for the diagnosis of sepsis in adult patients and compared the performance between presepsin, C-reactive protein (CRP), and procalcitonin (PCT).

Methods: A comprehensive systemic search was conducted in PubMed, EMBASE, and Google Scholar for studies that evaluated the diagnostic accuracy of presepsin for sepsis until January 2017. The hierarchical summary receiver operating characteristic method was used to pool individual sensitivity, specificity, diagnostic odds ratio (DOR), positive likelihood ratio (PLR), negative likelihood ratio (NLR), and area under the receiver operating characteristic curve (AUC).

Results: Eighteen studies, comprising 3470 patients, met our inclusion criteria. The pooled diagnosis sensitivity and specificity of presepsin for sepsis were 0.84 (95% CI 0.80–0.87) and 0.76 (95% CI 0.67–0.82), respectively. Furthermore, the pooled DOR, PLR, NLR, and AUC were 16 (95% CI 10–25), 3.4 (95% CI 2.5–4.6), 0.22 (95% CI 0.17–0.27), and 0.88 (95% CI 0.85–0.90), respectively. Significant heterogeneity was found in both sensitivities (Cochrane $Q = 137.43$, $p < 0.001$, $I^2 = 87.63\%$) and specificities (Cochrane $Q = 180.76$, $p < 0.001$, $I^2 = 90.60\%$). Additionally, we found no significant difference between presepsin and PCT (AUC 0.87 vs. 0.86) or CRP (AUC 0.85 vs. 0.85). However, for studies conducted in ICU, the pooled sensitivity of presepsin was found to be higher than PCT (0.88, 95% CI 0.82–0.92 vs. 0.75, 95% CI 0.68–0.81), while the pooled specificity of presepsin was lower than PCT (0.58, 95% CI 0.42–0.73 vs. 0.75, 95% CI 0.65–0.83).

Conclusion: Based on the results of our meta-analysis, presepsin is a promising marker for diagnosis of sepsis as PCT or CRP, but its results should be interpreted more carefully and cautiously since too few studies were included and those studies had high heterogeneity between them. In addition, continuing re-evaluation during the course of sepsis is advisable.

Keywords: Presepsin, sCD14, Sensitivity, Specificity, Meta-analysis, Sepsis, Adults

*Correspondence: drkfchen@gmail.com
[6] Clinical Informatics and Medical Statistics Research Center, Chang Gung University, 5 Fu-Shin Street, Gueishan Village, Taoyuan 333, Taiwan
Full list of author information is available at the end of the article

Background

Sepsis, a life-threatening disease, contributes to more than twenty thousand deaths in the USA each year, accounting for almost 1–2% of all patients admitted to the hospitals, and as much as 25% of intensive care unit (ICU) admissions [1]. Typically, patients with sepsis can be treated efficiently with early intravascular fluid and antibiotics in the ICU to avoid mortality development. However, it is difficult to decide early on whether to apply these methods due to the existence of non-infectious systemic inflammatory response syndrome (SIRS) [2]. Therefore, identifying a biomarker that can efficiently distinguish sepsis from non-infectious SIRS has become an important topic.

Recently, some studies investigated candidate biomarkers to detect sepsis reported such as procalcitonin (PCT), C-reactive protein (CRP), lipopolysaccharide-binding protein (LBP), interleukins, provasopressin, and myeloid cells expressing triggering receptor-1 (TREM-1) [3–7]. However, none of them have been proven to be accurate enough to distinguish sepsis from SIRS. The Surviving Sepsis Campaign further 'weakly' recommended the measurement of procalcitonin levels to be used to support shortening the duration or discontinuation of antimicrobial therapy in sepsis patients under low quality of evidence [8]. Although CRP and PCT are the preferred biomarkers to be used in clinical context currently [9, 10], some issues for their diagnostic accuracy still remain unsolved, which prevent clinicians from starting or withholding antimicrobial therapy. A previous review revealed that CRP performs relatively inaccurately in the diagnostic tasks of sepsis compared with PCT [11]. The results from three published reviews indicated that the sensitivity and specificity of both CRP (ranged from 35 to 100% and from 18 to 84%, respectively) and PCT vary (ranged from 42 to 100% and from 48 to 100%, respectively) [10–12]. In addition, studies suggested that the CRP level increases in 4–6 h and reaches the peak in 48–72 h after the inflammatory onset [13], while PCT level increases in 8–24 h and reaches the peak later than 24 h [14]. Therefore, both PCT and CRP might be still not reliable enough as early indicators for sepsis used in the clinical context.

CD14 is a free fragment of glycoprotein expressed on monocytes and macrophages. It is a receptor of lipopolysaccharide–lipopolysaccharide-binding protein (LPS–LBP) complexes, transducing the endotoxin signal from bacterial infection through the Toll-like receptor-4 with the help of thinositol lipid structure [15]. Its soluble form, soluble CD14 (sCD14), is produced from cell secretion or when membrane-bound, CD14 (mCD14) detaches from cells such as phagocytes. The N-terminal fragments of 13 kDa consist of sCD14 subtype (sCD14-ST), also called presepsin, are closely related to mediating the immune response to LPS [16] and could be detected easier than mCD14 in the blood. Similar to other reported biomarkers, the distribution of presepsin values is slightly different, with a small overlap between healthy controls (294.2 $\pm$ 121.4 pg/ml) and septic patients (817.9 $\pm$ 572.7 pg/ml) [17]. Moreover, the level of presepsin typically increases within 2 h and reaches the peak in 3 h after infection [14]. By using the chemiluminescence enzyme immunoassay as detecting tool, the result can be available in 1.5 h [18]. The above evidence indicates that presepsin might be a better biomarker for sepsis during the early stage of sepsis than in later stages.

Recently, more clinical trials assessing the diagnostic accuracy of presepsin have been published. Most reported better results compared to other biomarkers. Therefore, we conducted this systematic review and meta-analysis not only to pool the results from relevant studies, but also to compare the diagnostic accuracy of presepsin with other biomarkers in diagnosing sepsis. We aimed to generate a more comprehensive understanding of the diagnostic performance and potential influence factors of presepsin in distinguishing sepsis from non-infectious SIRS.

Methods

This study was performed and reported in accordance with the relevant reporting guideline (Preferred Reporting Items for Systematic Reviews and Meta-Analyses, PRISMA) [19].

Search strategy and literature selection

We developed a protocol prior to conducting this systematic review and meta-analysis. A comprehensive systemic search was carried out in PubMed and EMBASE for studies evaluating the diagnostic accuracy of presepsin for sepsis until January 2017. The following search terms were used: [('Systemic Inflammatory Response Syndrome' OR 'SIRS') AND 'Sepsis'] AND ('Early Diagnosis' OR 'Diagnosis') AND ('sCD14' OR 'presepsin') AND 'adult' in PubMed and [sensitivity OR diagnostic AND accuracy:lnk OR diagnostic AND ('sepsis'/exp OR sepsis) AND ('sCD14' OR sCD14) OR ('presepsin' OR presepsin) AND (English)/lim] in EMBASE, to search for original, English language, research articles that studied the diagnostic accuracy between septic and non-septic in adult patients. Additionally, we also conducted searches on Google Scholar and checked the reference lists to avoid potential missingness.

Two reviewers (CCW and HML) independently screened and decided the inclusion of the studies in the review after removing duplicated references. The inclusion criteria were: (1) sepsis-related studies; (2)

diagnostic instead of prognostic studies: i.e. diagnosing sepsis instead of predicting mortality; and (3) articles in English. On the other hand, studies were excluded according to the following criteria: (1) non-sepsis-related studies; (2) non-diagnostic studies; (3) non-original studies: e.g. literature review, editorial piece; (4) studies with no performance parameters given (i.e. sensitivity, specificity and 2 × 2 contingency tables); and (5) non-blood specimen. Agreement regarding study inclusion between the reviewers was assessed using the Cohen's kappa statistic [20].

Data extraction

All relevant information, such as study setting, material and method, statistical method, and the results, was extracted independently via a piloted electrical form (Microsoft Access) by two authors (CCW and HML). The results of their extraction were double-checked to ensure the accuracy and all discrepant results were solved by consensus meetings. We transformed the numbers of true positive, false positive, false negative, and true negative based on the provided indices of sensitivity, specificity, and sample size values for statistical calculation. If any information was not provided, we contacted the authors by emails.

Quality assessment

Two authors (CCW and HML) independently assessed the risk of bias of each study by the Quality Assessment of Diagnostic Accuracy Studies (QUADAS-2) checklist [21] recommended by the Cochrane collaboration for the quality assessment of diagnostic studies. The QUADAS-2 tool is constituted of four domains, including patient selection, index test, reference standard, and flow and timing. It assists authors of systematic reviews in rating the risk of bias and applicability in diagnostic accuracy from their studies. To judge the risk of bias of each study, signalling questions were provided. Agreement between the two reviewers for the assessment of methodological quality was evaluated using the Cohen's kappa statistic [20]. All disagreements were solved by consensus meetings.

Meta-analysis

All statistical tests were two-sided, and statistical significance was defined as p value <0.05. The Midas module for Stata 13.1 (Stata Corporation, College Station, TX, USA) was used for all statistical and meta-analysis. We used mada package in R (version 3.1.3) to do the bivariate binomial mixed-effect meta-regression model. Midas and the QUADAS modules for Stata were used for all graphical display of the quality of the included studies. Publication bias was tested by the Deek's effective sample size funnel plots versus the diagnostic odds ratio.

The pooled sensitivity, specificity, diagnostic odds ratio (DOR), positive likelihood ratio (PLR), negative likelihood ratio (NLR), and the area under the receiver operating characteristic curve (AUC) were calculated based on the hierarchical summary receiver operating characteristic (HSROC) method [22] for meta-analysis of diagnostic test data. The advantage of this approach was that it could maximize the use of available data from each study, irrespective of the threshold used. Additionally, the respective summary receiver operating characteristic curves (SROC) [23] and AUC, irrespective of the different cut-off points used, were also conducted.

We checked heterogeneity of these included studies, as well as in different subgroups, to further evaluate the performance of presepsin. Heterogeneity can be caused by two types of effects, threshold and non-threshold. For threshold effects, the heterogeneity was calculated by the Spearman correlation coefficient (ρ) between logarithms of sensitivity and (1-specificity) and visual inspection from the SROC curve. Chi-square (χ^2) test, Cochrane Q test, and the I^2 metric were used for non-threshold effect heterogeneity [24]. A value of I^2 greater than 50% was considered significant heterogeneity. When heterogeneity was present, univariable meta-regression analyses using bivariate binomial mixed-effect model and subgroup analyses were performed to find the source of variability by potentially influencing factors in sensitivity and specificity, including country of study, patient sources, types of specimen, sample sizes, proportions of patients with sepsis, cut-off values, and different compositions of control groups. Additionally, some of our included studies were direct comparisons between presepsin, PCT, and CRP. Subgroup analyses were conducted to compare the diagnostic accuracy and performance between these three biomarkers. We also used the information on cut-off from each study to determine an optimal cut-off by maximizing the Youden index (sensitivity + specificity-1) in this diagnostic test accuracy reviews.

Results

Our search in electronic databases yielded 86 published studies, 62 of which were excluded for various reasons based on screening the titles and abstracts (Fig. 1), leaving 24 studies that were assessed for full-text review. Among the 24 studies, we excluded another six studies; three were not related to diagnostic test, two did not report enough information to conduct a 2 × 2 contingency table, and one was not related to blood sample. Finally, 18 studies fulfilled our eligibility criteria and were included in the final meta-analyses [17, 25–41] (Fig. 1).

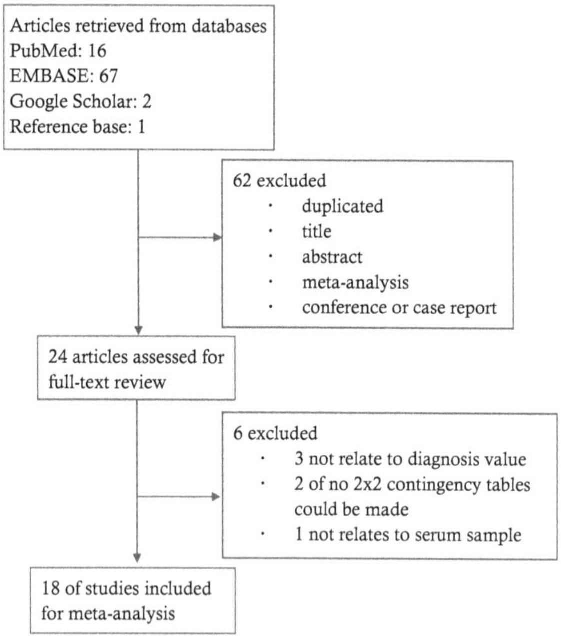

Fig. 1 Flow chart of study identification, inclusion, and exclusion for meta-analysis

Characteristics of included studies

The main characteristics and data of each included study are summarized in Tables 1 and 2. The 18 included studies were published between 2011 and 2017. Of the 3470 patients included in the 18 studies, 1904 (54.88%) were admitted to the emergency departments (ED), 783 (22.56%) were admitted to the ICU, and 783 (22.56%) were admitted in the ED and ICU. Among the 1338 patients included in the control group, 953 (71.23%) were categorized as non-infectious SIRS and 385 (28.77%) as normal healthy volunteers. The total proportion of patients with sepsis was 61.44%. There were 17 prospective studies and one retrospective. All were case–control design. Of these, 14 studies were defined as 'gold standard' by the criterions defined in the 1991 ACCP/SCCM consensus conference [42], two by the third international consensus definitions for sepsis and septic shock (sepsis-3) [43], one by Spanish Society of Infectious Diseases and Clinical Microbiology (SEIMC) [44], and another by American Burn Association (ABA) [45]. Among the types of specimen tested for presepsin detection, six studies used whole blood, ten studies used plasma, and two studies used serum. All studies used PATHFAST assay analysis system.

Results of quality assessment

The methodological quality assessments with the QUADAS-2 tool for the 18 included studies are summarized in Table 3 and Fig. 2. All studies scored 'low' in the domain of bias in the reference standard, since the guidelines of the ACCP/SCCM consensus conference [42], Sepsis-3 [43], SEIMC [44], and ABA [45] were used to diagnose sepsis in these studies. For the domain of risk of bias in patient selection, the 16 studies providing clear definition of exclusion criteria were scored 'low' risk. Two studies that did not show enough information about how they excluded patients was scored 'unclear'. Regarding the risk of bias in index tests, all studies not pre-specifying a threshold were scored 'high risk'. For patient flow and timing domain, 14 studies scored 'low' since they clearly defined the appropriate interval between the index test and reference standard in their studies. In relation to applicability, all included studies scored well for the reference standard domain except one [35], since the target condition as defined by the reference standard (SEIMC) which was used for definition of bacteremia does not match the review question. In the patient selection criteria, 11 studies were in accordance with our inclusion criteria and scored 'low'. In the quality assessment, the Cohen's kappa statistic for the inter-rater agreement was 0.34. Subsequently, all disagreeing evaluations were resolved after consensus meetings.

Meta-analysis

Deek's effective sample size funnel plot and the regression test of asymmetry of the included studies indicated that there was no direct evidence for publication bias (p value = 0.68) (Fig. 3). The sensitivity of presepsin ranged from 0.67 to 1.0 among the 18 included studies, while the specificity of presepsin ranged from 0.33 to 0.98 (Fig. 4). The pooled sensitivity and specificity obtained by the HSROC method were 0.84 (95% CI 0.80–0.87) and 0.76 (95% CI 0.67–0.84), respectively (Figs. 4, 5a). We also constructed summary ROC for presepsin, and the result showed that the AUC was 0.88 (95% CI 0.85–0.90, Fig. 5a). The pooled DOR, PLR, and NLR of presepsin were 16 (95% CI 10–25), 3.4 (95% CI 2.5–4.6), and 0.22 (95% CI 0.17–0.27), respectively. The median cut-off for presepsin in the included studies was 600 pg/ml (IQR 439–664). More cautiously, after excluding one study [39] because its individual sensitivity and specificity were outside the confidence region in the summary operating point, we summarized the pooled statistics for remaining 17 studies [17, 25–38, 40, 41]. However, the subsequently pooled performance indices were not significantly different [sensitivity: 0.83 (95% CI 0.79–0.86), specificity: 0.72 (95% CI 0.65–0.79), AUC: 0.86, and pooled DOR: 13 (95% CI 10–17)]. Our analysis indicated that presepsin could offer a good degree of accuracy to diagnose sepsis.

Table 1 Main characteristics of the included studies

References	Country	Mean age (years) total or case/control	Patient source	Sepsis/control (*n*)	Specimen tested	Inclusion criteria	Controls	Reference	Tests
Shozushima et al. [17]	Japan	62	CCU and ED	101/41	Whole blood	Presented to CCU and ED with ≥ 2 criteria for SIRS	SIRS (n = 41)	ACCP/SCCM 1991	PATHFAST
Endo et al. [29]	Japan	75/66	ICU and ED	115/70	Whole blood	Presented to ICU or ED with 1 criteria for SIRS	Non-infectious (n = 70)	Blood culture	PATHFAST
Liu et al. [33]	China	71/69	ED	680/279	Whole blood	Presented to ED with definition of sepsis by ACCP/SCCM	SIRS (n = 179) HC (n = 100)	ACCP/SCCM 2001	PATHFAST
Ulla et al. [38]	Italy	71/56	ED	106/83	Plasma	Presented to ED with ≥ 2 criteria for SIRS	SIRS (n = 83)	ACCP/SCCM 1991	PATHFAST
Vodnik et al. [39]	Serbia	56/55.15	ED	30/100	Plasma	Presented to ED with ≥ 2 criteria for SIRS and intra-abdominal infection	SIRS (n = 30) HC (n = 70)	ACCP/SCCM 1991	PATHFAST
Behnes et al. [25]	Germany	68/64	ICU	81/15	Serum	Presented to ICU with proven criteria of septic shock	SIRS (n = 15)	ACCP/SCCM 1991	PATHFAST
Brenner et al. [26]	Germany	70/44	ICU	60/60	Plasma	Presented to ICU with proven criteria of septic shock	HC (n = 30) Postoperative (n = 30)	ACCP/SCCM 2001	PATHFAST
Romualdo et al. [35]	Spain	71/67	ED	37/189	Plasma	Presented to ED with SIRS and suspected infection	Negative blood cultures in SIRS (n = 189)	SSIDCM	PATHFAST
Ishikura et al. [31]	Japan	67.2	ED	43/39	Whole blood	Presented to ED and CCM with ≥ 1 criteria for SIRS	Non-sepsis (n = 39)	ACCP/SCCM 1991	PATHFAST
Kweon et al. [32]	Korea	64.3/56.1	ED	73/45	Whole blood	Presented to ED with ≥ 2 criteria for SIRS	SIRS (n = 20) HC (n = 25)	ACCP/SCCM 1991	PATHFAST
Cakir Madenci et al. [27]	Turkey	38.5/44	ICU	26/11	Plasma	Presented to ICU with burn	Burn patients without sepsis (n = 11)	ABA	PATHFAST
Nakamura et al. [34]	Japan	70	ICU	37/75	Serum	ICU admission	Non-sepsis (n = 75)	ACCP/SCCM 1991	PATHFAST
Sargentini et al. [36]	Italy	55/53	CCU	60/44	Plasma	CCU admission	SIRS (n = 14) HC (n = 30)	ACCP/SCCM 1991	PATHFAST

Table 1 continued

References	Country	Mean age (years) total or case/control	Patient source	Sepsis/control (*n*)	Specimen tested	Inclusion criteria	Controls	Reference	Tests
Godnic et al. [30]	Slovenia	Not provided	ICU	40/7	Plasma	Presented to ICU with ≥ 2 criteria for SIRS	SIRS (n = 7)	Blood culture	PATHFAST
Takahashi et al. [37]	Japan	80	ED and ICU	359/97	Whole blood	Presented to ED with ≥ 1 criteria for SIRS	SIRS (n = 97)	ACCP/SCCM 1991	PATHFAST
Carpio et al. [28]	Peru	34/69	ICU	114/9	Plasma	Presented to ICU with SIRS and suspected infection	SIRS (n = 9)	ACCP/SCCM 1991	PATHFAST
Kada Klouche et al. [41]	France	58	ICU	100/44	Plasma	Presented to ICU with suspected infection	SIRS (n = 44)	Sepsis 3.0	PATHFAST
Romualdo et al. [40]	Spain	73/69	ED	70/130	Plasma	Presented to ED with suspected infection	Non-complicated infection (n = 130)	Sepsis 3.0	PATHFAST

ABA American Burn Association, *ACCP* American College of Chest Physicians, *ED* emergency department, *HC* healthy control, *ICU* intensive care unit, *postoperative control* major abdominal surgery without any evidence of infection, *SCCM* Society of Critical Care Medicine, *SIRS* systemic inflammatory response syndrome, *SSIDCM* Spanish Society of Infectious Diseases and Clinical Microbiology

Table 2 Diagnostic accuracy of the included studies

References	Thresholds (pg/mL)	AUC	Sensitivity	Specificity	TP	FP	FN	TN
Shozushima et al. [17]	415	0.85	0.80	0.81	81	8	20	33
Endo et al. [29]	600	0.91	0.88	0.81	101	13	14	57
Liu et al. [33]	317	0.82	0.71	0.86	481	40	199	239
Ulla et al. [38]	600	0.70	0.79	0.62	84	32	22	51
Vodnik et al. [39]	630	1.00	1	0.98	30	2	0	98
Behnes et al. [25]	700	0.84	0.90	0.60	73	6	8	9
Brenner et al. [26]	825	0.83	0.91	0.33	55	40	5	20
Romualdo et al. [35]	729	0.75	0.81	0.63	30	70	7	119
Ishikura et al. [31]	647	0.89	0.93	0.76	40	9	3	30
Kweon et al. [32]	430	0.94	0.88	0.82	64	8	9	37
Cakir Madenci et al. [27]	542	0.83	0.77	0.76	20	3	6	8
Nakamura et al. [34]	670	0.78	0.70	0.81	26	14	11	61
Sargentini et al. [36]	600	0.89	0.86	0.72	52	12	8	32
Godnic et al. [30]	413	0.71	0.85	0.63	34	3	6	4
Takahashi et al. [37]	685	0.89	0.80	0.83	285	16	74	81
Carpio et al. [28]	370	0.74	0.81	0.75	92	2	22	7
Kada Klouche et al. [41]	466	0.75	0.90	0.55	90	20	10	24
Romualdo et al. [40]	849	0.78	0.67	0.81	47	25	23	105

TP true positive, *FP* false positive, *FN* false negative, *TN* true negative, *AUC* area under the receiver operating characteristic curve

Table 3 Quality assessment for 18 studies (QUADAS-2)

Study	Risk of bias				Applicability concerns		
	Patient selection	Index test	Reference standard	Flow and timing	Patient selection	Index test	Reference standard
Shozushima [17]	?	☹	☺	☺	☺	☺	☺
Endo [29]	☺	☹	☺	?	☺	☺	☺
Liu [33]	☺	☹	☺	☺	☺	☺	☺
Ulla [38]	☺	☹	☺	?	☺	☺	☺
Vodnik [39]	☺	☹	☺	☺	☹	☺	☺
Behnes [25]	☺	☹	☺	☺	☹	☺	☺
Brenner [26]	☺	☹	☺	☺	☹	☺	☺
Romualdo [35]	☺	☹	☺	☺	☺	☺	☹
Ishikura [31]	☺	☹	☺	?	☺	☺	☺
Kweon [32]	☺	☹	☺	☺	☺	☺	☺
Cakir Madenci [27]	☺	☹	☺	☺	☹	☺	☺
Nakamura [34]	☺	☹	☺	☺	☹	☹	☺
Sargentini [36]	☺	☹	☺	?	?	☺	☺
Godnic [30]	?	☹	☺	☺	?	☺	☺
Takahashi [37]	☺	☹	☺	☺	☺	☺	☺
Carpio [28]	☺	☹	☺	☺	☺	☺	☺
Kada Klouche [41]	☺	☹	☺	☺	☺	☺	☺
Romualdo [40]	☺	☹	☺	☺	☺	☺	☺

☺ Low Risk ☹ High Risk ? Unclear Risk

Investigation of heterogeneity

From visual inspection of the SROC curve (Fig. 5a) and the estimation of the Spearman correlation coefficient ($\rho = -0.26$, $p = 0.31$), we concluded that heterogeneity was unlikely due to the diagnostic threshold effect. Significant heterogeneity in both sensitivities (Cochrane $Q = 137.43$, $p < 0.001$, $I^2 = 87.63\%$) and specificities (Cochrane $Q = 180.76$, $p < 0.001$, $I^2 = 90.60\%$) were found among all included studies for the non-threshold effect. The results of univariable meta-regression revealed that studies conducted in Asia, patients admitted in intensive care units, studies with whole blood specimens, sample sizes greater than 150, proportion of patients with sepsis greater than 0.5, and cut-off values greater than 700 accounted for the heterogeneity of sensitivity, whereas patient admitted in intensive care units, percentage of patients with sepsis great than 50%, and cut-off values great than 700 accounted for the heterogeneity of specificity (Table 4; Fig. 6).

Results of subgroup analyses

In subgroup analyses, we found lower pooled sensitivity and higher pooled specificity in the Asian countries (0.81 vs. 0.86, $p < 0.05$; 0.82 vs. 0.70, $p < 0.05$, respectively,

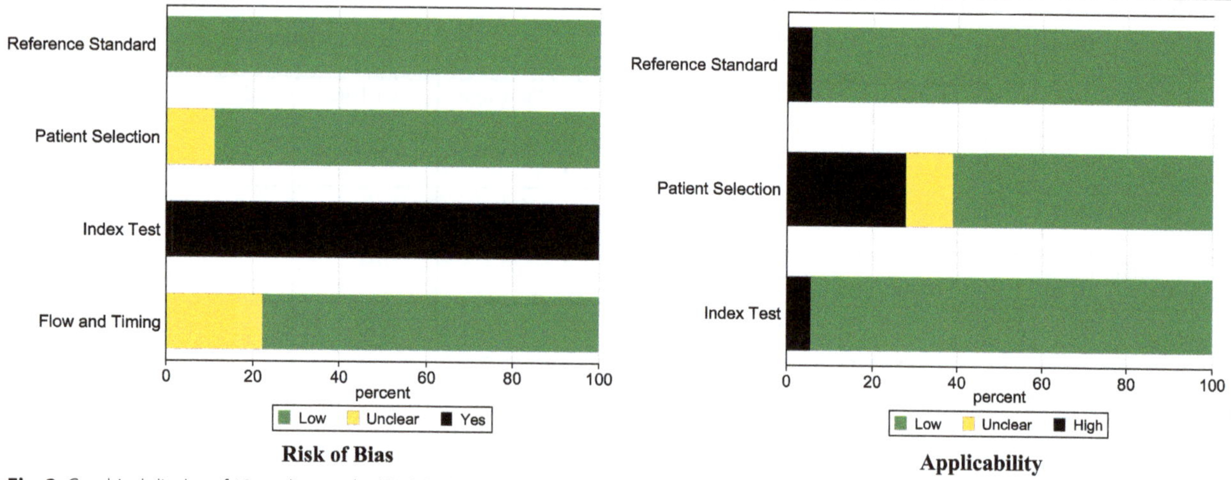

Fig. 2 Graphical display of 18 studies results (QUADAS-2)

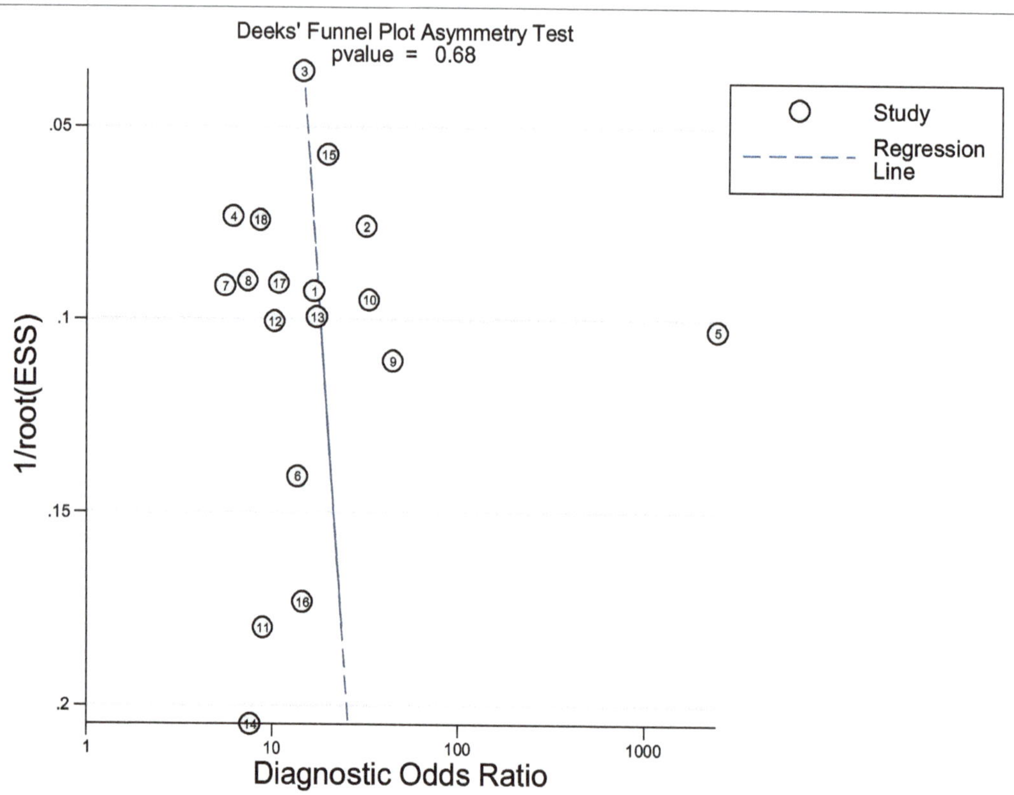

Fig. 3 Deeks' funnel plot asymmetry test for publication bias

Table 4). Furthermore, the higher pooled specificity in the non-ICU settings (0.82 vs. 0.64), whole blood specimens (0.82 vs. 0.71), lower than 50% of patients with sepsis (0.86 vs. 0.72), cut-off values great than 700 (0.80 vs. 0.59, all $p < 0.05$, Table 4) were found.

Seven of the included studies [31–33, 35, 38–40], comprising 1904 patients, were performed in ED, and eight [25–28, 30, 34, 36, 41], comprising 783 patients, were in ICU (Table 1). We performed a subgroup analysis restricted to these two groups because of the possibility

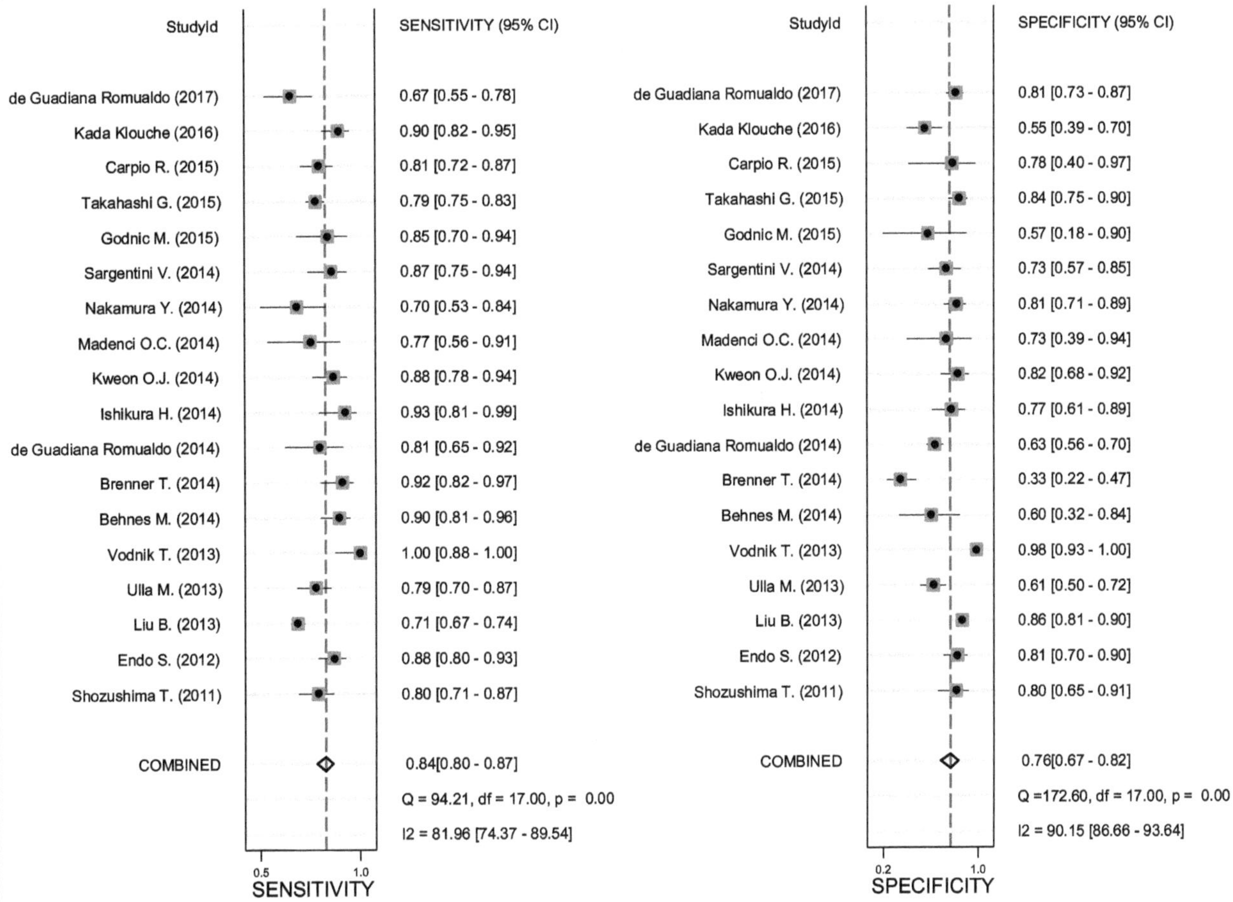

Fig. 4 Forest plots of the sensitivity and specificity for presepsin across all included studies

that different levels of severity existed between them. The pooled specificity was higher in ED versus ICU (0.82, 95% CI 0.69–0.91 vs. 0.64, 95% CI 0.51–0.76). The AUC indicated the possible better accuracy of presepsin in ED than in ICU (0.91 vs. 0.85).

Different compositions of control group

Among the included studies, five studies [27, 29, 31, 34, 39] recorded the diagnosis accuracy between healthy control and sepsis, eight studies [17, 28, 30, 35, 37, 38, 40, 41] recorded it between non-infectious SIRS and sepsis, and five studies [25, 26, 32, 33, 36] recorded it between mixed controls (SIRS and normal) and sepsis. We found the higher pooled sensitivity, specificity, AUC, and DOR for the first group (0.88, 0.82, 0.88, 26, respectively, Table 5). The cut-off values for presepsin used in these three groups ranged from 542–670, 370–849, and 317–825 pg/ml, respectively, and the median cut-off was 618 pg/ml (IQR 600–647), 533 pg/ml (IQR 415–696), and 574 pg/ml (IQR 430–700), respectively.

Performance comparison with PCT and CRP

The summary diagnostic accuracy of the included studies for biomarkers, presepsin, PCT, and CRP is summarized in Table 6. From Table 7 and Fig. 5b, c, we found no significant difference between presepsin and PCT in 13 studies comprising 2915 patients. Furthermore, the pooled sensitivity of presepsin was found to be higher than PCT in 5 studies conducted in ICU comprising 452 patients (0.88, 95% CI 0.82–0.92 vs. 0.75, 95% CI 0.68–0.81), while the pooled specificity of presepsin was lower than PCT (0.58, 95% CI 0.42–0.73 vs. 0.75, 95% CI 0.65–0.83). Additionally, the analysis results revealed that the AUC of presepsin was similar with CRP (0.85 vs. 0.85) in seven studies comprising 1204 patients.

Among these 13 studies that have a direct comparison between presepsin and PCT, seven studies defined the 'gold standard' by the criterions defined in the 1991 ACCP/SCCM consensus conference. The results revealed that the performance of presepsin was similar with PCT in these seven studies (Table 7). Similarly, among the

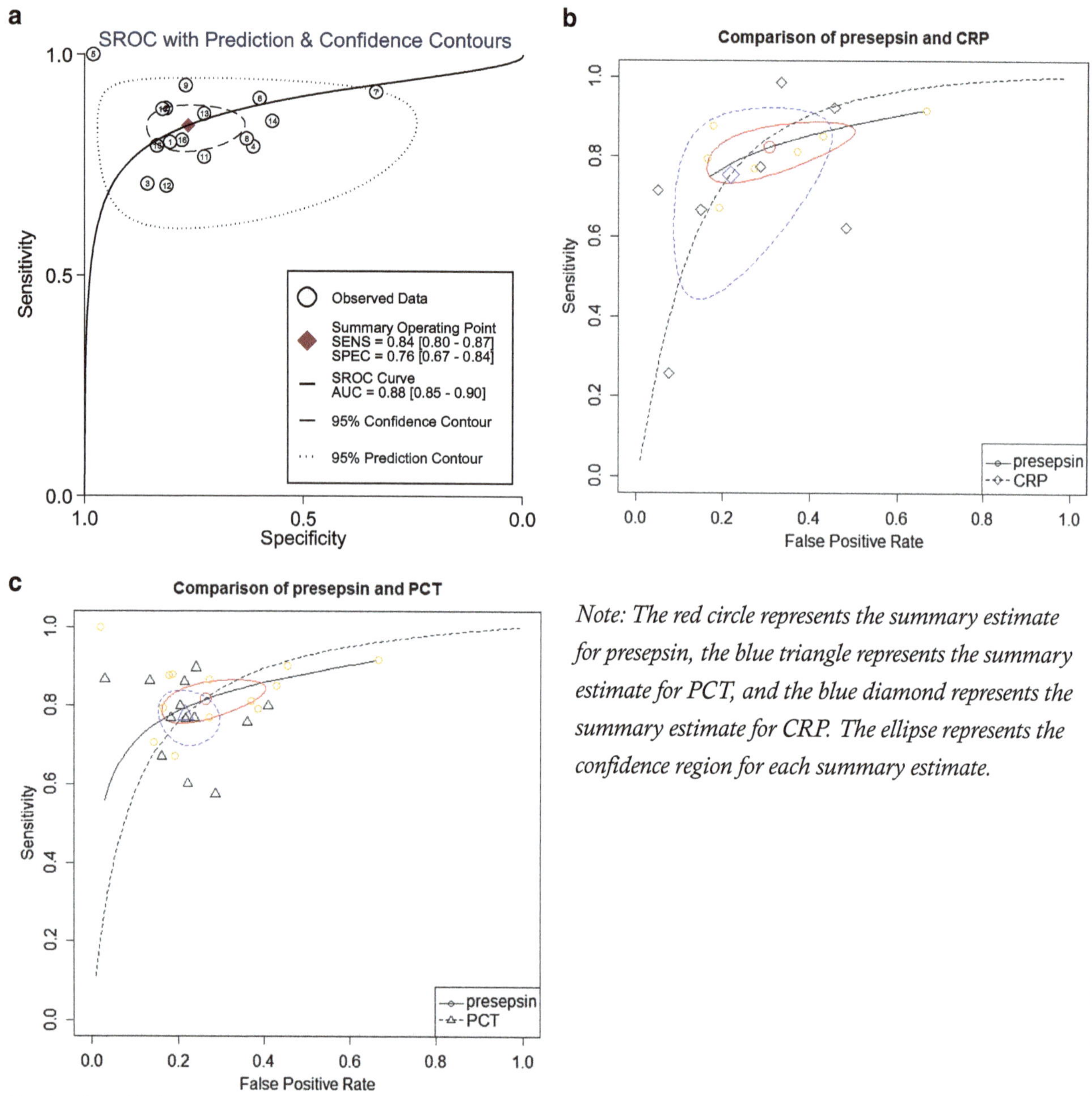

Fig. 5 **a** Hierarchical summary receiver operating characteristic plot of presepsin across all included studies. **b** Comparisons of presepsin and C-reactive protein with summary receiver operating characteristic curves. **c** Comparisons of presepsin and procalcitonin with summary receiver operating characteristic curves. *Note* the *red circle* represents the summary estimate for presepsin, the *blue triangle* represents the summary estimate for procalcitonin, and the *blue diamond* represents the summary estimate for C-reactive protein. The *ellipse* represents the confidence region for each summary estimate

seven studies that compared presepsin with CRP, there were three studies that utilized the criterions defined in the 1991 ACCP/SCCM consensus conference as 'gold standard', and the results revealed that CRP has higher pooled specificity (0.85 vs. 0.69) and AUC (0.91 vs. 0.87) than presepsin. However, the study numbers utilizing other criteria (sepsis 3.0, ABA, SEIMC) were too small to perform the subgroup meta-analysis.

Optimal cut-off

From Fig. 7, the difference between these two fitted lines, known as Youden index, varied by different cut-offs. The cut-off that maximized the Youden index was 600–650 pg/ml. Considering the varied cut-off values between studies, we calculated the pooled sensitivity and specificity for four studies [25, 26, 35, 40] with cut-off values great than 700 pg/ml and for the other 14 studies [17,

Table 4 Summary of subgroup analysis of the included studies by the potentially influencing variables

Variable	Category	Number of studies	Number of patients	Pooled sensitivity	Pooled specificity
Asian country	Yes	8	2091	0.81 (0.76–0.86)	0.82 (0.78–0.85)
	No	10	1379	0.86 (0.80–0.90)	0.70 (0.54–0.83)
Patients admitted in ICU	Yes	8	783	0.86 (0.80–0.90)	0.64 (0.51–0.76)
	No	10	2687	0.83 (0.76–0.89)	0.82 (0.73–0.88)
Whole blood specimen	Yes	6	1942	0.83 (0.73–0.88)	0.82 (0.78–0.86)
	No	12	1528	0.84 (0.79–0.89)	0.71 (0.58–0.82)
Sample sizes great than 150	Yes	6	2215	0.78 (0.72–0.83)	0.77 (0.68–0.84)
	No	12	1255	0.87 (0.82–0.90)	0.75 (0.62–0.84)
Proportions of patients with sepsis great than 0.5	Yes	14	2802	0.84 (0.80–0.88)	0.72 (0.63–0.79)
	No	4	668	0.85 (0.55–0.96)	0.86 (0.63–0.95)
Cut-off value great than 700	Yes	4	642	0.85 (0.70–0.93)	0.59 (0.37–0.78)
	No	14	2828	0.84 (0.79–0.87)	0.80 (0.72–0.85)

27–34, 36–39, 41] that cut-off value smaller than 700 pg/ml. We found the lower pooled specificity in the cut-off values greater than 700 pg/ml studies (0.59 vs. 0.80, $p < 0.05$, respectively, Table 4).

Discussion

As sepsis is the leading cause of death among critically ill patients, early diagnosis of sepsis is often essential for the following treatment to improve outcomes. Since clinical signs of sepsis often overlap with systemic inflammatory response syndrome (SIRS) [12], an effective biomarker is needed to distinguish sepsis from non-infectious SIRS. Presepsin, which is part of CD14, can be detected in the blood and its level elevates closely related to the immune response to LPS [16]. A previous study also found the level of presepsin measured from patients with infection could be well distinguished from those measured from patients without infection, which has indicated that presepsin might be a promising biomarker in diagnosing sepsis from the physiological aspect [29].

To our knowledge, there have been five meta-analyses published recently evaluating the diagnostic value of presepsin [46–50]. However, we found that some of them were designed sub-optimally regarding study eligibility. In addition, in their subgroup analyses revealed strong heterogeneity due to small samples sizes and lower percentages of patients with sepsis between studies. Moreover, most of them mentioned the requirement of comparison with other biomarkers. Our meta-analysis not only included more recently studies but also compared presepsin with other biomarkers (PCT and CRP). Additional subgroup analyses were also conducted due to high heterogeneity between studies. Besides, potential influences caused by different compositions of control groups and different timings when biomarkers were measured were also assessed.

After reviewing 18 studies, a total of up to 3470 patients were included. Our results suggested good overall diagnostic accuracy for presepsin according to the pooled sensitivity and specificity and AUC value. As it is often not easy to give a clinical explanation for a test result directly from the AUC value, which indicates an overall accuracy for diagnosis, we provided a more understandable clinical explanation of the results of the pooled positive likelihood ratio (PLR: 3.4) and the negative likelihood ratio (NLR: 0.22). The clinical explanation for PLR and NLR suggested that it could be nearly four times more likely for a patient to have sepsis with a positive presepsin result and only one-fourth for a patient with a negative presepsin result. However, further studies for the diagnostic performance of presepsin were still needed due to a few possible issues found for presepsin according to the results of our subgroup analyses.

The different definitions of control groups could be one of the possible sources of heterogeneity among those included studies. Instead of distinguishing sepsis from normal healthy controls, the methods to distinguish non-infectious SIRS from sepsis were truly necessary in the real world clinical situation. However, normal healthy controls might be included in the clinical trials for good diagnostic outcomes. From our result (see Table 5), we found lower diagnostic accuracy when leaving out the normal healthy controls from control groups (AUC value 0.84). Consequently, the reliability of the pooled result could be called into question. Therefore, we recommended that future studies avoid the case–control design as QUADAS-2 suggested [21].

Another possible source of heterogeneity came from the use of different specimen types. Our subgroup analysis result suggested that the use of whole blood had higher specificity than plasma, with statistical significance. Nevertheless, a simple adjustment might

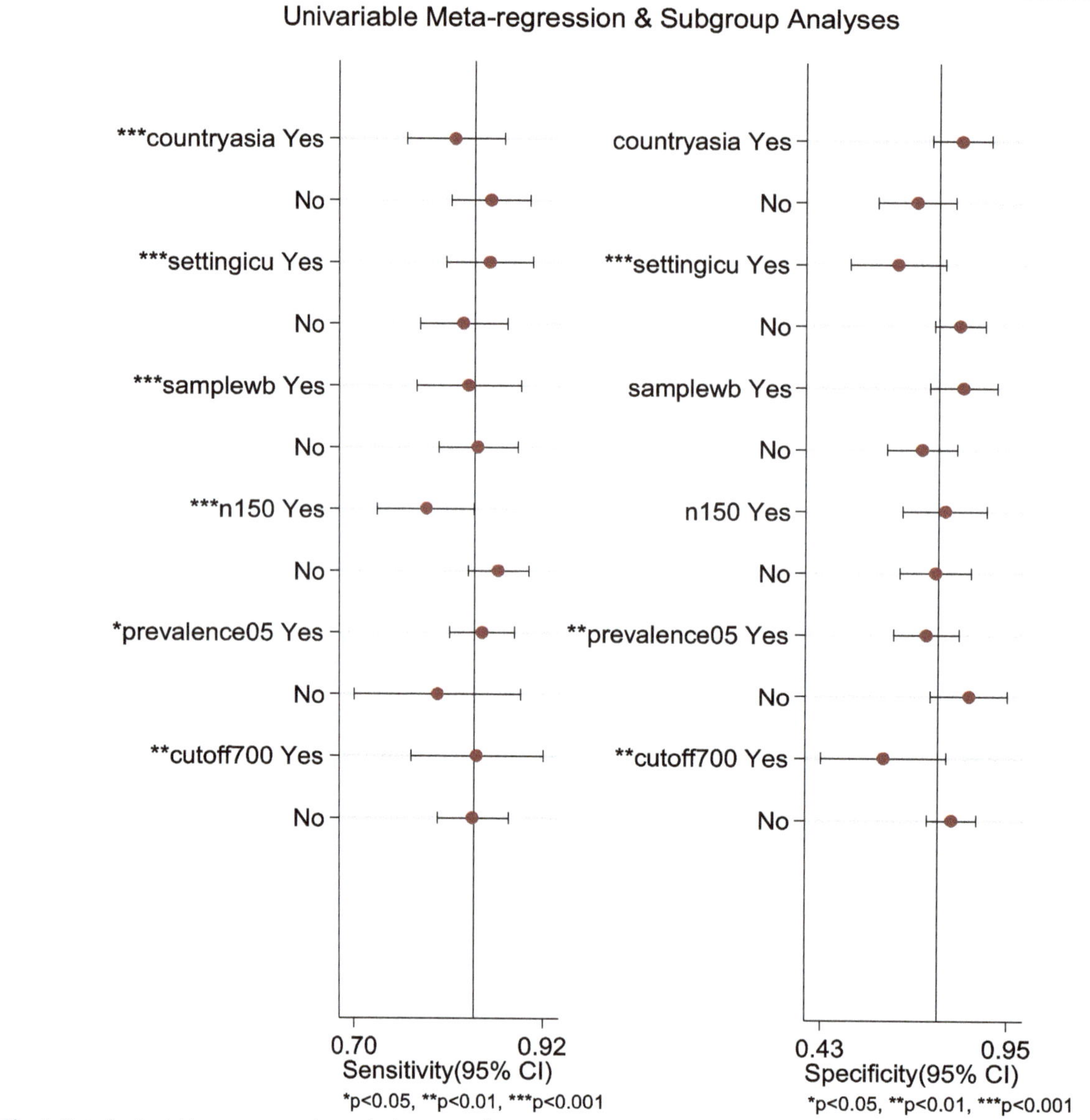

Fig. 6 Plot of univariable meta-regression and subgroup analysis

Table 5 Summaries of pooled sensitivity and specificity of presepsin to diagnose sepsis for different compositions of control group

Case	Control	Number of studies	Number of patients	Pooled sensitivity	Pooled specificity	AUC	Pooled DOR	Median cut-off
Sepsis	Healthy	5	546	0.88 (0.70–0.96)	0.82 (0.75–0.88)	0.88	26 (9–75)	618
Sepsis	Mixed	5	1397	0.86 (0.76–0.92)	0.68 (0.47–0.83)	0.86	15 (9–23)	574
Sepsis	Non-infectious SIRS	8	1527	0.81 (0.76–0.85)	0.71 (0.63–0.78)	0.84	10 (8–15)	533

be sufficient enough to eliminate the bias. A previous study revealed that, when measured using PATHFAST system, cardiac troponin I (cTnI), myoglobin, MB isoenzyme of creatine kinase (CK–MB), and N-terminal probrain natriuretic peptide (NT-proBNP) were shown to have a highly correlated linear relationship (correlation coefficients >0.9, calculated by Passing–Bablok regression analysis) between two types of samples [51].

Table 6 Summary diagnostic accuracy of the included studies for biomarkers, presepsin, procalcitonin, and C-reactive protein

References	Sepsis/control (*n*)	Presepsin			Procalcitonin			C-reactive protein		
		Sensitivity	Specificity	AUC	Sensitivity	Specificity	AUC	Sensitivity	Specificity	AUC
Shozushima et al. [17]	101/41	0.80	0.81	0.88	–	–	0.65	–	–	0.82
Endo et al. [29]	115/70	0.88	0.81	0.91	0.86	0.79	0.91	–	–	–
Liu et al. [33]	680/279	0.71	0.86	0.82	0.60	0.78	0.72	–	–	–
Ulla et al. [38]	106/83	0.79	0.62	0.70	0.89	0.76	0.88	–	–	–
Vodnik et al. [39]	30/100	1	0.98	0.99	0.87	0.97	0.96	–	–	0.96
Behnes et al. [25]	81/15	0.90	0.60	0.84	–	–	0.86	–	–	–
Brenner et al. [26]	60/60	0.91	0.67	0.83	0.77	0.78	0.84	0.67	0.85	0.79
Romualdo et al. [35]	37/189	0.81	0.63	0.75	0.76	0.64	0.79	0.62	0.52	0.60
Ishikura et al. [31]	43/39	0.93	0.76	0.89	–	–	–	–	–	–
Kweon et al. [32]	73/45	0.88	0.82	0.94	0.86	0.87	0.92	0.99	0.67	0.85
Cakir Madenci et al. [27]	26/11	0.77	0.76	0.83	0.76	0.79	0.85	0.92	0.58	0.82
Nakamura et al. [34]	37/75	0.70	0.81	0.78	–	–	–	–	–	–
Sargentini et al. [36]	60/44	0.86	0.72	0.89	0.80	0.80	0.91	–	–	–
Godnic et al. [30]	40/7	0.85	0.63	0.71	0.58	0.67	0.63	0.77	0.75	0.73
Takahashi et al. [37]	359/97	0.80	0.83	0.89	0.77	0.76	0.85	0.72	0.95	0.82
Carpio et al. [28]	114/9	0.81	0.75	0.83	–	–	–	–	–	–
Kada Klouche et al. [41]	100/44	0.90	0.55	0.75	0.80	0.59	0.80	–	–	–
Romualdo et al. [40]	70/130	0.67	0.81	0.78	0.67	0.84	0.82	0.26	0.92	0.59

AUC, area under the receiver operating characteristic curve; –, not report

Table 7 Summaries of performance statistics of presepsin, procalcitonin, and C-reactive protein for diagnosing sepsis

Category	Biomarkers	Number of studies	Number of patients	Pooled sensitivity	Pooled specificity	AUC	Pooled DOR
All	Presepsin	13	2915	0.84 (0.79–0.88)	0.75 (0.64–0.84)	0.87 (0.84–0.90)	16 (8–30)
	Procalcitonin	13	2915	0.78 (0.72–0.83)	0.79 (0.73–0.85)	0.86 (0.82–0.88)	14 (8–23)
All	Presepsin	7	1204	0.83 (0.76–0.88)	0.70 (0.55–0.81)	0.85 (0.81–0.88)	11 (7–18)
	C-reactive protein	7	1204	0.77 (0.53–0.91)	0.79 (0.62–0.89)	0.85 (0.82–0.88)	13 (5–36)
ED	Presepsin	6	1822	0.83 (0.68–0.92)	0.83 (0.67–0.92)	0.90 (0.87–0.92)	24 (5–113)
	Procalcitonin	6	1822	0.79 (0.68–0.87)	0.83 (0.72–0.91)	0.88 (0.85–0.90)	19 (7–52)
ICU	Presepsin	5	452	0.88 (0.82–0.92)	0.58 (0.42–0.73)	0.87 (0.84–0.90)	10 (5–18)
	Procalcitonin	5	452	0.75 (0.68–0.81)	0.75 (0.65–0.83)	0.82 (0.78–0.85)	9 (6–15)
Sepsis-1/2	Presepsin	7	2076	0.86 (0.76–0.91)	0.79 (0.60–0.91)	0.90 (0.87–0.92)	23 (7–77)
	Procalcitonin	7	2076	0.80 (0.72–0.87)	0.83 (0.75–0.89)	0.89 (0.86–0.91)	20 (9–45)
Sepsis-1/2	Presepsin	3	694	0.86 (0.75–0.93)	0.69 (0.33–0.90)	0.87 (0.83–0.91)	16 (6–38)
	C-reactive protein	3	694	0.86 (0.44–0.98)	0.85 (0.63–0.95)	0.91 (0.86–0.93)	34 (9–127)

However, whether there is also a linear relationship existing between two types of sampling methods for presepsin is still not confirmed. Therefore, we suggested future studies to examine the relationship for this possible bias.

Interestingly, we found lower pooled specificity among patients who were admitted to the ICUs. We suggest that higher proportion of critically ill patients in the ICU might be a possible source. However, this finding could be difficult to explain clinically, since it could come from numerous other possible sources. More information is needed to explore this result in more detail.

PCT is a biomarker currently used for diagnosis of sepsis [9, 10], and its diagnostic accuracy has been widely studied. From a meta-analysis of PCT in 2007 [11], PCT seemed to become widely studied since 1999 [52, 53], while the earliest study we found for presepsin was in 2011 [17]. This might indicate that presepsin was still not a well-studied biomarker compared to PCT. In

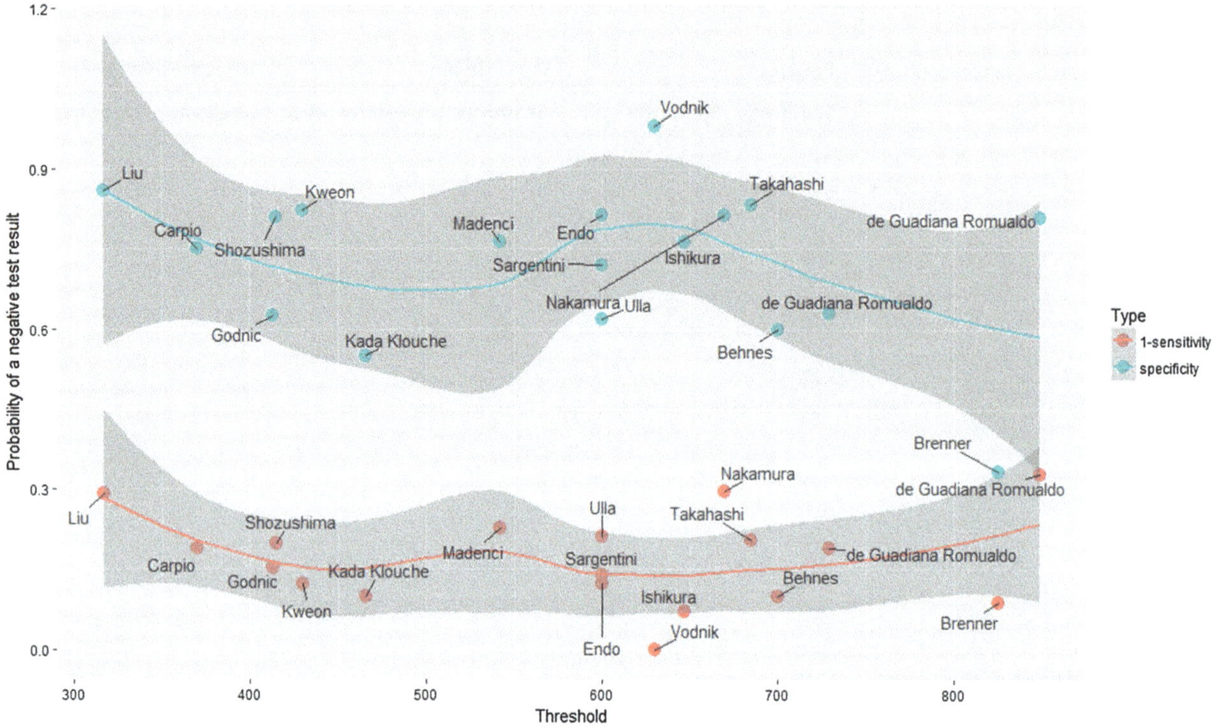

Fig. 7 Plot for solve the 'optimal cut-off'

addition, a previous study revealed that the presepsin level typically elevates earlier than PCT [14]. We have tried to replicate the result by performing a subgroup analysis to compare the diagnostic accuracy of presepsin with PCT in the ED, which approximately represented the earlier stage of sepsis. However, we did not find any significant difference between presepsin and PCT measured in either EDs (AUC 0.90 and 0.88) or ICUs (AUC 0.87 and 0.82). Besides, from our subgroup analysis result for these studies, we found similar diagnostic accuracy between presepsin (AUC 0.87) and PCT (AUC 0.86), which indicates that presepsin is a promising biomarker for study. Our current results suggested no obvious better performance of presepsin than PCT in the diagnosis of sepsis. Further studies focusing on the diagnostic accuracy difference between presepsin and PCT might still be needed.

Although CRP is another commonly used biomarker in the clinical context, previous studies revealed that its diagnostic accuracy for sepsis is significantly lower than PCT [11]. But, after comparing presepsin with CRP, we observed no significant difference between CRP (AUC 0.85) and presepsin (AUC 0.85). Furthermore, the confidence region overlapped from the sensitivity versus FPR curve is summarized in Fig. 5b, c. Our results supported that presepsin showed similar performance with CRP in sepsis diagnosis.

The strengths of this systematic review and meta-analysis include (1) the performance of presepsin was formally compared with PCT and CRP; (2) detailed subgroup analyses were utilized to solve the heterogeneity between the included studies; (3) different compositions of control groups (healthy control, non-infectious SIRS, and mixed) were compared in the subgroup analysis; (4) the timing of biomarker measurements and different specimen types were taken into account in the analysis; and (5) the optimal cut-off was attempted to be determined in this study.

There were some limitations for our study. First, most studies we included diagnosed sepsis using reference standard from ACCP/SCCM 1991 (10 studies) and 2001 (2 studies) (Sepsis 1.0 or 2.0) instead of the newly defined Sepsis 3.0 [43]. Clinical trials are still needed to re-evaluate the performance and the optimal cut-off of presepsin accordingly. Second, although we have included 18 studies in our study, the statistical power might still be not enough to confirm the diagnostic value of presepsin. Finally, as we only include studies written in English, there may be some language bias in our study.

Conclusions

Based on the results of our meta-analysis, presepsin is a promising marker for diagnosis of sepsis as PCT or CRP, but these results should be interpreted carefully and cautiously, since only a limited number of studies included and high heterogeneity between them. Additionally, it cannot be recommended as a single test for sepsis diagnosis, but may be useful in combination with some sensitive biological markers. In addition, continuing re-evaluation during the course of sepsis is advisable.

Abbreviations

ABA: American Burn Association; AUC: area under the receiver operating characteristic curve; CRP: C-reactive protein; CI: confidence interval; DOR: diagnostic odds ratio; ED: emergency department; HSROC: hierarchical summary receiver operating characteristic; ICU: intensive care unit; LBP: lipopolysaccharide-binding protein; LPS: lipopolysaccharide; LR: likelihood ratio; NLR: negative likelihood ratio; PCT: procalcitonin; PLR: positive likelihood ratio; QUADAS: Quality Assessment of Diagnostic Accuracy Studies; SEIMC: Spanish Society of Infectious Diseases and Clinical Microbiology; SIRS: systemic inflammatory response syndrome; SROC: summary receiver operating characteristic; TREM-1: myeloid cells expressing triggering receptor-1.

Authors' contributions

KFC, CCW, and HML contributed to manuscript preparation. KFC, CCW, and HML contributed to review and revision. KFC and CCW contributed to statistical analysis. CCW and HML contributed to quality assessment. CHC, STH, CFY, SHL, and CHL contributed to study selection and data extraction. All authors read and approved the final manuscript.

Author details

[1] Department of Emergency Medicine, Chang Gung Memorial Hospital, Keelung, Taiwan. [2] School of Medicine, Chang Gung University, Taoyuan, Taiwan. [3] Department of Emergency Medicine, Chang Gung Memorial Hospital, Linkou, Taiwan. [4] Division of Infectious Diseases, Department of Internal Medicine, Chang Gung Memorial Hospital at Linkou, Chang Gung University College of Medicine, Taoyuan, Taiwan. [5] Department of Family Medicine, Chang Gung Memorial Hospital, Linkou, Taiwan. [6] Clinical Informatics and Medical Statistics Research Center, Chang Gung University, 5 Fu-Shin Street, Gueishan Village, Taoyuan 333, Taiwan. [7] Community Medicine Research Center, Chang Gung Memorial Hospital, Keelung, Taiwan.

Acknowledgements

Not applicable.

Competing interests

The authors declare that they have no competing interests.

Funding

The study was supported by the National Science Council and Chang Gung Memorial Hospital in Taiwan (106-2314-B-182-028, CRRPG2B0125, CIRPG2E0022, CMRPG3F1851, and CMRPG2D0012). The funders had no role in study design, data collection and analysis, decision to publish, or preparation of the manuscript.

References

1. Zou Q, Wen W, Zhang XC. Presepsin as a novel sepsis biomarker. World J Emerg Med. 2014;5(1):16–9.
2. Mitaka C. Clinical laboratory differentiation of infectious versus non-infectious systemic inflammatory response syndrome. Clin Chim Acta. 2005;351(1–2):17–29.
3. Chen KF, Chaou CH, Jiang JY, Yu HW, Meng YH, Tang WC, Wu CC. Diagnostic accuracy of lipopolysaccharide-binding protein as biomarker for sepsis in adult patients: a systematic review and meta-analysis. PLoS ONE. 2016;11(4):e0153188.
4. Guignant C, Voirin N, Venet F, Poitevin F, Malcus C, Bohe J, Lepape A, Monneret G. Assessment of pro-vasopressin and pro-adrenomedullin as predictors of 28-day mortality in septic shock patients. Intensive Care Med. 2009;35(11):1859–67.
5. Lu YH, Liu L, Qiu XH, Yu Q, Yang Y, Qiu HB. Effect of early goal directed therapy on tissue perfusion in patients with septic shock. World J Emerg Med. 2013;4(2):117–22.
6. Seligman R, Papassotiriou J, Morgenthaler NG, Meisner M, Teixeira PJ. Prognostic value of midregional pro-atrial natriuretic peptide in ventilator-associated pneumonia. Intensive Care Med. 2008;34(11):2084–91.
7. Wu HP, Chen CK, Chung K, Jiang BY, Yu TJ, Chuang DY. Plasma transforming growth factor-beta1 level in patients with severe community-acquired pneumonia and association with disease severity. J Formos Med Assoc. 2009;108(1):20–7.
8. Rhodes A, Evans LE, Alhazzani W, Levy MM, Antonelli M, Ferrer R, Kumar A, Sevransky JE, Sprung CL, Nunnally ME, et al. Surviving Sepsis Campaign: international guidelines for management of sepsis and septic shock: 2016. Crit Care Med. 2017;45(3):486–552.
9. Julian-Jimenez A, Candel-Gonzalez FJ, Gonzalez Del Castillo J. Usefulness of inflammation and infection biomarkers in the Emergency Department. Enferm Infecc Microbiol Clin. 2014;32(3):177–90.
10. Kibe S, Adams K, Barlow G. Diagnostic and prognostic biomarkers of sepsis in critical care. J Antimicrob Chemother. 2011;66(Suppl 2):ii33–40.
11. Tang BM, Eslick GD, Craig JC, McLean AS. Accuracy of procalcitonin for sepsis diagnosis in critically ill patients: systematic review and meta-analysis. Lancet Infect Dis. 2007;7(3):210–7.
12. Wacker C, Prkno A, Brunkhorst FM, Schlattmann P. Procalcitonin as a diagnostic marker for sepsis: a systematic review and meta-analysis. Lancet Infect Dis. 2013;13(5):426–35.
13. Volanakis JE. Human C-reactive protein: expression, structure, and function. Mol Immunol. 2001;38(2–3):189–97.
14. Okamura Y, Yokoi H. Development of a point-of-care assay system for measurement of presepsin (sCD14-ST). Clin Chim Acta. 2011;412(23–24):2157–61.
15. Gong XW, Jiang Y. Structure, function and modulation of actin-related protein 2/3 complex. Sheng Li Ke Xue Jin Zhan. 2004;35(4):306–10.
16. Mussap M, Noto A, Fravega M, Fanos V. Soluble CD14 subtype presepsin (sCD14-ST) and lipopolysaccharide binding protein (LBP) in neonatal sepsis: new clinical and analytical perspectives for two old biomarkers. J Matern Fetal Neonatal Med. 2011;24(Suppl 2):12–4.
17. Shozushima T, Takahashi G, Matsumoto N, Kojika M, Okamura Y, Endo S. Usefulness of presepsin (sCD14-ST) measurements as a marker for the diagnosis and severity of sepsis that satisfied diagnostic criteria of systemic inflammatory response syndrome. J Infect Chemother. 2011;17(6):764–9.
18. Shirakawa K, Naitou K, Hirose J, Takahashi T, Furusako S. Presepsin (sCD14-ST): development and evaluation of one-step ELISA with a new standard that is similar to the form of presepsin in septic patients. Clin Chem Lab Med. 2011;49(5):937–9.
19. Moher D, Liberati A, Tetzlaff J, Altman DG, Group P. Preferred reporting items for systematic reviews and meta-analyses: the PRISMA statement. J Clin Epidemiol. 2009;62(10):1006–12.
20. Landis JR, Koch GG. The measurement of observer agreement for categorical data. Biometrics. 1977;33(1):159–74.
21. Whiting PF, Rutjes AW, Westwood ME, Mallett S, Deeks JJ, Reitsma JB, Leeflang MM, Sterne JA, Bossuyt PM. Group Q-: QUADAS-2: a revised tool for the quality assessment of diagnostic accuracy studies. Ann Intern Med. 2011;155(8):529–36.
22. Rutter CM, Gatsonis CA. A hierarchical regression approach to meta-analysis of diagnostic test accuracy evaluations. Stat Med. 2001;20(19):2865–84.

23. Moses LE, Shapiro D, Littenberg B. Combining independent studies of a diagnostic test into a summary ROC curve: data-analytic approaches and some additional considerations. Stat Med. 1993;12(14):1293–316.
24. Higgins JP, Thompson SG. Quantifying heterogeneity in a meta-analysis. Stat Med. 2002;21(11):1539–58.
25. Behnes M, Bertsch T, Lepiorz D, Lang S, Trinkmann F, Brueckmann M, Borggrefe M, Hoffmann U. Diagnostic and prognostic utility of soluble CD 14 subtype (presepsin) for severe sepsis and septic shock during the first week of intensive care treatment. Crit Care. 2014;18(5):507.
26. Brenner T, Fleming T, Uhle F, Silaff S, Schmitt F, Salgado E, Ulrich A, Zimmermann S, Bruckner T, Martin E, et al. Methylglyoxal as a new biomarker in patients with septic shock: an observational clinical study. Crit Care. 2014;18(6):683.
27. Cakir Madenci O, Yakupoglu S, Benzonana N, Yucel N, Akbaba D, Orcun Kaptanagasi A. Evaluation of soluble CD14 subtype (presepsin) in burn sepsis. Burns. 2014;40(4):664–9.
28. Carpio R, Zapata J, Spanuth E, Hess G. Utility of presepsin (sCD14-ST) as a diagnostic and prognostic marker of sepsis in the emergency department. Clin Chim Acta. 2015;450:169–75.
29. Endo S, Suzuki Y, Takahashi G, Shozushima T, Ishikura H, Murai A, Nishida T, Irie Y, Miura M, Iguchi H, et al. Usefulness of presepsin in the diagnosis of sepsis in a multicenter prospective study. J Infect Chemother. 2012;18(6):891–7.
30. Godnic M, Stubljar D, Skvarc M, Jukic T. Diagnostic and prognostic value of sCD14-ST–presepsin for patients admitted to hospital intensive care unit (ICU). Wien Klin Wochenschr. 2015;127(13–14):521–7.
31. Ishikura H, Nishida T, Murai A, Nakamura Y, Irie Y, Tanaka J, Umemura T. New diagnostic strategy for sepsis-induced disseminated intravascular coagulation: a prospective single-center observational study. Crit Care. 2014;18(1):R19.
32. Kweon OJ, Choi JH, Park SK, Park AJ. Usefulness of presepsin (sCD14 subtype) measurements as a new marker for the diagnosis and prediction of disease severity of sepsis in the Korean population. J Crit Care. 2014;29(6):965–70.
33. Liu B, Chen YX, Yin Q, Zhao YZ, Li CS. Diagnostic value and prognostic evaluation of Presepsin for sepsis in an emergency department. Crit Care. 2013;17(5):R244.
34. Nakamura Y, Ishikura H, Nishida T, Kawano Y, Yuge R, Ichiki R, Murai A. Usefulness of presepsin in the diagnosis of sepsis in patients with or without acute kidney injury. BMC Anesthesiol. 2014;14:88.
35. Romualdo LG, Torrella PE, Gonzalez MV, Sanchez RJ, Holgado AH, Freire AO, Acebes SR, Oton MD. Diagnostic accuracy of presepsin (soluble CD14 subtype) for prediction of bacteremia in patients with systemic inflammatory response syndrome in the Emergency Department. Clin Biochem. 2014;47(7–8):505–8.
36. Sargentini V, Ceccarelli G, D'Alessandro M, Collepardo D, Morelli A, D'Egidio A, Mariotti S, Nicoletti AM, Evangelista B, D'Ettorre G, et al. Presepsin as a potential marker for bacterial infection relapse in critical care patients. A preliminary study. Clin Chem Lab Med. 2015;53(4):567–73.
37. Takahashi G, Shibata S, Ishikura H, Miura M, Fukui Y, Inoue Y, Endo S. Presepsin in the prognosis of infectious diseases and diagnosis of infectious disseminated intravascular coagulation: a prospective, multicentre, observational study. Eur J Anaesthesiol. 2015;32(3):199–206.
38. Ulla M, Pizzolato E, Lucchiari M, Loiacono M, Soardo F, Forno D, Morello F, Lupia E, Moiraghi C, Mengozzi G, et al. Diagnostic and prognostic value of presepsin in the management of sepsis in the emergency department: a multicenter prospective study. Crit Care. 2013;17(4):R168.
39. Vodnik T, Kaljevic G, Tadic T, Majkic-Singh N. Presepsin (sCD14-ST) in preoperative diagnosis of abdominal sepsis. Clin Chem Lab Med. 2013;51(10):2053–62.
40. de Guadiana Romualdo LG, Torrella PE, Acebes SR, Oton MD, Sanchez RJ, Holgado AH, Santos EJ, Freire AO. Diagnostic accuracy of presepsin (sCD14-ST) as a biomarker of infection and sepsis in the emergency department. Clin Chim Acta. 2016;464:6–11.
41. Klouche K, Cristol JP, Devin J, Gilles V, Kuster N, Larcher R, Amigues L, Corne P, Jonquet O, Dupuy AM. Diagnostic and prognostic value of soluble CD14 subtype (Presepsin) for sepsis and community-acquired pneumonia in ICU patients. Ann Intensive Care. 2016;6(1):59.
42. Bone RC, Balk RA, Cerra FB, Dellinger RP, Fein AM, Knaus WA, Schein RM, Sibbald WJ. Definitions for sepsis and organ failure and guidelines for the use of innovative therapies in sepsis. The ACCP/SCCM Consensus Conference Committee. American College of Chest Physicians/Society of Critical Care Medicine. Chest. 1992;101(6):1644–55.
43. Singer M, Deutschman CS, Seymour CW, Shankar-Hari M, Annane D, Bauer M, Bellomo R, Bernard GR, Chiche JD, Coopersmith CM, et al. The third international consensus definitions for sepsis and septic shock (sepsis-3). JAMA. 2016;315(8):801–10.
44. Orta Mira N, Guna Serrano Mdel R, Perez JL, Gimeno Cardona C. Quality assessment program of the Spanish Society of Infectious Diseases and Clinical Microbiology. Analysis of results. 2005. Enferm Infecc Microbiol Clin. 2006;24(Suppl 1):1–7.
45. Greenhalgh DG, Saffle JR, Holmes JHT, Gamelli RL, Palmieri TL, Horton JW, Tompkins RG, Traber DL, Mozingo DW, Deitch EA, et al. American Burn Association consensus conference to define sepsis and infection in burns. J Burn Care Res. 2007;28(6):776–90.
46. Tong X, Cao Y, Yu M, Han C. Presepsin as a diagnostic marker for sepsis: evidence from a bivariate meta-analysis. Ther Clin Risk Manag. 2015;11:1027–33.
47. Wu J, Hu L, Zhang G, Wu F, He T. Accuracy of presepsin in sepsis diagnosis: a systematic review and meta-analysis. PLoS ONE. 2015;10(7):e0133057.
48. Zhang J, Hu ZD, Song J, Shao J. Diagnostic value of presepsin for sepsis: a systematic review and meta-analysis. Medicine (Baltimore). 2015;94(47):e2158.
49. Zhang X, Liu D, Liu YN, Wang R, Xie LX. The accuracy of presepsin (sCD14-ST) for the diagnosis of sepsis in adults: a meta-analysis. Crit Care. 2015;19:323.
50. Zheng Z, Jiang L, Ye L, Gao Y, Tang L, Zhang M. The accuracy of presepsin for the diagnosis of sepsis from SIRS: a systematic review and meta-analysis. Ann Intensive Care. 2015;5(1):48.
51. Kurihara T, Yanagida A, Yokoi H, Koyata A, Matsuya T, Ogawa J, Okamura Y, Miyamoto D. Evaluation of cardiac assays on a benchtop chemiluminescent enzyme immunoassay analyzer, PATHFAST. Anal Biochem. 2008;375(1):144–6.
52. Bossink AW, Groeneveld AB, Thijs LG. Prediction of microbial infection and mortality in medical patients with fever: plasma procalcitonin, neutrophilic elastase-alpha1-antitrypsin, and lactoferrin compared with clinical variables. Clin Infect Dis. 1999;29(2):398–407.
53. Ugarte H, Silva E, Mercan D, De Mendonca A, Vincent JL. Procalcitonin used as a marker of infection in the intensive care unit. Crit Care Med. 1999;27(3):498–504.

12

Cell-cycle arrest biomarkers in urine to predict acute kidney injury in septic and non-septic critically ill patients

M. Cuartero[1*], J. Ballús[2], J. Sabater[2], X. Pérez[2], N. Nin[3], J. Ordonez-Llanos[4] and A. J. Betbesé[1]

Abstract

Purpose: To analyse the usefulness of the composite index of the tissue inhibitor of metalloproteinases-2 (TIMP-2) and insulin-like growth factor-binding protein 7 (IGFBP7) as urinary biomarkers for the early prediction of AKI in septic and non-septic patients.

Methods: This is a prospective, observational study including patients admitted to ICU from acute care departments and hospital length of stay <48 h. The main exclusion criteria were pre-existing eGFR <30 mL/min/1.73 m^2 and hospitalisation 2 months prior to current admission. The [TIMP-2]·[IGFBP7] index was analysed twice, within the first 12 h of ICU admission.

Results: The sample included 98 patients. AKI incidence during ICU stay was 50%. Sepsis was diagnosed in 40.8%. Baseline renal variables were comparable between subgroups except for a higher baseline eGFR in non-septic patients. Patients were stratified based on the presence of AKI and their highest level of [TIMP-2]·[IGFBP7] within the first 12 h of stay. [TIMP-2]·[IGFBP7] index values were dependent on the incidence of AKI but not of sepsis. [TIMP-2]·[IGFBP7] values were significantly related to AKI severity according to AKIN criteria ($p < 0.0001$). The AUROC curve to predict AKI of the worst [TIMP-2]·[IGFBP7] index value was 0.798 (sensitivity 73.5%, specificity 71.4%, $p < 0.0001$). Index values below 0.8 ruled out any need for renal replacement (NPV 100%), whereas an index >0.8 predicted a rate of AKI of 71% and AKIN ≥ 2 of 62.9%.

Conclusions: In our study, urinary [TIMP-2]·[IGFBP7] was an early predictor of AKI in ICU patients regardless of sepsis. Besides, index values <0.8$(ng/mL)^2/1000$ ruled out the need for renal replacement.

Keywords: Acute kidney injury, Biomarkers, Tissue inhibitor of metalloproteinases-2, Insulin-like growth factor-binding protein 7, ICU patients, Sepsis

Background

Acute kidney injury (AKI) is a frequent complication in ICU patients [1]. AKI definitions based on serum creatinine (sCr) have shown a large variation in AKI incidence and associated outcomes [2]. However, it has been observed that AKI requiring renal replacement therapy (RRT) is an independent factor of poor outcome [3, 4], with an associated mortality rate of 50–60% [2, 3].

*Correspondence: mireia.cuartero@gmail.com; mcuartero@santpau.cat
[1] Intensive Care Department and Institut d'Investigacions Biomèdiques, Hospital de la Santa Creu i Sant Pau, Universitat Autònoma de Barcelona, Sant Quintí 89, 08041 Barcelona, Spain
Full list of author information is available at the end of the article

Sepsis is a relevant contributing factor to AKI development. AKI is present in >30% of those with sepsis [5, 6] and in >50% of those with septic shock [7, 8]. Pathogens producing sepsis and their toxins affect the whole body as well as specific organs. Damaging molecules can reach the proximal renal tubular cells in high concentrations and may trigger kidney injury followed by inflammation and oxidative stress and, finally, cell damage [9].

Diagnosis of AKI has changed in the last decade with the advent of RIFLE [10], AKIN [11] and KDIGO [12] classifications. These tools are based on sCr and diuresis. However, sCr is a late and non-specific AKI biomarker [13, 14]. Biomarkers that can rapidly and specifically recognise AKI are therefore needed. A few recent studies have shown that tissue inhibitor of metalloproteinases-2 (TIMP-2) and insulin-like growth factor-binding protein 7 (IGFBP7) are specific biomarkers of structural renal damage in critically ill patients [15, 16]. Renal tubular cells enter in G_1 cell arrest to block the effects of molecules contributing to cell-cycle promotion, such as cyclins. This mechanism prevents the extension of cell damage. TIMP-2 and IGFBP7 are protective molecules involved in G_1 cell-cycle arrest that moderate apoptotic, angiogenic [17], inflammatory [18, 19] and ischaemic processes [20]. Since renal cell arrest usually occurs 24–48 h before sCr rises due to a significant fall in the glomerular filtration rate, TIMP-2 and IGFBP7 are thought to be earlier AKI biomarkers than sCr.

TIMP-2 and IGFBP7 are detectable in urine. Previous studies in unselected ICU populations have shown that when analysed together as the index [TIMP-2]·[IGFBP7], they perform better than sCr, urine and plasma NGAL, plasma cystatin-C and KIM-1 for early detection of AKI and improved risk stratification for renal and general outcomes [15, 16]. The aim of this study was to assess whether values of the TIMP-2 and IGFBP7 index were early predictors of AKI in a selected ICU population free of the most frequent AKI risk factors. To date, the influence of sepsis on TIMP-2 and IGFBP7 expression in critically ill patients is not well defined. As a secondary objective, we thus also evaluated the potential usefulness of [TIMP-2]·[IGFBP7] index in septic ICU patients.

Methods

The study protocol was approved by the institutional review board at each participating centre. We obtained informed consent from patients or their guardians. The study prospectively included patients over 18 years of age with an expected ICU stay of at least 48 h. We included patients admitted to ICU either from the emergency department or after undergoing acute surgery. Exclusion criteria were pregnancy, established anuric AKI, pre-existing chronic kidney disease (CKD) with estimated glomerular filtration rate (eGFR) <30 mL/min/1.73 m^2 and current hospital length of stay >48 h. Medical management was left to the discretion of the attending physicians. All healthcare providers involved were blinded to the biomarkers results.

Sampling and measurement of the [TIMP-2]·[IGFBP7] index

Urine samples for biomarker analysis were collected twice: at ICU admission and up to 12 h later simultaneously with the morning blood work. Urine samples were centrifuged, and supernatants were frozen at ≤ -70 °C and stored until analysed. Before analysis in a central laboratory at Hospital de la Santa Creu i Sant Pau, aliquots were thawed at room temperature and centrifuged at 3000 rpm for 15 min. A previous study in the central laboratory showed there were no significant differences in the [TIMP-2]·[IGFBP7] index between fresh and frozen urine samples (data not shown). The [TIMP-2]·[IGFBP7] index was measured by a sandwich fluorescent quantitative immunoassay adapted to a portable device (Nephrocheck®, Astute Medical). All samples were analysed in the same batch to avoid between-batch variability. The portable device provides a [TIMP-2]·[IGFBP7] index in ((ng/mL)^2/1000) units. According to the manufacturer, an index $\leq$0.3 suggests a low risk of AKI, values between 0.3 and 2.0 suggest a high risk, and values >2.0 suggest a very high risk [15].

Data collection

Clinical data included patient demographics and comorbidities. The APACHE II score, the SAPS II and the SOFA score were recorded at ICU admission. Patients were classified following the AKIN classification [11], which includes changes in sCr and urine output. Baseline sCr was taken from patients' pre-admission records whenever possible and used to estimate eGFR before ICU admission using the Cockcroft–Gault formula. When baseline sCr was not available, AKI was defined only with AKIN urine output criterion. Sepsis and septic shock were defined according to standard criteria [1, 21].

Statistical analysis

IBM® SPSS® version 21 (IBM corp., Armonk, NY) was used. Variables with Gaussian distribution are reported as mean ± standard deviation and were compared with the Student's t test or one-way analysis of variance. Variables with a non-Gaussian distribution are reported as median and interquartile range (IQR) and were compared with Mann–Whitney's U or Kruskal–Wallis tests. Categorical data are reported as percentage and were compared using Chi-square test or Fisher exact test.

The primary outcome of the study was AKI prediction with the [TIMP-2]·[IGFBP7] index. For statistical analyses, we used the highest value observed during the first 12 h of ICU admission as the worst index. Reporting of results followed the Standards for Reporting Diagnostic Accuracy Studies (STARD) statement. As [TIMP-2]·[IGFBP7] index provides a quantitative result that it is interpreted with two cut-offs, analysis was performed to establish the diagnostic accuracy of the test in comparison with the reference standard, which is the AKIN definition of AKI. Diagnostic values, positive predictive values (PPV) and negative predictive values (NPV) were assessed a priori for AKI statistically relevant variables by the area under the receiver operator characteristic curve

(AUROC) and by the odds ratio (OR). Results were presented with a 95% confidence interval and probability (p). For selected thresholds of [TIMP-2]·[IGFBP7], sensitivities, specificities, PPV and NPV were reported for the worst [TIMP-2]·[IGFBP7] value within the first 12 h in the ICU. The ROC analysis was used to calculate the best [TIMP-2]·[IGFBP7] cut-off point for AKI and AKIN ≥ 2 prediction. A $p < 0.05$ was considered significant.

Results

We recruited 100 consecutive patients fulfilling the admission criteria in the ICU of two university hospitals, from June 2011 to April 2013. Two patients were excluded from the study because one of their samples was missing (Fig. 1). Table 1 includes the main characteristics and outcomes of the overall study population as well as in subgroups depending on the occurrence of AKI and sepsis at admission. Further epidemiological data are included in Additional file 1: Table S1.

At admission, 44 patients presented some grade of AKI, more frequently observed in septic patients; 19 fulfilled criteria for AKIN 1, 20 AKIN 2 and 5 AKIN 3. Throughout ICU admission AKI affected 49 of 98 patients. The incidence of AKIN ≥ 2 increased from 25.5 to 31.6% in those patients who presented AKI. Five of 98 patients required RRT within the first 48 h of admission. 40.8% had sepsis at ICU admission.

When comparing subgroups depending on the occurrence of AKI and sepsis in ICU (Table 1; Additional file 1: Table S1), those patients in AKI or sepsis categories were older and had a higher incidence of shock and higher severity scores. Although the incidence of shock in both subgroups was higher, there was no statistical difference in the incidence of septic shock between the non-AKI and AKI subgroups. Septic patients also showed a lower baseline eGFR. However, baseline sCr and the remaining patients' characteristics for both subgroups did not differ.

Overall mortality was 10.2% in ICU, and 12.2 and 13.3%, respectively, at 28 and 90 days (Table 1; Additional file 1: Table S1).

Composite index of [TIMP-2]·[IGFBP7]

[TIMP-2]·[IGFBP7] index values were significantly higher in patients with AKI (1.03, IQR 0.38–3.29) than

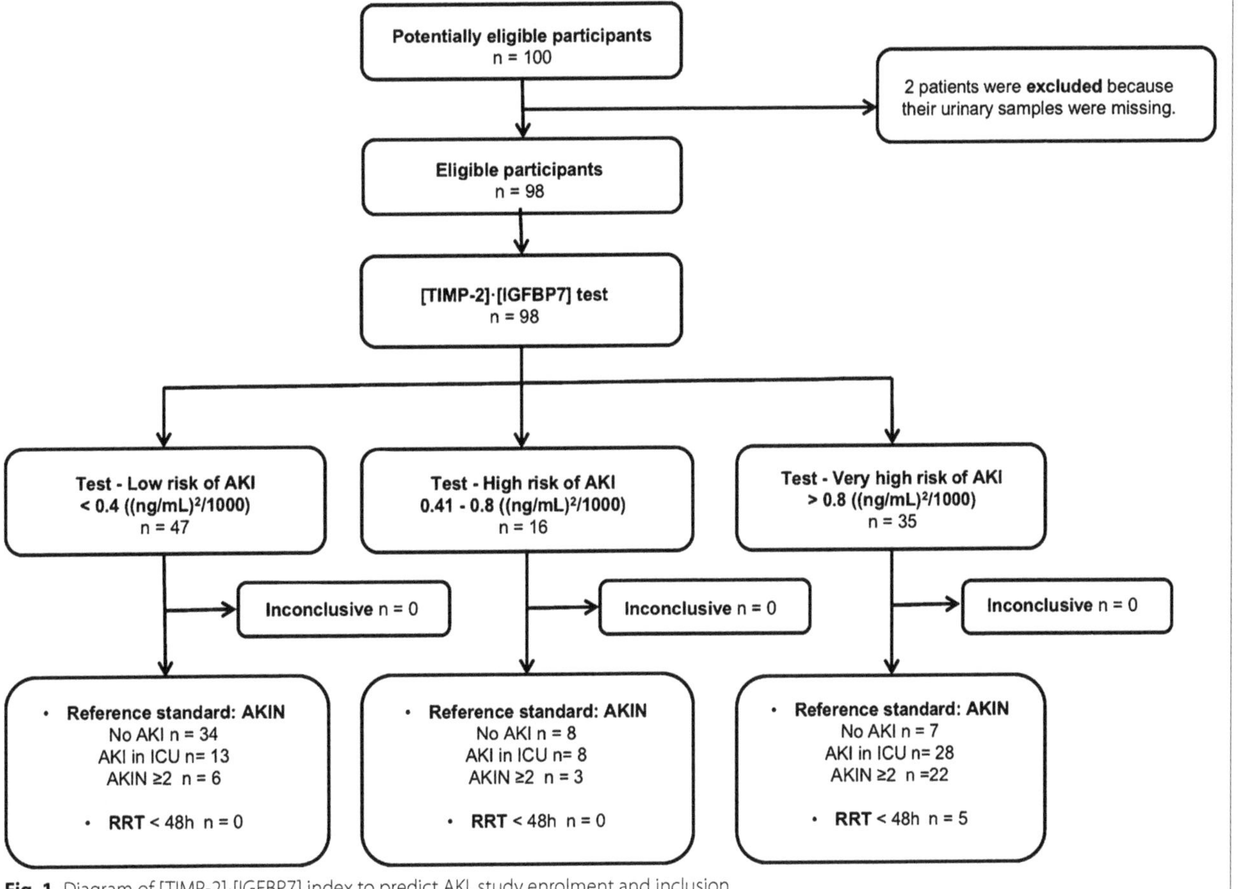

Fig. 1 Diagram of [TIMP-2]·[IGFBP7] index to predict AKI, study enrolment and inclusion

Table 1 Main characteristics of the study population in subgroups of AKI/non-AKI and septic/non-septic patients

	Total	Non-AKI	AKI	*p* value	Non-septic	Septic	*p* value
n	98	49	49	–	58	40	–
Men	65 (66.3%)	30 (61.2%)	35 (71.4%)	NS	38 (65.5%)	27 (67.5%)	NS
Age (years)	55 ± 17.3	50.4 ± 17.9	59.9 ± 15.5	0.006	50.9 ± 16.6	61.2 ± 16.8	0.003
Renal characteristics							
Baseline eGFR (mL/min) *n* = 86	110.6 ± 53.7	120.5 ± 60.5	100.7 ± 44.6	NS	121.9 ± 58.9	94.8 ± 41.2	0.020
Baseline creatinine (μmol/L) *n* = 86	79 ± 31.5	80.5 ± 32.3	78.1 ± 31.1	NS	79.6 ± 28.9	78.9 ± 35.1	NS
Creatinine upon ICU admission	94.1 ± 42.2	74.6 ± 30.2	113.1 ± 43.9	<0.001	85.0 ± 36.8	106.9 ± 46.5	0.015
AKI at admission	44 (44.9%)	–	44 (89.8%)	–	20 (34.5%)	24 (60%)	0.013
AKIN ≥ 2 upon ICU admission	25 (25.5%)	–	25 (51%)	–	9 (15.5%)	16 (40%)	0.009
Renal replacement <48 h	5 (5.1%)	0 (0%)	5 (10.2%)	0.056	4 (6.9%)	1 (2.5%)	NS
Worst value [TIMP-2]·[IGFBP7] ((ng/mL)^2/1000)	0.41 (0.20–1.36)	0.24 (0.11–0.48)	1.03 (0.38–3.29)	<0.001	0.36 (0.14–1.08)	0.56 (0.26–2.94)	NS
ICU epidemiological data							
Shock	35 (35.7%)	11 (22.5%)	24 (50%)	0.011	10 (17.2%)	25 (62.5%)	<0.001
Septic shock	19 (19.4%)	6 (12.3%)	13 (26.5%)	NS	–	19 (47.5%)	–
Mechanical ventilation	79 (80.6%)	39 (79.6%)	40 (81.6%)	NS	44 (75.9%)	35 (87.5%)	NS
SAPS II	37.4 ± 18.3	30.9 ± 14.9	43.9 ± 19.2	<0.001	30.9 ± 15.6	46.8 ± 18.1	<0.001
APACHE II	15.7 ± 8.2	13.5 ± 7.7	17.9 ± 8.2	0.007	14.2 ± 8.5	17.9 ± 7.3	0.024
SOFA at ICU admission	7.5 ± 3.7	6.1 ± 3.2	8.9 ± 3.7	<0.001	6.7 ± 3.7	8.7 ± 3.4	0.009
ICU LOS (days)	11.1 ± 14.6	10.0 ± 10.6	12.3 ± 18.8	NS	9.3 ± 11.0	13.9 ± 18.5	NS
Hospital LOS (days)	23.6 ± 25.0	23.4 ± 23.3	23.8 ± 27.0	NS	21.4 ± 21.3	26.9 ± 29.6	NS
ICU mortality	10 (10.2%)	4 (8.2%)	6 (12.3%)	NS	6 (10.3%)	4 (10%)	NS

Values expressed as either % per column, mean ± standard deviation or median and interquartile range. *p* value of statistical significance

NS no statistical significance, *AKI* acute kidney injury, *AKIN* acute kidney injury network definition, *APACHE II* acute physiology and chronic health evaluation II, *ICU* intensive care unit, *LOS* length of stay, *SAPS II* Simplified Acute Physiology Score II, *SOFA* sequential organ failure assessment score

in those without AKI (0.24, IQR 0.11–0.48) ($p < 0.001$) (Table 1). These differences were unrelated to the presence of sepsis (Table 2). Patients who developed AKI presented higher median index values (1.05, IQR 0.41–2.31 for patients without sepsis; 0.98, IQR 0.36–3.94 for septic patients) than those without AKI (0.21 IQR 0.10–0.40 in non-septic patients and 0.32 IQR 0.15–0.63 for those with sepsis) with $p < 0.001$ between subgroups with and without AKI (no statistical differences were found between septic and non-septic status).

Table 2 Worst [TIMP-2]·[IGFBP7] distribution within 12 h of ICU admission depending on AKI and sepsis

	AKI –	*p* value	AKI +
Sepsis –	0.21 (0.10–0.40) (*n* = 35)	⇐ *p* < 0.001 ⇒	1.05 (0.41–2.31) (*n* = 23)
p value	⇑ NS ⇓		⇑ NS ⇓
Sepsis +	0.32 (0.15–0.63) (*n* = 14)	⇐ *p* = 0.009 ⇒	0.98 (0.36–3.94) (*n* = 26)

(AKI + vs. AKI –) and (Sepsis + vs. Sepsis –) represent the presence or absence of either AKI during hospital stay or sepsis upon admission, respectively. Values show median and percentiles 25–75. *p* represents the statistical intra-group differences. [TIMP-2]·[IGFBP7] values given in ((ng/mL)^2/1000)

AKI acute kidney injury, *NS* no statistical differences

The index values were significantly related to AKI presence and severity according to AKIN criteria (Fig. 2). In contrast, index values did not appear to be influenced by sepsis, either in AKI or non-AKI patients (Table 2).

[TIMP-2]·[IGFBP7] values increased in 44% of patients within 12 h of ICU admission; index values decreased in all other patients. Overall, a repeated determination of [TIMP-2]·[IGFBP7] did not show any differences between non-AKI/AKI and non-septic/septic subgroups (Additional file 2: Figure S1).

We divided the patients into 3 subgroups depending on the cut-offs proposed in previous studies [15] (Table 3). Although baseline sCr showed no statistically significant difference between subgroups, baseline eGFR significantly declined at index values >2.0. AKI occurrence and AKIN ≥ 2 during ICU stay were significantly more frequent in the groups with index >0.31. However, the need for RRT did not differ according to the index values. There were also differences between subgroups in the incidence of shock, SAPS II score and ICU length of stay. Patients with high-risk values also had longer ICU length of stay but not hospital length of stay, both with

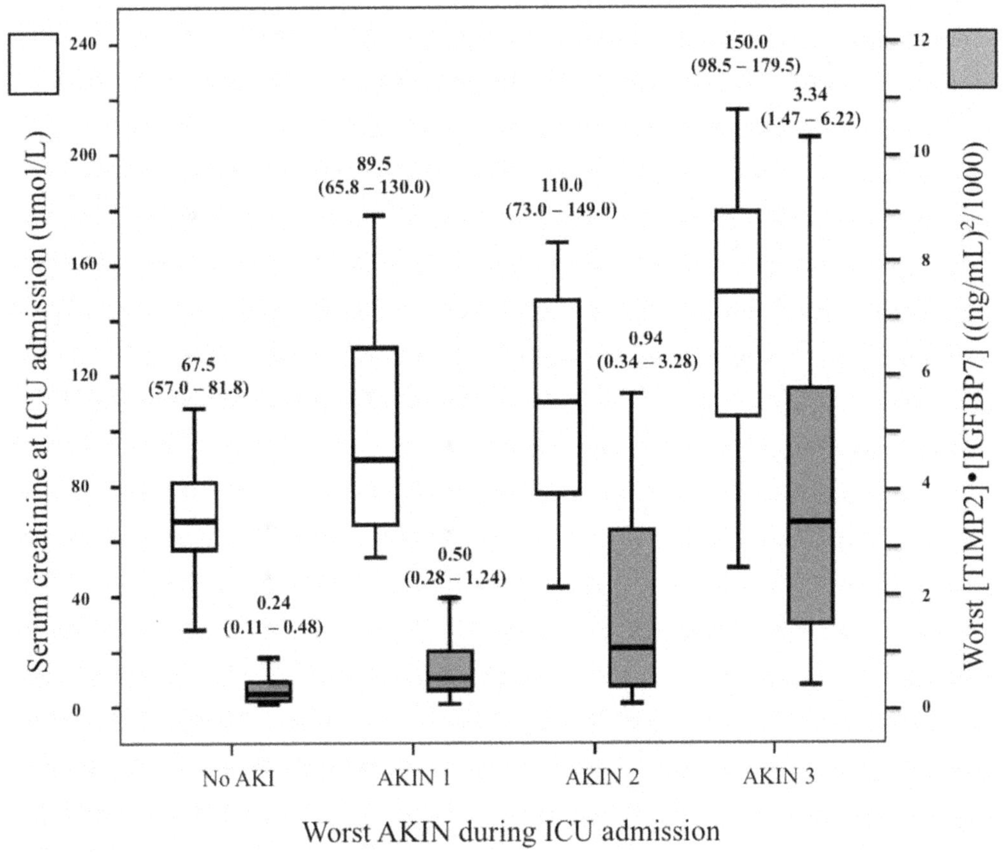

Fig. 2 Boxplot comparing the worst [TIMP-2]·[IGFBP7] index and sCr upon admittance with the worst AKIN. *Boxplots* indicate the median, 25th and 75th percentiles. Whiskers indicate the 5th and 95th percentiles. Statistical significance (*p*) comparing each biomarker index with AKIN and RIFLE categories. *p* was determined by Kruskal–Wallis test, not correlation. We found statistical differences in the worst [TIMP-2]·[IGFBP7] index concentrations when comparing the subgroup without AKI with any degree of AKI defined by AKIN. Between non-AKI and AKIN 1, p was 0.014 and $p < 0.001$ when comparing with AKIN 2 and AKIN 3. In between AKIN 1 and AKIN 3, $p = 0.004$, whereas in between AKIN 2 and AKIN 3 $p = 0.039$. When comparing sCr levels with AKIN, we found differences between the subgroup without AKI with AKIN 1 ($p = 0.008$), AKIN 2 and 3 (for both $p < 0.001$). In between AKIN 1 and 3, p was 0.048 and $p = 0.033$ in AKIN 2 versus AKIN 3

wide standard deviation. According to the manufacturer's [TIMP-2]·[IGFBP7] stratification, both subgroups of patients with high and very high-risk values needed RRT. There were no differences between subgroups regarding ICU mortality or mortality at 28 and 90 days.

We assessed the best predictive cut-off of [TIMP-2]·[IGFBP7] index to predict AKI and AKIN $\geq$ 2.0 in our population. Table 4 details the sensitivity and specificity of [TIMP-2]·[IGFBP7] test with increasing indexes, as well as the overall accuracy of the test to predict AKI and AKIN $\geq$ 2. The AUROC curve of the worst value [TIMP-2]·[IGFBP7] within the first 12 h of ICU admission for AKI prediction was 0.798 (0.709–0.886, $p < 0.0001$)) for an index value of 0.40, with sensitivity of 73.5% (95% CI 69.7–77.5%) and specificity of 71.4% (95% CI 67.4–75.4%) (Table 4; Fig. 3). To predict AKIN $\geq$ 2, the AUROC was 0.805 (0.700–0.909, $p < 0.0001$) with an index value of 0.80, sensitivity of 72.0% (95% CI 68.1–75.9%) and specificity of 78.1% (95% CI 74.6–81.8%).

Patients with index values $\geq$0.80 (ng/mL)^2/1000 were older (Table 3). Our threshold did not reveal differences in baseline sCr, baseline eGFR, ICU or hospital length of stay between subgroups. The incidence of shock was higher in patients with index values $\geq$0.8, although this difference was only marginally significant ($p = 0.053$). However, all patients requiring RRT showed an index value $\geq$0.8. Thus, compared with the values previously reported in other studies, the observed cut-offs identified 25 additional patients that would not require RRT.

We also evaluated PPV and NPV for both sets of cut-offs (data not shown). However, both sets were equally able to differentiate patients with AKI and AKIN $\geq$ 2. Although the low incidence of RRT per se increases the NPV, our own specific cut-offs better classified those

Table 3 Population characteristics depending on different cut-offs of [TIMP-2]·[IGFBP7] index for AKI diagnose

	Worst [TIMP-2]·[IGFBP7] index within the first 12 h in ((ng/mL)^2/1000)							
	≤0.3	0.31–2	>2	*p* value	≤0.4	0.41–0.8	>0.8	*p* value
n	38	40	20	–	47	16	35	–
Men (*n* = 65)	21 (55.3%)	30 (75%)	14 (70%)	NS	29 (61.7%)	12 (75%)	24 (68.6%)	NS
Age (years)	53 ± 18.4	54 ± 16.7	62 ± 15	NS	52 ± 18.5	52 ± 18.4	61 ± 13.7	0.043
Renal characteristics								
Baseline creatinine (μmol/L)	84 ± 31.9	72 ± 28.5	85 ± 34.9	NS	83 ± 30.1	66 ± 33.3	80 ± 32	NS
Baseline eGFR (mL/min) *n* = 86	117 ± 60.1 (*n* = 31)	123 ± 48.1 (*n* = 35)	79 ± 40.9 (*n* = 20)	0.008	112 ± 55.4 (*n* = 39)	128 ± 54.1 (*n* = 12)	103 ± 52.7 (*n* = 35)	NS
AKI while in ICU (*n* = 49)	9 (23.7%)	22 (55%)	18 (90%)	<0.001	13 (27.7%)	8 (50%)	28 (80%)	<0.001
AKIN ≥ 2 while in ICU (*n* = 31)	4 (10.5%)	13 (32.5%)	14 (70%)	<0.001	6 (12.8%)	3 (18.8%)	22 (62.9%)	<0.001
RRT <48 h (*n* = 5)	0 (0%)	3 (7.5%)	2 (10%)	NS	0 (0%)	0 (0%)	5 (14.3%)	0.007
ICU epidemiological data								
Sepsis at admission (*n* = 40)	11 (29%)	18 (45%)	11 (55%)	NS	16 (34%)	8 (50%)	16 (45.7%)	NS
Shock (*n* = 35)	11 (29%)	12 (30%)	12 (60%)	0.039	13 (27.7%)	4 (25%)	18 (51.4%)	0.053
Mechanical ventilation (*n* = 79)	32 (84.2%)	32 (80%)	15 (75%)	NS	39 (83%)	13 (81.3%)	27 (77.1%)	NS
SAPS II	35 ± 15.4	34 ± 17.4	49 ± 21.1	0.004	35 ± 16.2	28 ± 11.9	44 ± 21.1	0.006
APACHE II	16 ± 8.7	15 ± 7.5	17 ± 8.8	NS	15 ± 8.2	13 ± 6.0	18 ± 8.8	NS
SOFA at ICU admission	7 ± 3.5	7 ± 3.9	8 ± 3.8	NS	7 ± 3.8	7 ± 3.7	8 ± 3.5	NS
ICU LOS	8.6 ± 9.1	15.6 ± 20.1	7.0 ± 5.3	0.036	8.8 ± 8.7	12.6 ± 15.8	13.6 ± 19.6	NS
Hospital LOS	24.6 ± 25.9	24.9 ± 28.9	19.2 ± 12.5	NS	23.6 ± 24.9	20.8 ± 16.1	24.9 ± 28.7	NS
ICU mortality (*n* = 10)	4 (10.5%)	4 (10%)	2 (10%)	NS	4 (8.5%)	1 (6.3%)	5 (14.3%)	NS

Values expressed as either % of cases per row or mean ± standard deviation. *p* value of statistical significance

In our database, five patients had a much longer length of stay (51, 53, 60, 68 and 97 days) than the overall group (≤30 days). Four of these five patients presented index values 0.31–2 ((ng/mL)^2/1000), which may explain this finding

NS no statistical significance, *AKI* acute kidney injury, *AKIN* acute kidney injury network definition, *APACHE II* acute physiology and chronic health evaluation II, *ICU* intensive care unit, *LOS* length of stay, *SAPS II* Simplified Acute Physiology Score II, *SOFA* sequential organ failure assessment score

Table 4 Diagnostic and overall accuracy of [TIMP-2]·[IGFBP7] for AKI compared with gold standard AKIN classification

[TIMP-2]·[IGFBP7] cut-off value ((ng/mL)^2/1000)	Se %	95% CI	Sp %	95% CI	AUC	95% CI
0.3—to predict AKI	81.6	78.2–85.0	59.2	54.9–63.5	0.80	0.71–0.89
0.4—to predict AKI	73.5	69.7–77.5	71.4	67.4–75.4		
0.8—to predict AKIN ≥ 2	72.0	68.1–75.9	78.1	74.6–81.8	0.81	0.70–0.91
2.0—to predict AKIN ≥ 2	48.0	43.6–52.4	90.4	87.8–93.0		

AUC area under curve of ROC analysis; *CI* confidence interval; *Se* sensitivity; *Sp* specificity

patients who finally underwent RRT ($p = 0.007$), with a NPV of 100% (95% CI 96.4–100%) for a cut-off >0.8 ((ng/mL)^2/1000) versus 96.2% (95% CI 92–100%) for a cut-off >2 ((ng/mL)^2/1000). Values above 2 ((ng/mL)^2/1000) could only rule out the need of RRT in 40% of cases (95% CI 0–83%).

Taking into account the characteristics of our population (Tables 1, 3), we conducted stepwise logistic

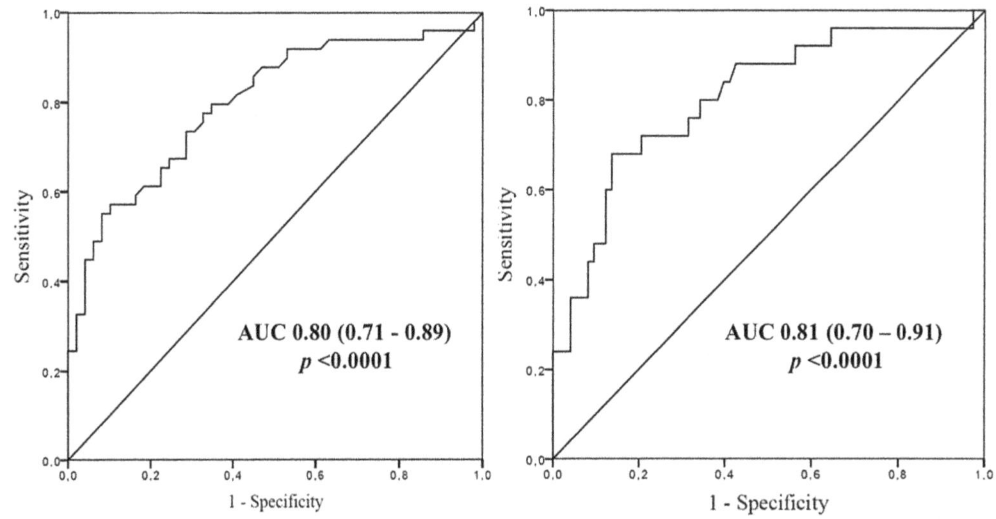

Best Cut-off 0.4 ((ng/mL)^2 / 1000) Sensitivity 73.5%; Specificity 71.4%

Best Cut-off 0.8 ((ng/mL)^2 / 1000) Sensitivity 72.0%; Specificity 78.1%

Fig. 3 ROC curve for the worst [TIMP-2]·[IGFBP7] index to predict AKI and AKIN ≥ 2. ROC curve and area under the curve (AUC) for the worst [TIMP-2]·[IGFBP7] index concentration within the first 12 h of ICU admission to predict AKI (*left*) and AKIN ≥ 2 (*right*)

regression analysis using as covariates age, sepsis, shock, previous hepatopathy, secondary ARDS, SAPS II, SOFA at admission and the worst value [TIMP-2]·[IGFBP7] for AKI and AKIN ≥ 2 prediction. In our equation, [TIMP-2]·[IGFBP7] index showed an OR of 3.15 (95% IC 1.60–6.17, $p = 0.001$) for AKI prediction and 1.85 (95% IC 1.33–2.57, $p = 0.001$) for AKIN ≥ 2 prediction.

Discussion

Our results showed that the [TIMP-2]·[IGFBP7] index is a useful predictor of AKI in the first 12 h of ICU admission in both septic and non-septic critically ill patients otherwise free of common AKI risk factors. Our AUROC curves of [TIMP-2]·[IGFBP7] for prediction of both AKI and AKIN ≥ 2 (0.798 and 0.805, respectively) agreed with the results already described in the literature [15, 22–25]. A recently published subgroup analysis of septic patients in sapphire and topaz studies shows similar results [26]. In our study, patients with high index values showed a 3.15- and a 1.85-fold risk to present AKI and AKIN ≥ 2, respectively. The most relevant finding in our study is that a cut-off [TIMP-2]·[IGFBP7] of 0.8 ((ng/mL)^2/1000) showed a NPV 100% for RRT requirement. Thus, beyond their AKI prognostic capacity, these biomarkers also ruled out the need for RRT below this threshold over the first 12 h of ICU admission.

Sepsis is a common feature in ICU patients [1]. In our study, 40.8% of patients were septic at ICU admission and had a higher incidence of AKIN ≥ 2. Gómez's unified theory of sepsis-induced AKI may explain why some critically ill patients can present AKI in hyperdynamic and/or non-hypotensive status [27]. AKI and sepsis are reciprocal risk factors. Sepsis triggers inflammation and oxidative stress, and promotes microvascular dysfunction, which can lead to AKI. On the other hand, AKI impairs monocyte cytokine production and elevates plasma cytokine levels [28], acting as a sepsis risk factor. The fact that [TIMP-2]·[IGFBP7] are independently associated with AKI in sepsis is a relevant advantage of these biomarkers compared with more widely described NGAL or cystatin-C [29–31].

Another important finding regards the timing to analyse [TIMP-2]·[IGFBP7]. Repeated determinations of any biomarker in a short period of time may reduce their intrinsic variability and increase their diagnostic or prognostic power. We performed two [TIMP-2]·[IGFBP7] determinations (admission and up to 12 h later) for each patient. In a post-operative cardiac surgery setting, Meersch [23, 32] showed that [TIMP-2]·[IGFBP7] rose as fast as 4 h after surgery (AUROC 0.84, Se 0.92 Sp 0.81) for the highest concentration of [TIMP-2]·[IGFBP7] within the first 24 h. However, in our study, repeated determinations did not improve prediction. This is relevant because a single analysis is easier to implement and decreases costs. The manufacturer recommends repeat testing of patients with an inconclusive result. We would only suggest considering repeating the test in those cases in which clinically their result is difficult to interpret.

Our study tested these biomarkers in a selected ICU population free of common AKI risk factors [33]. Most studies analysing the role of classical or emerging biomarkers in ICU subjects have been done in unselected populations. Accordingly, the number of patients presenting different degrees of renal dysfunction is variable, but usually high. AKI is a common complication of many non-renal hospitalisations [34, 35]; it has been estimated that the incidence of hospital-acquired renal insufficiency is about 7% [36]. Ideally, to describe the characteristics of a new AKI biomarker this incidence should be studied in subjects with a normal baseline renal function. Although our patients may not fully represent an average ICU population in view of our selective inclusion and exclusion criteria, our approach decreases the confounding effect of intra-hospital risk factors to develop AKI, such as exposure to nephrotoxics, hypotension and nosocomial sepsis.

Patients with AKI and/or sepsis showed higher severity scores, and ICU and hospital length of stay, although the latter did not reach statistical difference. Mortality rates remained very low. Thus, we did not find significant differences. This could be partially explained because of our study exclusion criteria. We excluded patients with established anuric AKI at admission, who had the highest risk for poor outcome related to AKI [2, 3], and patients with an expected ICU length of stay <2 days because of their severe condition. Besides, we did not recruit those subjects who had already been hospitalised. In a subanalysis of the PICARD study [37], which analysed the relationship between AKI and sepsis, septic patients either before or after AKI onset presented higher mortality rates than non-septic patients (48, 44 and 21%, respectively).

We also clinically assessed the cut-off values described in the literature. The sapphire and opal studies [15, 16] reported the same cut-off values for the risk of AKI development. In our cohort, the best cut-off index values were 0.4 and 0.8 ((ng/mL)^2/1000) to differentiate no AKI risk, high risk and very high risk (Table 4). The lower cut-off was very close to the 0.3 previously reported, and it is in keeping with the value cited in the FDA report [38]. Thus, the lower threshold may be helpful to consider before the indication of procedures involving nephrotoxics or to avoid starting RRT in oliguric patients. We also found a consistent NPV above 70% to exclude any degree of AKI. When using our own threshold for very high risk of AKI [0.8 ((ng/mL)^2/1000)], we did differentiate all patients who finally underwent RRT ($p = 0.007$). The controversy arises in the 0.41–0.8 ((ng/mL)^2/1000) range; although this subgroup of patients might benefit from a second sampling, this is not supported by our results.

The main limitations in our study are the small sample size and the enrolment in only two centres. Although the overall findings are consistent with recent studies, our thresholds do need further validation. The main strength of the study is the clinical design. The restricted inclusion criteria reduced the size of our cohort and the statistical power, which may also explain the low mortality rate. However, we obtained most baseline sCr and we ensured that patients who developed AKI did not have previous significant CKD. Unlike most observational studies, our proof of model selection of patients also ruled out the added effect of intra-hospital risk factors for AKI.

Conclusions

Unlike other renal biomarkers, [TIMP-2]·[IGFBP7] predict AKI in both septic and non-septic critically ill patients. These biomarkers are especially useful to promptly differentiate patients without AKI from those with a very high risk of developing AKI. Below the cut-off value of 0.8 ((ng/mL)^2/1000), the [TIMP-2]·[IGFBP7] index was able to exclude those patients who needed RRT in our study population.

Additional files

Additional file 1: Table S1. Main characteristics of study population in subgroups of AKI/non-AKI and septic/non-septic patients. Values expressed as either % per column or mean ± standard deviation; *NS* no statistical significance; *p* value of significance. Abbreviations in alphabetical order. *AKI* acute kidney injury, *AKIN* acute kidney injury definition, *APACHE II* acute physiology and chronic health evaluation II, *ARDS* acute respiratory distress syndrome, *BMI* body mass index, *COPD* chronic obstructive pulmonary disease, *DM* diabetes mellitus, *HTN* hypertension, *RRT* renal replacement technique, *SAPS II* Simplified Acute Physiology Score II, *SOFA* sequential organ failure assessment score. *Exposure to either nephrotoxic or diuretic prior to ICU admission. **Differences in medical admission are due to higher incidence of neurological admissions in subgroup of non-septic patients (24.1% in non-septic subgroup vs. 7.5% in septic patients) and higher incidence of respiratory admissions in septic patients (10.3% in non-septic vs. 47.5% in septic subgroup). As shown in the table, none of the trauma patients included presented concomitant sepsis at ICU admission.

Additional file 2: Figure S1. Boxplot for [TIMP-2]·[IGFBP7] index values at each determination and depending on AKI and sepsis occurrence. Boxplot represents index values upon admission and up to 12 h later for the overall study population as well as for the subgroups of patients with and without sepsis upon ICU admission. *BM* biomarker, *NS* no statistical significance.

Abbreviations

TIMP-2: tissue inhibitor of metalloproteinases-2; IGFBP7: insulin-like growth factor-binding protein 7; AKI: acute kidney injury; AKIN: acute kidney injury network definition; ICU: intensive care unit; RRT: renal replacement therapy; sCr: serum creatinine; RIFLE: risk–injury–failure–loss–end-stage renal disease classification; ED: emergency department; CKD: chronic kidney disease; CrCL: creatinine clearance; APACHE II: acute physiology and chronic health evaluation II; SAPS: Simplified Acute Physiology Score; SOFA: sequential organ failure assessment; SIRS: systemic inflammatory response syndrome; Md: median; IQR: interquartile range; PPV: positive predictive value; NPV: negative predictive value; AUROC: area under the receiver operator characteristic curve; OR: odds ratio; Se: sensitivity; Sp: specificity.

Authors' contributions

MC, JO-LI and AJB had full access to all data in the study. They take responsibility for both the integrity and the accuracy of the data analysis. Both authors JO-LI and AJB were equally directors of the work. MC, JO-LI, AJB, JB, JS and XP enrolled subjects and collected data from the two ICU involved in the study. All authors reviewed the data and participated in discussions related to interpretation. All authors read and approved the final manuscript.

Author details

[1] Intensive Care Department and Institut d'Investigacions Biomèdiques, Hospital de la Santa Creu i Sant Pau, Universitat Autònoma de Barcelona, Sant Quintí 89, 08041 Barcelona, Spain. [2] Intensive Care Department, Hospital Universitari Bellvitge, Hospitalet de Llobregat, Universitat de Barcelona, Feixa Llarga, 08907 L'Hospitalet de Llobregat, Barcelona, Spain. [3] Intensive Care Department, Hospital Universitario de Getafe, Km 12500 Madrid - Toledo Road, 28905 Getafe, Madrid, Spain. [4] Biochemistry Department and Institut d'Investigacions Biomèdiques, Hospital de la Santa Creu i Sant Pau, Universitat Autònoma de Barcelona, Sant Quintí 89, 08041 Barcelona, Spain.

Acknowledgements

The study sponsor (LaboratorisRubió) was responsible for providing the portable device (Nephrocheck®, Astute Medical). The study design, data analysis and interpretation were independently performed by MC, JO-LI and AJB. Carolyn Newey made the grammar review. The authors would like to thank the staff in the ICU and biochemistry departments who generously participated in sample processing and analysis and whose work is essential to the completion of this study.

Competing interests

MC has received congress fees from Laboratoris Rubió to present the preliminary results of this study at ISICEM 2015.

Availability of data and materials

The data supporting the study findings can be shared upon direct request to the authors in a collaborative research approach.

Funding

The study did not have any funding support.

References

1. Levy MM, Fink MP, Marshall JC, Abraham E, Angus D, Cook D, et al. 2001 SCCM/ESICM/ACCP/ATS/SIS international sepsis definitions conference. Crit Care Med. 2003;31(4):1250–6.
2. Hoste EAJ, Schurgers M. Epidemiology of acute kidney injury: how big is the problem? Crit Care Med. 2008;36(4 Suppl):S146–51.
3. Metnitz PGH, Krenn CG, Steltzer H, Lang T, Ploder J, Lenz K, et al. Effect of acute renal failure requiring renal replacement therapy on outcome in critically ill patients. Crit Care Med. 2002;30(9):2051–8.
4. Oppert M, Engel C, Brunkhorst F-M, Bogatsch H, Reinhart K, Frei U, et al. Acute renal failure in patients with severe sepsis and septic shock—a significant independent risk factor for mortality: results from the German Prevalence Study. Nephrol Dial Transplant. 2008;23(3):904–9.
5. Bagshaw SM, Uchino S, Bellomo R, Morimatsu H, Morgera S, Schetz M, et al. Septic acute kidney injury in critically ill patients: clinical characteristics and outcomes. Clin J Am Soc Nephrol. 2007;2(11):431–9.
6. Lopes JA, Jorge S, Resina C, Santos C, Pereira A, Neves J, et al. Acute renal failure in patients with sepsis. Crit Care. 2007;11:411.
7. Bagshaw SM, Lapinsky S, Dial S, Arabi Y, Dodek P, Wood G, et al. Acute kidney injury in septic shock: clinical outcomes and impact of duration of hypotension prior to initiation of antimicrobial therapy. Intensive Care Med. 2009;35:871–81.
8. Uchino S, Kellum JA, Bellomo R, Doig GS, Morimatsu H, Morgera S, et al. Acute renal failure in critically ill patients a multinational, multicenter study. J Am Med Assoc. 2005;294(7):813–8.
9. Gomez H, Ince C, De Backer D, Pickkers P, Payen D, Hotchkiss J. A unified theory of sepsis-induced acute kidney injury: inflammation, microcirculatory dysfunction, bioenergetics, and the tubular cell adaptation to injury. Shock. 2014;41:3–11.
10. Bellomo R, Ronco C, Kellum JA, Mehta RL, Palevsky P. Acute renal failure–definition, outcome measures, animal models, fluid therapy and information technology needs: the Second International Consensus Conference of the Acute Dialysis Quality Initiative (ADQI) Group. Crit Care. 2004;8(4):R204–12.
11. Mehta RL, Kellum JA, Shah SV, Molitoris BA, Ronco C, Warnock DG, et al. Acute Kidney Injury Network: report of an initiative to improve outcomes in acute kidney injury. Crit Care. 2007;11(2):R31.
12. Kellum JA, Lameire N, Aspelin P, Barsoum RS, Burdmann EA, KDIGO Group, et al. KDIGO clinical practice guideline for acute kidney injury. Kidney Int Suppl. 2012;2:1–138.
13. Dunn B, Anderson S, Brenner B. The hemodynamic basis of progressive renal disease. Semin Nephrol. 1986;6(2):122–38.
14. Brenner B, Rector F. The kidney. 6th ed. Philadelphia: Saunders; 2000.
15. Kashani K, Al-Khafaji A, Ardiles T, Artigas A, Bagshaw SM, Bell M, et al. Discovery and validation of cell cycle arrest biomarkers in human acute kidney injury. Crit Care BioMed Central Ltd. 2013;17(1):R25.
16. Hoste EAJ, McCullough PA, Kashani K, Chawla LS, Joannidis M, Shaw AD, et al. Derivation and validation of cutoffs for clinical use of cell cycle arrest biomarkers. Nephrol Dial Transplant. 2014;29(11):2054–61.
17. Rifai N, Gillette MA, Carr SA. Protein biomarker discovery and validation: the long and uncertain path to clinical utility. Nat Biotechnol. 2006;24(8):971–83.
18. Seo D-W, Li H, Qu C-K, Oh J, Kim Y-S, Diaz T, et al. Shp-1 mediates the antiproliferative activity of tissue inhibitor of metalloproteinase-2 in human microvascular endothelial cells. J Biol Chem. 2006;281(6):3711–21.
19. Bonventre J, Yang L. Cellular pathophysiology of ischemic acute kidney injury. J Clin Invest. 2011;121(11):4210–21.
20. Witzgall R, Brown D, Schwarz C, Bonventre JV. Localization of proliferating cell nuclear antigen, vimentin, c-Fos, and clusterin in the postischemic kidney. J Clin Invest. 1994;93(May):2175–88.
21. Singer M, Deutschman CS, Seymour CW, Shankar-Ari M, Annane D, Bauer M, et al. The third international consensus definition for sepsis and septic shock (Sepsis-3). J Am Med Assoc. 2016;315(8):801–10.
22. Yamashita T, Doi K, Hamasaki Y, Matsubara T, Ishii T, Yahagi N, et al. Evaluation of urinary tissue inhibitor of metalloproteinase-2 in acute kidney injury: a prospective observational study. Crit Care. 2014;18(6):1–9.
23. Meersch M, Schmidt C, Van Aken H, Martens S, Rossaint J, Singbartl K, et al. Urinary TIMP-2 and IGFBP7 as early biomarkers of acute kidney injury and renal recovery following cardiac surgery. PLoS ONE. 2014;9(3):e93460.
24. Bihorac A, Chawla LS, Shaw AD, Al-Khafaji A, Davison DL, DeMuth GE, et al. Validation of cell-cycle arrest biomarkers for acute kidney injury using clinical adjudication. Am J Respir Crit Care Med. 2014;189(8):932–9.
25. Gocze I, Koch M, Renner P, Zeman F, Graf BM, Dahlke MH, et al. Urinary biomarkers TIMP-2 and IGFBP7 early predict acute kidney injury after major surgery. PLoS ONE. 2015;10(3):e0120863.
26. Honore PM, Nguyen HB, Gong M, Chawla LS, Bagshaw SM, Artigas A, et al. Urinary tissue inhibitor of metalloproteinase-2 and insulin-like growth factor-binding protein 7 for risk stratification of acute kidney injury in patients with sepsis. Crit Care Med. 2016;44(10):1851–60. doi:10.1097/CCM.0000000000001827.
27. Gomez H, Ince C, De Backer D, Pickkers P, Payen D, Hotchkiss J, et al. A unified theory of sepsis-induced acute kidney injury: inflammation, microcirculatory dysfunction, bioenergetics, and the tubular cell adaptation to injury. Shock. 2014;41(1):3–11.
28. Himmelfarb J, Le P, Klenzak J, Freedman S, McMenamin ME, Ikizler TA. Impaired monocyte cytokine production in critically ill patients with acute reanl failure. Kidney Int. 2004;66:2354–60.

29. Mårtensson J, Bell M, Oldner A, Xu S, Venge P, Martling C-R, et al. Neutrophil gelatinase-associated lipocaline in adult septic patients with and without acute kidney injury. Intensive Care Med. 2010;36(8):1333–40.
30. Wheeler DS, Devarajan P, Ma Q, Harmon K, Monaco M, Cvijanovich N, et al. Serum neutrophil gelatinase-associated lipocalin (NGAL) as a marker of acute kidney injury in critically ill children with septic shock. Crit Care Med. 2008;36(4):1297–303.
31. Bagshaw SM, Bennett M, Haase M, Haase-Fielitz A, Egi M, Morimatsu H, et al. Plasma and urine neutrophil gelatinase-associated lipocalin in septic versus non-septic acute kidney injury in critical illness. Intensive Care Med. 2010;36(3):452–61.
32. Stege D, Meersch M, Schmidt C, Aken H Van, Rossaint J, Go D, et al. Validation of cell-cycle arrest biomarkers for acute kidney injury after pediatric cardiac surgery. PLoS One. 2014;9(10):e110865. doi:10.1371/journal.pone.0110865.
33. Bienholz A, Wilde B, Kribben A. From the nephrologist's point of view: diversity of causes and clinical features of acute kidney injury. Clin Kidney J. 2015;8(4):405–14.
34. Hou S, Bushinsky D, Wish J, Cohen J, Harrington J. Hospital-acquired renal insufficiency: a prospective study. Am J Med. 1983;74(2):243–8.
35. Wang HE, Muntner P, Chertow GM, Warnock DG. Acute kidney injury and mortality in hospitalized patients. Am J Nephrol. 2012;35(4):349–55.
36. Nash K, Hafeez A, Hou S. Hospital-acquired renal insufficiency. Am J Kidney Dis. 2002;39(5):930–6.
37. Mehta RL, Bouchard J, Soroko SB, Ikizler TA, Paganini EP, Chertow GM, et al. Sepsis as a cause and consequence of acute kidney injury: program to improve care in acute renal disease. Intensive Care Med. 2011;37(2):241–8.
38. U.S. Food and Drug Administration (2014). Evaluation of automatic class III designation for nephrocheck test system. Retrieved from: https://www.accessdata.fda.gov/cdrh_docs/pdf13/DEN130031.pdf.

13

Short-term effects of passive mobilization on the sublingual microcirculation and on the systemic circulation in patients with septic shock

Tuanny Teixeira Pinheiro, Flávio Geraldo Rezende de Freitas*, Karla Tuanny Fiorese Coimbra, Vanessa Marques Ferreira Mendez, Heloísa Baccaro Rossetti, Paulo Vinicius Talma, Antônio Tonete Bafi and Flávia Ribeiro Machado

Abstract

Background: Active mobilization is not possible in patients under deep sedation and unable to follow commands. In this scenario, passive therapy is an interesting alternative. However, in patients with septic shock, passive mobilization may have risks related to increased oxygen consumption. Our objective was to evaluate the impact of passive mobilization on sublingual microcirculation and systemic hemodynamics in patients with septic shock.

Methods: We included patients who were older than 18 years, who presented with septic shock, and who were under sedation and mechanical ventilation. Passive exercise was applied for 20 min with 30 repetitions per minute. Systemic hemodynamic and microcirculatory variables were compared before (T0) and up to 10 min after (T1) passive exercise. p values <0.05 were considered significant.

Results: We included 35 patients (median age [IQR 25–75%]: 68 [49.0–78.0] years; mean (±SD) Simplified Acute Physiologic Score (SAPS) 3 score: 66.7 ± 12.1; median [IQR 25–75%] Sequential Organ Failure Assessment (SOFA) score: 9 [7.0–12.0]). After passive mobilization, there was a slight but significant increase in proportion of perfused vessels (PPV) (T0 [IQR 25–75%]: 78.2 [70.9–81.9%]; T1 [IQR 25–75%]: 80.0 [75.2–85.1] %; $p = 0.029$), without any change in other microcirculatory variables. There was a reduction in heart rate (HR) (T0 (mean ± SD): 95.6 ± 22.0 bpm; T1 (mean ± SD): 93.8 ± 22.0 bpm; $p < 0.040$) and body temperature (T0 (mean ± SD): 36.9 ± 1.1 °C; T1 (mean ± SD): 36.7 ± 1.2 °C; $p < 0.002$) with no change in other systemic hemodynamic variables. There was no significant correlation between PPV variation and HR ($r = -0.010$, $p = 0.955$), cardiac index ($r = 0.218$, $p = 0.215$) or mean arterial pressure ($r = 0.276$, $p = 0.109$) variation.

Conclusions: In patients with septic shock after the initial phase of hemodynamic resuscitation, passive exercise is not associated with relevant changes in sublingual microcirculation or systemic hemodynamics.

Keywords: Sepsis, Shock, septic, Physical therapy specialty, Exercise therapy, Microcirculation, Intensive care

Background

Patients with sepsis who require intensive care usually receive interventions that promote immobilization, mainly the administration of sedative and analgesic drugs to facilitate invasive mechanical ventilation (MV) and reduce pain, agitation, and anxiety [1, 2]. Sepsis-induced metabolic and inflammatory changes can also lead to polyneuromyopathy characterized by a reduction in muscle force-generating capacity and atrophy and by alteration of bioenergetics [3] and sensitivity [4]. The combination of critical illness and bed rest may result in intensive care

*Correspondence: flaviogrf@yahoo.com.br
Anesthesiology, Pain and Intensive Care Department, Federal University of Sao Paulo, Napoleão de Barros 737, Sao Paulo, SP 04024002, Brazil

unit (ICU)-acquired weakness [5], which is associated with prolonged duration of MV, longer ICU length of stay, poor health-related quality of life, and reduced functional and cognitive capacity among survivors [4, 6–8].

Early mobilization in mechanically ventilated patients who are critically ill reduces the effects of ICU-acquired weakness [9–11]. This approach is feasible, appears to be safe [10, 12], and improves functional outcomes [10]. However, active mobilization is not possible in patients under deep sedation and unable to follow commands. In this scenario, passive therapy is an interesting alternative [13]. Passive mobilization can preserve joint mobility and muscle length [14], attenuate muscle atrophy [15], and reduce levels of inflammatory cytokines [16]. In sedated patients with septic shock, passive mobilization may have risks. In addition to accidental displacement of catheters, endotracheal tubes, enteral feeding tubes, and other supportive equipment [17], some studies have suggested that passive movements can result in a significant increase in oxygen consumption (VO_2) and a decrease in venous oxygen saturation (SvO_2) [18, 19]. Consequently, tissue hypoperfusion may ensue in patients with compromised cardiovascular status [18, 19]. Nonetheless, the impact of passive movements is debatable. Several other studies did not report significant effects on systemic hemodynamic variables [11, 13, 16, 17, 20–24].

No previous studies have explored the effects of mobilization on microcirculation. In these severely ill patients, it might be possible that passive mobilization can increase the blood flow to the working muscles and decrease splanchnic blood flow. These physiologic changes could lead to alterations in sublingual microvascular flow, density, and heterogeneity. However, as the relationship between systemic hemodynamics and microcirculation are not straightforward [25, 26], the assessment of microcirculation might also improve our understanding of the effects of passive mobilization beyond changes to systemic hemodynamics. We hypothesized that in patients with septic shock passive movements might be harmful by inducing significant changes in systemic hemodynamics. We also hypothesized that in these patients the changes induced by passive movements might lead to sublingual microcirculatory impairment. Thus, the objective of this study was to investigate the short-term effects of passive mobilization on sublingual microcirculation and on systemic hemodynamics variables in patients with septic shock and deep sedation.

Methods

This study was carried out in two medical-surgical ICUs within the same university hospital. The local ethics committee approved the study (number: 1056/11), and the patients' next of kin signed informed consent forms allowing their participation. This study was conducted according to the principles of the Declaration of Helsinki and the Brazilian National Council of Health Resolution 466/2012.

Patients

We included patients if they met all the following criteria: 18 years of age or older, septic shock [27] with noradrenaline requirement between 0.1 and 1.0 mcg/kg/min, sedation with a Ramsay scale of 6 [28], mechanical ventilation, an arterial line for blood pressure monitoring, and an indwelling subclavian or jugular central venous catheter. All patients were included after the resuscitation phase of shock.

The exclusion criteria were intracranial hypertension, status epilepticus, or cardiac arrhythmia at the time of the study; acute myocardial infarction (Killip classification 4); thrombocytopenia (<30,000 cells/μL); hemoglobin <7.0 g/dL; leukocytosis (>50,000 cells/μL), peripheral arterial disease, worsening oxygenation status in the last 6 h (oxygen partial pressure to oxygen inspired fraction ratio decrease of >50), circulatory shock of multiple causes, or pregnant and moribund patients. We also excluded patients with medical conditions that prevented the use of a mobilization protocol, such as bone tumors, unconsolidated or unstable bone fracture, amputation, postoperative period for placement or removal of upper and lower limbs bone prosthesis, deep vein thrombosis or phlebitis, musculoskeletal deformity, and compartment syndrome in the upper or lower limbs. In addition, we excluded patients with mucosal injury or recent maxillofacial surgery that interfered with imaging acquisition.

Study protocol

Patients were kept in a semi-recumbent position (30°). Passive movements of the upper limbs (flexion–extension of the wrist, elbow, and shoulder) and lower limbs (flexion–extension of the ankle, knee, and hip) were performed in a counter-clockwise direction starting from the upper right. The frequency of 30 movements per minute was assured by a digital metronome MA-1 BLBK® (KORG, Tokyo, Japan) with 5 min for each limb, totaling 20 min of exercise. One of the investigators (TTP), a trained physiotherapist, applied the passive mobilization protocol. Although this protocol is a standard of care in our unit, it is not routinely applied in those severely ill patients.

We observed all patients for 20 min before passive movement to assure that there were no significant variations in sedative and vasoactive medication infusions as well as hemodynamic and respiratory parameters. Before the intervention, the vasopressor dose was titrated by the attending physician targeting a mean arterial pressure of at least 65 mmHg. The protocol was interrupted if any of the following adverse events occurred: detection of active movement, hypoxemia (pulse oximetry <88%), hemodynamic instability (heart rate (HR) <45 bpm, mean arterial pressure (MAP) <60 mmHg or >120 mmHg), and changes in the doses of vasoactive or sedation drugs.

Variables

We recorded systemic hemodynamics and sublingual microcirculatory variables before (T0) and up to 10 min after (T1) passive movements. We assessed the sublingual microcirculation using sidestream dark field (SDF) imaging (Microscan®; MicroVision Medical, Amsterdam, Netherlands). To ensure image quality and adequate reproducibility, we adopted recommended techniques for video acquisition [29]. After removing saliva and oral secretions, the probe was applied over the mucosa. Special care was taken to avoid pressure artifacts, which was verified by checking ongoing flow in larger microvessels. We collected three high-quality steady images of at least 10 s in different sublingual regions using a portable computer and an analog-to-digital video converter (ADVC110, Canopus Co., San Jose, CA, USA). The image quality was checked before being stored at full size as DV-AVI files. Digital sequences were stored and we used the AVA 3.0® software (MicroVision Medical, Amsterdam, Netherlands) for automated vascular analysis. The correct procedure for vascular video analysis with AVA 3.0® software includes some manual analysis steps, including erasing incorrectly detected vessel segments and adding undetected vessel segments. Two investigators (TTP and ATB) analyzed the images off-line. The images were presented in a random order to prevent image pairing. Microcirculatory parameters included the microcirculatory flow index (MFI), the total vascular density (TVD), the De Backer score (DBS), the perfused vascular density (PVD), the proportion of perfused vessels (PPV), and the heterogeneity index (HI) [29]. To calculate the MFI score, the image was divided into four quadrants and the predominant type of flow was assessed in each quadrant using semiquantitative criteria and scored as continuous (continuous flow for at least 10 s = 3), sluggish (slow but continuous flow = 2), intermittent (no flow ≤ 50% of time = 1), or absent (no flow ≥ 50% of time = 0). The MFI score averaged the values of the four quadrants. The TVD was calculated as the length of vessels divided by total area of the image. After drawing three equidistant horizontal and three equidistant vertical lines on the screen, we calculated the De Backer score as the number of vessels crossing the lines divided by the total length of the lines. The PPV (%) can be calculated as follows: 100 × (total number of vessels − [no flow + intermittent flow])/total number of vessels. The PVD was calculated as the length of perfused vessels (flow scores of 2–3) divided by the total area of the image. We used the values generated by AVA software report. As microcirculation is heterogeneous, we calculated the HI defined as the difference between maximal and minimal PPV divided by the mean PPV value of all sublingual sites. All the variables were related to vessels with diameters less than 20 μm.

The cardiac index (CI) was measured by transpulmonary thermodilution (VolumeView/EV1000™ system, Edwards Lifesciences, Irvine, CA, USA), pulmonary thermodilution using the traditional bolus method (Edwards Lifesciences LLC, Irvine, CA, USA), or echocardiography (SonoAce R7 device, Samsung Medison, Seoul, Korea) in patients without invasive monitoring. We also collected data on age, gender, body mass index, severity scores such as Sequential Organ Failure Assessment (SOFA) and Simplified Acute Physiologic Score (SAPS) 3, admission diagnosis, Charlson index, comorbidities, source of infection, sedative drugs, vasoactive drugs, time on vasopressors, mechanical ventilation parameters, ICU length of stay, and ICU mortality.

Statistical analysis

To calculate the sample size, we hypothesize a mean decrease of 0.25 and a standard deviation of the difference of 0.5 in the MFI after passive mobilization using 0.05 as the significance level of 0.05 with a power of 80%. Using a paired sample *t* test, the required sample size was 34 patients.

The data are expressed as a number (percent), the mean ± standard deviation, or the median (interquartile range), as appropriate. Continuous data were tested for normality by Shapiro–Wilk's test. The systemic hemodynamic and microcirculatory variables were compared at T0 and T1 using a paired Wilcoxon test or paired *t* test, as appropriate. For the systemic hemodynamic variables, we defined post hoc as clinically relevant those changes greater than 10% using as reference the baseline [30]. As our primary hypothesis was that passive mobilization would potentially cause a worsening in the microcirculation we also hypothesize that this would occur mainly in patients using higher doses of noradrenaline. Thus, we analyzed our results according to the baseline noradrenaline dose. We classified as low-dose group dose those patients using less than 0.3 mcg/kg/min and as high-dose group those using ≥0.3 mcg/kg/min. We compared the microcirculatory variables at moments T0 and T1 within the groups, using *t* test or Wilcoxon test, as appropriate. We also measured the intensity of variation between T0 and T1 and compare the results of all microcirculatory variables between the groups using Mann–Whitney test or *t* test, as appropriate. The correlation between induced changes in systemic hemodynamics and microcirculatory variables was assessed using a Spearman correlation test.

We used SPSS version 22.0 for Windows (Armonk, NY: IBM Corp) for statistical analysis. The results with *p* values <0.05 were considered significant. For the sample size calculation, we used MedCalc software 14.12.0 (MedCalc Software bvba, Belgium).

Results

We collected data from October 2013 to May 2015. Over the study period, 2877 patients were admitted to the ICU, of whom 302 (10.5%) had septic shock and were mechanically ventilated. After the exclusion criteria were applied, 36 patients were included. However, one patient presented active movement during the protocol and was subsequently excluded (Fig. 1).

The patients included in our study were elderly (68; 49–78 years) and severely ill, as assessed by their SOFA (9; 7.0–12.0) and SAPS 3 (66.7 ± 12.1) scores. The lung was the main source of sepsis, and the mortality rate was high (60%). All patients were included after the initial phase of shock resuscitation. The patients were submitted to passive movements at approximately 39 h; 24.0–72.0 h after vasopressor infusion. The minimum duration of vasopressor infusion was 8 h. The baseline characteristics are listed in Table 1.

We obtained the cardiac index by pulmonary thermodilution ($n = 14$), transpulmonary thermodilution ($n = 8$), and transthoracic echocardiography ($n = 12$). In one patient, we were not able to record the velocity–time integral of flow through the left ventricular outflow tract. Systemic hemodynamic variables before and after passive movements are provided in Table 2. There was no significant change after exercise except for clinically non-relevant decreases in HR (T0: 95.6 ± 22.0 bpm; T1: 93.8 ± 22.0 bpm, $p < 0.040$) and body temperature (T0: 36.9 ± 1.1 °C; T1: 36.7 ± 1.2 °C, $p < 0.002$). There was no change in the lactate levels or in the central venous oxygen saturation levels.

After passive mobilization, there was a slight but significant increase in PPV (T0: 78.2 (70.9–81.9) %; T1: 80.0 (75.2–85.1) %, $p < 0.029$), without any change in other microcirculatory variables. The microcirculatory variables are provided in Table 3. However, when we analyzed the patients according to the baseline dose of noradrenaline, only those patients using high doses at baseline had a significant increase in PPV, while those in the low-dose group did not change their PPV after the intervention (see Additional file 1: eTable 1). We tried to better understand the association between the noradrenaline dose at baseline and the changes in PPV by assessing the intensity of PPV variation (T1–T0). However, there was no significant difference between the two groups, underscoring the relevance of our previous finding of an association between noradrenaline doses and the variation in PPV (see Additional file 1: eTable 2). There was no correlation between PPV variation and the variation in systemic hemodynamics (ΔHR: $r = -0.010$, $p = 0.955$, ΔCI: $r = 0.218$, $p = 0.215$, and ΔMAP: $r = 0.276$, $p = 0.109$) (see Additional file 1: eFigure 1). We did not observe adverse events during passive movements or in the recovery period.

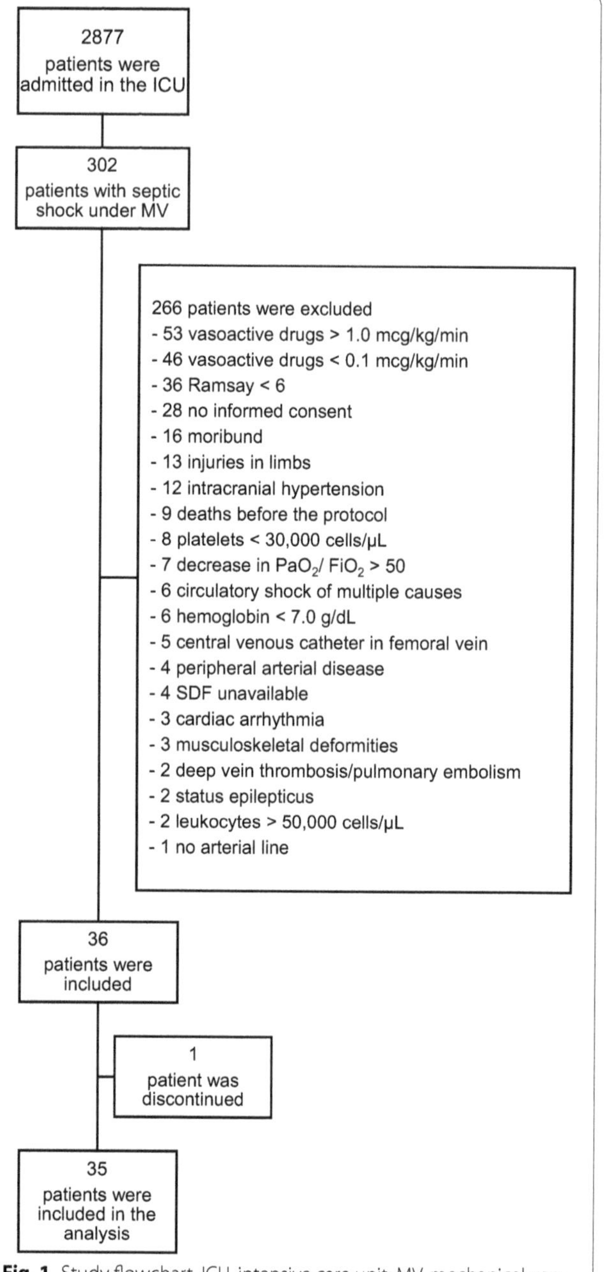

Fig. 1 Study flowchart. ICU, intensive care unit; MV, mechanical ventilation; PaO_2, arterial oxygen partial pressure; FiO_2, oxygen inspired fraction; SDF, sidestream dark field

Table 1 Baseline characteristics and clinical data of the study population

Characteristics	Results ($n = 35$)
Age (years)	68 (49.0–78.0)
Gender, male	16 (45.7)
BMI (kg/m^2)	24.6 ± 5.0
SOFA[a]	9 (7.0–12.0)
SAPS 3 score	66.7 ± 12.1
Admission diagnosis	
Surgical	19 (54.3)
Clinical	16 (45.7)
Charlson index	2.0 (1.0–6.0)
Comorbidities	
Hypertension	15 (42.9)
Diabetes mellitus	10 (28.6)
Liver failure	4 (11.4)
Source of infection	
Pulmonary	18 (51.4)
Abdominal	8 (22.9)
Blood flow	6 (17.1)
Others	3 (8.6)
Sedative drugs	
Propofol (mg/kg/h) ($n = 30$)	1.84 ± 0.83
Fentanyl (mcg/kg/h) ($n = 28$)	3.42 ± 1.41
Midazolam (mcg/kg/h) ($n = 5$)	0.08 (0.06–0.17)
Vasoactive drugs	
Norepinephrine (mcg/kg/min) ($n = 35$)	0.39 ± 0.20
Epinephrine (mcg/kg/min) ($n = 2$)	0.01 (0.01–0.01)
Dobutamine (mcg/kg/min) ($n = 1$)	2.85
Time on vasopressors pre-protocol (h)	39 (24.0–72.0)
Mechanical ventilation	
PEEP (cmH_2O)	8.0 (6.0–10.0)
FiO_2 (%)	40.0 (30.0–50.0)
PaO_2/FiO_2	239.0 ± 83.0
Cstat (mL/cmH_2O)	33.9 ± 13.7
Tidal volume (mL/kg)[b]	7.2 ± 1.4
Driving pressure (cmH_2O)	12.0 (9.0–16.0)
ICU LOS (days)	17.0 (12.0–25.0)
ICU mortality	21 (60.0)

The results are expressed as a number (%), the mean ± standard deviation or the median (25–75%)

BMI, body mass index; SOFA, Sequential Organ Failure Assessment; SAPS 3, Simplified Acute Physiology Score 3; PEEP, positive end-expiratory pressure; PaO_2, arterial oxygen partial pressure; FiO_2, oxygen inspired fraction; Cstat, static compliance; ICU, intensive care unit; LOS, length of stay

[a] SOFA was calculated on the study day, [b] based on predicted body weight

Table 2 Systemic hemodynamic and ventilation variables at baseline and after exercise

Variable	Baseline	After exercise	p value
HR (bpm)	95.6 ± 22.0	93.8 ± 22.0	0.040
MAP (mmHg)	75.0 (71.0–85.0)	74.0 (69.0–84.0)	0.859
CVP (mmHg)	9.3 ± 3.6	8.7 ± 3.2	0.077
CI (L/min m^2)	2.5 (1.7–3.6)	2.5 (1.7–3.3)	0.930
Lactate (mg/dL)	15.0 (12.0–24.0)	15.5 (11.7–23.5)	0.554
$SvcO_2$ (%)	73.4 ± 8.6	72.8 ± 9.3	0.315
ΔPCO_2 (torr)	5.3 ± 1.7	5.0 ± 2.1	0.450
Body temperature, (°C)	36.9 ± 1.1	36.7 ± 1.2	0.002
PaO_2 (torr)	91.0 (78.5–99.7)	93.3 (75.9–102.2)	0.973
$PaCO_2$ (torr)	40.1 (33.9–45.7)	39.7 (32.8–48.2)	0.977
Hb (g/dL)	9.7 (8.7–11.8)	10.2 (8.6–11.9)	0.493
BE	−4.2 ± 5.4	−4.0 ± 5.6	0.297

The results are expressed as the mean ± standard deviation or the median (25–75%). Paired t test or paired Wilcoxon test

HR, heart rate; MAP, mean arterial pressure; CVP, central venous pressure; CI, cardiac index; $SvcO_2$, central venous oxygen saturation; ΔPCO_2, carbon dioxide venoarterial gradient; PaO_2, arterial oxygen partial pressure; $PaCO_2$, carbon dioxide partial pressure; Hb, hemoglobin; BE, base excess

Discussion

Our data suggest that passive mobilization of patients with septic shock after an initial phase of hemodynamic resuscitation does not compromise the microcirculation or the systemic hemodynamics. Passive mobilization was associated with an isolated and discrete improvement in the PPV. We also observed significant, although clinically non-relevant, reductions in HR and temperature.

Although passive mobilization has been widely used in the ICU over the years [31, 32], few studies have evaluated the effects of passive mobilization on hemodynamic and tissue perfusion variables. Two studies reported an increase in VO_2 and a reduction in SvO_2 after passive cyclic movements of the lower limbs. In our study, we were not able to find this reduction in $SvcO_2$. However, one of the studies analyzed a small number of patients, which compromises the reproducibility of their results [19]. In the other, the patients were not under deep sedation; therefore, voluntary muscular activation may have occurred that could have caused the alterations. Electromyography was not performed to verify the absence of voluntary muscular contractions in these patients [18]. In contrast, in agreement with our findings, other studies showed stability or no-relevance clinical or systemic hemodynamic variables after passive exercise [11, 13, 16, 20–24].

The absence of significant changes in systemic hemodynamics can be explained by the deep sedation of our patients. Deep sedation would reduce the occurrence of adrenergic stimuli as a function of physical exercise. The passive movement applied in our study probably did not activate the exercise pressor reflex, activated by muscular ergoreceptors, which generally stimulate sympathetic autonomic activity, generating cardiovascular alterations [33]. In addition, sedation reduces the chance of

Table 3 Sublingual microcirculation variables at baseline and after exercise

Variable	Baseline	After exercise	p value
MFI	2.8 (2.3–3.0)	2.8 (2.6–3.0)	0.462
TVD (mm/mm^2)	25.6 ± 4.3	26.1 ± 4.2	0.354
DBS (n/mm)	16.0 ± 2.2	16.3 ± 1.9	0.489
PVD (mm/mm^2)	22.4 ± 3.9	23.2 ± 3.4	0.122
PPV (%)	78.2 (70.9–81.9)	80.0 (75.2–85.1)	0.029
HI	0.15 (0.11–0.32)	0.12 (0.07–0.22)	0.149

The results are expressed as the mean ± standard deviation or the median (25–75%). Paired *t* test or paired Wilcoxon test

MFI microcirculatory flow index, *TVD* total vascular density, *DBS* De Backer score, *PVD* perfused vascular density, *PPV* proportion of perfused vessels, *HI* heterogeneity index

voluntary muscle activity either assisting or resisting the movement performed by the physical therapist.

According to our results, microcirculatory indices were also not compromised by passive mobilization. These data are consistent with our results for systemic hemodynamics, suggesting that passive exercise does not harm patients with septic shock. We did not find previous studies that evaluated the impact of these maneuvers on microcirculation, which makes our results novel. We demonstrated that passive mobilization discretely increased the PPV, an important variable for microcirculation evaluation, since it has previously been shown as a marker of disease severity [34]. This finding was unexpected as our primary hypothesis was an impairment in the microcirculation secondary to our intervention. Although our study is underpowered to assess the potential explanations for this finding, we can provide some hypotheses. It is possible that slight changes in CI, MAP, and HR could have led to an improvement in perfusion and consequently to an improvement in PPV. However, we were unable to statistically show association between these variables. The venous return during lower extremity passive exercises usually is not sufficient to produce significant hemodynamic changes, because the patients are kept in a semi-recumbent position (30°), mobilizing less venous blood from the large splanchnic compartment. The passive leg raising hemodynamic effects also vanish after 1 min [35]. However, it is potentially possible that slight changes in the venous return, not detectable by the central venous pressure, might have contributed to a recruitment of previously closed vessels. As the intervention was made in the upper and lower limbs, a direct effect on the sublingual microcirculation is biological implausible. However, it is possible that exercise release substances, such as endorphins, have unknown effects in the microcirculation. Notwithstanding, due to our primary hypothesis, we believed that this might also be a type 1 error, and the significant difference was found only by chance, since others microcirculatory parameters did not significantly change.

Of notice, our microcirculatory variables, except the PPV, were only mildly affected, which are not a usual finding in severely ill septic shock patients with high SOFA and SAPS 3 scores and a high mortality rate. Some studies have shown that high levels of noradrenaline and the presence of hyperlactacidemia were associated with deranged microcirculatory parameters [36–38]. A possible explanation for our findings would be a dissociation between systemic hemodynamics and the microcirculation, which has already been described following resuscitation [25, 26], However, our systemic variables do not suggest this is the case. The vast majority of our patients had normal CO_2 gradient values, SvO_2 and lactate levels, although still using moderate doses of noradrenaline. This suggests that their mildly affected systemic variables parallel their mildly affected microcirculation. By contrary, this does not mean their survival rates would be lower. They are severely ill patients, and the determinants of sepsis survival in low- and middle-income countries are far beyond the factors analyzed in this study.

This study has some strengths. The inclusion of patients was consecutive. To the best of our knowledge, this is the first study to evaluate the impact of passive exercise on sublingual microcirculation using videomicroscopy. Microcirculation analysis is important, as studies in patients with sepsis have suggested that microcirculatory variables may remain altered despite the normalization of classic tissue perfusion variables [39]. Another relevant aspect was the technique used, as patient movement was reproduced manually by a single physical therapist, demonstrating that the protocol can be performed in places with limited resources. All four limbs were mobilized, not only the lower limbs, which is the most common practice in the ICU. In addition, all patients were severely ill and were administered vasoactive infusions and deep sedation. The use of passive mobilization in patients under minimal dose of vasopressor is already part of the current guidelines [40]. Usually, patients with higher doses would be considered by the multidisciplinary team excessively ill to be submitted to passive mobilization [41], which adds value to our findings and might stimulate its practice in this specific population. There are theoretical benefits with the use of passive mobilization [14–16]. Early mobilization in mechanically ventilated patients who are critically ill reduces the effects of ICU-acquired weakness [9–11], and this strategy includes the use of protocols of passive movements as adopted in our study.

This study also has some limitations. First, the single-center nature of our study might compromise the generalization of the results. Second, we analyzed systemic hemodynamics and microcirculation only in two periods, before and after exercise, and it is possible that changes occurred during mobilization. However, it is not possible to analyze the microcirculation during exercise. Third, our sample size does not allow a reliable analysis of the effects of different vasopressors on the microcirculation. Fourth, we found a high density and perfusion values in a very sick population and a bias in the software-assisted analysis cannot be rule out as we have consciously manually added undetected vessel segments during the analysis. However, our paired analysis minimizes the impact of this potential bias. Finally, three different methods were used to obtain CI due to ethical concerns. We used invasive monitoring only when the patient already required it for his own clinical condition. In patients without any invasive monitoring we used transthoracic echocardiography. However, we used the same technique before and after exercise in each patient, which attenuates this potential limitation as the patient was his own control and all the analysis were done using paired tests. Although cardiac output estimated by transthoracic echocardiography is not accurate and precise [42], it accurately tracks variations in CI [43] and transpulmonary thermodilution devices are comparable with the pulmonary artery catheter [44].

Conclusions

In patients with septic shock after the initial phase of hemodynamic resuscitation, passive exercise does not seem to be associated with relevant changes in microcirculation or in the systemic hemodynamics.

Abbreviations

BE: base excess; BMI: body mass index; CI: cardiac index; Cstat: static compliance; CVP: central venous pressure; DBS: De Backer score; FiO_2: oxygen inspired fraction; Hb: hemoglobin; HI: heterogeneity index; HR: heart rate; ICU: intensive care unit; LOS: length of stay; MAP: mean arterial pressure; MFI: microcirculatory flow index; MV: mechanical ventilation; $PaCO_2$: carbon dioxide partial pressure; PaO_2: arterial oxygen partial pressure; PEEP: positive end-expiratory pressure; PVD: perfused vascular density; PPV: proportion of perfused vessels; SAPS 3: Simplified Acute Physiology Score 3; SDF: sidestream dark field; SOFA: Sequential Organ Failure Assessment; $SvcO_2$: central venous oxygen saturation; SvO_2: venous oxygen saturation; TVD: total vascular density; VO_2: oxygen consumption; Δ: delta.

Authors' contributions

TTP, FGRF, ATB, and FRM contributed to conception and design; TTP, FGRF, ATB, and KFTC were involved in data acquisition; all authors analyzed and interpreted the data; TTP, FGRF, and FRM wrote the manuscript. All authors read and approved the final manuscript.

Authors' information

TTP, VMFM, HBR, PVT are physiotherapists working at the intensive care unit. FGRF, ATB, KTFC, and FRM are physicians involved in microcirculation research in the unit. FGRF and FRM are professors of Critical Care at the university. FRM is the chair of the Intensive Care department.

Acknowledgements

Not applicable.

Competing interests

The authors declare that they have no competing interests.

Funding

This study was supported by Fundação de Apoio a Pesquisa do Estado de São Paulo FAPESP (Grant No. 2012 19 051-1). FAPESP had no role in the study design; the collection, analysis and interpretation of the data; or the manuscript's authorship.

References

1. Vender JS, Szokol JM, Murphy GS, Nitsun M. Sedation, analgesia, and neuromuscular blockade in sepsis: an evidence-based review. Crit Care Med. 2004;32(Suppl 11):S554–61.
2. Barr J, Fraser GL, Puntillo K, Ely EW, Gélinas C, Dasta JF, et al. Clinical practice guidelines for the management of pain, agitation, and delirium in adult patients in the intensive care unit. Crit Care Med. 2013;41(1):263–306.
3. Callahan LA, Supinski GS. Sepsis-induced myopathy. Crit Care Med. 2009;37(10 Suppl):S354–67.
4. Hermans G, Van den Berghe G. Clinical review: intensive care unit acquired weakness. Crit Care. 2015;19:274.
5. Schweickert WD, Hall J. ICU-acquired weakness. Chest. 2007;131(5):1541–9.
6. De Jonghe B, Sharshar T, Lefaucheur JP, Authier FJ, Durand-Zaleski I, Boussarsar M, et al. Paresis acquired in the intensive care unit: a prospective multicenter study. JAMA. 2002;288(22):2859–67.
7. Hermans G, Van Mechelen H, Clerckx B, Vanhullebusch T, Mesotten D, Wilmer A, et al. Acute outcomes and 1-year mortality of intensive care unit-acquired weakness. A cohort study and propensity-matched analysis. Am J Respir Crit Care Med. 2014;90(4):410–20.
8. Latronico N, Bolton CF. Critical illness polyneuropathy and myopathy: a major cause of muscle weakness and paralysis. Lancet Neurol. 2011;10(10):931–41.
9. Morris PE, Goad A, Thompson C, Taylor K, Harry B, Passmore L, et al. Early intensive care unit mobility therapy in the treatment of acute respiratory failure. Crit Care Med. 2008;36(8):2238–43.
10. Schweickert WD, Pohlman MC, Pohlman AS, Nigos C, Pawlik AJ, Esbrook C, et al. Early physical and occupational therapy in mechanically ventilated, critically ill patients: a randomized controlled trial. Lancet. 2009;373(9678):1874–82.
11. Burtin C, Clerckx B, Robbeets C, Ferdinande P, Langer D, Troosters T, et al. Early exercise in critically ill patients enhances shot-term functional recovery. Crit Care Med. 2009;37(9):2499–505.
12. Bailey P, Thomsen GE, Spuhler VJ, Blair R, Jewkes J, Bezdjian L, et al. Early activity is feasible and safe in respiratory failure patients. Crit Care Med. 2007;35(1):139–45.
13. Pires-Neto RC, Kawaguchi YM, Hirota AS, Fu C, Tanaka C, Caruso P, et al. Very early passive cycling exercise in mechanically ventilated critically ill patients: physiological and safety aspects—a case series. PLoS One. 2013;8(9):e74182:1–7.
14. Salter RB. The biologic concept of continuous passive motion of synovial joints. The first 18 years of basic research and its clinical application. Clin Orthop Relat Res. 1989;242:12–25.
15. Griffiths RD, Palmer TE, Helliwell T, MacLennan P, MacMillan RR. Effect of passive stretching on the wasting of muscle in the critically ill. Nutrition. 1995;11(5):428–32.
16. Amidei C, Sole ML. Physiological responses to passive exercise in adults receiving mechanical ventilation. Am J Crit Care. 2013;22(4):337–48.
17. Adler J, Malone D. Early mobilization in the intensive care unit: a systematic review. Cardiopulm Phys Ther J. 2012;23(1):5–13.

18. Norrenberg M, Backer D, Freidman G, Moraine JJ, Vincent JL. Cardiovascular response to passive leg movement in critically ill patients. Clin Intensive Care. 1999;10(1):1–6.
19. Savi A, Maia CP, Dias AS, Teixeira C. Efeitos hemodinâmicos e metabólicos da movimentação passiva dos membros inferiores em pacientes sob ventilação mecânica. Rev bras ter intensiva. 2010;22(4):315–20.
20. Hickmann CE, Roeseler J, Castanares-Zapatero D, Herrera EI, Mongodin A, Laterre PF. Energy expenditure in the critically ill performing early physical therapy. Intensive Care Med. 2014;40(4):548–55.
21. Genc A, Koca U, Gunerli A. What are the hemodynamic and respiratory effects of passive limb exercise for mechanically ventilated patients receiving low-dose vasopressor/inotropic support? Crit Care Nurs Q. 2014;37(2):152–8.
22. Thelandersson A, Volkmann R, Cider A. Blood flow velocity and vascular resistance during passive leg exercise in the critically ill patient. Clin Physiol Funct Imaging. 2012;32(5):338–42.
23. Thelandersson A, Cider Å, Volkmann R. Cerebrovascular and systemic haemodynamic parameters during passive exercise. Adv Physiother. 2010;12(1):58–63.
24. Berney S, Denehy L. The effect of physiotherapy treatment on oxygen consumption and haemodynamics in patients who are critically ill. Aus J Physiother. 2003;49(2):99–105.
25. Dubin A, Pozo MO, Casabella CA, Pálizas F Jr, Murias G, Moseinco MC, et al. Increasing arterial blood pressure with norepinephrine does not improve microcirculatory blood flow: a prospective study. Crit Care. 2009;13(3):R92.
26. De Backer D, Ortiz JA, Salgado D. Coupling microcirculation to systemic hemodynamics. Curr Opin Crit Care. 2010;16(3):250–4.
27. Bone RC, Balk RA, Cerra FB, Dellinger RP, Fein AM, Knaus WA, et al. Definitions for sepsis and organ failure and guidelines for the use of innovative therapies in sepsis. The ACCP/SCCM Consensus Conference Committee. American College of Chest physicians/Society of Critical Care Medicine. Chest. 1992;101(6):1644–55.
28. Ramsay MA, Savage TM, Simpson BR, Goodwin R. Controlled sedation with alphaxalone-alphadolone. Br Med J. 1974;2(5920):656–9.
29. De Backer D, Hollenberg S, Boerma C, Goedhart P, Büchele G, Ospina-Tascon G, et al. How to evaluate the microcirculation: report of a round table conference. Crit Care. 2007;11(5):R101.
30. Michard F, Boussat S, Chemla D, Anguel N, Mercat A, Lecarpentier Y, et al. Relation between respiratory changes in arterial pulse pressure and fluid responsiveness in septic patients with acute circulatory failure. Am J Respir Crit Care Med. 2000;162(1):134–8.
31. Hodgin KE, Nordon-Craft A, McFann KK, Mealer ML, Moss M. Physical therapy utilization in intensive care units: results from a national survey. Crit Care Med. 2009;37(2):561–6.
32. Stockley RC, Hughes J, Morrison J, Rooney J. An investigation of the use of passive movements in intensive care by UK physiotherapists. Physiotherapy. 2010;96(3):228–33.
33. Kaufman MP, Hayes SG. The exercise pressor reflex. Clin Auton Res. 2002;12(6):429–39.
34. De Backer D, Donadello K, Sakr Y, Ospina-Tascon G, Salgado D, Scolletta S, et al. Microcirculatory alterations in patients with severe sepsis: impact of time of assessment and relationship with outcome. Crit Care Med. 2013;41(3):791–9.
35. Monnet X, Teboul J-L. Passive leg raising: five rules, not a drop of fluid! Crit Care. 2015;19(1):18.
36. De Backer D, Creteur J, Preiser JC, Dubois MJ, Vincent JL. Microvascular blood flow is altered in patients with sepsis. Am J Respir Crit Care Med. 2002;166(1):98–104.
37. Hernandez G, Boerma EC, Dubin A, Bruhn A, Koopmans M, Edul VK, et al. Severe abnormalities in microvascular perfused vessel density are associated to organ dysfunctions and mortality and can be predicted by hyperlactatemia and norepinephrine requirements in septic shock patients. J Crit Care. 2013;28(4):538.e9–14.
38. Edul VS, Enrico C, Laviolle B, Vazquez AR, Ince C, Dubin A. Quantitative assessment of the microcirculation in healthy volunteers and in patients with septic shock. Crit Care Med. 2012;40(5):1443–8.
39. Trzeciak S, McCoy JV, Phillip Dellinger R, Arnold RC, Rizzuto M, Abate NL, et al. Early increases in microcirculatory perfusion during protocol-directed resuscitation are associated with reduced multi-organ failure at 24 h in patients with sepsis. Intensive Care Med. 2008;34(12):2210–7.
40. Sommers J, Engelbert RH, Dettling-Ihnenfeldt D, Gosselink R, Spronk PE, Nollet F, et al. Physiotherapy in the intensive care unit: an evidence-based, expert driven, practical statement and rehabilitation recommendations. Clin Rehabil. 2015;29(11):1051–63.
41. Brown SM, Lanspa MJ, Jones JP, Kuttler KG, Li Y, Carlson R, et al. Survival after shock requiring high-dose vasopressor therapy. Chest. 2013;143(3):664–71.
42. Wetterslev M, Møller-Sørensen H, Johansen RR, Perner A. Systematic review of cardiac output measurements by echocardiography vs. thermodilution: the techniques are not interchangeable. Intensive Care Med. 2016;42(8):1223–33.
43. Mercado P, Maizel J, Beyls C, Titeca-Beauport D, Joris M, Kontar L, et al. Transthoracic echocardiography: an accurate and precise method for estimating cardiac output in the critically ill patient. Crit Care. 2017;21(1):136.
44. Monnet X, Teboul JL. Transpulmonary thermodilution: advantages and limits. Crit Care. 2017;21(1):147.

14

Effects of combination therapy using antithrombin and thrombomodulin for sepsis-associated disseminated intravascular coagulation

Toshiaki Iba[1*], Akiyoshi Hagiwara[2], Daizoh Saitoh[3], Hideaki Anan[4], Yutaka Ueki[5], Koichi Sato[6] and Satoshi Gando[7]

Abstract

Background: No single anticoagulant has been proven effective for sepsis-associated disseminated intravascular coagulation (DIC). Thus, the concomitant use of antithrombin concentrate and recombinant thrombomodulin has been conceived. This observational study was conducted to investigate the efficacy and safety of this combination therapy.

Methods: A total of 510 septic DIC patients who received antithrombin substitution were retrospectively analyzed. Among them, 228 were treated with antithrombin and recombinant thrombomodulin (combination therapy) and the rest were treated with antithrombin alone (monotherapy). Propensity score matching created 129 matched pairs, and 28-day all-cause mortality, DIC scores, the sequential organ failure assessment (SOFA) scores, and the incidence of bleeding were compared.

Results: A log-rank test revealed a significant association between combination therapy and a lower 28-day mortality rate (hazard ratio 0.49, 95% confidence interval 0.29–0.82, $P = 0.006$) in the matched pairs. The DIC scores and the SOFA scores in the combination therapy group were significantly lower than those in the monotherapy group on Day 4 and Day 7. The incidence of bleeding did not differ between the groups (2.11 vs. 2.31%, $P = 1.000$).

Conclusions: The current study demonstrated the potential benefit of adding recombinant thrombomodulin to antithrombin. The co-administration of these two anticoagulants was associated with reduced mortality among patients with sepsis-induced DIC without increasing the risk of bleeding.

Keywords: Disseminated intravascular coagulation, Sepsis, Antithrombin, Thrombomodulin, Propensity analysis

Background

Anticoagulant therapy for sepsis-associated disseminated intravascular coagulation (DIC) is widely performed in Japan [1], and antithrombin concentrate and recombinant thrombomodulin are the two most popular agents utilized for this treatment [2]. However, not a single anticoagulant has proven to be effective. Furthermore, neither of the above-mentioned agents has been recommended for use outside Japan [3, 4]. To examine the effects of recombinant thrombomodulin, Hayakawa et al. [5] conducted a retrospective multicenter survey examining 1784 sepsis-associated DIC cases. They created 452 propensity score-matched pairs and performed a logistic regression analysis. As a result, a significant association between recombinant thrombomodulin use and lower mortality (odds ratio [OR] 0.757; 95% confidence interval [CI] 0.574–0.999, $P = 0.049$) was recognized. The same group also performed a similar analysis on antithrombin

*Correspondence: toshiiba@cf6.so-net.ne.jp
[1] Department of Emergency and Disaster Medicine, Juntendo University Graduate School of Medicine, 2-1-1 Hongo Bunkyo-ku, Tokyo 113-8421, Japan
Full list of author information is available at the end of the article

concentrate and reported that the inverse probability of a treatment-weighted propensity score analysis indicated a statistically significant association between antithrombin supplementation and lower mortality (OR 0.748, 95% CI 0.572–0.978, $P = 0.034$). However, a propensity score-matched analysis did not show a significant association in a latter analysis [6]. In contrast to the situation in Japan, the international guidelines for sepsis do not recommend the use of antithrombin, and recombinant thrombomodulin is still not available outside Japan [7]. Despite the lack of robust evidence, the concomitant use of antithrombin and recombinant thrombomodulin has become popular in clinics, and recent post-marketing surveys have reported that combination therapy is now used in 50% of cases, at present [8]. Regarding the efficacy of combination therapy, available information remains sparse and the results are inconsistent. We formerly performed a logistic regression analysis among septic DIC patients who had undergone antithrombin supplementation and reported that the co-administration of recombinant thrombomodulin was a significant factor affecting survival [9]. Since the number of patients who received combination therapy was relatively small in that study, we repeated the survey and accumulated 159 patients in the second study [10]. This second survey demonstrated that the 28-day survival outcome in the combination therapy group was 80.5%, while it was only 63.9% in the antithrombin monotherapy group; this difference was statistically significant. Regarding the bleeding incidence, combination therapy is reportedly not associated with a risk of bleeding [10]. Since information regarding the effects and adverse effects of combination therapy is still limited [11], we planned to examine these issues in the third survey.

Methods

Patient selection

This post-marketing surveillance was performed as a multi-institutional, post-marketing survey. A total of 570 sepsis-associated DIC patients with an antithrombin activity ≦70% who were treated between June 2014 and June 2016 were registered. For the diagnosis of DIC, the Japanese Association for Acute Medicine (JAAM)-DIC criteria (Additional file 1: Supplement Table 1) [12] were utilized. Patients with a history of an allergic shock reaction to antithrombin, with major bleeding, an age of younger than 18 years old, or who were pregnant were excluded.

Ethics, consent and permissions and consent to publish

The survey was performed under the supervision of the Japanese Ministry of Health, Labour and Welfare (JMHW) and was conducted in accordance with the Declaration of Helsinki and Good Vigilance Practice and Good Post-marketing Study Practice. Since the complete anonymization of personal data was performed upon data collection, the ethical committee of Juntendo University waived the need to obtain informed consent and the patients' agreement. In the same reason, the institutional committee judged that the consent to publish was not required.

Treatment

When the patients met the JAAM-DIC criteria and had an antithrombin activity level of ≦ 70%, antithrombin concentrate (Nihon Pharmaceutical Co. Ltd, Tokyo, Japan) was administered for up to 3 consecutive days unless the patient died or treatment was stopped for any justifiable reason. The concomitant use of other anticoagulants was not prohibited, and recombinant thrombomodulin (TM-α; Asahi Kasei Parma Corporation, Tokyo, Japan) was administered intravenously according to the drug manufacturer's recommendation (0.06 mg/kg/day for 6 days by either intravenous bolus injection or intravenous infusion over 15 min via a catheter). Standard sepsis care was performed, and platelet concentrate and fresh-frozen plasma were used as substitution therapy, if necessary [13].

Data collection

The baseline data for the coagulation markers including fibrinogen/fibrin degradation products (FDP), D-dimer, prothrombin time (PT) ratio, platelet counts and antithrombin activity were measured before the treatment. Systemic inflammatory response syndrome (SIRS) score, sequential organ failure assessment (SOFA) score, and JAAM-DIC score were also calculated. Serial data for each coagulation marker, SIRS score, SOFA score and JAAM-DIC were also measured after the start of treatment (Day 2, Day 4, Day 7).

Survival was recorded until Day 28. The bleeding events were recorded throughout the observation period. Major bleeding was defined as bleeding that was either fatal, involved the failure of a critical organ, or was associated with a decrease in the hemoglobin level of 2.0 g/dL or more or required the infusion of 2 or more units of blood. The platelet count and other coagulation profiles were measured in local laboratories.

Statistical analysis

Student's t test, Mann–Whitney test, and Fisher's exact test were used to compare covariates between patients who received antithrombin alone (monotherapy group) versus antithrombin and recombinant thrombomodulin (combination therapy group). Bonferroni's correction was used to compare DIC score and SOFA score between two groups.

Cox's proportional hazards model (Cox hazard) was applied to evaluate the effectiveness of combination therapy. We selected some possible confounding covariates from the baseline characteristics and calculated a variance inflation factor (VIF). Finally, we set age, sex, baseline SOFA score, baseline DIC score, and antithrombin activity at baseline as confounding covariates. Then, a propensity score matching (PSM) was performed with these covariates.

A caliper width of s propensity score matching was set 0.06. Using this caliper width, we performed one-to-one nearest-neighbor matching without replacement between two groups.

To evaluate an effect size in the two matched groups, we calculated the standardized difference for continuous data and phi coefficient for categorical data. Log-rank test was used to compare two survival curves between monotherapy group and combination group. Data are expressed as a number (%), mean ± standard deviation (SD), or median (interquartile range), as appropriate. For all the reported results, $P < 0.05$ or $P < 0.017$ (0.05/3, Bonferroni's correction) was considered to denote statistical significance. R version 3.1.3 was used for all analysis, and SPSS 24.0 for Windows (IBM SPSS Inc., Chicago, IL) was validated for these analyses.

Results

Baseline characteristics

A total of 570 patients were registered in this survey; however, 60 cases were excluded because their treatments did not meet the study's criteria. Twenty-eight cases had an antithrombin activity > 70% when the treatment was initiated. In 16 cases, antithrombin activity was not measured. In the other 16 cases, antithrombin was not administered on the day of diagnosis. Data from 510 cases were used in the following analyses. Among them, 228 were treated with antithrombin and recombinant thrombomodulin (combination therapy group), and the remaining 282 were treated using antithrombin alone (monotherapy group). As for the infection focus, the respiratory system was the most frequent (29.6% 151/510). The baseline characteristics of the unmatched combination therapy and monotherapy groups are presented in Table 1. Propensity score matching created 129 matched pairs (Fig. 1). All the effect sizes of confounding covariates used by the propensity score were ≦ 0.1 for the matched patients, and the characteristics of the two groups were appropriately balanced (Table 2).

Effects on survival among the patients after propensity score matching

The Kaplan–Meier survival curves for the two groups are shown in Fig. 2. The hazard ratios (HRs) for 28-day mortality for combination therapy were 0.62 (95% CI 0.40–0.98, $P = 0.043$ [Cox's proportional hazards model) and 0.55 (95% CI 0.34–0.89, $P = 0.014$ [propensity score matching]), and significant associations were observed between the combination therapy and a lower 28-day mortality (Table 3).

Effects on coagulation markers, DIC score and SOFA score

The FDP level was significantly lower in the combination therapy group on Day 7 ($P = 0.002$). A significant difference in the PT ratio was observed on Day 7 between the groups ($P = 0.014$). The relative changes in JAAM-DIC score were significantly larger for the combination therapy group than for the monotherapy group on Day 4 and Day 7 ($P = 0.004$, 0.003, respectively). The relative changes in SOFA scores were significantly larger in the combination therapy group on Day 4 ($P = 0.011$) (Fig. 3).

Bleeding events

Eighty-four cases presented with bleeding at the time of the diagnosis of DIC were not included among the bleeding events. Twenty cases which have no bleeding records before or after treatment were also excluded from the analysis. Bleeding events observed after diagnosis occurred in 4 out of 190 cases (2.11% [major: 1 case, 0.53%]) in the combination therapy group and in 5 out of 216 cases (2.31% [major: 3 case, 1.39%]) in the monotherapy group. The difference in the bleeding rate was not significant between the two groups ($P = 1.000$ [major: $P = 0.626$]). The details of the bleeding events are summarized in Table 4.

Discussion

Though this study was conducted to examine the effect of combination therapy, the comparison was performed between a combination therapy group and an antithrombin monotherapy group. Hence, the effect of recombinant thrombomodulin as an addition to antithrombin treatment was examined practically. However, since previous studies have demonstrated the possible efficacy of antithrombin substitution for sepsis-associated DIC [9, 10], we think that the results of the current study support the favorable effects of combination therapy. As for the effect of antithrombin substitution, a study using real-world data from a nationwide administrative database in Japan reported a beneficial effect [14]. A total of 9075 patients with severe pneumonia-associated DIC were

Table 1 The baseline characteristics of the enrolled patients ($n = 510$)

Factors	Monotherapy group $n = 282$	Combination therapy group $n = 228$	*P* value	Missing value
Survival at day 28 (%)				
No	81 (28.7)	51 (22.4)	0.127	0
Yes	201 (71.3)	177 (77.6)		
Age (mean [SD])	71.7 (14.7)	72.3 (15.6)	0.663	0
Sex (%)				
Female	115 (40.8)	88 (38.6)	0.682	0
Male	167 (59.2)	140 (61.4)		
Infection focus (*n*, %)				
Respiratory system	91 (32.3)	60 (26.3)	0.172	0
Gastrointestinal system	69 (24.5)	66 (28.9)	0.268	0
Biliary system	35 (12.4)	28 (12.3)	1.000	0
Urinary system	36 (12.8)	39 (17.1)	0.208	0
Musculoskeletal	17 (6.0)	7 (3.1)	0.142	0
Skin and soft tissue	10 (3.5)	7 (3.1)	0.809	0
Central nerve system	2 (0.7)	2 (0.9)	1.000	0
Other	13 (4.6)	15 (6.6)	0.337	0
Unknown	35 (12.4)	20 (8.8)	0.199	0
Surgical intervention	23 (8.2)	34 (14.9)	0.023	0
Non-surgical drainage[#]	5 (1.8)	10 (4.4)	0.113	0
Baseline SOFA score median [25, 75%]				
Total SOFA	10.0 [7.0, 13.0]	11.0 [8.0, 13.0]	0.062	120
Coagulation	2.0 [1.0, 3.0]	2.0 [1.0, 3.0]	0.402	15
Hepatic	0.0 [0.0, 2.0]	0.0 [0.0, 1.0]	0.020	33
Cardiovascular	2.0 [0.0, 4.0]	3.0 [0.3, 4.0]	0.001	19
CNS system	2.0 [0.0, 3.0]	2.0 [1.0, 3.0]	0.312	60
Renal system	1.0 [0.0, 2.0]	1.0 [0.0, 2.0]	0.140	21
Respiratory system	2.0 [1.0, 3.0]	2.0 [1.0, 3.0]	0.038	88
Baseline DIC score median [25, 75%]				
Total DIC score	5.0 [4.0, 6.0]	5.0 [4.0, 7.0]	0.039	29
SIRS score (*n*, %)				
0 point	130 (46.4)	77 (34.4)		
1 point	150 (53.6)	147 (65.6)	0.006	6
Platelet score	3.0 [1.0, 3.0]	3.0 [1.0, 3.0]	0.182	1
FDP score	3.0 [1.0, 3.0]	3.0 [1.0, 3.0]	0.242	14
PT ratio score (*n*, %)				
0 point	53 (19.9)	33 (14.5)		
1 point	214 (80.1)	195 (85.5)	0.123	15
Baseline laboratory score median (SD)				
Platelet count ($\times 10^9$/L)	99.5 (77.6)	89.6 (68.1)	0.130	1
FDP (μg/mL)	56.6 (150.3)	48.8 (66.7)	0.526	110
D-dimer (μg/mL)	26.8 (46.7)	19.7 (29.1)	0.053	121
PT ratio	1.97 (6.08)	1.55 (0.52)	0.298	15
Antithrombin activity (%)	49.6 (13.8)	47.3 (12.7)	0.058	17

The data were shown as mean (standard deviation; SD) or median [25th percentile, 75th percentile]

As the SIRS score and the PT ratio score were composed of binary data, Fisher's exact test was performed

Non-surgical interventions are as follows: percutaneous transcatheter abscess drainage, urinary tract stenting, biliary tract stenting

n number, *SOFA* sequential organ failure assessment, *CNS* central nervous system, *DIC* disseminated intravascular coagulation, *SIRS* systemic inflammatory response syndrome, *FDP* fibrinogen/fibrin degradation products, *PT* prothrombin time

[#] For the selection of covariates, a variance inflation factor (VIF) was calculated and the covariates with VIF ≧ 5 were excluded. Finally, age, sex, baseline SOFA score, baseline DIC score, and antithrombin activityused were selected.

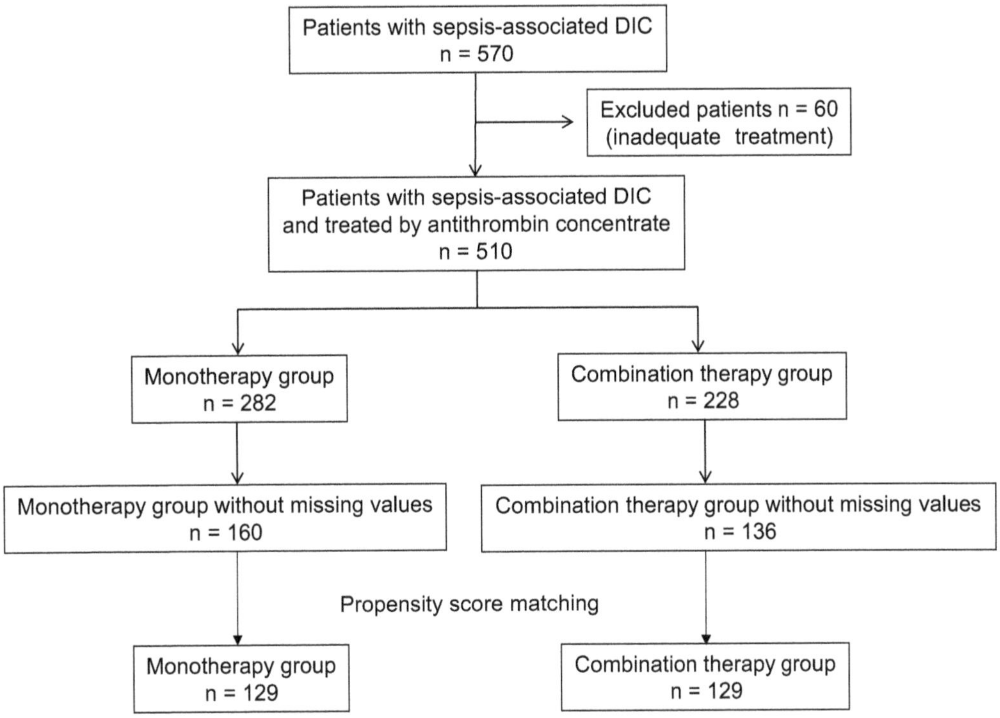

Fig. 1 Patient selection for the evaluation of antithrombin concentrate and recombinant thrombomodulin combination therapy. *DIC* disseminated intravascular coagulation

categorized into an antithrombin group (2663 cases) and a control group (6412 cases). Propensity score matching created a matched cohort of 2194 pairs of patients with and without antithrombin treatment. The results demonstrated that standard antithrombin supplementation (1500 IU/day × 3 days) was associated with a 9.9% (95% CI 3.5–16.3%) reduction in the 28-day mortality rate (with antithrombin vs. without antithrombin: 40.6 vs. 44.2%). In addition, multiple logistic regression analyses showed an association between antithrombin use and the 28-day mortality rate. Similar results in peritonitis-associated DIC patients have also been reported [15]. Based on these reports, we think that the results of the current study suggested the additive effects of recombinant thrombomodulin to antithrombin therapy in patients with sepsis-associated DIC.

With respect to the effect of recombinant thrombomodulin, a phase 3 randomized controlled trial (RCT) comparing recombinant thrombomodulin and heparin in 234 patients with DIC associated with hematologic malignancy or infection was performed in Japan [16], and a subgroup analysis for infection-based DIC revealed that although the mortality difference was 10.2% (recombinant thrombomodulin: 21.4 vs. heparin: 31.6%), the difference was not statistically significant (95% CI − 9.1 to 29.4%) [17]. Since then, the effectiveness of this new agent has been repeatedly evaluated. For example, Yamakawa et al. [18] reported a trend toward favorable outcomes in their systematic review based on a meta-analysis. They collated data from 12 studies (838 patients from 3 RCTs and 571 patients from 9 observational studies) and reported that the relative risk of death was 0.81 (95% CI 0.62–1.06) in the RCTs and 0.59 (95% CI 0.45–0.77) in the observational studies. In contrast, Tagami et al. [19] performed propensity score and instrumental variable analyses using a Japanese nationwide administrative database (matched cohort of 1140 pairs) and reported that treatment with recombinant thrombomodulin did not reduce mortality among patients with pneumonia-associated DIC. More recently, Hagiwara et al. [20] performed an RCT at a single institute with 92 cases and reported an improved DIC resolution rate but almost identical mortality rates. The reason for these contradictory results has not yet been clarified; however, the severity of the subjects might affect the discrepancy. The beneficial effect of anticoagulants generally increases along with the severity of sepsis, and the reported effect was more evident if the study targeted severer cases [21, 22]. Yoshimura et al. [23] performed a post hoc analysis using data from a multicenter retrospective cohort study and reported that the administration of recombinant thrombomodulin was significantly

Table 2 The baseline characteristics of the patients after propensity score matching ($n = 258$)

Factors	Monotherapy group $n = 129$	Combination therapy group $n = 129$	*P* value	Effect size
Age, mean (SD)	73.3 (12.0)	73.8 (11.5)	0.723	0.044[a]
Sex (*n*, %)				
Female	54 (41.9)	52 (40.3)	0.899	0.064[a]
Male	75 (58.1)	77 (59.7)		
Infection focus (*n*, %)				
Respiratory system	58 (45.0)	38 (29.5)	0.014	0.160
Gastrointestinal system	22 (17.1)	34 (26.4)	0.096	0.113
Biliary system	19 (14.7)	15 (11.6)	0.581	0.046
Urinary system	12 (9.3)	23 (17.8)	0.068	0.125
Musculoskeletal	8 (6.2)	4 (3.1)	0.376	0.074
Skin and soft tissue	5 (3.9)	3 (2.3)	0.722	0.045
Central nerve system	0	1 (0.8)	1.000	0.062
Others	3 (2.3)	8 (6.2)	0.216	0.096
Unknown	14 (10.9)	12 (9.3)	0.837	0.026
Surgical intervention	8 (6.2)	19 (14.7)	0.040	0.139
Non-surgical drainage[#]	1 (0.8)	4 (3.1)	0.370	0.084
Baseline SOFA score median [25, 75%]				
Total SOFA	10.7 [2.0, 22.0]	10.8 [3.0, 19.0]	0.849[a]	0.025[a]
Hepatic	1.0 [0.0, 3.0]	0.0 [0.0, 3.0]	0.015	0.182
Cardiovascular	3.0 [0.0, 4.0]	3.0 [0.0, 4.0]	0.266	0.151
CNS system	2.0 [0.0, 4.0]	2.0 [0.0, 4.0]	0.678	0.026
Renal system	1.0 [0.0, 4.0]	1.0 [0.0, 4.0]	0.656	0.028
Respiratory system	2.0 [0.0, 4.0]	2.0 [0.0, 4.0]	0.266	0.069
Baseline DIC score Median [25, 75%]				
Total DIC score	5.7 [2.0, 8.0]	5.7 [2.0, 8.0]	0.935[a]	0.013[a]
SIRS score (*n*, %)				
0 point	51 (39.5)	37 (28.7)		
1 point	78 (60.5)	92 (71.3)	0.088	0.114
Platelet score	3.0 [0.0, 3.0]	3.0 [0.0, 3.0]	0.778	0.048
FDP score	3.0 [0.0, 3.0]	3.0 [0.0, 3.0]	0.829	0.105
PT ratio score (*n*, %)				
0 point	15 (11.6)	21 (16.3)		
1 point	114 (88.4)	108 (83.7)	0.369	0.067
Baseline laboratory score mean (SD)				
Platelet count ($\times 10^9$/L)	8.60 (6.29)	8.47 (5.04)	0.853	0.023
FDP (μg/mL)	73.9 (191.1)	51.11 (73.35)	0.206	0.158
D-dimer (μg/mL)	28.3 (48.9)	21.1 (24.3)	0.166	0.185
PT ratio	2.42 (8.68)	1.50 (0.41)	0.232	0.150
Antithrombin activity (%)	45.6 (14.1)	47.7 (11.7)	0.928	0.011[a]

[#] For the selection of covariates, a variance inflation factor (VIF) was calculated and the covariates with VIF ≧ 5 were excluded. Finally, age, sex, baseline SOFA score, baseline DIC score, and antithrombin activityused were selected.

[a] Confounding covariates used by the propensity score (age, sex, baseline SOFA score, baseline DIC score, and antithrombin activity)

Non-surgical interventions are as follows: percutaneous transcatheter abscess drainage, urinary tract stenting, biliary tract stenting

When the basic assumptions of Student's *t* test were satisfied, data were shown mean (standard deviation) and the effect size was calculated using Cohen's *d*. When the basic assumptions of Student's *t* test were not satisfied, Mann–Whitney *U* test was performed and data were shown median [25 percentiles, 75 percentiles]. And the effect size was calculated using the following formula, *Z*-scores/a square root of sample number. For two-by-two contingency table, phi coefficient was used

n number, *SD* standard deviation, *SOFA* sequential organ failure assessment, *DIC* disseminated intravascular coagulation

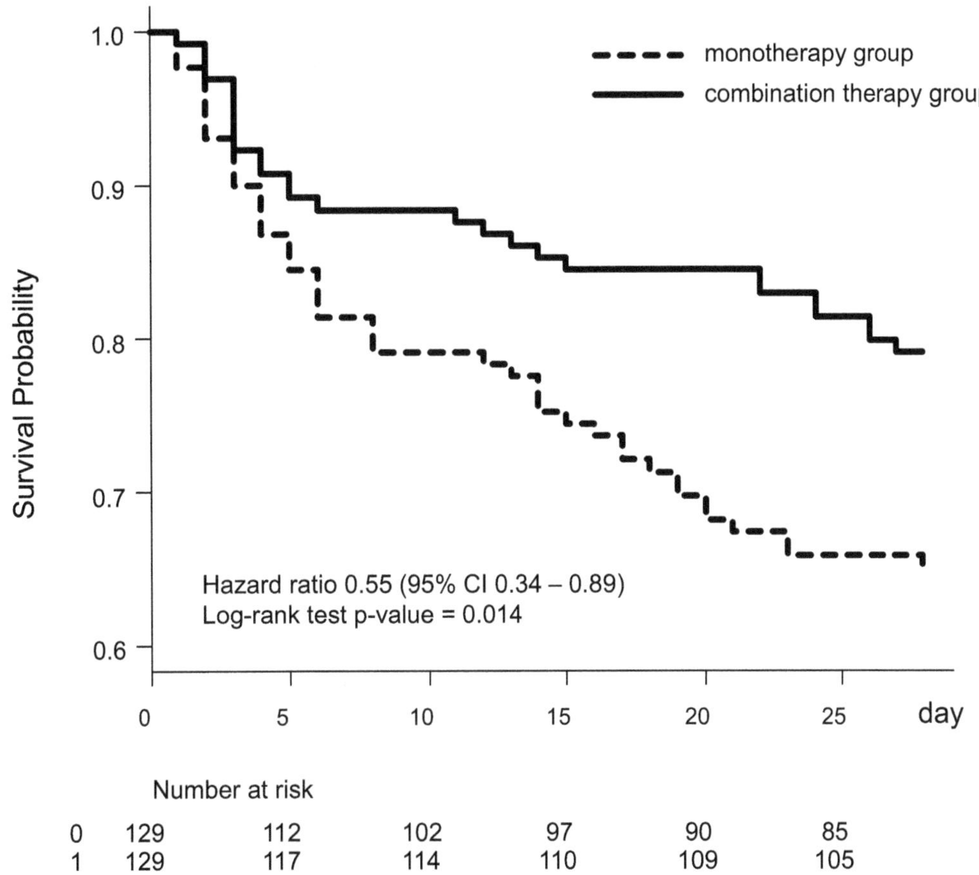

Fig. 2 Survival plots for patients in the propensity score-matched combination therapy and monotherapy groups. The 28-day survival rate was significantly higher in the combination therapy group (79.8%) than in the monotherapy group (70.0%) ($P = 0.014$, log-rank test). Hazard ratio 0.55 (0.34–0.89).

Table 3 Hazards ratio analysis in patients treated with combination therapy

Case number	Model	Hazard ratio (95% CI)	*P* value
510	Unadjusted	0.71 (0.45–1.11)	0.131
296[a]	Cox hazard	0.62 (0.40–0.98)	0.043
258	PS matching	0.49 (0.29–0.82)	0.006[$]

CI confidence interval, *Cox hazard* Cox's proportional hazards model, *PS* propensity score

[a] Complete case number without missing values

[$] *P* values were calculated using a log-rank test

associated with reduced mortality among patients with a high risk of death (APACHE II score: 24–29). Other than the above-mentioned studies, the largest RCT was conducted in 233 ICUs in 17 countries. A total of 750 patients with septic coagulopathy were randomized, and the results revealed a 3.8% reduction in the absolute risk of death (recombinant thrombomodulin group: 17.8% vs. placebo group: 21.6%, $P = 0.273$) [24]. This phase 2b study demonstrated a nonsignificant preferable effect of recombinant thrombomodulin. Regarding this study, one must keep in mind that not all patients had sepsis-associated DIC and the greatest benefit from the treatment was seen in patients with at least one organ system dysfunction and an PT international normalized ratio of greater than 1.4. In the current study, all the patients had DIC, the PT time was 1.61 ± 0.85 in the monotherapy group and 1.56 ± 0.54 in the combination therapy group, and the baseline SOFA scores were over 10 in both groups. Indeed, this was the first report to analyze matching data. As a result, a significant association between combination therapy and the 28-day mortality was recognized, and the mortality rate was significantly lower in the combination therapy group. In addition, both the JAAM-DIC score and the SOFA score were significantly lower in the combination therapy group than in the monotherapy group after the treatment (Days 4 and 7).

Regarding the safety features of recombinant thrombomodulin, a post-marketing surveillance of 2516 septic patients with DIC demonstrated that the frequency of critical bleeding was 2.6% [25], which did not differ from

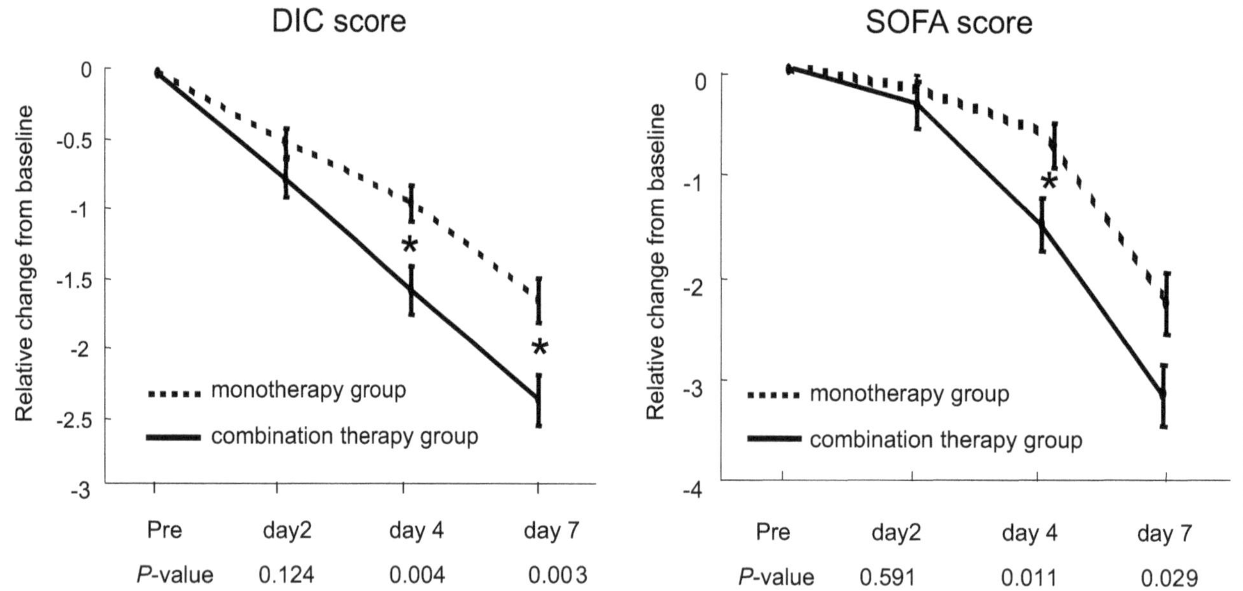

Fig. 3 Changes in JAAM-DIC score and SOFA score in the propensity score-matched combination therapy and monotherapy groups. The JAAM-DIC scores were significantly lower in the combination therapy group than in the monotherapy group on Day 4 and Day 7 ($P = 0.004$, 0.003, respectively). The SOFA scores were significantly lower in the combination therapy group on Day 4 ($P = 0.011$) and Day 7 ($P = 0.029$), *DIC* disseminated intravascular coagulation, *SOFA* sequential organ failure assessment; $^*P < 0.017$

Table 4 Bleeding complications

No.	Treatment group	Bleeding site	Major/minor
Unmatched group			
1	Combination therapy	Mesenterium and intraperitoneal space	Major
2	Combination therapy	Abdominal wall, port site	Minor
3	Combination therapy	Intraperitoneal space, abdominal drain	Minor
4	Combination therapy	Urinary tract	Minor
5	Monotherapy	Intracranial space	Major
6	Monotherapy	Intraperitoneal space	Major
7	Monotherapy	Cervical spinal cord tumor	Major
8	Monotherapy	Urinary tract	Minor
9	Monotherapy	Nasal mucosa	Minor
Matched group			
5	Monotherapy	Intracranial space	Major
7	Monotherapy	Cervical spinal cord tumor	Major
9	Monotherapy	Nasal mucosa	Minor

the results of the current study, suggesting that combination therapy might not increase the incidence of bleeding. However, since a significant number of patients were excluded from this analysis, this issue should be re-examined.

The theoretical rationale for combination therapy remains to be elucidated. However, a fundamental concept is that both antithrombin and thrombomodulin activities are significantly reduced and anticoagulatory function is disrupted during sepsis. Second, antithrombin and thrombomodulin–protein C are the two major anticoagulant systems and their mechanisms of action are independent. Third, both agents are expected to have anti-inflammatory actions [26, 27]. We think that the results obtained from the current study may support the above ideas. As for preclinical studies, we have examined the additive effects of combination therapy in a lipopolysaccharide-induced rat model of septic DIC. As a result, combination therapy attenuated organ damage and histologic changes and led to an improvement in survival [28, 29]. Additional studies are required to clarify the mechanism of action.

Limitations

First, we only compared the effect between a combination therapy group and an antithrombin monotherapy group. To examine the true effect of the combination therapy, a combination therapy group, a monotherapy group, and a control group treated without anticoagulant are needed. Second, the median age of the patients was relatively higher and over 70-year-old, and thus, it might be difficult to generalize to the other countries. Finally, this was a retrospective observational study. Since the beneficial effect of combination therapy was hypothesized by the current study, a prospective randomized study is necessary as the next stage of inquiry.

Conclusion

The potential benefits of the co-administration of antithrombin and recombinant thrombomodulin were examined in a multi-institutional observation study. A propensity score-matched analysis demonstrated that the combination therapy was associated with a reduced mortality among patients with sepsis-induced DIC. Furthermore, the bleeding incidence seemed sufficiently low and the addition of recombinant thrombomodulin did not appear to increase the risk of bleeding.

Abbreviations

DIC: disseminated intravascular coagulation; OR: odds ratio; JAAM: Japanese Association for Acute Medicine; JMHW: Japanese Ministry of Health, Labour and Welfare; FDP: fibrinogen/fibrin degradation products; PT: prothrombin time; SIRS: systemic inflammatory response syndrome; SOFA: sequential organ failure assessment; VIF: variance inflation factor; IPW: inverse probability of treatment-weighted; SD: standard deviation; HR: hazard ratios; RCT: randomized controlled trial.

Authors' contributions

TI and SG conceived the study and participated in its design. TI and AH participated in the sequence alignment and drafted the manuscript. AH performed the statistical analysis. AA and KS revised the manuscript. DS and YU helped to collect and arrange the data. All authors read and approved the final manuscript.

Author details

[1] Department of Emergency and Disaster Medicine, Juntendo University Graduate School of Medicine, 2-1-1 Hongo Bunkyo-ku, Tokyo 113-8421, Japan. [2] National Center for Global Health and Medicine, Emergency Medicine and Critical Care, Tokyo, Japan. [3] Division of Traumatology, Research Institute, National Defense Medical College, Tokyo, Japan. [4] Emergency Medical Center, Fujisawa City Hospital, Fujisawa, Japan. [5] Department of Acute Critical Care and Disaster Medicine, Tokyo Medical and Dental University, Tokyo, Japan. [6] Department of Surgery, Juntendo Shizuoka Hospital, Juntendo University Graduate School of Medicine, Izunokuni-shi, Japan. [7] Division of Acute and Critical Care Medicine, Department of Anesthesiology and Critical Care Medicine, Hokkaido University Graduate School of Medicine, Sapporo, Japan.

Acknowledgements

The authors also thank all the institutes that participated in the post-marketing surveillance.

Funding

This work was supported by Ministry of Education, Culture, Sports, Science and Technology (Supported Program for the Strategic Research Foundation at Private Universities).

Competing interests

The authors declare that they have no competing interests.

References

1. Iba T, Thachil J. Present and future of anticoagulant therapy using antithrombin and thrombomodulin for sepsis-associated disseminated intravascular coagulation: a perspective from Japan. Int J Hematol. 2016;103:253–61.
2. Murata A, Okamoto K, Mayumi T, Muramatsu K, Matsuda S. Recent change in treatment of disseminated intravascular coagulation in Japan: an epidemiological study based on a National Administrative Database. Clin Appl Thromb Hemost. 2016;22:21–7.
3. Levi M, Toh CH, Thachil J, Watson HG. Guidelines for the diagnosis and management of disseminated intravascular coagulation. British Committee for Standards in Haematology. Br J Haematol. 2009;145:24–33.
4. Di Nisio M, Baudo F, Cosmi B, D'Angelo A, De Gasperi A, Malato A, et al. Diagnosis and treatment of disseminated intravascular coagulation: guidelines of the Italian Society for Haemostasis and Thrombosis (SISET). Thromb Res. 2012;129:e177–84.
5. Hayakawa M, Yamakawa K, Saito S, Uchino S, Kudo D, Iizuka Y, et al. Recombinant human soluble thrombomodulin and mortality in sepsis-induced disseminated intravascular coagulation. A multicentre retrospective study. Thromb Haemost. 2016;115:1157–66.
6. Hayakawa M, Kudo D, Saito S, Uchino S, Yamakawa K, Iizuka Y, et al. Antithrombin supplementation and mortality in sepsis-induced disseminated intravascular coagulation: a multicenter retrospective observational study. Shock. 2016;46:623–31.
7. Rhodes A, Evans LE, Alhazzani W, Levy MM, Antonelli M, Ferrer R, et al. Surviving sepsis campaign: international guidelines for management of sepsis and septic shock: 2016. Crit Care Med. 2017;45:486–552.
8. Iba T, Gando S, Saitoh D, Ikeda T, Anan H, Oda S, et al. Efficacy and bleeding risk of antithrombin supplementation in patients with septic disseminated intravascular coagulation: a third survey. Clin Appl Thromb Hemost. 2017;23:422–8.
9. Iba T, Saitoh D, Wada H, Asakura H. Efficacy and bleeding risk of antithrombin supplementation in septic disseminated intravascular coagulation: a secondary survey. Crit Care. 2014;18:497.
10. Iba T, Gando S, Saitoh D, Wada H, Di Nisio M, Thachil J. Antithrombin supplementation and risk of bleeding in patients with sepsis-associated disseminated intravascular coagulation. Thromb Res. 2016;145:46–50.
11. Yasuda N, Goto K, Ohchi Y, Abe T, Koga H, Kitano T. The efficacy and safety of antithrombin and recombinant human thrombomodulin combination therapy in patients with severe sepsis and disseminated intravascular coagulation. J Crit Care. 2016;36:29–34.
12. Gando S, Iba T, Eguchi Y, Ohtomo Y, Okamoto K, Koseki K, et al. A multicenter, prospective validation of disseminated intravascular coagulation diagnostic criteria for critically ill patients: comparing current criteria. Crit Care Med. 2006;34:625–31.
13. Wada H, Asakura H, Okamoto K, Iba T, Uchiyama T, Kawasugi K, et al. Expert consensus for the treatment of disseminated intravascular coagulation in Japan. Thromb Res. 2010;125:6–11.
14. Tagami T, Matsui H, Horiguchi H, Fushimi K, Yasunaga H. Antithrombin and mortality in severe pneumonia patients with sepsis-associated disseminated intravascular coagulation: an observational nationwide study. J Thromb Haemost. 2014;12:1470–9.
15. Tagami T, Matsui H, Fushimi K, Yasunaga H. Supplemental dose of antithrombin use in disseminated intravascular coagulation patients after abdominal sepsis. Thromb Haemost. 2015;114:537–45.
16. Saito H, Maruyama I, Shimazaki S, Yamamoto Y, Aikawa N, Ohno R, et al. Efficacy and safety of recombinant human soluble thrombomodulin (ART-123) in disseminated intravascular coagulation: results of a phase III, randomized, double-blind clinical trial. J Thromb Haemost. 2007;5:31–41.
17. Aikawa N, Shimazaki S, Yamamoto Y, Saito H, Maruyama I, Ohno R, et al. Thrombomodulin alfa in the treatment of infectious patients complicated by disseminated intravascular coagulation: subanalysis from the phase 3 trial. Shock. 2011;35:349–54.
18. Yamakawa K, Aihara M, Ogura H, Yuhara H, Hamasaki T, Shimazu T. Recombinant human soluble thrombomodulin in severe sepsis: a systematic review and meta-analysis. J Thromb Haemost. 2015;13:508–19.
19. Tagami T, Matsui H, Horiguchi H, Fushimi K, Yasunaga H. Recombinant human soluble thrombomodulin and mortality in severe pneumonia patients with sepsis-associated disseminated intravascular coagulation: an observational nationwide study. J Thromb Haemost. 2015;13:31–40.

20. Hagiwara A, Tanaka N, Uemura T, Matsuda W, Kimura A. Can recombinant human thrombomodulin increase survival among patients with severe septic-induced disseminated intravascular coagulation: a single-center, open-label, randomized controlled trial. BMJ Open. 2016;30:e012850.
21. Freeman BD, Zehnbauer BA, Buchman TG. A meta-analysis of controlled trials of anticoagulant therapies in patients with sepsis. Shock. 2003;20:5–9.
22. Dhainaut JF, Yan SB, Joyce DE, Pettilä V, Basson B, Brandt JT, et al. Treatment effects of drotrecogin alfa (activated) in patients with severe sepsis with or without overt disseminated intravascular coagulation. J Thromb Haemost. 2004;2:1924–33.
23. Yoshimura J, Yamakawa K, Ogura H, Umemura Y, Takahashi H, Morikawa M, et al. Benefit profile of recombinant human soluble thrombomodulin in sepsis-induced disseminated intravascular coagulation: a multicenter propensity score analysis. Crit Care. 2015;19:810.
24. Vincent JL, Ramesh MK, Ernest D, LaRosa SP, Pachl J, Aikawa N, et al. A randomized, double-blind, placebo-controlled, Phase 2b study to evaluate the safety and efficacy of recombinant human soluble thrombomodulin, ART-123, in patients with sepsis and suspected disseminated intravascular coagulation. Crit Care Med. 2013;41:2069–79.
25. Mimuro J, Takahashi H, Kitajima I, Tsuji H, Eguchi Y, Matsushita T, et al. Impact of recombinant soluble thrombomodulin (thrombomodulin alfa) on disseminated intravascular coagulation. Thromb Res. 2013;131:436–43.
26. Wiedermann CJ. Clinical review: molecular mechanisms underlying the role of antithrombin in sepsis. Crit Care. 2006;10:209.
27. Abeyama K, Stern DM, Ito Y, Yoshimoto Y, Tanaka M, Uchimura T, et al. The N-terminal domain of thrombomodulin sequesters high-mobility group-B1 protein, a novel antiinflammatory mechanism. J Clin Invest. 2005;15:1267–74.
28. Iba T, Nakarai E, Takayama T, Nakajima K, Sasaoka T, Ohno Y. Combination effect of antithrombin and recombinant human soluble thrombomodulin in an LPS induced rat sepsis model. Crit Care. 2009;13:R203–9.
29. Iba T, Miki T, Hashiguchi N, Yamada A, Nagaoka I. Combination of antithrombin and recombinant thrombomodulin attenuates leukocyte-endothelial interaction and suppresses the increase of intrinsic damage-associated molecular patterns in endotoxemic rats. J Surg Res. 2014;187:581–6.

Pharmacogenomic biomarkers do not predict response to drotrecogin alfa in patients with severe sepsis

Djillali Annane[1], Jean-Paul Mira[2], Lorraine B. Ware[3], Anthony C. Gordon[4], Charles J. Hinds[5], David C. Christiani[6], Jonathan Sevransky[7], Kathleen Barnes[8], Timothy G. Buchman[7], Patrick J. Heagerty[9], Robert Balshaw[10], Nadia Lesnikova[10], Karen de Nobrega[10], Hugh F. Wellman[11], Mauricio Neira[11], Alexandra D. J. Mancini[11], Keith R. Walley[12] and James A. Russell[12*]

Abstract

Purpose: To explore potential design for pharmacogenomics trials in sepsis, we investigate the interaction between pharmacogenomic biomarkers and response to drotrecogin alfa (activated) (DrotAA). This trial was designed to validate whether previously identified improved response polymorphisms (IRPs A and B) were associated with an improved response to DrotAA in severe sepsis.

Methods: Patients with severe sepsis at high risk of death, who received DrotAA or not, with DNA available were included and matched to controls adjusting for age, APACHE II or SAPS II, organ dysfunction, ventilation, medical/surgical status, infection site, and propensity score (probability that a patient would have received DrotAA given their baseline characteristics). Independent genotyping and two-phase data transfer mitigated bias. The primary analysis compared the effect of DrotAA in IRP+ and IRP− groups on in-hospital 28-day mortality. Secondary endpoints included time to death in hospital; intensive care unit (ICU)-, hospital-, and ventilator-free days; and overall DrotAA treatment effect on mortality.

Results: Six hundred and ninety-two patients treated with DrotAA were successfully matched to 1935 patients not treated with DrotAA. Genotyping was successful for 639 (DrotAA) and 1684 (nonDrotAA) matched patients. The primary hypothesis of a genotype-by-treatment interaction (assessed by conditional logistic regression analysis) was not significant ($P = 0.30$ IRP A; $P = 0.78$ IRP B), and there was no significant genotype by treatment interaction for any secondary endpoint.

Conclusions: Neither IRP A nor IRP B predicted differential response to DrotAA on in-hospital 28-day mortality.

ClinicalTrials.gov registration NCT01486524

Keywords: Drotrecogin alfa (activated), Activated protein C, Pharmacogenomics biomarker, Propensity score, Severe sepsis

Background

Pharmacogenomic biomarkers identify patients who have altered drug response according to their genotype. For example, use of pharmacogenomics of warfarin decreases risk of adverse events (severe hemorrhage) and increases efficacy [1–3]. Similarly, pharmacogenomics could be used to predict how patients with sepsis may respond to adjunctive therapies.

Treatment with DrotAA led to variable clinical responses in patients with sepsis. Then, one trial conducted in both severe sepsis and septic shock found a significant absolute

*Correspondence: jrussell@mrl.ubc.ca
[12] Critical Care Research Laboratories, Centre for Heart Lung Innovation, St. Paul's Hospital, University of British Columbia, Burrard Building, Rm 166 - 1081 Burrard St, Vancouver, BC V6Z 1Y6, Canada
Full list of author information is available at the end of the article

risk reduction (ARR) of 6.1% in the 28-day mortality rate [4]. Other trials including only severe sepsis [5] or only septic shock [6, 7] failed to find survival benefit. One reason for the highly variable responses to DrotAA treatment observed in clinical trial may be related to genetic predisposition. In previous analyses, a combination of single nucleotide polymorphisms (SNPs) that defined two improve response polymorphisms (IRPs) was associated with a significant genotype-by-treatment interaction for effect of DrotAA on mortality.

Though DrotAA was withdrawn from the market by Ely Lilly, our overarching goal was to elaborate a pharmacogenomic approach using DrotAA as a practical example. Accordingly, the primary hypothesis was that IRP A and/or IRP B predict a differential DrotAA treatment effect in patients with severe sepsis and high risk of death.

Methods

This is an abbreviated presentation of the methods of the current study because the details were published prior to undertaking analyses [8].

Prior studies—background on selection of pharmacogenomic biomarkers for current study

To screen for genomic biomarkers, a Genome Wide Association Study (GWAS) of the PROWESS study [4] was performed (unpublished data) using DNA from 1446 patients to genotype approximately 1.2 million SNPs (Illumina® Human1 M-Duo BeadChip). These results were taken forward to an independent cohort of patients who had septic shock, some of whom were treated with DrotAA and some of whom were not. This small replication cohort was drawn from St. Paul's Hospital (SPH) and the Vasopressin and Septic Shock Trial (VASST) [9].

The replication cohort was used to confirm two IRPs. Two-SNP composite improved response polymorphisms (IRPs), A and B, were constructed. Patients were classified as IRP A+ or − and IRP B+ or − if they had one of both of the responsive genotype. For each IRP, individual patients were considered biomarker positive if they had the responsive genotype for either of the SNPs or for both of the SNPs in the IRP. The individual SNPs in each IRP were associated with a differential DrotAA treatment effect in PROWESS (derivation cohort) and replicated in the replication cohort (unpublished).

The two SNPs comprising IRP A were chosen based first on the alignment of direction and strength of their signals by analyzing the interaction of SNP and treatment effect on mortality in both the PROWESS study and the replication cohort. Secondly, these two SNPs were chosen based on biological plausibility linking the proteins coded by these genes to pathways of sepsis or pathways regarding mechanisms of action of DrotAA. The two SNPs of IRP A are RYR2 (ryanodine receptor 2 gene) rs684923 on chromosome 1 and ACIN1 (apoptotic chromatin condensation inducer 1 gene) rs3751501 on chromosome 14. The SNP of RYR2 could act to enhance efficacy of activated protein C on protection of endothelial permeability via its effects on endothelial protein C receptor and sphingosine-1-phosphate receptor 1 (S1P). When activated protein C (APC) binds to PAR1, this triggers more conversion of sphingosine to S1P, and this could decrease the amount of sphingosine and thus disinhibit the ryanodine receptor. We also suggest that this disinhibition of the ryanodine receptor by the actions of APC varies according to the genotype of the ryanodine receptor.

Phosphorylation of a residue (S422) inACIN1 (Acinus-S variant) by AKT (prosurvival kinase) completely inhibits cleavage of Acinus-S by caspase-3, abrogating the formation of fragment p17 which is essential for chromatin condensation during apoptosis. Apoptosis is increased in some tissues and cells (lymphocytes, dendritic cells, pulmonary and gut epithelial cells) and is decreased in other tissues and cells (neutrophils) in sepsis. This gene modulates apoptosis and activated protein C has anti-apoptotic actions apoptosis so we suggest that there could be an interaction between polymorphisms of ACIN1 and response to DrotAA. More specifically, the genetic variants rs3751501 (AA|AG), associated with increased ARR (absolute risk reduction) and coding for amino acid 478 F in ACIN1, would render ACIN1 constitutively non-phosphorylated at residue 478 F and hence constitutively nonphosphorylated at S422, leading to AKT-independent regulation of chromatin condensation by Acinus-S during apoptosis, because nonphosphorylated acinus-S would be constitutively cleavable by caspase-3.

The two SNPs comprising IRP B were chosen based solely on the strength of their signals in the PROWESS and replication cohorts. These two SNPs are SPATA7 (spermatogenesis associated 7 gene) rs3179969 on chromosome 14 and FLI1 (Friend leukemia virus integration 1 gene) rs640098 on chromosome 11.

For the replication cohort, the ARR was 19.7% for IRP A+ patients (95% confidence interval (CI) 2.2–37.1%), whereas for the IRP A − patients the ARR was −8.9% (95% CI −22.6–4.9%)($p = 0.018$ unadjusted). The ARR was 21.2% for IRP B+ patients (95% CI 3.2–39.2%), whereas for the IRP B − patients the ARR was −5% (95% CI −18.2–8.2%)($p = 0.04$ unadjusted).

The current study—overall design

This was an international, multicenter, retrospective, controlled, outcome-blinded, genotype-blinded, and matched-patients study [8]. Retrospectively accessed DNA and clinical data were analyzed to validate the pre-specified IRPs. Prospective aspects of this study were the genotyping of patients with regard to the IRPs and the statistical testing of the prespecified genotype hypothesis. Eight academic centers contributed the data and DNA from 10 cohorts (5 EU, 4 US, 1 Canada).

Study population and treatment groups

Patients included in the current study (the INDICATED population) met prespecified eligibility criteria [8] and DrotAA-treated patients were matched to DrotAA-free patients. Eligibility criteria (aligned with the approved use of DrotAA in the USA and EU) were used to select the primary study population (INDICATED). Such patients with high risk of death represented common practice for use of DrotAA [10–14]. No patient in this study was part of a prospective randomized trial of DrotAA. Patients were treated according to standard care at their sites, and data and DNA samples collected at that time were retrospectively accessed for this study. All patients were enrolled after the Food and Drug Administration (FDA) or European Medicines Agency (EMA) approval of DrotAA.

Matching DrotAA-treated to control patients

The current study incorporated a robust, well-accepted matching strategy. A propensity score of the estimated probability that a patient would have received DrotAA given their key baseline characteristics was calculated, and patients were selected as matches had to be within a prespecified tolerance on this score. Combining the use of propensity scores with covariate matching is superior to the use of either strategy alone [15]. The intended clinical variables for the calculation of the Mahalanobis distance and the reasons why these variables were chosen were described previously [8].

Syreon Corporation (a clinical research organization) conducted the study. A two-phase transfer of data from each center was performed to ensure that the selection of matched control patients was blinded and unbiased. Data transfer 1 included variables to confirm eligibility and to conduct the matching. Once the matching was achieved, the matched sets of treated and control patients were "locked" together. Then data transfer 2 (outcomes and genotypic data) was sent to Syreon.

Genotyping

Genotyping for the IRP SNPs was done using a validated Taqman®-based analytical method and the laboratory was blinded to treatment and outcome. A 91-SNP ancestry informative marker (AIM) panel was genotyped by the GoldenGate® analytical method.

Statistical analysis

As previously noted [8], this study had 90% power to detect a treatment-by-IRP interaction assuming an absolute mortality reduction of 15% in the DrotAA-treated group compared to control in IRP + patients and with 1–2% difference in mortality between the treated and control groups in IRP- patients.

The primary analysis was done on the Matched-INDICATED population (comparing the effect of treatment in the IRP + and IRP- groups) by testing for the effect of the interaction between IRP and DrotAA treatment on the primary endpoint in a conditional logistic regression model, conditioning on the matching while incorporating the principal component scores from the 91-SNP AIM panel data (as covariates to control for potential population stratification). The primary endpoint was in-hospital mortality through Day 28 (i.e., patients were followed until hospital discharge or Day 28, whichever came first). Each of the primary analyses, one for IRP A and one for IRP B, was done as a two-sided test with $\alpha = 2.5\%$ for an overall, Bonferroni-corrected, type I error rate of 5%.

Results

Prior to matching patients treated with DrotAA differed significantly from nonDrotAA patients in many important baseline clinical respects (Additional file 1: Supplement Tables 1–6). After applying the eligibility criteria for the INDICATED population, there were 11,018 patients not treated with DrotAA from whom to choose matched controls for the 738 DrotAA-treated patients (ratio 15:1) (Fig. 1). Suitable matches were not available for 46 (6.2%) of the 738 INDICATED DrotAA-treated patients. Thus, after matching, the number of matched-INDICATED DrotAA-treated patients was 692. Overall the matched ratio was 2.8 control patients for every DrotAA-treated patient. Baseline clinical characteristics of the matched 692 DrotAA patients were similar to the 1,935 matched control patients (Table 1). The DrotAA group had higher proportion of coagulation dysfunction and a higher use of vasopressors (Table 1). Matching was done before genotype was known so it is relevant to observe that within the IRP A + and IRP A- and the IRP B+ and IRP B− genotype subgroups, DrotAA-treated patients were similar to matched control patients (Additional file 1: Supplement Tables 8–19). The Primary Analysis Population (PAP) included 639 DrotAA-treated patients and 1684 matched controls. The primary reasons why patients could not be included in the PAP were insufficient quantity of DNA or unsuccessful genotyping (Fig. 1, Additional file 1: Supplement Table 7).

Effect of DrotAA on mortality

Irrespective of genotype, the ARR was in favor of DrotAA (estimated weighted mortality: DrotAA 25.1%, nonDrotAA 30.5%) ($P = 0.006$, Additional file 1: Supplement Table 21).

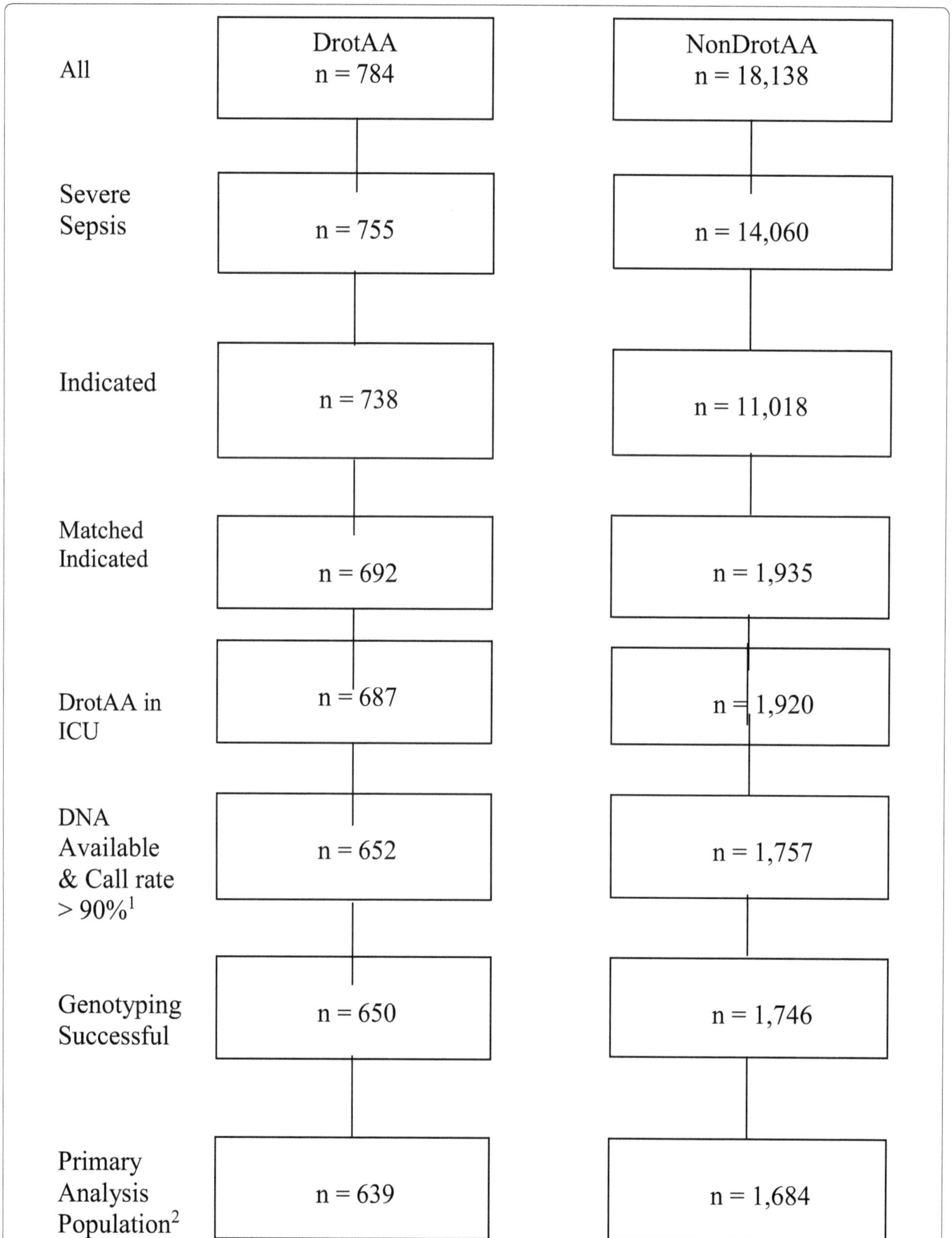

Fig. 1 Patient enrollment in DrotAA and nonDrotAA groups. Superscript notes: [1]Based on GoldenGate genotyping for AIM panel SNPs and research SNPs. [2]Each matched set required 1 DrotAA-treated patient and 1–3 nonDrotAA-treated patients

Table 1 Baseline characteristics for ALL and matched-INDICATED populations by treatment

Baseline characteristics[a]	ALL patients		Matched-INDICATED	
	DrotAA ($n = 784$)	NonDrotAA ($n = 18,138$)	DrotAA ($n = 692$)	NonDrotAA ($n = 1935$)
Age (Mean)	58.4	60.4	59.0	59.1
SD	16.1	16.9	15.4	9.2
P value[b]	0.001		0.69	
Male (%)	59.7	59.9	60.1	61.2
P value	0.93		0.65	
APACHE II (mean)	26.1	21.1	25.8	25.5
SD	8.2	7.7	7.9	4.7
P value	< 0.0001		0.02	
SAPS II (mean)	58.1	47.8	59.1	58.5
SD	19.2	19.1	18.8	10.9
P value	< 0.0001		0.77	
Origin of sepsis (%)				
Nosocomial	8.4	4.7	7.2	12.3
Community acquired	38.6	14.3	39.7	34.7
Unknown	52.9	81.0	53.0	53.0
P value	0.003		< 0.0001	
Anatomic site of primary infection (%)				
Lung	51.5	23.4	52.9	46.8
Abdomen	12.2	6.9	13.2	12.7
CNS	1.3	0.6	0.9	0.7
Blood	3.4	2.0	3.0	3.5
Urinary tract	4.1	2.7	3.8	3.3
Unknown	22.1	60.2	21.1	29.0
Other	5.4	4.2	5.2	4.1
P value	0.0004		0.55	
Use of vasopressors (%)				
Yes	91.2	54.7	91.8	81.2
No	8.3	39.2	7.8	17.8
Unknown	0.5	6.1	0.4	1.0
P value	< 0.0001		< 0.0001	
Mechanical ventilation (%)				
Yes	76.3	72.3	75.7	76.4
No	6.4	19.5	6.2	5.2
Unknown	17.3	8.2	18.1	18.4
P value	< 0.0001		0.08	
Number of organ systems with dysfunction (%)				
0	1.4	9.9	0.0	0.0
1	2.2	23.8	0.1	0.8
2	20.7	30.8	21.0	22.0
3	33.0	19.4	35.1	34.0
4	24.9	11.3	26.3	29.4
5	13.6	4.1	13.9	11.7
6	4.2	0.7	3.6	2.2
P value	< 0.0001		0.82	
Cardiovascular dysfunction (%)				
Yes	96.0	66.9	98.7	98.3

Table 1 continued

Baseline characteristics[a]	ALL patients		Matched-INDICATED	
	DrotAA ($n = 784$)	NonDrotAA ($n = 18,138$)	DrotAA ($n = 692$)	NonDrotAA ($n = 1935$)
No	2.4	30.2	1.0	1.0
Unknown	1.5	2.9	0.3	0.7
P value	< 0.0001		0.36	
Pulmonary dysfunction (%)				
Yes	92.6	69.5	95.4	95.3
No	5.1	18.8	3.9	3.4
Unknown	2.3	11.7	0.7	1.3
P value	< 0.0001		0.34	
CNS dysfunction (%)				
Yes	28.4	21.0	27.7	31.4
No	33.2	34.5	33.8	30.9
Unknown	38.4	44.5	38.4	37.7
P value	0.0003		0.01	
Coagulation dysfunction (%)				
Yes	31.4	14.0	31.8	25.0
No	65.4	68.7	66.3	72.6
Unknown	3.2	17.3	1.9	2.4
P value	< 0.0001		< 0.0001	
Renal dysfunction (%)				
Yes	63.3	29.4	65.6	61.7
No	33.9	54.1	32.4	36.6
Unknown	2.8	16.6	2.0	1.7
P value	< 0.0001		< 0.01	
Hepatic dysfunction (%)				
Yes	23.9	13.0	24.4	23.8
No	66.8	66.7	67.6	68.5
Unknown	9.3	20.3	7.9	7.7
P value	< 0.0001		0.71	

[a] Summary statistics for the NonDrotAA group were weighted to reflect the unequal numbers of DrotAA and NonDrotAA patients in each of the matched sets

[b] Descriptive *P* values are from clustered regression analysis using linear regression (numeric variables) or binary logistic regression (categorical variables) comparing the proportion of patients in the most frequent category between DrotAA vs NonDrotAA, clustering on the matched sets and with weights based on the number of patients in DrotAA and NonDrotAA matched sets. Patients in the unknown categories were excluded from the tests. No adjustments were made to account for multiple inference

Primary endpoint: genotype-by-DrotAA treatment interaction

The primary hypothesis of a genotype by DrotAA treatment interaction assessed by conditional logistic regression analysis for IRP A was not significant ($P = 0.30$, Table 2), and the direction of the effect was opposite to what had been expected as shown by the negative parameter estimate for the interaction term (Additional file 1: Supplement Tables 20–21). The IRP B result was also not significant ($P = 0.78$, Table 2), and the direction of effect was opposite to what had been expected. There was a

Table 2 Primary efficacy analysis—conditional logistic regression model including AIM Panel PCs

Factor/effect	Estimate	SE	Odds ratio (OR) estimate	OR 95% CI		*P* value[c]
				Lower	Upper	
Primary efficacy analysis for IRP A						
IRP A*Treatment Interaction[a]	− 0.31	0.303	0.731	0.403	1.324	0.30
IRP A+: DrotAA versus NonDrotAA	0.11	0.245	1.112	0.688	1.799	0.66
IRP A−: DrotAA versus NonDrotAA	0.42	0.145	1.522	1.145	2.024	< 0.01
DrotAA: IRP A+ versus IRP A−	− 0.30	0.258	0.740	0.446	1.228	0.24
NonDrotAA: IRP A+ versus IRP A−	0.01	0.150	1.013	0.755	1.359	0.93
AIM Panel PCs[b]						0.14
Primary efficacy Analysis for IRP B						
IRP B*Treatment Interaction[a]	− 0.09	0.325	0.912	0.482	1.722	0.78
IRP B+: DrotAA versus NonDrotAA	0.23	0.277	1.257	0.730	2.162	0.41
IRP B−: DrotAA versus NonDrotAA	0.32	0.138	1.379	1.052	1.807	0.02
DrotAA: IRP B+ versus IRP B−	− 0.19	0.285	0.829	0.475	1.449	0.51
NonDrotAA: IRP B+ versus IRP B−	− 0.09	0.156	0.910	0.670	1.236	0.55
AIM Panel PCs[b]						0.14

Analysis for IRP A involved 376 discordant matched sets from a total of 637 matched sets

Analysis for IRP B involved 372 discordant matched sets from a total of 634 matched sets

[a] The interaction odds ratio is a ratio of odds ratios

[b] A total of 10 AIM Panel PCs were included which accounted for 33.9% of the variance in the AIM Panel data for the Matched-INDICATED Primary Analysis Population based on all cohorts

[c] *P* values from conditional logistic regression partial likelihood ratio tests for the IRP*Treatment Interaction and the combined AIM Panel PCs; all other *P* values are from Wald Chi-square tests

therapeutic benefit of DrotAA treatment in IRP A- negative and IRP B- negative patients.

Neither IRP A nor IRP B predicted ICU and hospital survival rates or the destination at hospital discharge. At hospital discharge, the mortality rates were 32.2 and 36.2% for DrotAA group and nonDrotAA groups, respectively. Approximately 19% of patients were discharged home, 13% went to long-term care facilities, 9% went to another acute care hospital, and discharge location was unknown for the remainder (24–27%).

Sensitivity analyses with common matching variables included as covariates

The inclusion of the common matching variables as covariates in the conditional logistic regression model did not change any of the conclusions regarding IRP A, IRP B, or the overall DrotAA effect (Table 3). We used conditional logistic regression and included common matching variables (age, APACHE II score or SAPS II score, and respiratory dysfunction (yes/no)) as covariates to correct for residual imbalances across IRP genotype subgroups. Neither self-reported race nor genetically determined continent of origin impacted the overall DrotAA treatment effect or the IRP*Treatment interactions in conditional logistic regression models.

Sensitivity analyses according to high APACHE II/SAPS II scores

As in PROWESS [4] the overall effect of DrotAA differed according to severity of illness (Table 4). Greater severity of illness was defined by APACHE II ≥25 and by SAPS II ≥54. ARR based on crude mortality rates was 10.3% in the high severity of illness and—1.8% in the low severity of illness subgroups.

Sensitivity analyses of individual IRP A and IRP B SNPs

None of the IRP A nor IRP B SNPs was significantly associated with treatment effect when analyzed individually.

Secondary endpoints

Time to death in hospital analyses showed a beneficial DrotAA treatment effect but no additional benefit to knowing IRP A or IRP B genotype (Fig. 2). None of the secondary efficacy endpoints analyses (time to death in hospital, ICU-free days, hospital-free days, and mechanical-ventilator-free days) showed a significant genotype-by-treatment interaction (Additional file 1: Supplement Tables 22–26).

Discussion

This international, multicenter, retrospective, non-randomized, controlled, outcome-blinded, genotype-blinded, and matched-patients study found that neither

Table 3 Secondary analysis with common matching variables included as covariates—conditional logistic regression for differential treatment effects of IRP A and IRP B on mortality

Factor/effect	Estimate	SE	Odds Ratio (OR) estimate	OR 95% CI		*P* value[c]
				Lower	Upper	
Analysis for IRP A						
IRP A*Treatment Interaction[a]	−0.34	0.304	0.710	0.391	1.289	0.26
IRP A+ : DrotAA versus NonDrotAA	0.08	0.246	1.087	0.671	1.761	0.74
IRP A−: DrotAA versus NonDrotAA	0.43	0.146	1.532	1.151	2.039	< 0.01
DrotAA: IRP A+ versus IRP A−	−0.32	0.259	0.725	0.436	1.205	0.22
NonDrotAA: IRP A+ versus IRP A−	0.02	0.150	1.022	0.761	1.372	0.89
AIM Panel PCs[b]						0.13
Common covariates used in matching						0.74
Age (per year)	−0.02	0.024	0.976	0.930	1.023	0.30
APACHE II (per point)[d]	0.05	0.080	1.054	0.901	1.233	0.51
SAPS II (per point)[d]	0.01	0.041	1.006	0.929	1.091	0.88
Respiratory dysfunction (Yes vs. No)	0.86	0.778	2.371	0.515	10.90	0.27
Analysis for IRP B						
IRP B*Treatment Interaction[a]	−0.10	0.325	0.908	0.480	1.719	0.77
IRP B+: DrotAA versus NonDrotAA	0.22	0.278	1.251	0.726	2.155	0.42
IRP B−: DrotAA versus NonDrotAA	0.32	0.138	1.377	1.050	1.806	0.02
DrotAA: IRP B+ vs IRP B−	−0.19	0.285	0.826	0.472	1.443	0.50
NonDrotAA: IRP B+ vs IRP B−	−0.10	0.157	0.909	0.668	1.236	0.54
AIM panel PCs[b]						0.15
Common covariates used in matching						0.75
Age (per year)	−0.02	0.024	0.976	0.931	1.024	0.32
APACHE II (per point)[d]	0.04	0.080	1.045	0.894	1.223	0.58
SAPS II (per point)[d]	−0.00	0.041	0.997	0.919	1.081	0.94
Respiratory dysfunction (Yes vs. No)	0.12	0.935	1.127	0.180	7.050	0.90

Analysis for IRP A involved 376 discordant matched sets from a total of 637 matched sets

Analysis for IRP B involved 372 discordant matched sets from a total of 634 matched sets

[a] The interaction odds ratio is a ratio of odds ratios

[b] A total of 10 AIM Panel PCs were included which account for 33.9% of the variance in the AIM Panel data for the Matched-INDICATED Primary Analysis Population based on all cohorts

[c] *P* values from conditional logistic regression partial likelihood ratio tests for the IRP*Treatment Interaction and the combined AIM Panel PCs; all other *P* values are from Wald Chi-square tests

[d] Sites with APACHE II scores were analyzed with 0's for SAPS II scores, and vice versa

IRP A nor IRP B predicted differential DrotAA treatment effects on in-hospital mortality through Day 28 in patients with severe sepsis. Furthermore, there was no significant genotype by treatment interaction for any of the secondary endpoints. Nonetheless, as yet undiscovered, other genotypes might accurately predict response to DrotAA.

Despite the negative results of the genotype by DrotAA treatment interaction, we suggest that this study provided a potential design for future evaluations of pharmacogenomic biomarkers of drugs and devices for use in sepsis. Most recent and ongoing sepsis trials include DNA biobanking. We propose that these trials systematically explore potential experimental treatment interaction with genomic biomarkers. If any positive interaction, a confirmatory RCT with biomarker-based stratification of randomization would then be conducted.

The possible explanations for the negative findings are that the prior discovery studies were false positive results that did not validate because the biology assumptions were incorrect for the biology SNPs and that the statistics were misleading for the statistically chosen SNPs. The lessons to be learned for future biomarker trials include need for greater validation in prior studies before the pivotal trials are done, perhaps focus only on statistically chosen SNPs, and access to prior trials in which SNPs were assessed (such as PROWESS in the current example).

We believe that this is the largest study of predictive genomic biomarkers for any drug used in sepsis. DrotAA

Table 4 Secondary analyses for effects of high APACHE II/SAPS II scores on differential treatment effects of IRP A and IRP B on mortality—conditional logistic regression models including AIM panel PCs

Factor/effect	Estimate	SE	Odds Ratio (OR) estimate	OR 95% CI		*P* value[c]
				Lower	Upper	
Analysis for IRP A						
Treatment	−0.15	0.258	0.861	0.519	1.427	0.56
IRP A	−0.08	0.278	0.926	0.537	1.597	0.78
IRP A by treatment interaction[a]	−0.01	0.535	0.989	0.347	2.819	0.98
High APACHE II/SAPS II Scores	−0.06	0.352	0.940	0.472	1.872	0.86
High APACHE II/SAPS II scores by treatment interaction[a]	0.82	0.315	2.273	1.226	4.215	< 0.01
High APACHE II/SAPS II scores by IRP A Interaction[a]	0.15	0.329	1.164	0.611	2.218	0.65
IRP A by treatment by high APACHE II/SAPS II Scores	−0.42	0.651	0.659	0.184	2.360	0.52
AIM Panel PCs[b]						< 0.01
Analysis for IRP B						
Treatment	−0.13	0.251	0.880	0.538	1.438	0.61
IRP B	0.14	0.280	1.153	0.666	1.999	0.61
IRP B by treatment interaction[a]	−0.09	0.541	0.912	0.316	2.635	0.87
High APACHE II/SAPS II Scores	0.10	0.344	1.100	0.561	2.157	0.78
High APACHE II/SAPS II Scores by Treatment[a]	0.63	0.302	1.869	1.033	3.379	0.04
High APACHE II/SAPS II Scores by IRP B Interaction[a]	−0.35	0.338	0.704	0.363	1.366	0.30
IRP B by treatment by high APACHE II/SAPS II Scores	0.09	0.677	1.092	0.290	4.118	0.90
AIM Panel PCs[b]						< 0.01

Analysis for IRP A involves 376 discordant matched sets from a total of 637 matched sets. Analysis for IRP B involves 372 discordant matched sets from a total of 634 matched sets

[a] The interaction odds ratio is a ratio of odds ratios

[b] A total of 10 AIM Panel PCs have been included which account for 33.9% of the variance in the AIM Panel data for the Matched-INDICATED Primary Analysis Population based on all cohorts

[c] *P* values are from Wald Chi-square tests; the test of the combined AIM Panel PCs is the sum of the individual Wald Chi-square tests

treatment was associated with similar survival benefit in the IRP + and IRP- genotype subgroups. Self-reported ethnicity, genetically assigned continent of origin, and high APACHE II/SAPS II analyses did not show predictive genetic IRP effects in any subgroup. Exploratory analyses of the four individual IRP SNPs also did not show any predictive biomarker effects. Similarly, neither IRP A nor IRP B was predictive of differential DrotAA treatment effects on secondary efficacy endpoints. Only the IRP B + genotype was associated with significantly longer duration in hospital in DrotAA-treated patients compared with the IRP B- genotype.

Strengths of this study were first, identification of a well-defined and clinically appropriate patient population (on-label as defined by the approved indications for DrotAA in both the EU and the USA). Secondly, we minimized patient selection bias by using matching to select appropriate patients for the control group to overcome the lack of randomization to DrotAA treatment. DrotAA was typically given to younger patients with greater severity of disease in clinical practice. Therefore, simply comparing the mortality rates in all DrotAA-treated patients to all nonDrotAA-treated patients in the 10 cohorts would have been invalid. The considerations in designing this study were to use either design-based or analysis-based methods to control for characteristics that differed at baseline between treatment groups. We chose to use a design-based approach of matching to tightly control for key measures, so that the control group was comparable to the treated group. This also permitted efficient use of resources since only a subsample of all possible controls would be needed for detailed genotypic evaluation. The low use of DrotAA in clinical practice for patients with severe sepsis in the included cohorts permitted this matched-patients study to be conducted. If the drug had been used most of the time in the eligible patients, then it would have been very difficult to match appropriate nonDrotAA-treated patients as matched controls. The matching process was successful in achieving well-balanced study groups, and balance between the two study groups was achieved across IRP genotype subgroups (IRP+, IRP−), thus minimizing confounding of any biomarker effects (IRP*treatment interaction) by baseline differences.

The third strength of the study was quality of data, genotyping, and ancestry-control. Extensively reviewed

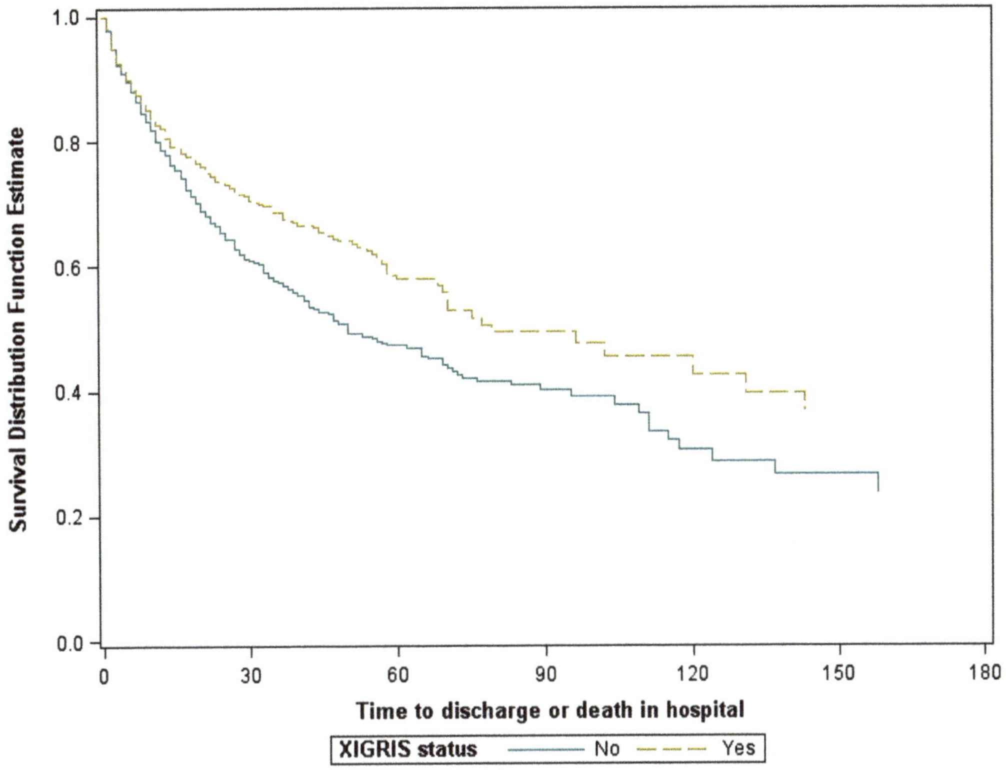

Fig. 2 Kaplan–Meier curves showing estimated 28-day mortality rates of approximately 28% for the DrotAA (Xigris) group and 38% for the nonDrotAA group

phenotypic data from all 10 cohorts were combined in a common database. Genotyping of the IRP SNPs was conducted using a validated Taqman-based method. A panel of ancestry informative markers (AIM panel with 91 SNPs) was genotyped using a qualified GoldenGate genotyping method. Quality criteria were applied to the genomic data based on per-sample and per-SNP call rates and Hardy–Weinberg equilibrium testing. These strengths are confirmed by finding similar results to PROWESS in that we were successful in overcoming the patient selection bias that can occur in a retrospective, nonrandomized study.

DrotAA has been suggested to be beneficial in the most severe patients, and especially in those with advanced coagulopathy. Coagulation dysfunction was diagnosed in only 31.8% of the treated patients, which might partly explain the negative results. However, we clarify that we chose our inclusion criteria to align with the drug label and indicated use of DrotAA. Our overall hypothesis was that a genomic marker(s) would identify responders to DrotAA and that a diagnostic kit could then be developed to help clinicians decide whom to treat with DrotAA.

The SNP selection and interaction test results of the prior studies could have been influenced by the so-called winner's curse. If adequate methods had been taken to deal with the winner's curse, then the sample size requirement for adequate power may have increased because we would not have over-estimated the assumed effect size of the IRP.

Although the present results are negative, it is useful to discuss the feasibility of IRP detection (including time and cost) and treatment allocation based on the presence of such IRPs. The genotype can be measured now in 40–60 min (Cepheid for example), even in the Emergency or ICU setting, and location(s) a time frame reasonable for IRP detection in sepsis and septic shock. The cost would depend upon the technology platform cost, the reagent costs, and the clinical value of the test results based on studies of cost–benefit of the test versus not having the test.

Limitations of our study were that the treatment assignment of DrotAA was not blinded nor randomized, outcomes were obtained retrospectively from databases, and we could not assess safety due to lack of adequate data. Examples of some confounders that we could not control for are physician and judgement regarding patient prognosis and eligibility for treatment with DrotAA, individual ICU or hospital policies regarding use of DrotAA, and other underlying disease that we did not capture. We did not specifically select patients that were randomized in DrotAA trials because we did not have access to the trials of DrotAA that collected DNA such as PROWESS [4, 16]. Sepsis is a complex trait, so it is likely that future research regarding better patient selection for treatment will consider several phenotypic biomarkers (not just focusing on genetic diversity) with or without genotype assessments.

Why were our IRP A and IRP B genotypes not predictive? It is possible that our method of selection of SNPs for IRP A and IRP B was inadequate. We used an underpowered replication cohort to refine SNPs of interest from the PROWESS study and we incorporated both SNPs based on pure statistical signal in the replication cohort as well as SNPs that were chosen based on both strength of signal in the replication cohort as well as biological plausibility. Our study highlights the importance and difficulty of validation of predictive genotype-base biomarkers in severe sepsis.

Our finding of a beneficial treatment effect of DrotAA in the current study differs from PROWESS SHOCK [6] and from the APROCCHS trial [7] (in which there was no treatment effect) and may reflect selection bias. Additionally, our study was not randomized, included an earlier era of patients, and we found higher mortality rates than in PROWESS SHOCK.

Conclusions

Neither IRP A nor IRP B predicted a differential DrotAA treatment effect in patients with severe sepsis and high risk of death.

Abbreviations

PROWESS: prospective recombinant human activated protein C worldwide evaluation in severe sepsis; IRP: improved response polymorphism; DROTAA: drotrecogin alfa (activated); APACHE II: acute physiology and chronic health evaluation; SAPS: simplified acute physiology score; SNP: single nucleotide polymorphism; ICU: intensive care unit; ARR: absolute risk reduction; GWAS: Genome Wide Association Study; SPH: St. Paul's Hospital; VASST: vasopressin and septic shock trial; RYR2: ryanodine receptor 2 gene; ACIN1: apoptotic chromatin condensation inducer 1 gene; S1P: sphingosine-1-phosphate receptor 1; APC: activated protein C; PAR1: protease-activated receptor 1; AKT: prosurvival kinase; SPATA7: spermatogenesis associated 7 gene; FLI1: friend leukemia virus integration 1 gene; FDA: food and drug administration; EMA: European medicines agency; AIM: ancestry informative marker; PAP: primary analysis population; APROCCHS: activated protein C and corticosteroids for human septic shock.

Authors' contributions

DA, PJH, RB, NL, HFW, MN, ADJM, and JAR contributed to conception and design. DA, JP M, LBW, ACG, CJH, DCC, JS, KB, TGB, PJH, RB, NL, KN, HFW, MN, ADJM, KRW, and JAR contributed to analysis and interpretation, and drafted the manuscript for important intellectual content. All authors read and approved the final manuscript.

Authors' information

Not applicable.

Author details

[1] Service de Reanimation Medicale, Hopital R. Poincare, 104 Bd Raymond Poincare, 92380 Garches, France. [2] Sorbonne Paris Cité, Cochin Hotel-Dieu University Hospital Medical Intensive Care Unit, AP-HP, Université Paris Descartes, 75014 Paris, France. [3] Departments of Medicine and Pathology, Microbiology and Immunology, Vanderbilt University School of Medicine, 1161 21st Avenue South T1218 MCN, Nashville, TN 37232-2650, USA. [4] Section of Anaesthetics, Pain Medicine, and Intensive Care, Charing Cross Hospital, Imperial College London, Fulham Palace Road, London W6 8RF, UK. [5] Barts and The London School of Medicine, Queen Mary University of London, London, UK. [6] Harvard Medical School and School of Public Health, 665 Huntington Avenue, Building I Room 1401, Boston, MA 02115, USA. [7] Emory Center for Critical Care, Woodruff Health Sciences Center, Emory University, Atlanta, GA, USA. [8] Division of Allergy and Clinical Immunology, Department of Medicine, Johns Hopkins University, Baltimore, MD, USA. [9] Department of Biostatistics, University of Washington, F-600, Health Sciences Building, Office: H-665D HSB, Box 357232, Seattle, WA 98195-7232, USA. [10] Syreon Corporation, Vancouver, BC, Canada. [11] Formerly with Sirius Genomics Inc, Vancouver, BC, Canada. [12] Critical Care Research Laboratories, Centre for Heart Lung Innovation, St. Paul's Hospital, University of British Columbia, Burrard Building, Rm 166 - 1081 Burrard St, Vancouver, BC V6Z 1Y6, Canada.

Acknowledgements

We thank all the patients who are part of this study and their families. We also thank the caregivers of the patients in these centers. Dr Gordon is a UK National Institute for Health Research (NIHR) Clinician Scientist award holder and is grateful for funding from the NIHR comprehensive Biomedical Research Centre funding stream. Dr. Ware is funded by an American Heart Association Established Investigator Award.

Competing interests

Dr. Russell was a consultant, founder, and shareholder of Sirius Genomics at the time of this study. Dr. Russell reports patents owned by the University of British Columbia (UBC) that are related to PCSK9 inhibitor (s) and sepsis and related to the use of vasopressin in septic shock. Dr. Russell is an inventor on these patents. Dr. Russell is a founder, Director, and shareholder in Cyon Therapeutics Inc. (developing a sepsis therapy). Dr. Russell has share options in Leading Biosciences Inc. Dr. Russell is a shareholder in Molecular You Corp. Dr. Russell reports receiving consulting fees from: (1) Cubist Pharmaceuticals (now owned by Merck; formerly was Trius Pharmaceuticals; developing antibiotics), (2) Leading Biosciences (developing a sepsis therapeutic), (3) Ferring Pharmaceuticals (manufactures vasopressin and is developing selepressin), (4) Grifols (sells albumin), (5) La Jolla Pharmaceuticals (developing angiotensin II; Dr. Russell chairs the DSMB of a trial of angiotensin II), (6) CytoVale Inc. (developing a sepsis diagnostic), (7) Asahi Kesai Pharmaceuticals of America (AKPA)(developing recombinant thrombomodulin). Dr. Russell reports having received an investigator-initiated grant from Grifols that is provided to and administered by UBC. Ms. Mancini and Mr. Wellman were employees and shareholders of Sirius Genomics at the time of the study. Anthony C. Gordon and Patrick J. Heagerty were consultants to Sirius Genomics at the time of this study. Dr. Walley was a founder and shareholder of Sirius Genomics at the time of this study. Robert Balshaw, Nadia Lesnikova, and Karen de Nobrega were employees of Syreon Corp. at the time of this study.

Funding
This study was funded by Sirius Genomics Inc.

References

1. Wang L, McLeod HL, Weinshilboum RM. Genomics and drug response. N Engl J Med. 2011;364(12):1144–53.
2. Schwarz UI, Ritchie MD, Bradford Y, et al. Genetic determinants of response to warfarin during initial anticoagulation. N Engl J Med. 2008;358(10):999–1008.
3. Rieder MJ, Reiner AP, Gage BF, et al. Effect of VKORC1 haplotypes on transcriptional regulation and warfarin dose. N Engl J Med. 2005;352(22):2285–93.
4. Bernard GR, Vincent JL, Laterre PF, et al. Efficacy and safety of recombinant human activated protein C for severe sepsis. N Engl J Med. 2001;344(10):699–709.
5. Abraham E, Laterre PF, Garg R, et al. Drotrecogin alfa (activated) for adults with severe sepsis and a low risk of death. N Engl J Med. 2005;353(13):1332–41.
6. Ranieri VM, Thompson BT, Barie PS, et al. Drotrecogin alfa (activated) in adults with septic shock. N Engl J Med. 2012;366(22):2055–64.
7. Annane D, Timsit JF, Megarbane B, et al. Recombinant human activated protein C for adults with septic shock: a randomized controlled trial. Am J Respir Crit Care Med. 2013;187(10):1091–7.
8. Annane D, Mira JP, Ware LB, et al. Design, conduct, and analysis of a multicenter, pharmacogenomic, biomarker study in matched patients with severe sepsis treated with or without drotrecogin Alfa (activated). Ann Intensive Care. 2012;2(1):15.
9. Russell JA, Walley KR, Singer J, et al. Vasopressin versus norepinephrine infusion in patients with septic shock. N Engl J Med. 2008;358(9):877–87.
10. Rowan KM, Welch CA, North E, Harrison DA. Drotrecogin alfa (activated): real-life use and outcomes for the UK. Crit Care. 2008;12(2):R58.
11. Bertolini G, Rossi C, Anghileri A, Livigni S, Addis A, Poole D. Use of Drotrecogin alfa (activated) in Italian intensive care units: the results of a nationwide survey. Intensive Care Med. 2007;33(3):426–34.
12. Wheeler A, Steingrub J, Schmidt GA, et al. A retrospective observational study of drotrecogin alfa (activated) in adults with severe sepsis: comparison with a controlled clinical trial. Crit Care Med. 2008;36(1):14–23.
13. Kanji S, Perreault MM, Chant C, Williamson D, Burry L. Evaluating the use of Drotrecogin alfa (activated) in adult severe sepsis: a Canadian multicenter observational study. Intensive Care Med. 2007;33(3):517–23.
14. Vincent JL, Laterre PF, Decruyenaere J, et al. A registry of patients treated with drotrecogin alfa (activated) in Belgian intensive care units: an observational study. Acta Clin Belg. 2008;63(1):25–30.
15. Rosenbaum PR, Rubin DB. The bias due to incomplete matching. Biometrics. 1985;41(1):103–16.
16. Man M, Close SL, Shaw AD, et al. Beyond single-marker analyses: mining whole genome scans for insights into treatment responses in severe sepsis. Pharmacogenomics J. 2013;13(3):218–26.

16

Predictors of response to fixed-dose vasopressin in adult patients with septic shock

Gretchen L. Sacha[1*], Simon W. Lam[1], Abhijit Duggal[2], Heather Torbic[1], Stephanie N. Bass[1], Sarah C. Welch[1], Robert S. Butler[3] and Seth R. Bauer[1]

Abstract

Background: Vasopressin is often utilized for hemodynamic support in patients with septic shock. However, the most appropriate patient to initiate therapy in is unknown. This study was conducted to determine factors associated with hemodynamic response to fixed-dose vasopressin in patients with septic shock.

Methods: Single-center, retrospective cohort of patients receiving fixed-dose vasopressin for septic shock for at least 6 h with concomitant catecholamines in the medical, surgical, or neurosciences intensive care unit (ICU) at a tertiary care center. Patients were classified as responders or non-responders to fixed-dose vasopressin. Response was defined as a decrease in catecholamine dose requirements and achievement of mean arterial pressure ≥ 65 mmHg at 6 h after initiation of vasopressin.

Results: A total of 938 patients were included: 426 responders (45%), 512 non-responders (55%). Responders had lower rates of in-hospital (57 vs. 72%; $P < 0.001$) and ICU mortality (50 vs. 68%; $P < 0.001$), and increased ICU-free days at day 14 and hospital-free days at day 28 (2.3 ± 3.8 vs. 1.6 ± 3.3; $P < 0.001$ and 4.2 ± 7.2 vs. 2.8 ± 6.0; $P < 0.001$, respectively). On multivariable analysis, non-medical ICU location was associated with increased response odds (OR 1.70; $P = 0.0049$) and lactate at vasopressin initiation was associated with decreased response odds (OR 0.93; $P = 0.0003$). Factors not associated with response included APACHE III score, SOFA score, corticosteroid use, and catecholamine dose.

Conclusion: In this evaluation, 45% responded to the addition of vasopressin with improved outcomes compared to non-responders. The only factors found to be associated with vasopressin response were ICU location and lactate concentration.

Keywords: Sepsis, Septic shock, Vasopressors, Vasopressin, Norepinephrine, Catecholamines

Background

Due to its vasoconstrictive properties, arginine vasopressin (AVP) is often utilized in practice for patients with shock requiring hemodynamic support. The Surviving Sepsis Campaign guidelines suggest AVP as an adjunct to norepinephrine (NE) at a fixed dosage of 0.03 units/min to achieve mean arterial pressure (MAP) goals or decrease NE requirements [1]. However, due to limited data these recommendations have a weak grading. In the landmark Vasopressin and Septic Shock Trial (VASST), patients were randomized to either AVP plus NE or NE monotherapy, with no mortality difference detected between treatment approaches [2]. However, further analyses have suggested that patients with less severe forms of septic shock may benefit from AVP [2, 3]. Despite limited data supporting the efficacy of this agent and weak guideline recommendations, clinicians commonly utilize AVP in practice.

The importance of targeting and maintaining goal MAP along with early initiation of vasoactive agents in patients with septic shock has been associated with reduced mortality rates [4, 5]. In fact, delays in vasoactive initiation were associated with increased mortality [5]. Conversely, the importance of limiting catecholamines (CA)

*Correspondence: sachag@ccf.org
[1] Department of Pharmacy, Cleveland Clinic, 9500 Euclid Avenue (Hb-105), Cleveland, OH 44195, USA
Full list of author information is available at the end of the article

and utilizing non-CA vasoactive agents, such as AVP, is becoming more apparent and may ultimately improve patient outcomes [6–8]. Similarly, initiating AVP early in shock presentation may yield beneficial results [9, 10].

Unfortunately, there are still many unknowns regarding the most appropriate management strategy in patients with septic shock and the choice of vasoactive agent (especially second line) involves the weighing of a dynamic interplay of mechanisms and resultant responses of these agents. Specifically, one such agent is AVP and the ideal patient population to initiate AVP is unknown. There are limited data that may indicate a benefit in patients that are less severely ill [2, 3], have renal dysfunction [11, 12], or are receiving corticosteroids [13–15]. This study was designed to describe the impact of fixed-dose AVP on hemodynamic response and determine factors associated with response to AVP in a large cohort of adult patients with septic shock. The primary objective was to ascertain patient-specific factors at AVP initiation associated with a higher likelihood of response to AVP therapy. Secondary objectives included comparing clinical outcomes between responders and non-responders, and evaluating clinical characteristics over time, including MAP, lactate and CA dosage.

Methods

This was a retrospective, single-center evaluation of fixed-dose AVP at a large tertiary care academic medical center. Adults over the age of 18 with active orders for AVP between September 2011 and August 2015 were screened for inclusion. Patients with septic shock, receiving adjunctive, fixed-dose AVP for at least 6 h in the medical intensive care unit (ICU), surgical ICU, or neurosciences ICU were included. Patients must have received one or more CA agent for at least 1 h prior to AVP initiation and only the first course of AVP was included. Patients were excluded if they had incomplete electronic data or AVP was initiated in the operating room.

Patients were classified as responders to AVP if they achieved both a decrease in CA dosage and MAP ≥ 65 mmHg 6 h after AVP initiation. Six hours was chosen based on an evaluation showing MAP during the first 6 h was independently associated with mortality in patients with septic shock [16]. CA dosage was described in NE-equivalent dosage requirements from the following formula [NE (mcg/min)] + [Epinephrine (mcg/min)] + [Dopamine (mcg/kg/min)/2] + [Phenylephrine (mcg/min)/10] [2]. Septic shock was defined as meeting two or more systemic inflammatory response syndrome criteria with the presence of antibiotics and hypotension requiring CAs. The presence of acute kidney injury (AKI) was determined and patients were categorized into one of the risk, injury, failure, loss, and end-stage kidney disease (RIFLE) categories based on serum creatinine increase at ICU admission and AVP initiation [11]. Total fluid bolus volume was calculated as crystalloid volume, with colloid equivalent doses [17, 18] and defined as total volume of fluids given 6 h prior to NE initiation until AVP initiation. Corticosteroid receipt was defined as receiving at least one dose of corticosteroids at AVP initiation up to 6 h after initiation.

Outcomes collected included in-hospital and ICU mortality, alive ICU-free days at day 14, alive hospital-free days at day 28, duration of mechanical ventilation, SOFA score change 48 h after AVP initiation, CA dosage change at 6 h after AVP initiation, need for continuous renal replacement therapy (CRRT) initiation, and CA duration. Cohorts of interest were defined a priori based on previous literature suggesting beneficial outcomes with AVP: NE-equivalent CA dose < 15 mcg/min at AVP initiation [2], lactate concentration ≤ 1.4 mmol/L at AVP initiation [2], receipt of corticosteroids [13, 15] obesity category [19, 20], the use of > 1 vasoactive agent at AVP initiation [2], and renal insufficiency per RIFLE category [11].

Data are presented as mean ± SD for continuous variables and *n* (%) for categorical variables. Univariate analyses between responders and non-responders were tested using either Chi-Square or Fisher's exact test, as appropriate, for categorical variables or ANOVA for continuous variables. Between-group differences in change in MAP, lactate concentration, CA dosage requirements, and central venous oxygen saturation ($ScvO_2$) were assessed at consecutive time intervals from AVP initiation to 72 h. A Bonferroni correction was applied to the pairwise comparisons. The effect of baseline variables on AVP response and ICU mortality were assessed using stepwise multivariable logistic regression. Statistically significant and variables with biologic plausibility for influencing the outcome were considered for the model and tested for colinearity using variance inflation factors and condition indices. If two variables were determined to be collinear [21], only one was included in the multivariable regression analysis. *P* values < 0.05 were considered to be statistically significant. All statistical analyses were performed with SAS 9.4 Software (SAS Institute Inc., Cary, NC) and StataIC 14 (StataCorp LLC, College Station, Tx). This study was approved by the Cleveland Clinic institutional review board (Study Number 15-2100).

Results

Of the 2555 screened, 938 (36.7%) met criteria for inclusion and of these, 426 (45.4%) were classified as responders to AVP and 512 (54.6%) as non-responders (Fig. 1). The average age was 62 ± 14 years, most patients were Caucasian (69.5%) and treated in the medical ICU (75.9%;

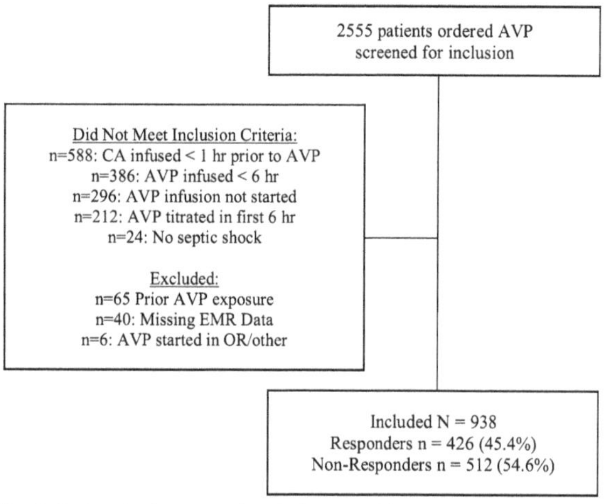

Fig. 1 Patient inclusion and exclusion tree. There were 2555 patients screened for inclusion into the study. Of the screened patients, 1506 patients did not meet initial inclusion criteria and 111 met exclusion criteria leaving 938 patients included in the evaluation. *AVP* arginine vasopressin; *CA* catecholamine; *EMR* electronic medical record; *OR* operating room

Table 1). When compared to responders, non-responders had higher rates of hepatic failure (19.3 vs. 14.3%; $P = 0.04$), lower MAP values (65 ± 12 vs. 69 ± 12 mmHg; $P < 0.001$) and higher lactate concentrations (5.4 ± 4.8 vs. 4.0 ± 3.6 mmol/L; $P < 0.001$) at AVP initiation. The average AVP initial dose was 0.03 units/min (range 0.01–0.08 units/min).

Responders had lower rates of in-hospital and ICU mortality (56.6 vs. 71.7%; $P < 0.001$ and 50.2 vs. 67.8%; $P < 0.001$, respectively), more ICU-free days at day 14 (2.3 ± 3.8 vs. 1.6 ± 3.3 days; $P < 0.001$), more hospital-free days at day 28 (4.2 ± 7.2 vs. 2.8 ± 6.0 days; $P < 0.001$) and less frequent need for CRRT within 72 h after AVP initiation (20.2 vs. 30%; $P = 0.002$) (Table 2). There was a significant difference between groups in the change in SOFA score from AVP initiation until 48 h (responders 0.30 ± 2.9 vs. non-responders 0.83 ± 2.9; $P = 0.02$) and CA dose change from AVP initiation until 6 h (responders -12.8 ± 9.6 mcg/min vs. non-responders $+13.8 \pm 51.2$ mcg/min; $P < 0.001$). Responders also had more CA-free and MV-free days on day 14 compared to non-responders (both $P < 0.001$). On multivariable logistic regression, treatment in the surgical or neurosciences ICU compared to the medical ICU and lower lactate concentrations was independently associated with higher odds of response to AVP ($P = 0.005$ and $P < 0.001$, respectively). Additionally, a positive hemodynamic response to AVP was independently associated with lower ICU mortality (Table 3).

In the predefined cohorts of interest, there was no association between the cohort designation and hemodynamic response in patients whether classified on the receipt of corticosteroids, obesity category, number of vasopressors required at AVP initiation, or RIFLE-defined AKI. Patients with lactate concentrations ≤ 1.4 mmol/L had higher odds of response to AVP while patients with NE-equivalent CA doses < 15 had a decreased odds of response to AVP (Table 4).

There was a significant difference in CA dosage between responders and non-responders at every time point from AVP initiation through 48 h (Fig. 2a). There was also a significant difference in MAP change from AVP initiation in the responders compared to the non-responders at 3 and 24 h: +5.4 versus +2.6 mmHg ($P < 0.001$) and +2.0 versus − 2.0 mmHg ($P < 0.001$) (Fig. 2b). Finally, lactate concentration differed significantly between responders and non-responders at every time point evaluated from AVP initiation through 48 h (Fig. 2c). There was no difference in $ScvO_2$ at any time point (Fig. 2d).

Discussion

This evaluation identified 938 patients in which 45% had a positive hemodynamic response to AVP which was associated with decreased mortality, increased ICU- and hospital-free days, and decreased CA dosage requirements. The improvement in outcomes in responders indicates the definition used for hemodynamic response may be an appropriate pharmacodynamic marker of response to AVP therapy and should be further evaluated in future studies. Furthermore, on multivariable analyses, non-medical ICU treatment and decreasing lactate concentrations were independently associated with a positive response to AVP and AVP response was independently associated with decreased ICU mortality. It is important to understand that the clinical utilization of AVP and its place in therapy relies on imperfect data, clinical experience, and weak guideline recommendations. Regardless of this, it is commonly used in clinical practice as an adjunct to NE in patients with refractory septic shock [22]. Its proposed mechanism of action is twofold, by causing V1 receptor-mediated vasoconstriction in some vascular smooth muscle beds [23], AVP can be utilized as a vasopressor similar to CAs. Additionally, in patients with septic shock, a relative endogenous vasopressin deficiency may exist and fixed, low dose exogenous AVP can be utilized as an endocrine supplement with resultant improvements in hemodynamics [12, 24–27]. Clinicians are often put in challenging situations in which they must determine if AVP should be initiated for an individual patient with few data available to inform the decision. The results of this study identify patient characteristics associated with response to AVP and can assist with decision-making regarding AVP initiation.

Table 1 Baseline characteristics

Characteristic	Total (N=938)	Non-responders (N=512)	Responders (N=426)	P value
Characteristics at ICU admission				
Age, years	62±14	61±15	62±14	0.17
Male, n (%)	493 (52.6)	272 (53.1)	221 (51.9)	0.70
Race, n (%)				0.10
Caucasian	652 (69.5)	357 (69.7)	295 (69.2)	
African American	241 (25.7)	124 (24.2)	117 (27.5)	
Other	45 (4.8)	31 (6.1)	14 (3.3)	
ICU type, n (%)				0.06
Medical	712 (75.9)	401 (78.3)	311 (73.0)	
Neurological	65 (6.9)	27 (5.3)	38 (8.9)	
Surgical	161 (17.2)	84 (16.4)	77 (18.1)	
Weight, kg	90.5±34.0	92.0±37.1	88.6±29.9	0.13
BMI, kg/m^2	31.5±11.7	31.9±12.6	31.0±10.4	0.22
ESRD, n (%)	119 (12.7)	58 (11.3)	61 (14.3)	0.17
APACHE III	106±34	107±36	104±30	0.09
APS	90±32	92±35	88±29	0.14
Comorbid conditions, n (%)				
Diabetes mellitus	286 (30.5)	152 (29.7)	134 (31.5)	0.56
Hepatic failure	160 (17.1)	99 (19.3)	61 (14.3)	0.04
Immune suppression	196 (20.9)	109 (21.3)	87 (20.4)	0.75
Leukemia/myeloma	65 (6.9)	38 (7.4)	27 (6.3)	0.52
Moderate COPD	13 (1.4)	9 (1.8)	4 (0.9)	0.45
Severe COPD	85 (9.1)	42 (8.2)	43 (10.1)	0.45
No chronic health issues, n (%)	232 (24.7)	118 (23.0)	114 (26.8)	0.19
Characteristics at time of AVP initiation				
Appropriate antibiotics, n (%)[a]	887 (94.6)	487 (95.1)	400 (93.9)	0.41
Fluids prior to AVP, mL/kg	30.7±34.4	30.6±35.1	30.8±33.6	0.95
MAP, mmHg	67±12	65±12	69±12	< 0.001
Lactate, mmol/L	4.8±4.4	5.4±4.8	4.0±3.6	< 0.001
SOFA score	13±4	12±3	13±4	0.49
Total CA dose				
mcg/min	28.2±19.9	27.8±21.9	28.6±17.3	0.54
mcg/kg/min	0.34±0.26	0.33±0.27	0.35±0.25	0.18
Catecholamine agent, n (%)				
Norepinephrine	937 (99.9)	511 (99.8)	426 (100.0)	0.99
Phenylephrine	66 (7.0)	31 (6.1)	35 (8.2)	0.20
Epinephrine	25 (2.7)	11 (2.1)	14 (3.3)	0.28
Dopamine	4 (0.4)	2 (0.4)	2 (0.5)	0.99
AVP dose				
Units/min	0.0314±0.0063	0.0317±0.0064	0.0312±0.0062	0.24
Units/kg/h	0.0226±0.0084	0.0224±0.0084	0.0227±0.0083	0.66
Corticosteroids, n (%)	571 (60.9)	320 (62.5)	251 (58.9)	0.26
AKI, n (%)				0.21
Risk	79 (8.4)	50 (9.8)	29 (6.8)	
Injury	32 (3.4)	21 (4.1)	11 (2.6)	
Failure	142 (15.1)	75 (14.6)	67 (15.7)	
Loss	0 (0)	0 (0)	0 (0)	
CRRT, n (%)	159 (17.0)	81 (15.8)	78 (18.3)	0.31

AKI acute kidney injury, *AVP* arginine vasopressin, *APS* acute physiology score, *BMI* body mass index, *CA* catecholamine, *COPD* chronic obstructive pulmonary disease, *CRRT* continuous renal replacement therapy, *ESRD* end-stage renal dysfunction, *MAP* mean arterial pressure, *SOFA* sequential organ failure assessment

[a] Antibiotics were considered to be appropriate if patients received antibiotics described in the Centers for Medicare & Medicaid Services sepsis measure or received an appropriately de-escalated antibiotic regimen for an isolated pathogen on the day of AVP initiation

Table 2 Patient outcomes

Outcome	Total ($N=938$)	Non-responders ($N=512$)	Responders ($N=426$)	P value
In-hospital mortality, n (%)	608 (64.8)	367 (71.7)	241 (56.6)	< 0.001
ICU mortality, n (%)	561 (59.8)	347 (67.8)	214 (50.2)	< 0.001
ICU-free days at day 14	1.9 ± 3.6	1.6 ± 3.3	2.3 ± 3.8	< 0.001
Hospital-free days at day 28	3.4 ± 6.6	2.8 ± 6.0	4.2 ± 7.2	< 0.001
MV-free days at day 14	2.8 ± 4.9	2.2 ± 4.5	3.6 ± 5.3	< 0.001
SOFA score change[a]	0.6 ± 2.9	0.8 ± 2.9	0.3 ± 2.9	0.02
Respiration score change	2.3 ± 1.5	2.0 ± 1.5	2.5 ± 1.4	< 0.001
Coagulation score change	0.46 ± 1.0	0.5 ± 0.9	0.4 ± 1.0	0.19
Liver score change	0.1 ± 0.7	0.1 ± 0.8	0.7 ± 0.6	0.90
Neurological score change	− 0.1 ± 1.1	0.1 ± 1.1	− 0.2 ± 1.0	< 0.001
Cardiovascular score change	− 1.9 ± 1.7	− 1.6 ± 1.7	− 2.1 ± 1.7	< 0.001
CRRT initiation between AVP start and 72 h, n (%)[b]	190 (25.0)	112 (30.0)	78 (20.2)	0.002
CA dose change[c], mcg/min	+1.7 ± 40.6	+13.8 ± 51.2	− 12.8 ± 9.6	< 0.001
CA-free days at day 14	5.0 ± 5.8	3.9 ± 5.5	6.3 ± 6.0	< 0.001

CA catecholamine, *CRRT* continuous renal replacement therapy, *MV* mechanical ventilation, *SOFA* sequential organ failure assessment

[a] Evaluated at hour 48 after vasopressin initiation

[b] Evaluated only in patients who survived at least 24 h after vasopressin initiation

[c] Evaluated at hour 6 after vasopressin initiation

VASST is the largest trial of AVP in septic shock and randomized patients to either AVP plus NE or NE monotherapy [2]. While no mortality difference was detected between groups in the main analysis, several subsequent analyses have suggested benefit in specific subgroups of patients. In a priori-defined subgroup analyses, VASST showed improved 28- and 90-day outcomes in patients allocated to AVP with "less severe septic shock" (CA requirements < 15 mcg/min) and patients receiving one vasopressor at baseline (compared to two or more) [2], findings which were not corroborated in the current study. Furthermore, in contrast to VASST, the current study found patients with CA doses < 15 mcg/min had lower odds of response to AVP. The cutoff of 15 mcg/min was based on the results of VASST; however, it is unknown if an optimal CA dose threshold for achieving hemodynamic response with AVP exists and 15 mcg/min may not be the ideal threshold to evaluate. In fact, in a recent retrospective cohort study, increasing the AVP initiation threshold from a NE dose of 10 mcg/min to 50 mcg/min was not associated with increased mortality [28]. It should be noted that in clinical practice, AVP is frequently initiated in patients with NE dosage requirements exceed 15 mcg/min. In fact, the average NE dose at AVP initiation was 28 mcg/min in the current study which is similar to VASST (20 mcg/min) [2].

In an additional VASST post hoc subgroup analysis, patients receiving AVP with baseline lactate concentration ≤ 1.4 mmol/L had lower 28-day mortality rates than those receiving NE [2]. A subsequent re-analysis of VASST based on the updated definitions for septic shock also found improved survival in patients initiated on AVP with a lactate concentration ≤ 2 mmol/L [3]. The current study parallels these findings, with lower lactate concentrations independently associated with higher odds of hemodynamic response. Altogether, low lactate concentrations appear to be a useful biomarker for initiation of AVP. In comparison with VASST, which found no effect on renal replacement therapy, the current evaluation showed that fewer responders required a new initiation of CRRT compared to non-responders. These findings corroborate those from the Vasopressin versus Norepinephrine as Initial Therapy in Septic Shock (VANISH) trial which showed a decreased rate of renal replacement therapy initiation in patients who received vasopressin (when compared to NE) [29].

In addition, this study found no association with corticosteroid use and hemodynamic response; a combination previously thought to have a positive interaction [13]. The lack of an effect observed in this evaluation compared to previous studies could be due to differences of corticosteroid use. In the VASST analysis, the use of corticosteroids was regarded as receipt of at least one dose within the 28-day observation period, whereas the current study ensured corticosteroids were used concomitantly with AVP. However, it is important to note that patients could have received corticosteroids up to 6 h after AVP initiation, potentially affecting their ability to detect a response

Table 3 Results of multivariable analyses

Outcome	OR (95% CI)	P value
Multivariable analysis and association with response to vasopressin[a]		
Non-medical ICU	1.70 (1.18–2.46)	0.005
Lactate at AVP initiation, mmol/L	0.93 (0.89–0.97)	< 0.001
Multivariable analysis and association with ICU mortality		
Hemodynamic response to AVP	0.51 (0.35–0.76)	0.001
Catecholamine dose, mcg/kg/min	3.14 (1.36–7.28)	0.008
Lactate at AVP initiation, mmol/L	1.10 (1.04–1.18)	0.002
AKI presence		
Rifle versus no AKI	3.64 (1.77–7.49)	< 0.001
Injury versus no AKI	5.80 (1.13–29.60)	0.035
Failure versus no AKI	2.63 (1.38–5.01)	0.003
ESRD versus no AKI	2.37 (1.27–4.43)	0.007
APACHE III score	1.01 (1.01–1.02)	< 0.001
SOFA score	1.16 (1.08–1.25)	< 0.001
Medical ICU	1.58 (1.02–2.45)	0.040
Race (Caucasian)	1.72 (1.14–2.60)	0.010
Age	1.01 (1.00–1.03)	0.036
Hepatic failure	0.89 (0.48–1.62)	0.696

AKI acute kidney injury, *AVP* vasopressin, *ESRD* end-stage renal dysfunction, *SOFA* sequential organ failure assessment

[a] Variables entered into the model but without a statistically significant association with vasopressin response include RIFLE-defined AKI category, corticosteroid use, SOFA score, APACHE III score, hepatic failure, race, age, and catecholamine dosage (in mcg/kg/min)

to corticosteroids in the evaluated time frame. Furthermore, the lack of detected benefit with corticosteroids could be due to differences in the outcomes evaluated in the current study (hemodynamic response) versus historical studies (mortality) [2, 13–15]. However, the lack of association seen in the current evaluation corroborates the findings seen in VANISH which detected no interaction between AVP and corticosteroid use on 28-day mortality [29]. Additional studies are needed to determine the relationship between corticosteroid use and hemodynamic response to AVP in patients with septic shock.

An additional finding of the current study was the CA-sparing effect, in that CA dosages decreased in responders at every time point from AVP initiation until 48 h. In fact, because the MAP was > 65 mmHg when AVP was added, a CA-sparing effect was likely the intended goal of AVP initiation. Responders also had more CA-free days at day 14 compared to non-responders, further showing the CA-sparing effect observed in this group. The benefit of sparing CAs in patients with septic shock has recently become more apparent [6–8]. One analysis found that raising MAP values above 70 mmHg with increasing vasoactive doses resulted in increased organ failure events [6]. Additionally, excess CAs can have a negative effect on the immune system and can cause tachyarrhythmias, hyperglycemia, splanchnic hypoperfusion, and myocardial depression. This new perspective emphasizes the importance of limiting CA doses while maintaining goal MAP, a method that can be achieved through AVP utilization.

Upon multivariable logistic regression, treatment in the medical ICU was associated with lower odds of response to AVP. Patients with sepsis secondary to medical (vs. surgical) conditions have higher mortality [30], which may influence AVP response. Additionally, these patient populations can present with a differing mix of comorbidities, which may alter patient outcomes differently [31], and medical patients may have lower frequencies of infectious source control (due to the prevalence of in-operable infections, i.e., pneumonia), which could decrease their response to treatment, including vasoactive therapies. It is also possible that there were residual confounders between medical ICU and non-medical ICU patients unable to be controlled for in the multivariable model. This finding of differing AVP response by treatment ICU and the potential mechanisms should be explored further.

This study has important implications for practice and future research. Regardless of the patients' CA dose, the association between low lactate concentration and hemodynamic response with AVP suggests that this marker of "less severe septic shock" is a useful indicator for AVP initiation. Furthermore, because of the improved outcomes in patients who had a positive hemodynamic response to

Table 4 Predefined cohorts of interest

Cohort of interest	Responders *N* (%)	Non-responders *N* (%)	*P* value	OR (95% CI) hemodynamic response	OR (95% CI) ICU mortality
Corticosteroids					
Yes	251 (58.9)	320 (62.5)	0.26	0.86 (0.66–1.12)	1.01 (0.77–1.32)
No[a]	175 (41.1)	192 (37.5)			
Lactate concentration					
> 1.4 mmol/L[a]	211 (78.4)	321 (88.7)	< 0.001	2.15 (1.39–3.32)^	0.39 (0.25–0.60)^
≤ 1.4 mmol/L	58 (21.6)	41 (11.3)			
BMI classification					
Underweight[a]	18 (4.2)	20 (3.9)	0.98		
Normal	94 (22.1)	106 (20.7)		0.99 (0.50–1.97)	1.09 (0.53–2.12)
Overweight	114 (26.8)	140 (27.3)		0.90 (0.46–1.79)	1.02 (0.51–2.05)
Obesity class I	81 (19.0)	101 (19.7)		0.89 (0.44–1.80)	0.91 (0.45–1.86)
Obesity class II	48 (11.3)	53 (10.4)		1.01 (0.48–2.12)	1.13 (0.52–2.43)
Obesity class III	71 (16.7)	92 (18.0)		0.86 (0.42–1.74)	0.77 (0.37–1.57)
CA equivalent dose					
≥ 15 mcg/min[a]	370 (86.9)	424 (82.8)	0.087	0.57 (0.36–0.92)^	0.62 (0.44–0.89)^
< 15 mcg/min	56 (13.1)	88 (17.2)			
Total vasopressor quantity					
1 Vasopressor[a]	370 (86.9)	463 (90.4)	0.084	1.43 (0.95–2.15)	1.98 (1.26–3.12)^
> 1 Vasopressor	56 (13.1)	49 (9.6)			
Renal insufficiency					
Yes	220 (51.6)	268 (52.3)	0.83	0.97 (0.75–1.26)	1.59 (1.23–2.07)^
No[a]	206 (48.4)	244 (47.7)			
AKI class					
No AKI presence[a]	258 (60.6)	308 (60.2)	0.21		
AKI-risk	29 (6.8)	50 (9.8)		0.69 (0.43–1.13)	2.40 (1.43–4.03)^
AKI-injury	11 (2.6)	21 (4.1)		0.63 (0.30–1.32)	3.30 (1.41–7.76)^
AKI-failure	67 (15.7)	75 (14.6)		1.07 (0.74–1.54)	3.06 (2.00–4.66)^
AKI-end stage	61 (14.3)	58 (11.3)		1.26 (0.85–1.87)	1.64 (1.09–2.46)^

AKI acute kidney injury, *BMI* body mass index, *CA* catecholamine

^ $P < 0.05$

[a] The reference group used for the odds ratio result

AVP at 6 h, monitoring for the achievement of hemodynamic stability can be an important early warning sign for the bedside clinician. Specifically, in patients who do not achieve hemodynamic stability within 6 h of starting AVP, alternative therapeutic interventions such as epinephrine [32], corticosteroids [33, 34], angiotensin II [35] (if available), or increasing AVP dose (especially when NE requirements exceed 0.6 mcg/kg/min) [36] should be considered. The use of this trigger and the next best step should be further investigated. Future trials should incorporate the observed factors associated with AVP response into their design, which may improve their likelihood of finding a target population for AVP use. Additionally, trials should evaluate when to initiate additional adjunctive agents and also compare efficacy between adjunctive agents.

Strengths of this evaluation include its a priori-defined cohorts for analysis, and evaluation of fixed-dose AVP (which removes the potential confounder of titrated doses on AVP response). Limitations of this evaluation include the fact that it was a single-center, retrospective study with no randomization and relied on medical record charting that may not instantaneously capture exact medication administration timing and hemodynamic change. Secondly, the definition of AVP response was not developed based on previous literature or able to be validated in this current study, but was created in an attempt to reflect hemodynamic response to this agent. However, based on the observed differences between responders and non-responders, it appears to accurately reflect a clinically meaningful response. Albeit, with this definition, patients who were already in the recovery

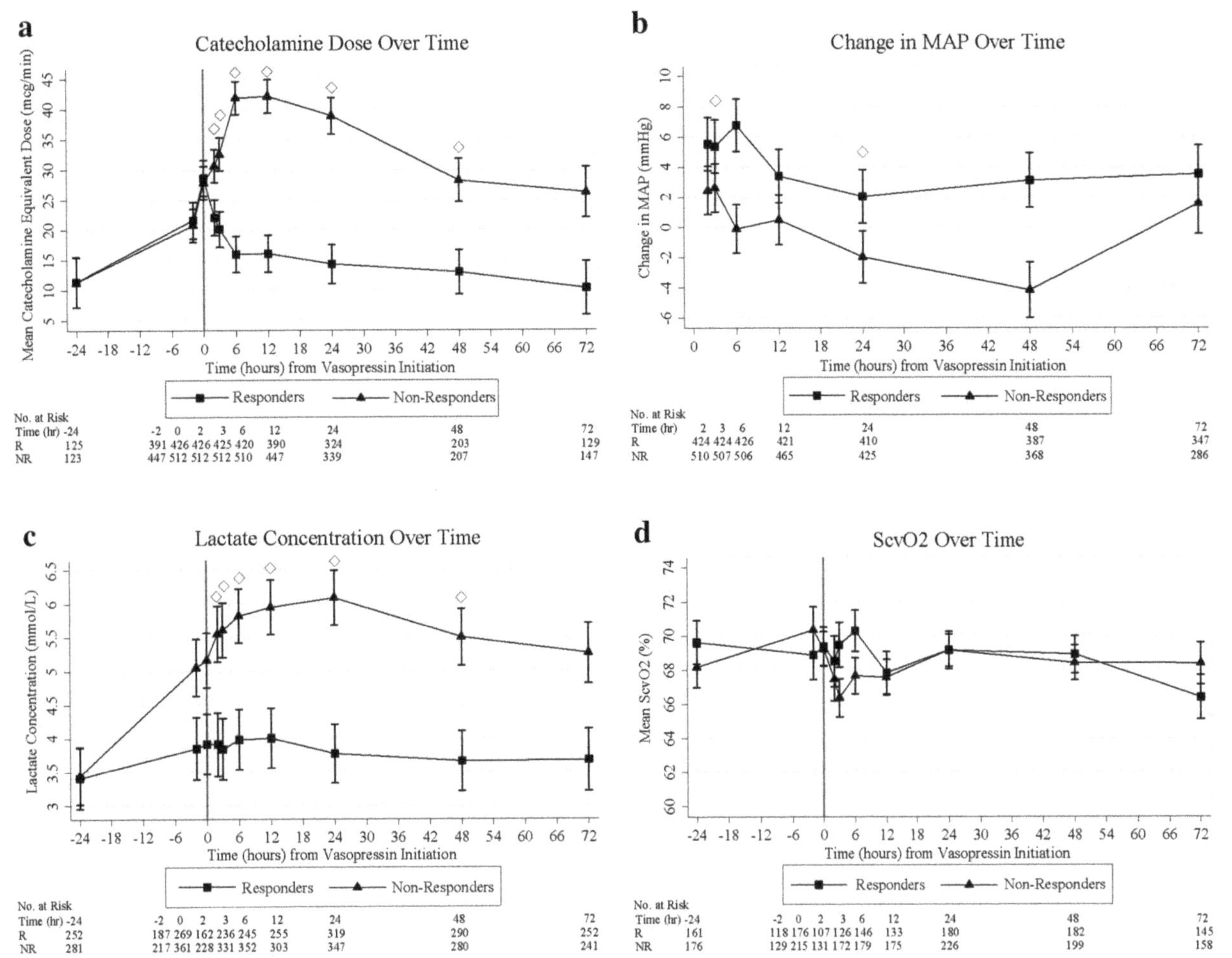

Fig. 2 Patient results over time for vasopressin responders and non-responders. **a** Catecholamine dose from -24 h to 72 h after vasopressin initiation. Responders had significantly lower catecholamine doses at 2, 3, 6, 12, 24 and 48 h after vasopressin initiation compared to non-responders. **b** Change in MAP from time 0 to 72 h after vasopressin initiation. Responders had significantly higher degrees of MAP change at 3 and 24 h after vasopressin initiation compared to non-responders. **c** Changes in lactate concentration from -24 h to 72 h after vasopressin initiation. Responders had significantly lower lactate concentrations at 2, 3, 6, 12, 24, and 48 h compared to nonresponders. **d** $ScvO_2$ from -24 h to 72 h after vasopressin initiation. There was no difference in $ScvO_2$ between responders and non-responders at any time point evaluated. *MAP* mean arterial pressure; *NR* non-responders; *R* responders; *ScvO2* central venous oxygen saturation. Data are means, with error bars indicating standard deviation. ◇ $P < 0.001$

phase of septic shock with decreasing CA dosage at AVP initiation were regarded as "responders." Additionally, patients classified as "non-responders" may have had decreased overall CA exposure with AVP than if they were not started on AVP, which was not accounted for in our definition of response. This study was also unable to incorporate markers of tissue perfusion (e.g., lactate, urine output, pH) into the definition of hemodynamic response, because these parameters were not consistently or frequently monitored and documented for every included patient. The importance of markers of tissue perfusion should not be overlooked as patients could potentially be at goal MAP, with reductions in CA doses as a result, but still have tissue hypoperfusion. This study also classified patients as having septic shock based on the previous definition and not the updated 2016 definition [1] which may result in more patients being included than those who had septic shock per the newest definition. Furthermore, cardiac output data were not available for most patients and therefore not collected. Although $ScvO_2$ values were elevated at baseline and not significantly different between responders and non-responders, we cannot adequately compare cardiac output between response groups. Additionally, the retrospective nature of this study makes identifying patients with true septic shock difficult, and as such, patients may have been included or excluded inadvertently. Finally, excluding patients who did not receive AVP for at least 6 h may have influenced the rates of response to therapy, as there may have been patients who responded earlier than 6 h and no longer needed vasoactive support with AVP (true responders) or patients who died within 6 h (true non-responders) and subsequently were excluded from the evaluation.

Conclusion

The current evaluation identified a large cohort of patients receiving fixed-dose AVP in which 45% responded to therapy. AVP response was associated with improved mortality and ICU and hospital-free days, indicating the definition used for hemodynamic response may be an appropriate pharmacodynamic marker of AVP therapy that can be used in future trials. In agreement with historical trials, patients with less severe forms of septic shock (lower lactate concentrations at baseline) appear to benefit more from AVP in comparison with patients with more severe forms. Future studies should incorporate the observed factors related to AVP response into their subsequent design to definitively identify the most appropriate patient population that would benefit from AVP.

Abbreviations

AKI: acute kidney injury; AVP: arginine vasopressin; CA: catecholamine; CRRT: continuous renal replacement therapy; ICU: intensive care unit; NE: norepinephrine; MAP: mean arterial pressure; RIFLE: risk, injury, failure, loss, end-stage kidney disease category; $ScVO_2$: central venous oxygen saturation; SOFA: sequential organ failure assessment; VASST: vasopressin and septic shock trial.

Authors' contributions

GLS contributed to study design, acquisition of data, analysis and interpretation of data, statistical analysis, drafting of the manuscript, critical revision of the manuscript for important intellectual content and provided final approval of the version to be published. SWL contributed to study conception and design, acquisition of data, analysis and interpretation of data, critical revision of the manuscript for important intellectual content and provided final approval of the version to be published. AD contributed to study conception, critical revision of the manuscript for important intellectual content and provided final approval of the version to be published. HT, SNB, and SCW contributed to study design, critical revision of the manuscript for important intellectual content and provided final approval of the version to be published. RSB contributed to statistical analysis and interpretation of data and provided intellectual input to the research and manuscript. SRB contributed to study conception and design, acquisition of data, analysis and interpretation of data, statistical analysis, drafting of the manuscript, critical revision of the manuscript for important intellectual content and provided final approval of the version to be published. All authors agree to be accountable for all aspects of work in ensuring that questions related to the accuracy or integrity of any part of the work are appropriately investigated and resolved. The authors would like to thank Eric Vogan for his assistance with this project. All authors read and approved the final manuscript.

Author details

[1] Department of Pharmacy, Cleveland Clinic, 9500 Euclid Avenue (Hb-105), Cleveland, OH 44195, USA. [2] Respiratory Institute, Cleveland Clinic, Cleveland, OH, USA. [3] Department of Quantitative Health Sciences, Cleveland Clinic, Cleveland, OH, USA.

Acknowledgements

The results of this evaluation were presented in abstract form at the Society of Critical Care Medicine's 2017 Critical Care Congress on January 23rd, 2017 in Honolulu, Hawaii.

Competing interests

The authors declare that they have no competing interests.

Funding

No funding was received for this project.

References

1. Rhodes A, Evans LE, Alhazzani W, Levy MM, Antonelli M, Ferrer R, et al. Surviving sepsis campaign: international guidelines for management of sepsis and septic shock: 2016. Intensive Care Med. 2017;43(3):304–77.
2. Russell JA, Walley KR, Singer J, Gordon AC, Hebert PC, Cooper DJ, et al. Vasopressin versus norepinephrine infusion in patients with septic shock. N Engl J Med. 2008;358(9):877–87.
3. Russell JA, Lee T, Singer J, Boyd JH, Walley KR, Vasopressin, et al. The septic shock 3.0 definition and trials: a vasopressin and septic shock trial experience. Crit Care Med. 2017;45(6):940–8.
4. Beck V, Chateau D, Bryson GL, Pisipati A, Zanotti S, Parrillo JE, et al. Timing of vasopressor initiation and mortality in septic shock: a cohort study. Crit Care. 2014;18(3):R97.
5. Bai X, Yu W, Ji W, Lin Z, Tan S, Duan K, et al. Early versus delayed administration of norepinephrine in patients with septic shock. Crit Care. 2014;18(5):532.
6. Dunser MW, Ruokonen E, Pettila V, Ulmer H, Torgersen C, Schmittinger CA, et al. Association of arterial blood pressure and vasopressor load with septic shock mortality: a post hoc analysis of a multicenter trial. Crit Care. 2009;13(6):R181.
7. Rudiger A, Singer M. Decatecholaminisation during sepsis. Crit Care. 2016;20(1):309.
8. Andreis DT, Singer M. Catecholamines for inflammatory shock: a Jekyll-and-Hyde conundrum. Intensive Care Med. 2016;42(9):1387–97.
9. Hammond DA, Cullen J, Painter JT, McCain K, Clem OA, Brotherton AL, et al. Efficacy and safety of the early addition of vasopressin to norepinephrine in septic shock. J Intensive Care Med. 2017. https://doi.org/10.1177/0885066617725255.
10. Clem OPJ, Cullen J, McCain K, Kakkera K, Meena N, Hammond D. Norepinephrine and vasopressin vs norepinephrine alone for septic shock: randomized controlled trial [abstract]. Crit Care Med. 2016;44(12 Suppl 1):1350.
11. Gordon AC, Russell JA, Walley KR, Singer J, Ayers D, Storms MM, et al. The effects of vasopressin on acute kidney injury in septic shock. Intensive Care Med. 2010;36(1):83–91.
12. Holmes CL, Walley KR, Chittock DR, Lehman T, Russell JA. The effects of vasopressin on hemodynamics and renal function in severe septic shock: a case series. Intensive Care Med. 2001;27(8):1416–21.
13. Russell JA, Walley KR, Gordon AC, Cooper DJ, Hebert PC, Singer J, et al. Interaction of vasopressin infusion, corticosteroid treatment, and mortality of septic shock. Crit Care Med. 2009;37(3):811–8.
14. Bauer SR, Lam SW, Cha SS, Oyen LJ. Effect of corticosteroids on arginine vasopressin-containing vasopressor therapy for septic shock: a case control study. J Crit Care. 2008;23(4):500–6.
15. Torgersen C, Luckner G, Schroder DC, Schmittinger CA, Rex C, Ulmer H, et al. Concomitant arginine-vasopressin and hydrocortisone therapy in severe septic shock: association with mortality. Intensive Care Med. 2011;37(9):1432–7.
16. Varpula M, Tallgren M, Saukkonen K, Voipio-Pulkki LM, Pettila V. Hemodynamic variables related to outcome in septic shock. Intensive Care Med. 2005;31(8):1066–71.
17. Finfer S, Bellomo R, Boyce N, French J, Myburgh J, Norton R, et al. A comparison of albumin and saline for fluid resuscitation in the intensive care unit. N Engl J Med. 2004;350(22):2247–56.

18. Brunkhorst FM, Engel C, Bloos F, Meier-Hellmann A, Ragaller M, Weiler N, et al. Intensive insulin therapy and pentastarch resuscitation in severe sepsis. N Engl J Med. 2008;358(2):125–39.
19. Wacharasint P, Boyd JH, Russell JA, Walley KR. One size does not fit all in severe infection: obesity alters outcome, susceptibility, treatment, and inflammatory response. Crit Care. 2013;17(3):R122.
20. Miller JT, Welage LS, Kraft MD, Alaniz C. Does body weight impact the efficacy of vasopressin therapy in the management of septic shock? J Crit Care. 2012;27(3):289–93.
21. DA Belsley KE, Welsch RE. Regression diagnostics: identifying influential data and sources of collinearity. Hoboken: Wiley; 1980.
22. Vail EA, Gershengorn HB, Hua M, Walkey AJ, Wunsch H. Epidemiology of vasopressin use for adults with septic shock. Ann Am Thorac Soc. 2016;13(10):1760–7.
23. Russell JA. Bench-to-bedside review: vasopressin in the management of septic shock. Crit Care. 2011;15(4):226.
24. Landry DW, Levin HR, Gallant EM, Ashton RC Jr, Seo S, D'Alessandro D, et al. Vasopressin deficiency contributes to the vasodilation of septic shock. Circulation. 1997;95(5):1122–5.
25. Landry DW, Levin HR, Gallant EM, Seo S, D'Alessandro D, Oz MC, et al. Vasopressin pressor hypersensitivity in vasodilatory septic shock. Crit Care Med. 1997;25(8):1279–82.
26. Holmes CL. Vasopressin in septic shock: does dose matter? Crit Care Med. 2004;32(6):1423–4.
27. Holmes CL, Patel BM, Russell JA, Walley KR. Physiology of vasopressin relevant to management of septic shock. Chest. 2001;120(3):989–1002.
28. Wu JY, Stollings JL, Wheeler AP, Semler MW, Rice TW. Efficacy and outcomes after vasopressin guideline implementation in septic shock. Ann Pharmacother. 2016. https://doi.org/10.1177/1060028016669163.
29. Gordon AC, Mason AJ, Thirunavukkarasu N, Perkins GD, Cecconi M, Cepkova M, et al. Effect of early vasopressin vs norepinephrine on kidney failure in patients with septic shock: the VANISH randomized clinical trial. JAMA. 2016;316(5):509–18.
30. Angus DC, Linde-Zwirble WT, Lidicker J, Clermont G, Carcillo J, Pinsky MR. Epidemiology of severe sepsis in the United States: analysis of incidence, outcome, and associated costs of care. Crit Care Med. 2001;29(7):1303–10.
31. Esper AM, Martin GS. The impact of comorbid [corrected] conditions on critical illness. Crit Care Med. 2011;39(12):2728–35.
32. Annane D, Vignon P, Renault A, Bollaert PE, Charpentier C, Martin C, et al. Norepinephrine plus dobutamine versus epinephrine alone for management of septic shock: a randomised trial. Lancet. 2007;370(9588):676–84.
33. Sligl WI, Milner DA Jr, Sundar S, Mphatswe W, Majumdar SR. Safety and efficacy of corticosteroids for the treatment of septic shock: a systematic review and meta-analysis. Clin Infect Dis. 2009;49(1):93–101.
34. Annane D, Sebille V, Charpentier C, Bollaert PE, Francois B, Korach JM, et al. Effect of treatment with low doses of hydrocortisone and fludrocortisone on mortality in patients with septic shock. JAMA. 2002;288(7):862–71.
35. Khanna A, English SW, Wang XS, Ham K, Tumlin J, Szerlip H, et al. Angiotensin II for the treatment of vasodilatory shock. N Engl J Med. 2017;377(5):419–30.
36. Torgersen C, Dunser MW, Wenzel V, Jochberger S, Mayr V, Schmittinger CA, et al. Comparing two different arginine vasopressin doses in advanced vasodilatory shock: a randomized, controlled, open-label trial. Intensive Care Med. 2010;36(1):57–65.

17

Occurrence of marked sepsis-induced immunosuppression in pediatric septic shock

Solenn Remy[1], Karine Kolev-Descamps[1], Morgane Gossez[2], Fabienne Venet[2,3], Julie Demaret[2], Etienne Javouhey[1] and Guillaume Monneret[2,3*]

Abstract

Background: While the process of sepsis-induced immunosuppression is now well described in adults, very little information is available on immune functions in pediatric sepsis. The current study investigated this in children with septic shock by performing immunomonitoring, including both innate (monocyte human leukocyte antigen-DR, mHLA-DR, expression) and adaptive immunity (lymphocyte subsets count), as well as cytokine concentrations (IL-6, IL-8, IL-10, IL-1Ra, TNF-α, IFN-γ). Subsequent objectives were to assess the associations between inflammatory response, potential immunosuppression and secondary acquired infection occurrence.

Methods: Single-center prospective observational study, including children aged between 1 month and 18 years admitted to pediatric intensive care unit (PICU) for septic shock. Age-matched controls were children hospitalized for elective surgery without any infectious criteria. Blood was sampled at day 1–2, 3–5, and 7–9 after sepsis onset. mHLA-DR and lymphocyte subsets count were measured by flow cytometry and cytokine concentrations by Luminex technology.

Results: A total of 26 children and 30 controls were included. Patients had lymphopenia, and mHLA-DR levels were significantly lower than controls at each time point ($p < 0.0001$). All cytokines peaked at day 1–2. Children with secondary acquired infection had lower day 3–5 mHLA-DR and higher pro-inflammatory cytokine concentrations (IL-6, IL-8 and TNF-α) at day 1–2 compared to children without secondary acquired infection.

Conclusions: The higher initial inflammatory cytokine production was, the more innate immunity was altered, while evaluated by low mHLA-DR expression. Children with decreased mHLA-DR expression developed more secondary acquired infections. Upon confirmation in multicenter cohorts, these results pave the way for immunostimulation for the most immunosuppressed children in order to prevent nosocomial infections in PICU.

Trial registration PedIRIS study NCT02848144. Retrospectively registered 28 July 2016

Keywords: Septic shock, Immunosuppression induced, Children

Background

Despite advances in critical care management, septic shock remains one of the most important causes of mortality and morbidity in children worldwide [1]. As for adults, the inability of adjunctive therapies to mitigate the deleterious effects of this condition indicates that it is likely that initial hypotheses for sepsis pathophysiology have been inadequately addressed [2]. In adults, it is now agreed that sepsis deeply perturbs immune balance by inducing a strong systemic inflammatory response and a concomitant anti-inflammatory process, acting as a negative feedback. This compensatory response may secondarily become harmful as most immune functions are compromised, and thus sepsis-induced immune alterations may play a major role in the decreased resistance

*Correspondence: guillaume.monneret@chu-lyon.fr
[2] Hospices Civils de Lyon, Immunology Laboratory, E. Herriot Hospital, 69003 Lyon, France
Full list of author information is available at the end of the article

to secondary acquired infections in patients who initially survive [3]. This immunosuppressive state is characterized by both abnormal innate and adaptive immune responses. In particular, patients mostly present with marked lymphopenia and decreased expression in monocyte human leukocyte antigen-DR (mHLA-DR). The latter remains, to date, the key parameter of patient monitoring and its diminished expression has been reported to be associated with increased mortality and nosocomial infection rate in adults [4–6]. In this context, and as it is already the case for cancer immunotherapy, targeted treatments aimed at rejuvenating immune responses in adult septic patients (e.g., GM-CSF, Interleukin-7, anti-PD-1/-L1) are now envisaged [7–10]. In comparison with adults, data are very scarce in children with septic shock. The impact of this altered immune response on secondary infections is poorly reported in children affected by septic shock. In order to envisage therapeutic interventions to restore immune function in children, a reliable biomarker is required to identify children at highest risk of secondary acquired infection or mortality. Such a marker is currently lacking in children. Most pediatric results are rarely specific of septic shock. They refer, as a whole, to various pediatric intensive care unit (PICU) admission causes (surgery, organ dysfunctions) [11–14], or are limited to particular cases of preterm neonates [15, 16]. Thus, the objective of the present prospective observational study was to investigate whether pediatric septic shock patients present immune alterations similar to those seen in adults. For this, immunomonitoring was performed during the first week after sepsis onset. This monitoring included mHLA-DR, lymphocyte subsets count, and phenotyping as well as measurement of plasma cytokine concentrations: interleukin-6 (IL-6), interleukin-8 (IL-8), interleukin-10 (IL-10), tumor necrosis factor-α (TNF-α), interferon-γ (IFN-γ), and interleukin-1 receptor antagonist (IL-1Ra). As control values may depend on age, and in the absence of mHLA-DR reference range in pediatrics, healthy children were also investigated to explore mHLA-DR expression during the first years of life.

Methods

Study population

This single-center, prospective study was held in PICU from a tertiary academic hospital (23 beds mixed medical-surgical unit, > 1100 admissions/year). Children, aged from 1 month to 18 years, were included prospectively during 24 h of PICU admission, if they presented septic shock, defined by "Surviving Sepsis Campaign" and Goldstein's criteria [17, 18]. Exclusion criteria were: non-septic shock, chronic inflammatory disease, long-term corticosteroid treatment, transplantation and/or immunosuppressive therapy, immunodeficiency syndrome, malignant tumors. Opposition from the child and/or parent/holder of parental authority also constituted exclusion criteria. Controls were age-matched to the case group and identified among outpatients admitted for a scheduled surgery, without any criteria of infection. Exclusion criteria were the same as the case group. Three age subgroups were defined: 1 month to 2, 2–8, and > 8 years, according to the physiological age-based development of immunity in children [19].

Clinical data and definitions

Clinical data were collected prospectively and obtained from the electronic medical record. At admission (day 1), severity of illness was evaluated using the pediatric index of mortality 2 (PIM2) [20]. Organ failure was assessed by the measurement of PEdiatric Logistic Organ Dysfunction Score, version 2 (PELOD-2) at day 1, 3, and 7 [21]. Vasoactive treatments during hospitalization in PICU were determined by the cumulative vasopressor index (CVI) [22]. We also collected incidence of secondary acquired infection, mortality (death occurring within 28 days after the onset of shock), number of mechanical ventilation-free days, and number of PICU-free days in the first 30 days. Secondary acquired infection was defined by Center for Disease Control criteria, included any new bacterial or fungal infection, distinct from initial infection, occurring more than 48 h after sepsis onset, during the first 30 days after sepsis onset [23]. Determination of secondary acquired infection was performed prospectively by one physician (SR), blinded to immunological data.

Blood sampling for immunomonitoring

Blood samples were collected within the first 48 h after the onset of infection, again between day 3–5, and day 7–9. Samples were not available if patients were no longer in PICU. Blood was collected in EDTA tubes, transported rapidly at 4 °C to the Cellular Immunology Laboratory, and analyzed within less than 4 h. The amount of blood sample did not exceed 2.4 ml/kg, in accordance with European recommendations. At each time point, the following parameters were determined by flow cytometry: mHLA-DR, total lymphocytes and lymphocytes subpopulations ($CD4^+$ and $CD8^+$ T cells, natural killer [NK] cells, regulatory T cells [Treg], and B cells). In addition, after completion of cellular analysis, plasma was obtained after centrifugation and stored at − 80 °C for subsequent quantification of following circulating cytokines: IL-6, IL-8, IL-10, IL-1RA, TNF-α, and IFN-γ. For the control group, blood was sampled in the operating room immediately after induction of general anesthesia with sevoflurane, before start of surgery.

Flow cytometry

Quantification of mHLA-DR on circulating monocytes was performed using a standardized flow cytometric assay as previously described [24.] The median fluorescence intensity of the entire monocyte population was then transformed to number of antibodies bound per cell (ABC) using calibrated PE beads (BD QuantiBRITE™ PE Beads, Becton–Dickinson San Jose, CA, USA). The following lymphocyte subsets were analyzed by flow cytometry as previously described [25, 26]: total T lymphocytes ($CD45^+$ $CD3^+$), $CD4^+$ T lymphocytes ($CD45^+$ $CD4^+$ $CD3^+$), $CD8^+$ T lymphocytes ($CD45^+$ $CD8^+$ $CD3^+$), total B cells ($CD45^+$ $CD19^+$), NK cells ($CD45^+$ $CD3^-$ $CD56^+$), and Treg ($CD4^+$ $CD25^+$ $CD127^-$). Results were expressed as numbers of cells per microliter of blood for lymphocyte subsets and as percentage of positive cells among total $CD4^+$ lymphocyte population for Treg.

Cytokine measurement

IL-6, IL-8, IL-10, IL-1RA, TNF-α, and IFN-γ were quantified with a single panel (Milliplex® MAP Human Cytokine/Chemokine Magnetic Bead Panel, Merck Millipore) using the fluorescent bead-based multiplexed Luminex xMAP technology [27]. Analyses were performed on Bio-Plex 200 Luminex instrument using Bio-Plex software (Bio-Rad, Hercules, CA, USA).

Statistical analysis

Results are expressed as median and interquartile range [IQR]. Comparisons between groups were analyzed using the Man–Whitney *U* test for continuous nonparametric variables; the independent paired *t* test for continuous parametric variables and the Chi-square test for categorical data. Correlation analyses were performed using the Pearson test for variables following a normal distribution, and Spearman for nonparametric variables. Kaplan–Meier analyses were performed using Youden's index to stratify groups of patients. A p value <0.05 was considered to represent significant statistical difference. Data were analyzed by using Prism6 software (GraphPad Inc., La Jolla, CA, USA).

Results

Subjects

Between September 2014 and July 2016, 73 children were screened for septic shock. Among these, 47 were excluded (toxic shock syndrome, non-infectious shock, known immunosuppression, or chronic inflammatory disease). A total of 26 children were included and analyzed (Fig. 1). Demographic data are presented in Table 1. Nine children (35%) presented a complex chronic condition. The most frequent was prematurity ($n=4$), but all children presented a corrected age greater than 1 month.

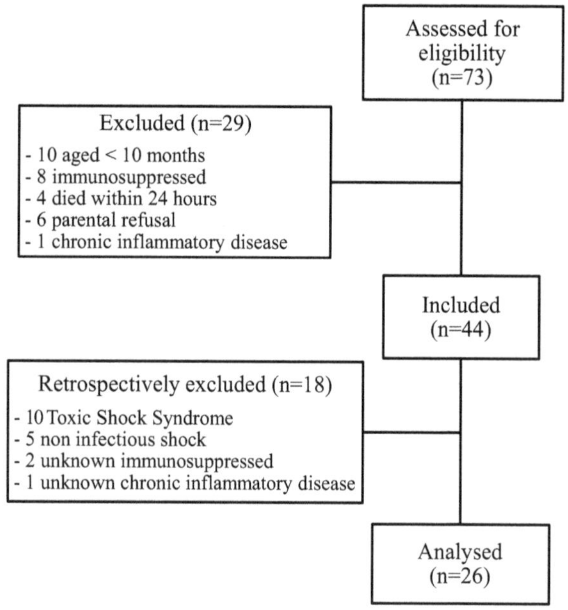

Fig. 1 Flowchart

Others presented psychomotor delay ($n=2$), polymalformative disease ($n=2$), and sickle cell disease ($n=1$). Two children died: one precociously at day 2, due to refractory shock with multi-organ failure; and the second one at day 32, with withdrawal treatment for major brain damage after meningitis. A total of 30 healthy children were included as controls. They were age-matched with children in septic shock ($p=0.3$, Mann–Whitney): 11 were aged between 1 month and 2 years, 14 between 2 and 8 years, and 5 > 8 years.

mHLA-DR expression

In healthy control children, mHLA-DR was > 25,000 ABC; among those aged between 1 month to 2 years it was (median [IQR]) 25,477 ABC [20,478–39,143], among those aged 2–8 years it was 34,295 ABC [25,763–43,368], and among those older than 8 years it was 29,597 ABC [26,636–41,939]; there was no significant difference between age subgroups ($p=0.35$; ANOVA, Fig. 2a). There was also no correlation between age and mHLA-DR ($r=0.018$).

In children with septic shock, mHLA-DR was 6066 ABC [3737–16,310] at day 1–2, 6308 ABC [3185–8965] at day 3–5, and 9323 ABC [6384–12,738] at 7–9; at each time point values were significantly different to that found in healthy control children ($p<0.0001$; Fig. 2b). There was no correlation between mHLA-DR and PIM2 or PELOD-2 scores, at any time point, while a significant correlation was found between day 3–5 mHLA-DR and CVI ($r=-0.50$; $p=0.031$; Fig. 2c).

Table 1 Characteristics of the 26 children with septic shock included in the study

	Septic shock ($n=26$)
Age (years)	2.12 [0.47–4.60]
Male gender [*n* (%)]	11 (42)
Complex chronic conditions [*n* (%)]	9 (35)
Primary nosocomial infection	1 (3.9)
Site of initial infection [*n* (%)]	
Blood	3 (11.5)
Lung	4 (15.4)
Abdomen	8 (30.8)
Multi-site	9 (34.6)
Others	1 (3.9)
No documentation	1 (3.9)
Microbiology	
Gram-negative bacteria	
Neisseria meningitidis	8 (30.8)
Escherichia coli	3 (11.5)
Klebsiella species	2 (7.7)
Enterobacter species	2 (7.7)
Campylobacter jejuni	1 (3.8)
Haemophilus influenzae	1 (3.8)
Gram-positive bacteria	
Streptococcus pneumoniae	3 (11.5)
Streptococcus pyogenes	2 (7.7)
Staphylococcus aureus	1 (3.8)
Viruses	
Parainfluenzae virus	1 (3.8)
PIM2 admission (%)	8.1 [3.2–17.4]
PELOD-2	
Day 1	9.5 [2.75–12.0]
Day 3	4.0 [0.0–10.0]
Day 7	0.0 [0.0–5.0]
CVI	4.0 [0.0–7.0]
ICU-free days in 30 days	23.0 [19.0–26.0]
Secondary acquired infections [*n* (%)]	8 (30)
Mortality [*n* (%)]	2 (7)

Values are expressed as median [interquartile range], or a number (percentage)

PIM2 pediatric index of mortality 2, *PELOD-2* PEdiatric Logistic Organ Dysfunction score, version 2, *CVI* cumulative vasopressor index

Cytokines

For all cytokines, maximal elevated values were measured on early time point. Then, they presented a gradual decrease on following days but remained significantly elevated in comparison with normal values (Table 2). At day 1–2, IL-6 and IL-8 levels were significantly correlated with PELOD-2 ($r=0.52$, $p=0.012$ and $r=0.43$, $p=0.048$, respectively) and with CVI ($r=0.65$, $p=0.001$ and $r=0.51$, $p=0.015$, respectively). No correlation between initial cytokines concentrations and PIM2 score was found. Also, there was no correlation between initial cytokines levels and mHLA-DR at day 1–2. However, IL-8, IL-10, IL-1ra and TNF-α levels at day 1–2 were significantly negatively correlated with mHLA-DR at day 3–5 ($r=-0.84$, $p<0.0001$; $r=-0.59$, $p=0.0198$; $r=-0.58$, $p=0.023$; $r=-0.69$, $p=0.0042$, respectively).

Lymphocyte subsets

Lymphocyte subsets from healthy control children are presented in Table 3. Among septic patients the total lymphocyte count was significantly lower than in healthy control children at day 1–2 and day 3–5; there was no significant difference at day 7–9 (Fig. 3a). Similar results were observed for $CD4^+$ (Fig. 3b) and $CD8^+$ T cell (Fig. 3c) subsets. The median total NK cell count was significantly lower as compared to healthy control children over the whole monitoring period (Fig. 3d). In contrast and, although diminished, B cells were modestly affected (Fig. 3e). The median proportion of Treg was initially similar to that found in healthy control children; this increased at day 3–5, and became significantly greater at day 7–9 (Fig. 3f). Of note, we did not find any correlation between lymphocytes subsets and CVI (data not shown).

Secondary acquired infections

A secondary acquired infection was diagnosed in eight children (Additional file 1: Tables S1 and S2). The median time to onset of these infections was 13.5 days (range: [9–25]). Compared to children who did not developed secondary acquired infection, the sole difference was a longer length of hospital stay for children who presented secondary acquired infection ($p=0.009$; Additional file 1: Table S1). Between these two groups, no difference was observed concerning duration of invasive equipment, PICU staying, complex chronic condition and severity scores. No significant difference in lymphocyte subset was observed between children with or without secondary acquired infections. No association was found between persistent lymphopenia (defined as an absolute lymphocyte count of <1000 cells/µl for 3 days) and development of secondary acquired infection. At day 1–2, there was no significant difference in mHLA-DR values; at day 3–5 those with secondary acquired infection had a significantly lower level of mHLA-DR (4398 ABC [2437–6212]) than those without (8474 ABC [5904–10,844], $p=0.022$; Fig. 2d). At day 1–2, children with secondary acquired infection had higher concentrations of IL-6, IL-8, and TNF-α than those without (Additional file 1: Table S1). There was no significant difference in cytokine concentrations at other time points. The area under the curve from receiver operating curve (ROC) analysis for the risk to develop a secondary acquired infection were all significantly >0.8 for these four significant parameters

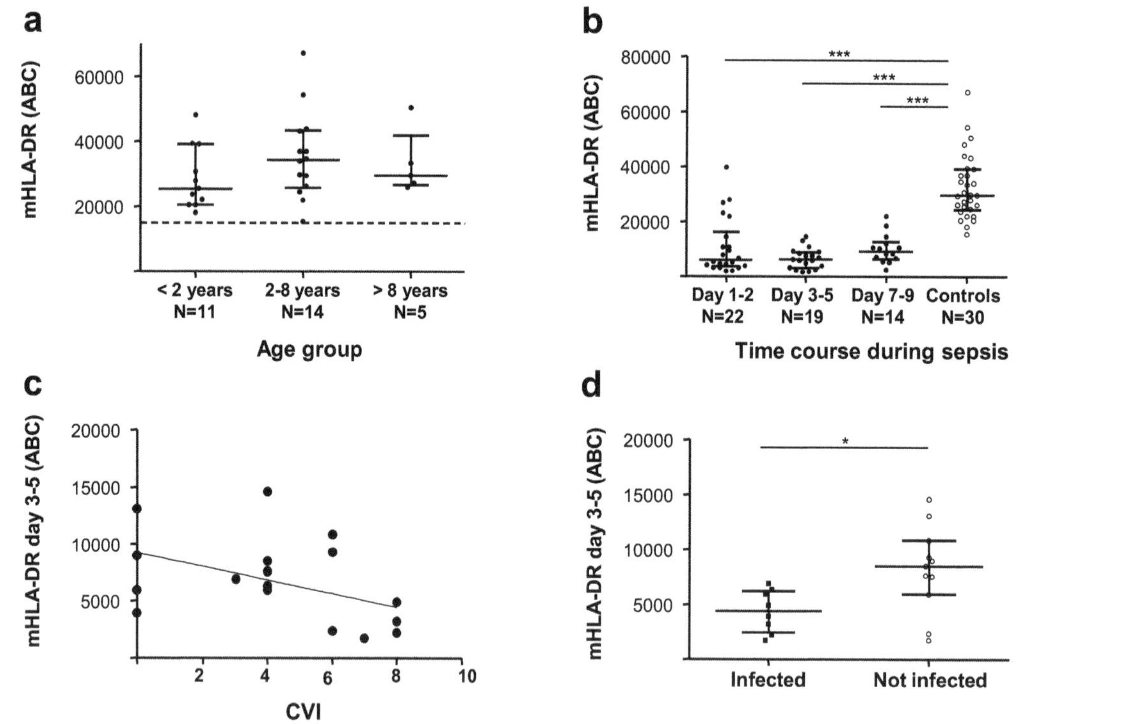

Fig. 2 mHLA-DR measurements in pediatric septic shock. **a** mHLA-DR expression in healthy children: no difference according to age groups ($p = 0.35$; ANOVA). Dashed line depicts usual threshold to define normal values in adults. **b** mHLA-DR was significantly decreased at each time point during septic shock, than controls ($p < 0.001$; Mann–Whitney). **c** mHLA-DR at day 3–5 was significantly negatively correlated with cumulative vasopressor index, CVI ($r = -0.50$; $p = 0.031$; Spearman). **d** mHLA-DR was significantly lower in children with secondary acquired infection than those without ($p = 0.022$; Student *t* test)

Table 2 Plasma cytokines levels from healthy children and children with septic shock

	Healthy controls	Children with septic shock		
		Day 1–2	Day 3–5	Day 7–9
IL-6	0.0 [0.0–0.36]	178.5 [25.77–3311]	18.13 [12.92–172.5]	17.97 [3.30–33.08]
IL-8	2.05 [0.43–5.06]	51.72 [19.07–145.7]	21.45 [11.42–56.36]	15.00 [7.98–37.98]
IL-10	0.36 [0.0–4.44]	43.37 [17.11–331.6]	8.26 [3.44–21.66]	11.83 [1.70–23.73]
IL1-RA	0.0 [0.0–17.16]	136.9 [23.72–647.8]	48.02 [0.0–153.2]	56.54 [0.0–121.3]
TNF-α	4.91 [3.35–7.11]	25.13 [14.52–40.47]	8.37 [5.34–14.62]	10.15 [4.10–15.43]
INF-γ	4.98 [1.82–6.45]	15.81 [6.55–24.22]	8.07 [2.78–11.45]	10.92 [4.65–23.70]

Values (pg/ml) are expressed as median [IQR]. All cytokine values in children with septic shock at all-time points were different from those of healthy controls

(mHLA-DR at day 3–5, and IL-6, IL-8 and TNF-α at day 1–2, Additional file 1: Table S3). In line with this, mHLA-DR at day 3–5 was negatively correlated with cytokines (except IFN-γ). Owing to the sample size, no multivariate regression could be performed to test independence between mHLA-DR and cytokines for the prediction of risk of secondary acquired infection occurrence.

We next performed Kaplan–Meier analyses associating mHLA-DR values and each cytokine level separately, which found that children with lowest values of mHLA-DR and highest cytokine levels were significantly more likely to be infected. Those with mHLA-DR above the threshold remained uninfected, independently of cytokine level (Additional file 1: Fig. S1).

Table 3 mHLA-DR and lymphocytes subsets depending on age in healthy and septic children

	0–2 years		2–8 years		>8 years	
	Healthy ($n=11$)	Septic ($n=11$)	Healthy ($n=14$)	Septic ($n=6$)	Healthy ($n=5$)	Septic ($n=2$)
mHLA-DR (ABC)	25,477 [20,478–39,143]	6302 [2187–9278]	34,295 [25,763–43,368]	5913 [2977–8911]	29,597 [26,636–41,939]	7927 [6888–8965]
Total lymphocytes (absolute count; cells/μl)	5934 [4148–8572]	2736 [1962–3550]	3623 [2940–4358]	1680 [897–2453]	2374 [1831–3298]	1047 [403–1691]
$CD4^+$ T cells (absolute count; cells/μl)	2187 [1566–2738]	1186 [939–1640]	1184 [968–1583]	574 [236–478]	895 [682–1100]	332 [187–478]
$CD8^+$ T cells (absolute count; cells/μl)	1033 [910–1380]	487 [311–591]	758 [631–1264]	365 [155–608]	689 [467–924]	161 [51–270]
NK cells (absolute count; cells/μl)	645 [392–753]	58 [25–124]	424 [295–576]	96 [35–156]	315 [191–645]	60 [4–117]
B cells (absolute count; cells/μl)	1811 [1326–2750]	901 [648–1397]	729 [563–988]	622 [288–791]	352 [273–508]	422 [150–693]
Regulatory T cells (% among $CD4^+$)	7.67 [5.39–8.24]	7.72 [5.1–9.0]	6.29 [5.29–8.31]	8.83 [7.1–10.3]	6.80 [6.10–8.48]	7.9 [5.8–10.1]

Values are expressed as median [IQR] according to age group. Septic children values were obtained at day 3

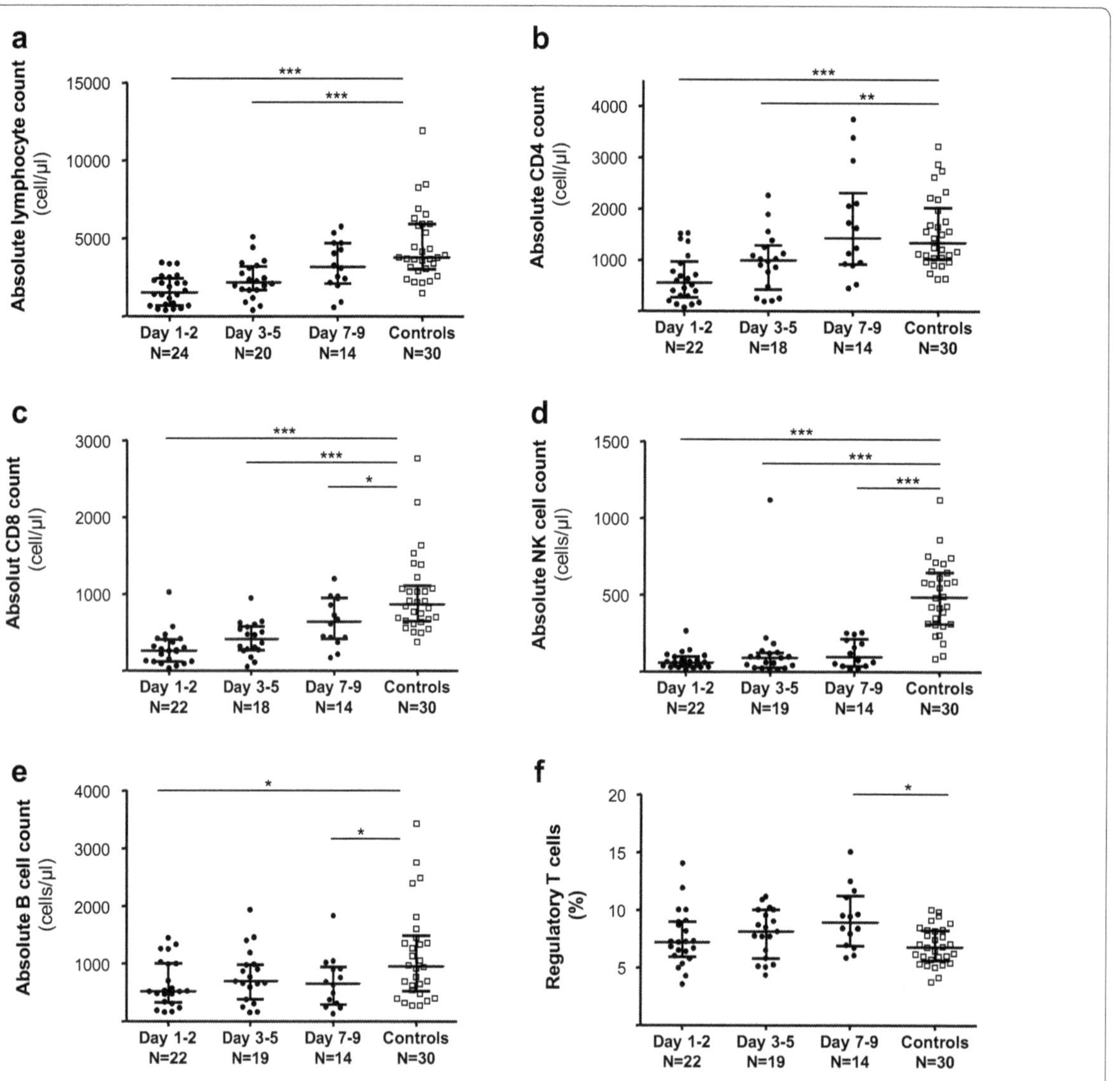

Fig. 3 Time course of lymphocytes' subsets during septic shock. **a** Total lymphocytes, **b** $CD4^+$ T cells, **c** $CD8^+$ T cells, **d** NK cells, **e** B cells (from **a** to **e**, results as cell number/µl), **f** proportion of regulatory T cells (among CD4+ lymphocytes). $^*p < 0.05$; $^{**}p < 0.01$; $^{***}p < 0.0001$

Discussion

The present investigation is, to the best of our knowledge, the first prospective pediatric study reporting a wide immune monitoring, specifically in septic shock. However, the first important result of this study is the values of mHLA-DR expression in healthy children. There was no variation according to age (between 6 months and 17 years) and, furthermore, the values are not different to those reported in adults [28]. These results strongly suggest that there is no difference between healthy adults and children in terms of mHLA-DR expression. Important fall in mHLA-DR during pediatric septic shock seems to be similar to those observed during adult septic shock.

The cytokine storm reported herein, involving both pro and anti-inflammatory cytokines, was found in the initial period after shock (day 1–2). At the same time, children who later developed a secondary acquired infection had higher plasma cytokine concentrations (i.e., IL-6, IL-8, and TNF-α). This is in agreement with observations from genomic studies that have found that early mRNA expression modulations of cytokines and apoptotic genes were associated with deleterious outcomes (mortality, secondary infections) [29, 30]. Moreover, to the best of our knowledge, this is the first pediatric study which reported correlation between initial cytokine storm and alteration of innate immunity, represented by loss of mHLA-DR.

Concerning adaptive immunity, B and T lymphocytes were diminished initially, but less impacted and corrected faster than mHLA-DR alteration. The modest diminution of B cells constitutes a difference with that found in adults, for instance Monserrat et al. [31] described severe abnormality of circulating B lymphocytes associated with mortality. Concerning NK cells, Halstead et al. [32] observed a decrease at the beginning of sepsis in children. The present study provides supplementary data since a deep and prolonged alteration of circulating NK cells was found. Although we did not explore this side, NK cell alterations could promote infections by opportunistic viral pathogens [33]. In contrast with the study reported by Muszynski et al. [14], an increase in Treg proportion during the first week was observed herein. This kinetic seems similar to that described in adult septic shock, where an increased proportion of Treg was associated with poor outcome [34]. Here, as for other lymphocyte parameters, no association with nosocomial infections was found. Additional functional testing (proliferation, intracellular cytokine production) would be likely informative and deserves to be further investigated. At this stage, the present lymphocyte data seem to indicate that altered lymphocyte count rapidly self-resolves, in contrast with observations made in adults.

With regards to innate immunity, loss of mHLA-DR has emerged as a gold standard biomarker owing to its association with altered monocyte functionality, increased mortality, and nosocomial infection rate after adult septic shock [6, 35]. In accordance, we report here a significant fall in mHLA-DR in children. Importantly, the lowest values at day 3–5 were found in patients who developed secondary acquired infections. At this time point, all patients with forthcoming infections presented mHLA-DR below 8000 ABC (i.e., the usual threshold for defining the most severely immunosuppressed adult patients [36]). Most pediatric studies have used ex vivo LPS-induced TNF-α production by monocytes to assess innate immunity function. However, Drewry et al. [35] presented recently mHLA-DR as a better predictor of deleterious outcomes than LPS-stimulated TNF-α production. Add to our results, these data reinforced the idea to use mHLA-DR as biomarker of altered innate immunity in pediatric studies. Due to low number of deaths in the present cohort, we did not investigate the potential association with mortality. Although not all obtained using a standardized measurement protocol, the pediatric mHLA-DR data available in the literature are in agreement with that reported herein. For example, Manzoli et al. [13] found the extent of mHLA-DR level reduction during the first week after sepsis onset to be associated with mortality (23% mortality), and Genel et al. [16] also reported lower levels of mHLA-DR among infected neonates who did not survive compared to those who did (20% mortality). Decreased mHLA-DR has also been described in pediatric surgery and was associated with later sepsis and pneumonia [37, 38]. In addition, Hall et al. [11] reported that, in children with multiple organ dysfunction syndrome, persistent decreased TNF-α release (that reflects monocyte functionality) over 5 days was associated with development of secondary infection. In addition, some in vitro and animal studies suggest potential role of norepinephrine in the development of sepsis-induced immunosuppression [39]. These data reinforced our significant correlation between day 3-5 mHLA-DR and CVI.

Collectively, this indicates that, as in adults, mHLA-DR presents potential for the identification of the most severe immunosuppressed children. The next step would, of course, be to perform multivariate analysis in a larger patient sample to explore the independence of each parameter in predicting deleterious outcomes. That given, Kaplan–Meier analyses found that although different markers (i.e., day 3–5 mHLA-DR and early elevated cytokines) were associated with secondary acquired infections, the weight of mHLA-DR was more important. Interestingly, as observed in adult trauma patients, association between early cytokines production and low day 3–5 mHLA-DR appeared as the poorest scenario in pediatric septic shock [40].

Furthermore, secondary acquired infections represent a major economic burden by significantly extending length of hospital stay [41, 42], and concordantly herein the length of hospitalization in those with secondary infection doubled (and this difference was significant). Taken together, these data reinforce the idea that most immunosuppressed septic children might benefit from immunostimulation as an adjunctive therapy [43]. Clinical trials are in progress with GM-CSF (NCT02361528) or IL-7 (NCT02640807/NCT02797431) in adults, and standardized tools are currently used to stratify patients in those trials. This progressively paves the way for this kind of approach in pediatrics, especially for innate immunity that seems to be more affected.

The study does, however, have some limitations. First, the relatively small number of included children precluded multivariate analyses to be performed. Second, some children were discharged from PICU before all samples were obtained, and therefore the time course of different immune parameters in less severe children was not determined. Due to the relatively short follow-up period, we cannot conclude on the long-term outcome of these children treated for septic shock. In addition, functional testing should be performed in next studies. Theses aspects need to be further explored, and ideally in a multicenter study.

Conclusion

As in adults, septic shock in pediatric patients induced marked alterations in immune parameters in accordance with the occurrence of a state of immunosuppression. The present results, in particular the association between low mHLA-DR expression and deleterious outcomes, deserves to be assessed and confirmed in multicenter studies.

Abbreviations

ABC: antibodies bound per cell; CVI: cumulative vasopressor index; IFN-γ: interferon-γ; IL-1Ra: interleukine-1 receptor antagonist; IL-6: interleukine-6; IL-8: interleukine-8; IL-10: interleukine-10; mHLA-DR: monocyte human leukocyte antigen-DR; NK cells: natural killer cells; PELOD-2: PEdiatric Logistic Organ Dysfunction Score, version 2; PICU: pediatric intensive care unit; PIM2: pediatric index of mortality 2; TNF-α: tumor necrosis factor-α; Treg: regulatory T cells.

Authors' contribution

EJ and GM conceptualized and designed the study, and reviewed and revised each draft of the manuscript. SR collected clinical data, performed biological analysis, designed and conducted the statistical analysis, drafted the initial manuscript and reviewed and revised the manuscript. KK-D collected clinical data, reviewed and revised the manuscript. JD, MG and FV performed biological analysis, participated in statistical analysis, and reviewed and revised the manuscript. All authors read and approved the final manuscript.

Author details

[1] Hospices Civils de Lyon, Paediatric Intensive Care Unit, Mother and Children University Hospital, 59 Boulevard Pinel, 69500 Bron, France. [2] Hospices Civils de Lyon, Immunology Laboratory, E. Herriot Hospital, 69003 Lyon, France. [3] EA 7426, Pathophysiology of Injury-Induced Immunosuppression, University Claude Bernard Lyon 1, BioMérieux Hospices Civils de Lyon, E. Herriot Hospital, 69003 Lyon, France.

Acknowledgements

The authors acknowledge technical staff from Cellular Immunology Laboratory for realization of biological analysis. The authors also thank the Clinical Investigation Center, EPICIME – Lyon, for help in study's organization.

Competing interests

The authors declare that they have no competing interests.

Funding

This study was supported by Hospices Civils de Lyon and University of Lyon. In addition, it was also funded by a research grant from the French Intensive Care Society (Société de Réanimation de Langue Française, SRLF) awarded to KKD. The sponsors of the study had no role in study design, data collection, analysis and interpretation, or writing of the report.

References

1. Schlapbach LJ, Straney L, Alexander J, MacLaren G, Festa M, Schibler A, et al. Mortality related to invasive infections, sepsis, and septic shock in critically ill children in Australia and New Zealand, 2002–13: a multicentre retrospective cohort study. Lancet Infect Dis. 2015;15(1):46–54.
2. Bilgin K, Yaramiş A, Haspolat K, Taş MA, Günbey S, Derman O. A randomized trial of granulocyte-macrophage colony-stimulating factor in neonates with sepsis and neutropenia. Pediatrics. 2001;107(1):36–41.
3. Hotchkiss RS, Monneret G, Payen D. Immunosuppression in sepsis: a novel understanding of the disorder and a new therapeutic approach. Lancet Infect Dis. 2013;13(3):260–8.
4. Venet F, Lukaszewicz A-C, Payen D, Hotchkiss R, Monneret G. Monitoring the immune response in sepsis: a rational approach to administration of immunoadjuvant therapies. Curr Opin Immunol. 2013;25(4):477–83.
5. Landelle C, Lepape A, Voirin N, Tognet E, Venet F, Bohé J, et al. Low monocyte human leukocyte antigen-DR is independently associated with nosocomial infections after septic shock. Intensive Care Med. 2010;36(11):1859–66.
6. Monneret G, Lepape A, Voirin N, Bohé J, Venet F, Debard A-L, et al. Persisting low monocyte human leukocyte antigen-DR expression predicts mortality in septic shock. Intensive Care Med. 2006;32(8):1175–83.
7. Hotchkiss RS, Monneret G, Payen D. Sepsis-induced immunosuppression: from cellular dysfunctions to immunotherapy. Nat Rev Immunol. 2013;13(12):862–74.
8. Hotchkiss RS, Moldawer LL. Parallels between cancer and infectious disease. N Engl J Med. 2014;371(4):380–3.
9. Delano MJ, Ward PA. The immune system's role in sepsis progression, resolution, and long-term outcome. Immunol Rev. 2016;274(1):330–53.
10. Meisel C, Schefold JC, Pschowski R, Baumann T, Hetzger K, Gregor J, et al. Granulocyte-macrophage colony-stimulating factor to reverse sepsis-associated immunosuppression: a double-blind, randomized, placebo-controlled multicenter trial. Am J Respir Crit Care Med. 2009;180(7):640–8.
11. Hall MW, Knatz NL, Vetterly C, Tomarello S, Wewers MD, Volk HD, et al. Immunoparalysis and nosocomial infection in children with multiple organ dysfunction syndrome. Intensive Care Med. 2011;37(3):525–32.
12. Muszynski JA, Nofziger R, Greathouse K, Nateri J, Hanson-Huber L, Steele L, et al. Innate immune function predicts the development of nosocomial infection in critically injured children. Shock (Augusta Ga.). 2014;42(4):313–21.
13. Manzoli TF, Troster EJ, Ferranti JF, Sales MM. Prolonged suppression of monocytic human leukocyte antigen-DR expression correlates with mortality in pediatric septic patients in a pediatric tertiary Intensive Care Unit. J Crit Care. 2016;33:84–9.
14. Muszynski JA, Nofziger R, Greathouse K, Steele L, Hanson-Huber L, Nateri J, et al. Early adaptive immune suppression in children with septic shock: a prospective observational study. Crit Care Lond Engl. 2014;18(4):R145.
15. Wisgrill L, Groschopf A, Herndl E, Sadeghi K, Spittler A, Berger A, et al. Reduced TNF-α response in preterm neonates is associated with impaired nonclassic monocyte function. J Leukoc Biol. 2016;100(3):607–12.
16. Genel F, Atlihan F, Ozsu E, Ozbek E. Monocyte HLA-DR expression as predictor of poor outcome in neonates with late onset neonatal sepsis. J Infect. 2010;60(3):224–8.
17. Dellinger RP, Levy MM, Rhodes A, Annane D, Gerlach H, Opal SM, et al. Surviving Sepsis Campaign: international guidelines for management of severe sepsis and septic shock, 2012. Intensive Care Med. 2013;39(2):165–228.
18. Goldstein B, Giroir B, Randolph A, International Consensus Conference on Pediatric Sepsis. International pediatric sepsis consensus conference: definitions for sepsis and organ dysfunction in pediatrics. Pediatr Crit Care Med J Soc Crit Care Med World Fed Pediatr Intensive Crit Care Soc. 2005;6(1):2–8.
19. Shearer WT, Rosenblatt HM, Gelman RS, Oyomopito R, Plaeger S, Stiehm ER, et al. Lymphocyte subsets in healthy children from birth through 18 years of age: the pediatric AIDS clinical trials group P1009 study. J Allergy Clin Immunol. 2003;112(5):973–80.
20. Slater A, Shann F, Pearson G, Paediatric Index of Mortality (PIM) Study Group. PIM2: a revised version of the Paediatric Index of Mortality. Intensive Care Med. 2003;29(2):278–85.
21. Leteurtre S, Duhamel A, Deken V, Lacroix J, Leclerc F, Groupe Francophone de Réanimation et Urgences Pédiatriques. Daily estimation of the severity of organ dysfunctions in critically ill children by using the PELOD-2 score. Crit Care Lond Engl. 2015;19:324.
22. Trzeciak S, McCoy JV, Phillip Dellinger R, Arnold RC, Rizzuto M, Abate NL, et al. Early increases in microcirculatory perfusion during protocol-directed resuscitation are associated with reduced multi-organ failure at 24 h in patients with sepsis. Intensive Care Med. 2008;34(12):2210–7.

23. Horan TC, Andrus M, Dudeck MA. CDC/NHSN surveillance definition of health care-associated infection and criteria for specific types of infections in the acute care setting. Am J Infect Control. 2008;36(5):309–32.
24. Demaret J, Walencik A, Jacob M-C, Timsit J-F, Venet F, Lepape A, et al. Inter-laboratory assessment of flow cytometric monocyte HLA-DR expression in clinical samples. Cytometry B Clin Cytom. 2013;84(1):59–62.
25. Venet F, Davin F, Guignant C, Larue A, Cazalis M-A, Darbon R, et al. Early assessment of leukocyte alterations at diagnosis of septic shock. Shock (Augusta Ga.). 2010;34(4):358–63.
26. Saison J, Maucort-Boulch D, Chidiac C, Demaret J, Malcus C, Cotte L, et al. Increased regulatory T-cell percentage contributes to poor CD4(+) lymphocytes recovery: a 2-year prospective study after introduction of antiretroviral therapy. Open Forum Infect Dis. 2015;2(2):ofv063.
27. de Jager W, te Velthuis H, Prakken BJ, Kuis W, Rijkers GT. Simultaneous detection of 15 human cytokines in a single sample of stimulated peripheral blood mononuclear cells. Clin Diagn Lab Immunol. 2003;10(1):133–9.
28. Döcke W-D, Höflich C, Davis KA, Röttgers K, Meisel C, Kiefer P, et al. Monitoring temporary immunodepression by flow cytometric measurement of monocytic HLA-DR expression: a multicenter standardized study. Clin Chem. 2005;51(12):2341–7.
29. Wong HR, Cvijanovich N, Wheeler DS, Bigham MT, Monaco M, Odoms K, et al. Interleukin-8 as a stratification tool for interventional trials involving pediatric septic shock. Am J Respir Crit Care Med. 2008;178(3):276–82.
30. Peronnet E, Nguyen K, Cerrato E, Guhadasan R, Venet F, Textoris J, et al. Evaluation of mRNA biomarkers to identify risk of hospital acquired infections in children admitted to paediatric intensive care unit. PLoS ONE. 2016;11(3):e0152388.
31. Monserrat J, de Pablo R, Diaz-Martín D, Rodríguez-Zapata M, de la Hera A, Prieto A, et al. Early alterations of B cells in patients with septic shock. Crit Care Lond Engl. 2013;17(3):R105.
32. Halstead ES, Carcillo JA, Schilling B, Greiner RJ, Whiteside TL. Reduced frequency of CD56 dim CD16 pos natural killer cells in pediatric systemic inflammatory response syndrome/sepsis patients. Pediatr Res. 2013;74(4):427–32.
33. von Muller L, Klemm A, Durmus N, Weiss M, Suger-Wiedeck H, Schneider M, et al. Cellular immunity and active human cytomegalovirus infection in patients with septic shock. J Infect Dis. 2007;196(9):1288–95.
34. Monneret G, Debard A-L, Venet F, Bohe J, Hequet O, Bienvenu J, et al. Marked elevation of human circulating CD4+CD25+regulatory T cells in sepsis-induced immunoparalysis. Crit Care Med. 2003;31(7):2068–71.
35. Drewry AM, Ablordeppey EA, Murray ET, Beiter ER, Walton AH, Hall MW, et al. Comparison of monocyte human leukocyte antigen-DR expression and stimulated tumor necrosis factor alpha production as outcome predictors in severe sepsis: a prospective observational study. Crit Care Lond Engl. 2016;20(1):334.
36. Bo L, Wang F, Zhu J, Li J, Deng X. Granulocyte-colony stimulating factor (G-CSF) and granulocyte-macrophage colony stimulating factor (GM-CSF) for sepsis: a meta-analysis. Crit Care Lond Engl. 2011;15(1):R58.
37. Gessler P, Pretre R, Bürki C, Rousson V, Frey B, Nadal D. Monocyte function-associated antigen expression during and after pediatric cardiac surgery. J Thorac Cardiovasc Surg. 2005;130(1):54–60.
38. Hoffman JA, Weinberg KI, Azen CG, Horn MV, Dukes L, Starnes VA, et al. Human leukocyte antigen-DR expression on peripheral blood monocytes and the risk of pneumonia in pediatric lung transplant recipients. Transpl Infect Dis. 2004;6(4):147–55.
39. Stolk RF, van der Poll T, Angus DC, van der Hoeven JG, Pickkers P, Kox M. Potentially inadvertent immunomodulation: norepinephrine use in sepsis. Am J Respir Crit Care Med. 2016;194(5):550–8.
40. Gouel-Chéron A, Allaouchiche B, Guignant C, Davin F, Floccard B, Monneret G, et al. Early interleukin-6 and slope of monocyte human leukocyte antigen-DR: a powerful association to predict the development of sepsis after major trauma. PLoS ONE. 2012;7(3):e33095.
41. Field-Ridley A, Dharmar M, Steinhorn D, McDonald C, Marcin JP. ICU-acquired weakness is associated with differences in clinical outcomes in critically ill children. Pediatr Crit Care Med J Soc Crit Care Med World Fed Pediatr Intensive Crit Care Soc. 2016;17(1):53–7.
42. Carcillo JA, Dean JM, Holubkov R, Berger J, Meert KL, Anand KJS, et al. Inherent risk factors for nosocomial infection in the long stay critically ill child without known baseline immunocompromise: a post hoc analysis of the crisis trial. Pediatr Infect Dis J. 2016;35(11):1182–6.
43. Pfortmueller CA, Meisel C, Fux M, Schefold JC. Assessment of immune organ dysfunction in critical illness: utility of innate immune response markers. Intensive Care Med Exp. 2017;5(1):49.

18

Development and performance of a novel vasopressor-driven mortality prediction model in septic shock

Saraschandra Vallabhajosyula[1,2,3*], Jacob C. Jentzer[1,2], Aditya A. Kotecha[3,4], Dennis H. Murphree Jr.[5], Erin F. Barreto[3,5,6], Ashish K. Khanna[7,8] and Vivek N. Iyer[2,3]

Abstract

Background: Vasoactive medications are essential in septic shock, but are not fully incorporated into current mortality prediction risk scores. We sought to develop a novel mortality prediction model for septic shock incorporating quantitative vasoactive medication usage.

Methods: Quantitative vasopressor use was calculated in a cohort of 5352 septic shock patients and compared using norepinephrine equivalents (NEE), cumulative vasopressor index and the vasoactive inotrope score models. Having best discrimination prediction, $\log_{10}$NEE was selected for further development of a novel prediction model for 28-day and 1-year mortality via backward stepwise logistic regression. This model termed 'MAVIC' (Mechanical ventilation, Acute Physiology And Chronic Health Evaluation-III, Vasopressors, Inotropes, Charlson comorbidity index) was then compared to Acute Physiology And Chronic Health Evaluation-III (APACHE-III) and Sequential Organ Failure Assessment (SOFA) scores in an independent validation cohort for its accuracy in predicting 28-day and 1-year mortality.

Measurements and main results: The MAVIC model was superior to the APACHE-III and SOFA scores in its ability to predict 28-day mortality (area under receiver operating characteristic curve [AUROC] 0.73 vs. 0.66 and 0.60) and 1-year mortality (AUROC 0.74 vs. 0.66 and 0.60), respectively.

Conclusions: The incorporation of quantitative vasopressor usage into a novel 'MAVIC' model results in superior 28-day and 1-year mortality risk prediction in a large cohort of patients with septic shock.

Keywords: Septic shock, Vasopressors, Inotropes, Norepinephrine, MAVIC model

Introduction

Sepsis is a leading public health problem with an increasing incidence in recent epidemiological data [1]. Despite recent advances, the mortality with sepsis and septic shock remains as high as 30–50% [2, 3]. Current prognostication systems for critical illness, such as the Acute Physiology And Chronic Health Evaluation-III (APACHE-III) and Sequential Organ Failure Assessment (SOFA) scores, assess end-organ damage, laboratory and physiological derangements and chronic comorbidities to aid in accurate mortality prediction [4]. The recent Sepsis-3 definitions emphasize the incorporation of the SOFA score into defining sepsis severity, including septic shock [4]. However, since the initial development of the SOFA score, advances in cardiovascular critical care have resulted in changes to the types, doses and combinations of vasoactive medications warranting a refinement of the SOFA score [5–7]. Previous work from our institution has shown that refining the cardiovascular component of the SOFA score results in significantly improved prediction of intensive care unit (ICU), hospital and 28-day mortality in patients with critical illness [5]. More importantly, their modified cardiovascular SOFA score was as reliable as the total SOFA score for mortality prediction. This highlights the critical importance of cardiovascular

*Correspondence: Vallabhajosyula.Saraschandra@mayo.edu
[1] Department of Cardiovascular Medicine, Mayo Clinic, 200 First Street SW, Rochester, MN 55905, USA
Full list of author information is available at the end of the article

integrity in overall prognostication. We have previously reported that nearly 60–70% of septic patients in the ICU have concomitant cardiac and renal end-organ damage [8, 9]. Cardiovascular dysfunction in sepsis is associated with poor short-term and long-term outcomes, and the use of high-dose vasopressors appears to further worsen prognosis in these situations [2, 3, 6, 8, 10]. Circulatory failure and shock remain the most widely noted forms of cardiovascular dysfunction in patients with sepsis. Given the importance and ubiquity of vasopressor use in septic shock, we sought to develop a novel risk prognostication system using a quantitative vasoactive medication scoring system approach. [6, 7]

Using a contemporary cohort of septic shock patients, we thus sought to develop and validate a novel risk prognostication model for 28-day mortality incorporating the best discriminative ability of three contemporary vasoactive medication scoring systems. This model was then compared to existing SOFA and APACHE-III prognostic risk scores.

Materials and methods

This was a retrospective cohort study of adult septic shock patients admitted to all ICUs at the Mayo Clinic in Rochester, Minnesota from January 1, 2010 to December 31, 2015. The characteristics of these ICUs and patient population included in this study have been described previously [11]. Briefly, the Mayo Clinic is a 2059 bed hospital over two campuses in Rochester Minnesota and has 14 sub-specialty ICUs that are staffed continually by board-certified intensivists. This study was approved by the Mayo Clinic Institutional Review Board. The Sepsis-3 criteria was used to define septic shock as sepsis requiring vasopressor use to maintain mean arterial pressure $\geq$ 65 mm Hg and blood lactate $\geq$ 2 mmol/L despite fluid resuscitation [4]. Adult (> 18 years) patients diagnosed with septic shock admitted to the ICU for $\geq$ 24 h were included in this study. We excluded patients who declined Minnesota research authorization and also those with repeat ICU admissions, end-of-life treatment limiting decisions and patients without post-ICU follow-up.

Data: definitions, sources and management

Demographics, comorbidities and clinical data were automatically abstracted from the Multidisciplinary Epidemiology and Translational Research in Intensive Care Laboratory (METRIC) DataMart as previously described [2, 3, 8, 10, 12]. This customized iterative data repository automatically abstracts vital signs, infusion rates, fluid balance, urine output data, ventilator parameters, hemodynamic variables and laboratory parameters every 15 min in real time. All patients with sepsis and septic shock have blood cultures and lactate levels checked and receive 30 ml/kg intravenous fluid and antimicrobial therapy within 3 h of sepsis onset as detected by electronic search algorithm. This is a part of an ongoing quality improvement initiative in the ICUs at Mayo Clinic [13, 14]. Acute kidney injury was electronically abstracted by a customized, validated search algorithm that screens all ICU patients [15]. Total and peak vasopressor doses for the first 24 h were abstracted from the METRIC DataMart. The SOFA and APACHE-III scores are calculated at admission and at 24 h using customized algorithms. We used the 24-h SOFA and APACHE-III scores in this study. Mortality data were abstracted from the Mayo Clinic databases, the State of Minnesota electronic death certificates and the Rochester Epidemiology Project death data system [16]. Two independent reviewers (SV and AAK) reviewed the electronically abstracted variables and, when needed, performed manual chart reviews to ensure accuracy and fidelity of data.

The primary aim was to develop a novel risk stratification model incorporating vasoactive medication scoring systems in the prediction of 28-day mortality in patients with septic shock. This novel model was then compared to currently existing standard severity of illness scoring systems, i.e., SOFA and APACHE-III scores. The secondary aim was to evaluate the ability of this model to predict 1-year mortality.

Vasoactive medication scoring systems

Total and peak simultaneous doses of vasoactive medications in the first 24-h were abstracted from the METRIC DataMart. We used the following scoring systems to quantify overall peak vasoactive medication requirements: (a) norepinephrine equivalents (NEE) [7], (b) vasoactive inotropic score (VIS) [17, 18] and (c) cumulative vasopressor index (CVI) [19]. The dose equivalency and calculations for these scoring systems are presented in Fig. 1. Peak simultaneous doses during the first 24 h of the ICU stay were used to develop these indices that were used for further analysis.

Model development, validation and statistical analysis

Continuous and categorical data are presented as median (interquartile range [IQR]) and total (percentage), respectively. Kruskal–Wallis and Fisher's exact tests were used to evaluate continuous and categorical outcomes. Odds ratios (OR) with 95% confidence intervals (CI) were used to report univariable and multivariable analysis results. Because of the skewed nature of NEE, VIS and CVI values, these values were converted to $\log_{10}$NEE, $\log_{10}$VIS and $\log_{10}$CVI, respectively, for continuous analyses. Area under the receiver operating characteristic curve (AUROC) analysis was utilized to evaluate discrimination

a

Vasoactive Agent	Dose	NEE
Epinephrine	0.1	0.1
Norepinephrine	0.1	0.1
Dopamine	15	0.1
Phenylephrine	1	0.1
Vasopressin	0.04	0.1

b

Vasoactive Inotrope Score
Dopamine + Dobutamine + [100 x Epinephrine] + [100 x Norepinephrine] + [10 x Milrinone] + [10,000 x Vasopressin]

c

Vasoactive Agent	Dose Range			
	1 point	2 points	3 points	4 points
Dopamine	0 < dose ≤ 5	5 < dose ≤ 10	10 < dose ≤ 15	>15
Epinephrine	---	0 < dose ≤ 0.05	0.05 < dose ≤ 0.1	>0.1
Norepinephrine	---	0 < dose ≤ 0.05	0.05 < dose ≤ 0.1	>0.1
Phenylephrine	---	0 < dose ≤ 0.4	0.4 < dose ≤ 0.8	>0.8
Vasopressin	---	---	---	Any dose

Fig. 1 Vasoactive medication scoring systems. Conversion and scoring systems used in norepinephrine equivalents (1A), vasoactive inotrope score (1B) and cumulative vasopressor index (1C). All doses in mcg/kg/min except vasopressin, which is U/min. *NEE* norepinephrine equivalents

of $\log_{10}$NEE, $\log_{10}$VIS and $\log_{10}$CVI for 28-day mortality on a derivation subset of the cohort. The scoring system with the highest discrimination was used further for model development in the multivariate analyses.

Using an outcome-agnostic sampling algorithm, the cohort was divided into derivation (75%) and validation (25%) subsets. As seen in Table 1, the outcomes for both 28-day and 1-year mortality are relatively balanced, thus no specific resampling approach was required. For the multivariable modeling, regression analysis with backward stepwise variable selection was conducted in order to derive a model for predicting 28-day and 1-year mortality using variables generated in the first 24 h of ICU stay. The variable selection component of this model was based on a liberal $p<0.20$ for inclusion [20]. Following training on the derivation subset, model performance was assessed on the 25% holdout set. Two-tailed $p<0.05$ was considered statistically significant. All statistical analyses were performed with JMP version 10.0.1 (SAS Institute, Cary, NC).

Results

During the period from January 1, 2010 through December 31, 2010, there were a total of 7516 ICU admissions for septic shock, of which 5352 (71.3%) patients were included (Fig. 2). The derivation and validation cohorts comprised 4033 (75.4%) and 1319 (24.6%) patients, respectively. Baseline characteristics for the total population and the individual cohorts are detailed in Table 1. The median vasopressor doses and vasoactive medication scores were comparable between the two cohorts (Tables 1, 2). In the total population, 28-day and 1-year mortalities were 45.1% and 49.7%, respectively, there were no significant differences in mortality between the

Table 1 Characteristics of the population at baseline and within 24 h of ICU admission

Parameter	Total cohort ($n=5352$)	Derivation cohort ($n=4033$)	Validation cohort ($n=1319$)	p
Age (years)	65.7 (56–75.3)	65.7 (55.8–75.3)	65.9 (56.4–75.1)	0.79
Caucasian race	4879 (91.2)	3677 (91.2)	1202 (91.1)	0.49
Male sex	3297 (61.6)	2512 (62.2)	785 (59.5)	0.07
Body mass index (kg/m^2)	28.5 (24.4–33.7)	28.5 (24.4–33.7)	28.6 (24.3–33.8)	0.88
Charlson comorbidity index	6 (4–8)	6 (4–8)	6 (3–8)	0.41
Heart failure	999 (18.7)	731 (18.1)	268 (20.3)	0.08
Diabetes mellitus, type II	1561 (29.2)	1196 (29.7)	365 (27.7)	0.17
Chronic kidney disease	1216 (22.7)	910 (22.6)	306 (23.2)	0.65
APACHE-III score (24 h)	83 (67–103)	83 (68–103)	82 (66–102)	0.39
SOFA score (24 h)	9 (7–12)	9 (7–12)	9 (8–12)	0.81
Peak lactate (mmol/L)	4.4 (2.8–7.9)	4.4 (2.8–8)	4.3 (2.8–7.8)	0.49
Invasive mechanical ventilation	4381 (81.9)	3283 (81.4)	1098 (83.2)	0.14
Acute kidney injury within 24 h	4226 (82.9)	3174 (82.5)	1052 (83.9)	0.28
Cumulative fluid balance (L) (h)				
3	6.2 (2.9–10.4)	6.2 (2.9–10.4)	6.3 (3–10.4)	0.32
6	7.1 (3.6–11.5)	7 (3.6–11.5)	7.3 (3.8–11.7)	0.27
24	9.3 (5.4–14.9)	9.6 (5.7–15.6)	9.6 (5.8–15.6)	0.23
ICU length of stay (days)	3.8 (2–7.7)	3.7 (2–7.7)	3.9 (2.1–7.7)	0.09
Hospital length of stay (days)	11.1 (6.5–21.7)	11 (6.5–21.5)	11.6 (6.6–22.2)	0.16
Peak 24-h vasopressor doses				
Norepinephrine (mcg/kg/min)	0.1 (0.16–0.25)	0.1 (0.05–0.25)	0.1 (0.05–0.25)	0.53
NEE (mcg/kg/min)	0.2 (0.1–0.32)	0.2 (0.1–0.32)	0.2 (0.1–0.32)	0.82
Vasoactive medication scores				
Log_{10}NEE	−0.7 (−1, −0.5)	−0.7 (−1, −0.5)	−0.7 (−1, −0.5)	0.82
Log_{10}VIS	1.3 (1–1.5)	1.2 (1–1.5)	1.2 (1–1.5)	0.95
Log_{10}CVI	0.7 (0.6–0.9)	0.7 (0.6–0.9)	0.8 (0.6–0.9)	0.25
≥ 2 vasoactive medications	3245 (60.6)	2412 (60.5)	833 (60.9)	0.80
28-day mortality	2416 (45.1)	1842 (45.7)	574 (43.5)	0.18
One-year mortality	2660 (49.7)	2026 (50.2)	634 (48.1)	0.17

Count (percentage) or median (interquartile range)

APACHE Acute Physiology And Chronic Health Evaluation, *CVI* cumulative vasopressor index, *ICU* intensive care unit, *NEE* norepinephrine equivalents, *SOFA* Sequential Organ Failure Assessment, *VIS* vasoactive inotropic score

derivation and validation cohorts (Table 1). All three vasoactive medication scoring systems were associated with unadjusted 28-day mortality in the derivation cohort—log_{10}NEE (OR 2.3 [95% CI 2.1–2.6]; $p<0.001$), log_{10}VIS (OR 2.9 [95% CI 2.5–3.3]; $p<0.001$) and log_{10}CVI (OR 1.2 [95% CI 1.1–1.2]; $p<0.001$). Log_{10}NEE and log_{10}VIS demonstrated fair discrimination (0.63, 0.61) prediction and log_{10}CVI demonstrated poor discrimination (0.52) for 28-day mortality in derivation cohort (Fig. 3). Log_{10}NEE was used for further analysis in the multivariate model and for the development of a prediction model.

Model development, validation and comparison

Using univariable analysis, significant predictors of 28-day mortality in the derivation cohort are identified as noted in Table 3. After adjusting for age, sex, severity of illness, comorbidity and use of mechanical ventilation, log_{10}NEE was an independent predictor of 28-day mortality (OR 1.6 [95% CI 1.4–1.9]; $p<0.001$). The multivariate model was reduced using a stepwise backward elimination process based on a liberal $p<0.20$. The final model incorporated Mechanical ventilation, APACHE-III, Vasopressors and Inotropes (log_{10}NEE) and Charlson comorbidity index (MAVIC) as significant predictors of 28-day mortality in patients with septic shock. This model demonstrated good discrimination of 28-day mortality (AUROC 0.73) in the validation cohort (Fig. 4). In comparison with the MAVIC model, standardized severity of illness scoring systems such as the APACHE-III (AUROC 0.66) and SOFA score (AUROC 0.59) showed

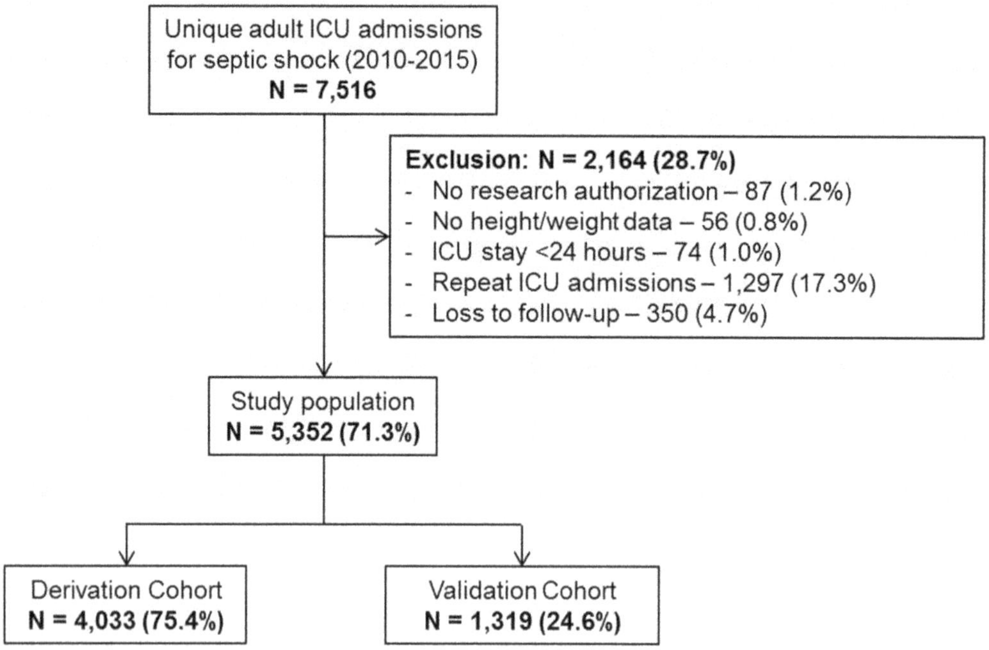

Fig. 2 Study population. *ICU* intensive care unit

Table 2 Peak vasoactive medication dosing in first 24 h

Vasoactive medication	Total cohort ($n = 5352$)	Derivation cohort ($n = 4033$)	Validation cohort ($n = 1319$)	p
Vasopressin				
Total patients	2200 (41.1)	1644 (40.8)	556 (42.2)	0.38
Peak dose (U/min)	0.04 (0.04–0.04)	0.04 (0.04–0.04)	0.04 (0.04–0.04)	0.98
Epinephrine				
Total patients	1633 (30.5)	1207 (29.9)	426 (32.3)	0.11
Peak dose (mcg/kg/min)	0.05 (0.04–0.1)	0.05 (0.04–0.1)	0.05 (0.04–0.1)	0.47
Phenylephrine				
Total patients	355 (6.6)	280 (6.9)	75 (5.7)	0.13
Peak dose (mcg/kg/min)	0.6 (0.1–1.3)	0.6 (0.3–1.2)	0.8 (0.4–1.4)	0.10
Dobutamine				
Total patients	271 (5.1)	201 (5.0)	70 (5.3)	0.66
Peak dose (mcg/kg/min)	5 (5–10)	5 (5–10)	5 (5–7.5)	0.38
Dopamine				
Total patients	208 (3.9)	150 (3.7)	58 (4.4)	0.29
Peak dose (mcg/kg/min)	5 (3–10)	5 (3–10)	5 (3–13)	0.29
Milrinone				
Total patients	700 (13.1)	522 (12.9)	178 (13.5)	0.61
Peak dose (mcg/kg/min)	0.25 (0.25–0.37)	0.25 (0.25–0.38)	0.25 (0.2–0.3)	0.12

Total (percentage) or median (interquartile range)

lower discrimination for 28-day mortality. Formal comparisons of all model AUROCs via DeLong test found all $p < 0.001$, indicating statistically significant differences.

The MAVIC model, likewise, demonstrated superiority in discrimination for 1-year mortality (AUROC 0.73) as compared to APACHE-III (AUROC 0.66) and SOFA scores (AUROC 0.60) in the validation cohort. As with

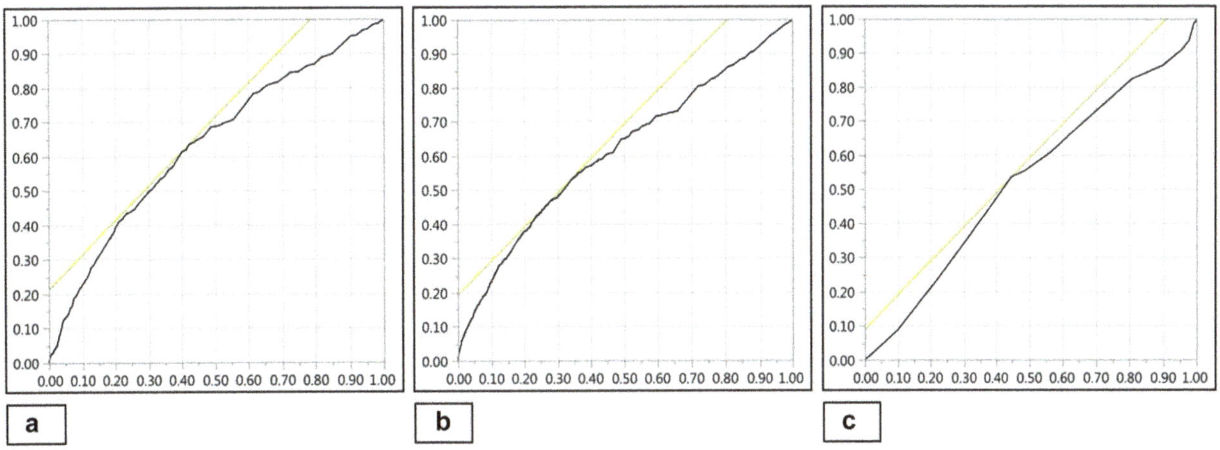

Fig. 3 Discrimination of vasoactive scoring systems for 28-day mortality. AUROC curve for log_{10}NEE = 0.63 (**a**); log_{10}VIS = 0.61 (**b**); and log_{10}CVI = 0.52 (**c**). *AUROC* area under receiver operating characteristic, *CVI* cumulative vasopressor index, *NEE* norepinephrine equivalents, *VIS* vasoactive inotrope score

Table 3 28-day mortality predictors in the derivation cohort

Parameter	Univariable analysis		Multivariable analysis		MAVIC model	
	OR (95% CI)[a]	*p*	OR (95% CI)[a]	*p*	OR (95% CI)[a]	*p*
Age	1.1 (1.1–1.1)	< 0.001	1.0 (0.9–1.0)	0.88	–	–
Male sex	0.8 (0.7–0.9)	0.001	0.9 (0.8–0.9)	0.03	–	–
BMI (kg/m^2)	0.9 (0.9–0.9)	0.02	0.9 (0.9–0.9)	< 0.001	–	–
CCI	1.2 (1.2–1.2)	< 0.001	1.2 (1.1–1.2)	< 0.001	1.1 (1.1–1.2)	< 0.001
APACHE-III score	1.1 (1.1–1.1)	< 0.001	1.1 (1.1–1.1)	< 0.001	1.1 (1.1–1.1)	< 0.001
Peak lactate (mmol/L)	1.1 (1.1–1.1)	< 0.001	1.1 (1.1–1.1)	< 0.001	–	–
Acute kidney injury	2.1 (1.7–2.5)	< 0.001	1.9 (1.6–2.3)	< 0.001	–	–
IMV	1.6 (1.4–1.9)	< 0.001	1.8 (1.5–2.2)	< 0.001	1.8 (1.5–2.2)	< 0.001
24-h cumulative fluids	1.0 (0.9–1.0)	0.77	–	–	–	–
Log_{10}24-h peak NEE	2.3 (2.1–2.6)	< 0.001	1.6 (1.4–1.9)	< 0.001	2.0 (1.7–2.3)	< 0.001

APACHE-III Acute Physiology And Chronic Health Evaluation-III, *BMI* body mass index, *CCI* Charlson comorbidity index, *CI* confidence interval, *IMV* invasive mechanical ventilation, *NEE* norepinephrine equivalents, *OR* odds ratio

[a] Unit odds ratios are represented for continuous variables

28-day mortality, comparison via DeLong test found all differences to be statistically significant.

Discussion

To the best of our knowledge, this is the first large observational study to use vasoactive scoring systems for prediction of mortality in adult patients with septic shock. Norepinephrine equivalents had superior discrimination for 28-day mortality compared to either the CVI or VIS in septic shock patients. Using data available within the first 24 h, NEE and three other independent predictors of 28-day mortality were combined to develop a parsimonious 4-component prognostic model (MAVIC). This MAVIC model was subsequently validated in a randomly generated validation cohort from the same population. The MAVIC model demonstrated superior discriminatory ability compared to the APACHE-III and SOFA scores for 28-day and 1-year mortality in septic shock.

Historically, in adult patients with sepsis and cardiogenic shock, vasoactive medication scoring systems have predominantly been used to classify the extent of hemodynamic support [21–23]. Vasoactive medications are used in an empiric fashion and often there are limited bedside data on cumulative vasopressor requirements [24]. Vasoactive medications are a severity of illness indicator; however, they are incompletely accounted for in scoring systems. More recent data have shown vasoactive medication requirements to be an independent

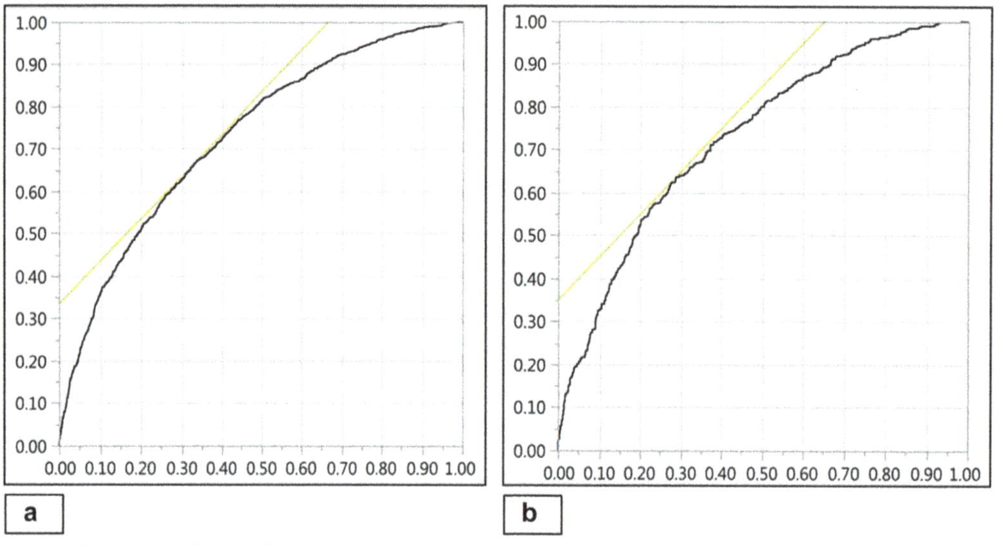

Fig. 4 Discriminatory ability of MAVIC model for 28-day mortality. AUROC curve for derivation (**a**) and validation cohorts (**b**) = 0.73. *AUROC* area under receiver operating characteristic, *MAVIC* Mechanical ventilation, APACHE-III, Vasopressors, Inotropes and Charlson comorbidity index

predictor of adverse outcomes [11, 25–27]. The need for high-dose vasopressors reflects a potentially fatal underlying condition with a high risk of complications, but the direct association remains to be proven. Though the VIS has been used to prognosticate in a smaller cohort of 138 pediatric patients with sepsis [28], this is the first large study using existing vasoactive scoring systems in the prognostication of adult septic shock patients. Prior studies have used either norepinephrine or cumulative vasopressor requirements to demonstrate higher mortality in patients with septic shock [27, 29]. In about 20–40% of septic patients, persistent vasoplegia results in refractory shock necessitating high-dose vasoactive medications, with a very high attributable mortality [29]. Refractory vasoplegia in sepsis is multi-factorial and usually fatal, leading investigators to evaluate alternate mechanisms of restoring vascular tone in these patients [6, 30]. High doses of vasopressors are associated with significant adverse events such as arrhythmias, myocardial infarctions, digital injury/ischemia and acute kidney injury [26, 27].

Existing prognostic scores (APACHE and SOFA) have several limitations [31]. The APACHE-III does not incorporate either vasopressor use or myocardial dysfunction in sepsis, both of which have mortality implications [2, 3, 8, 11]. The SOFA score also has some similar limitations as shown in the study by Yadav et al. [5]. They modified the cardiovascular component of the SOFA score and incorporated more detailed vasoactive medication dosage as well as organ failure assessment using serum lactate and the shock index. Their modified cardiovascular SOFA showed superior discriminatory power for ICU, in-hospital as well as 28-day mortality [5]. This study was limited in its ability to prognosticate in septic shock patients since it included all ICU patients. We performed an exploratory analysis using the modified cardiovascular SOFA in this population and it showed a poor discrimination for 28-day mortality (AUROC 0.51). This can partly be explained by the high modified cardiovascular SOFA score of 3 and 4 in this population reflective of their cardiovascular morbidity. Furthermore, the NEE model uses a more granular scoring system compared to the modified cardiovascular SOFA that might explain these differences. In another study, Johnson et al. [32] used a simplified version of the APACHE-IV score and developed a similar parsimonious scoring system in unselected critically ill patients without compromising the accuracy; however, it lacked adequate vasopressor data.

It is noteworthy that our model appears to further enhance risk assessment in patients with septic shock, who by definition comprise a high-risk cohort with a cardiovascular SOFA score of 3–4. Thus, our model appears to capture additional prognostic information than the individual SOFA component scores. Furthermore, with the advent of real-time sophisticated critical-illness computational algorithms, our model appears capable of incorporating real-time vasopressor use to provide clinicians with reliable and up-to-date prognostic information [12, 33].

The vasoactive scoring systems used in this study have been previously been used in the evaluation of septic shock patients; however, they have not been compared head-to-head [7, 17, 19]. In this study, we demonstrate NEE to have superior predictive performance for 28-day mortality relative to the VIS and CVI. This can be explained by multiple hypotheses. First, given the ubiquitous use of norepinephrine as the first-line vasopressor in septic shock it is likely that norepinephrine usage dominates the various scoring systems [34]. As noted in Table 1, individual peak norepinephrine doses formed nearly 40% of the peak total dose of NEE lending credence to this hypothesis. Second, the VIS scoring system was used and validated primarily to define inotrope requirements in pediatric and cardiac surgery populations, both of which significantly differ from the current population [17, 28]. Finally, the dose equivalency in the literature differs on the optimal conversion factors for vasoactive medications resulting in varied calibration with outcomes. The NEE conversion system used in this study is consistent with recent high-impact trials including the angiotensin II for the treatment of vasodilatory shock and vasopressin versus norepinephrine infusion in patients with septic shock trials [7, 35]. However, the NEE used by Brown et al. [29] to report high-dose vasopressors differs from our study.

This study has certain limitations. The use of a retrospective design is subject to selection and information bias that could have confounded the results. These patients were identified using the Sepsis-3 criteria retroactively during the study duration when the 2001 consensus criteria were in use; and this may have impacted case selection. All treatment decisions, including choice of vasoactive medication and arterial pressure goal, were at the discretion of the treating physician and no universal protocol for hemodynamic management of septic patients was in place during the study period. Despite protocoled hemodynamic management, a significant portion of the patients had a positive fluid balance at the end of day 1 suggestive of higher acuity of illness in this population. Alternate endpoints to critical illness such as functional status, disposition and return to work were not assessed in this study that could provide a greater emphasis on patient-centered outcomes and quality of life. We focused on early risk prognostication and thus could have overlooked late cardiovascular deterioration in these patients that could have contributed to 28-day mortality. Finally, the single-institution nature of this study limits external generalizability in the absence of validation studies at other centers. Strengths of the study include the large patient population studied and the use of a well-validated electronic database with 15-min data capture capabilities.

Conclusions

We report the development and validation of a novel MAVIC mortality prediction model for septic shock patients admitted to the ICU. The MAVIC model incorporates cumulative vasoactive medication usage within the first 24 h and outperforms both APACHE-III and SOFA scores for 28-day mortality prediction in septic shock patients. Vasopressor burden during early critical illness appears to be a marker for unfavorable outcomes. Newer scoring systems for critically ill patients with septic shock are needed that emphasize cardiovascular morbidity and vasoactive medication use to aid in early and reliable prognostication. Further validation of this model externally and in non-septic shock populations is desirable prior to acceptance in clinical practice.

Abbreviations

APACHE-III: Acute Physiology And Chronic Health Evaluation-III; AUROC: area under receiver operating characteristic curve; CI: confidence interval; CVI: cumulative vasopressor index; ICU: intensive care unit; MAVIC: Mechanical ventilation, APACHE-III, Vasopressors, Inotropes, Charlson comorbidity index; METRIC: Multidisciplinary Epidemiology and Translational Research in Intensive Care Laboratory; NEE: norepinephrine equivalents; OR: odds ratio; SOFA: Sequential Organ Failure Assessment; VIS: vasoactive inotrope score.

Authors' contributions

SV, JCJ, AKK and DHM contributed to study design, literature review, data analysis and statistical analysis. SV, JCJ, AAK and DHM contributed to data management, data analysis and drafting manuscript. SV, JCJ, AAK, DHM, EFB, AKK and VNI contributed to access to data. JCJ, EFB, AKK and VNI contributed to manuscript revision, intellectual revisions and mentorship. All authors read and approved the final manuscript.

Author details

[1] Department of Cardiovascular Medicine, Mayo Clinic, 200 First Street SW, Rochester, MN 55905, USA. [2] Division of Pulmonary and Critical Care Medicine, Department of Medicine, Mayo Clinic, Rochester, MN, USA. [3] Multidisciplinary Epidemiology and Translational Research in Intensive Care (METRIC) Laboratory, Mayo Clinic, Rochester, MN, USA. [4] Division of Pulmonary and Critical Care Medicine, Department of Medicine, Henry Ford Hospital/Wayne State University, Detroit, MI, USA. [5] Department of Health Sciences Research, Robert D. and Patricia E. Kern Center for the Science of Health Care Delivery, Mayo Clinic, Rochester, MN, USA. [6] Department of Pharmacy, Mayo Clinic, Rochester, MN, USA. [7] Center for Critical Care, Anesthesiology Institute, Cleveland Clinic, Cleveland, OH, USA. [8] Department of Outcomes Research, Cleveland Clinic, Cleveland, OH, USA.

Acknowledgements

None.

Competing interests

All authors report no financial or intellectual conflicts of interest related to this manuscript.

Funding
This research did not receive any specific grant from funding agencies in the public, commercial or not-for-profit sectors.

Prior presentation
Slide Presentation, 47th Critical Care Congress, Society of Critical Care Medicine, San Antonio TX (February 2018)

References

1. Kumar G, Kumar N, Taneja A, Kaleekal T, Tarima S, McGinley E, et al. Nationwide trends of severe sepsis in the 21st century (2000–2007). Chest. 2011;140(5):1223–31.
2. Vallabhajosyula S, Kumar M, Pandompatam G, Sakhuja A, Kashyap R, Kashani K, et al. Prognostic impact of isolated right ventricular dysfunction in sepsis and septic shock: an 8-year historical cohort study. Ann Intensive Care. 2017;7(1):94.
3. Vallabhajosyula S, Sakhuja A, Geske JB, Kumar M, Poterucha JT, Kashyap R, et al. Role of admission troponin-T and serial troponin-T testing in predicting outcomes in severe sepsis and septic shock. J Am Heart Assoc. 2017;6(9):e005930.
4. Singer M, Deutschman CS, Seymour CW, Shankar-Hari M, Annane D, Bauer M, et al. The third international consensus definitions for sepsis and septic shock (sepsis-3). JAMA. 2016;315(8):801–10.
5. Yadav H, Harrison AM, Hanson AC, Gajic O, Kor DJ, Cartin-Ceba R. Improving the accuracy of cardiovascular component of the sequential organ failure assessment score. Crit Care Med. 2015;43(7):1449–57.
6. Jentzer JC, Vallabhajosyula S, Khanna AK, Chawla LS, Busse LW, Kashani KB. Management of refractory vasodilatory shock. Chest. 2018;154(2):416–26.
7. Khanna A, English SW, Wang XS, Ham K, Tumlin J, Szerlip H, et al. Angiotensin II for the treatment of vasodilatory shock. N Engl J Med. 2017;377(5):419–30.
8. Vallabhajosyula S, Sakhuja A, Geske JB, Kumar M, Kashyap R, Kashani K, et al. Clinical profile and outcomes of acute cardiorenal syndrome type-5 in sepsis: an eight-year cohort study. PLoS ONE. 2018;13(1):e0190965.
9. Plataki M, Kashani K, Cabello-Garza J, Maldonado F, Kashyap R, Kor DJ, et al. Predictors of acute kidney injury in septic shock patients: an observational cohort study. Clin J Am Soc Nephrol. 2011;6(7):1744–51.
10. Vallabhajosyula S, Jentzer JC, Geske JB, Kumar M, Sakhuja A, Singhal A, et al. New-onset heart failure and mortality in hospital survivors of sepsis-related left ventricular dysfunction. Shock. 2018;49(2):144–9.
11. Kotecha A, Vallabhajosyula S, Apala DR, Frazee E, Iyer VN. Clinical outcomes of weight-based norepinephrine dosing in underweight and morbidly obese patients: a propensity-matched analysis. J Intensive Care Med. 2018. https://doi.org/10.1177/0885066618768180.
12. Herasevich V, Pickering BW, Dong Y, Peters SG, Gajic O. Informatics infrastructure for syndrome surveillance, decision support, reporting, and modeling of critical illness. Mayo Clin Proc. 2010;85(3):247–54.
13. Harrison AM, Thongprayoon C, Kashyap R, Chute CG, Gajic O, Pickering BW, et al. Developing the surveillance algorithm for detection of failure to recognize and treat severe sepsis. Mayo Clin Proc. 2015;90(2):166–75.
14. Siontis B, Elmer J, Dannielson R, Brown C, Park J, Surani S, et al. Multifaceted interventions to decrease mortality in patients with severe sepsis/septic shock-a quality improvement project. PeerJ. 2015;3:e1290.
15. Ahmed A, Vairavan S, Akhoundi A, Wilson G, Chiofolo C, Chbat N, et al. Development and validation of electronic surveillance tool for acute kidney injury: a retrospective analysis. J Crit Care. 2015;30(5):988–93.
16. Rocca WA, Yawn BP, St Sauver JL, Grossardt BR, Melton LJ 3rd. History of the Rochester Epidemiology Project: half a century of medical records linkage in a US population. Mayo Clin Proc. 2012;87(12):1202–13.
17. Gaies MG, Jeffries HE, Niebler RA, Pasquali SK, Donohue JE, Yu S, et al. Vasoactive-inotropic score is associated with outcome after infant cardiac surgery: an analysis from the Pediatric Cardiac Critical Care Consortium and Virtual PICU System Registries. Pediatr Crit Care Med. 2014;15(6):529–37.
18. Nguyen HV, Havalad V, Aponte-Patel L, Murata AY, Wang DY, Rusanov A, et al. Temporary biventricular pacing decreases the vasoactive-inotropic score after cardiac surgery: a substudy of a randomized clinical trial. J Thorac Cardiovasc Surg. 2013;146(2):296–301.
19. Trzeciak S, McCoy JV, Phillip Dellinger R, Arnold RC, Rizzuto M, Abate NL, et al. Early increases in microcirculatory perfusion during protocol-directed resuscitation are associated with reduced multi-organ failure at 24 h in patients with sepsis. Intensive Care Med. 2008;34(12):2210–7.
20. Bedogni G. Clinical prediction models—a practical approach to development, validation and updating. J R Stat Soc Ser A (Stat Soc). 2009;172(4):944.
21. Janiczek JA, Winger DG, Coppler P, Sabedra AR, Murray H, Pinsky MR, et al. Hemodynamic resuscitation characteristics associated with improved survival and shock resolution after cardiac arrest. Shock. 2016;45(6):613–9.
22. Du Z, Jia Z, Wang J, Xing Z, Jiang C, Xu B, et al. Effect of increasing mean arterial blood pressure on microcirculation in patients with cardiogenic shock supported by extracorporeal membrane oxygenation. Clin Hemorheol Microcirc. 2018;70(1):27–37.
23. Erwin BL, Denaburg MA, Barker AB, McArdle PJ, Windham ST, Morgan CJ. Evaluation of vasopressin for septic shock in patients on chronic renin-angiotensin-aldosterone system inhibitors. Crit Care Med. 2017;45(12):e1226–32.
24. Jentzer JC, Coons JC, Link CB, Schmidhofer M. Pharmacotherapy update on the use of vasopressors and inotropes in the intensive care unit. J Cardiovasc Pharmacol Ther. 2015;20(3):249–60.
25. Dunser MW, Ruokonen E, Pettila V, Ulmer H, Torgersen C, Schmittinger CA, et al. Association of arterial blood pressure and vasopressor load with septic shock mortality: a post hoc analysis of a multicenter trial. Crit Care. 2009;13(6):R181.
26. Schmittinger CA, Torgersen C, Luckner G, Schroder DC, Lorenz I, Dunser MW. Adverse cardiac events during catecholamine vasopressor therapy: a prospective observational study. Intensive Care Med. 2012;38(6):950–8.
27. Sviri S, Hashoul J, Stav I, van Heerden PV. Does high-dose vasopressor therapy in medical intensive care patients indicate what we already suspect? J Crit Care. 2014;29(1):157–60.
28. McIntosh AM, Tong S, Deakyne SJ, Davidson JA, Scott HF. Validation of the vasoactive-inotropic score in pediatric sepsis. Pediatr Crit Care Med. 2017;18(8):750–7.
29. Brown SM, Lanspa MJ, Jones JP, Kuttler KG, Li Y, Carlson R, et al. Survival after shock requiring high-dose vasopressor therapy. Chest. 2013;143(3):664–71.
30. Kotecha A, Vallabhajosyula S, Coville HH, Kashani K. Cardiorenal syndrome in sepsis: a narrative review. J Crit Care. 2018;43:122–7.
31. Keegan MT, Gajic O, Afessa B. Comparison of APACHE III, APACHE IV, SAPS 3, and MPM0III and influence of resuscitation status on model performance. Chest. 2012;142(4):851–8.
32. Johnson AE, Kramer AA, Clifford GD. A new severity of illness scale using a subset of Acute Physiology And Chronic Health Evaluation data elements shows comparable predictive accuracy. Crit Care Med. 2013;41(7):1711–8.
33. Aakre C, Franco PM, Ferreyra M, Kitson J, Li M, Herasevich V. Prospective validation of a near real-time EHR-integrated automated SOFA score calculator. Int J Med Inform. 2017;103:1–6.
34. Rhodes A, Evans LE, Alhazzani W, Levy MM, Antonelli M, Ferrer R, et al. Surviving Sepsis Campaign: international guidelines for management of sepsis and septic shock: 2016. Intensive Care Med. 2017;43(3):304–77.
35. Russell JA, Walley KR, Singer J, Gordon AC, Hebert PC, Cooper DJ, et al. Vasopressin versus norepinephrine infusion in patients with septic shock. N Engl J Med. 2008;358(9):877–87.

19

Effects of the timing of administration of IgM- and IgA-enriched intravenous polyclonal immunoglobulins on the outcome of septic shock patients

Giorgio Berlot[1*], Michele Claudio Vassallo[2], Nicola Busetto[1], Margarita Nieto Yabar[1], Tatiana Istrati[1], Silvia Baronio[1], Giada Quarantotto[1], Mattia Bixio[2], Giulia Barbati[3], Roberto Dattola[1], Irene Longo[1], Antonino Chillemi[1], Alice Scamperle[1], Fulvio Iscra[1] and Ariella Tomasini[1]

Abstract

Background: The administration of endovenous immunoglobulins in patients with septic shock could be beneficial and preparations enriched with IgA and IgM (ivIgGAM) seem to be more effective than those containing only IgG. In a previous study Berlot et al. demonstrated that early administration of ivIgGAM was associated with lower mortality rate. We studied a larger population of similar patients aiming either to confirm or not this finding considering also the subgroup of patients with septic shock by multidrug-resistant (MDR) pathogens.

Methods: Adult patients with septic shock in intensive care unit (ICU) treated with ivIgGAM from August 1999 to December 2016 were retrospectively examined. Collected data included the demographic characteristics of the patients, the diagnosis at admission, SOFA, SAPS II and Murray Lung Injury Score (LIS), characteristics of the primary infection, the adequacy of antimicrobial therapy, the delay of administration of ivIgGAM from the ICU admission and the outcome at the ICU discharge. Parametric and nonparametric tests and logistic regression were used for statistic analysis.

Results: During the study period 107 (30%) of the 355 patients died in ICU. Survivors received the ivIgGAM earlier than nonsurvivors (median delay 12 vs 14 h), had significantly lower SAPS II, SOFA and LIS at admission and a lower rate of MDR- and fungal-related septic shock. The appropriateness of the administration of antibiotics was similar in survivors and nonsurvivors (84 vs 79%, respectively, p: n.s). The delay in the administration of ivIgGAM from the admission was associated with in-ICU mortality (odds ratio per 1-h increase = 1.0055, 95% CI 1.003–1.009, $p < 0.001$), independently of SAPS II, LIS, cultures positive for MDR pathogens or fungi and onset of septic shock. Only 46 patients (14%) had septic shock due to MDR pathogens; 21 of them (46%) died in ICU. Survivors had significantly lower SAPS II, SOFA at admission and delay in administration of ivIgGAM than nonsurvivors (median delay 18 vs 66 h). Even in this subgroup the delay in the administration of ivIgGAM from the admission was associated with an increased risk of in-ICU mortality (odds ratio 1.007, 95% CI 1.0006–1.014, $p = 0.048$), independently of SAPS II.

Conclusions: Earlier administration of ivIgGAM was associated with decreased risk of in-ICU mortality both in patients with septic shock caused by any pathogens and in patients with MDR-related septic shock.

Keywords: Severe sepsis, Septic shock, Immunoglobulins, IgM, Multiple drug resistance, Intensive care unit

*Correspondence: berlot@inwind.it
[1] Department of Anesthesia, Resuscitation and Pain Therapy, Cattinara Hospital, University of Trieste, Strada di Fiume 447, 34149 Trieste, Italy
Full list of author information is available at the end of the article

Background

In the last few years it became clear that septic shock can occur in two different forms: the first is characterized by an excessive pro-inflammatory response due to the interaction between the host and the infecting germ whereas the other is associated with the progressive exhaustion of both the innate and adaptive immune system; the consequent decrease in the number of B-cells and of the production of immunoglobulins (Ig) often leads to secondary infections which can negatively affect the clinical outcome [1, 2]. The role of endogenous Ig has been enlightened by a number of investigations which demonstrated that (a) the concentrations of different classes of Ig were decreased both in community- and ICU-acquired septic shock; and that (b) these findings were associated with a greater vasopressor requirement, higher incidence of ARDS and increased mortality [3–5]. The protective effects of Ig are ascribed to their pleiotropic actions, including the enhancement of bacterial and viral clearance, the decreased synthesis of several pro-inflammatory cytokines and the scavenging of apoptotic cells [6].

Despite a better knowledge of their mechanisms of action and some meta-analyses demonstrating that (a) the administration of polyclonal intravenous Ig (ivIg) was associated with an improved outcome in septic patients; and (b) this effect was more marked when the preparation used in the trial contained increased amount of IgA and IgM (12% each one) (ivIgGAM) [7–10], the previous as well as the current guidelines of the Surviving Sepsis Campaign (SSC) recommend against their use; this statement is based on either the lack of randomized clinical trials (RCT) satisfying the evidence-based medicine (EBM) standards and to the different composition of the ivIg used [11]. Independently by the SSC, not only the ivIgGAM are widely used but a new preparation containing almost double concentrations of IgM (~23%) and IgA (~21%) has been developed whose use has been associated with an improved survival in patients with community-acquired pneumonia enrolled in a recent RCT (CIGMA) [12]; noteworthy, this effect was more marked in patients with baseline elevated levels of C-reactive protein, low levels of IgM or a combination of these abnormalities, possibly indicating a subset of patients who could take the maximal advantage from this approach.

The beneficial effect of IgM could be ascribed to its pentameric structure, including the neutralization of exo- and endotoxins, the enhancement of opsonization and phagocytosis and the increased bacterial lysis obtained via the activation of the alternative pathway of the complement system [12–21]; moreover, besides these anti-infective actions, IgM molecules have also some immunomodulatory effects such as the scavenging of excessive complement factors and the blunting of the production of some sepsis mediators [22].

As in a previous study Berlot et al. [23] demonstrated that in a group of severe sepsis and septic shock patients survivors were given ivIgGAM earlier than nonsurvivors and that each 24-h delay was associated with > 2% increase in the mortality rate, we studied a much larger population of similar patients aiming either to confirm or not this finding considering also the site of infection and the responsible germs.

Patients and methods

The hospital pharmacy provided names of all patients with septic shock admitted in the intensive care unit (ICU) of the University of Trieste since August 1999 to December 2016 and treated with ivIgGAM (Pentaglobin®; Biotest, Dreieich, Germany). The medical records of these patients were retrospectively examined except for patients who died within 24 h from admission in ICU and patients who did not meet SEPSIS 3 criteria for septic shock [24] (see flowchart Fig. 1). As ivIgGAM are routinely used in our ICU, the study did not imply any active intervention other than the standard medical care, so that the local Ethical committee deemed the patients' informed consent unnecessary. Critically ill adult patients with trauma, medical and surgical critical illnesses are admitted in this ICU, whereas patients with noncomplicated acute cardiac diseases and following cardiac surgery are treated in another department; pediatric and obstetric patients are admitted to another hospital.

The overall treatment was based on the SSC guidelines [11]. In particular in our ICU, the antimicrobial therapy was and is currently based on local guidelines which are periodically updated according to the microbiological reports; low-dose steroids at a dose not exceeding 200 mg/day were administered in patients not responding

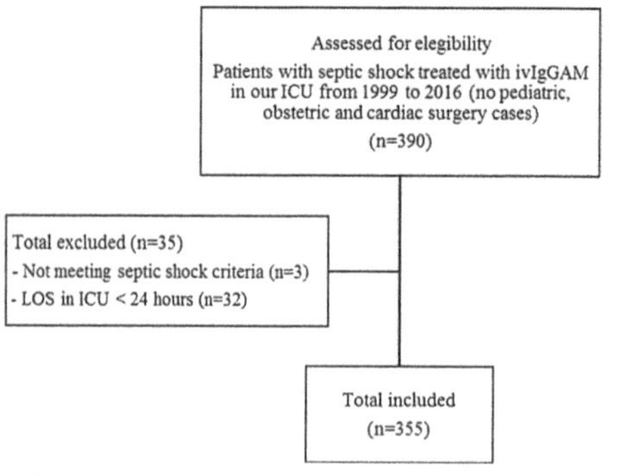

Fig. 1 Flowchart with inclusion and exclusion criteria. ivIgGAM, intravenous IgM- and IgA-enriched immunoglobulins; ICU intensive care unit; LOS length of stay

to fluids and vasoactive drugs. According to the international guidelines, fluids were administered respecting 3-h bundles. As an adjunctive treatment, every patient received the selective digestive tract decontamination (SDD) for the whole length of stay in ICU associated with iv cefotaxime for the initial 3 days. Oral and rectal swabs were obtained at admission and twice a week subsequently. Patients with a life expectancy < 3 months, with known immune depression (i.e., AIDS, acute leukemia.) and/or treated with immunosuppressant agents were not included in the study.

Septic shock was considered to be caused by MDR bacteria when cultures obtained within 12 h from the diagnosis were positive for at least one of the following: methicillin-resistant *Staphylococcus aureus* (MRSA), methicillin-resistant *Staphylococcus epidermidis* (MRSE), extended-spectrum beta-lactamase (ESBL)-producing *Enterococcus faecium,* vancomycin-resistant Enterococci (VRE), multidrug-resistant *Acinetobacter,* ESBL-producing Enterobacteriaceae, carbapenem-resistant Enterobacteriaceae and multidrug-resistant *Pseudomonas.*

The ivIgGAM were administered as adjunctive therapy at the dose of 250 mg/kg/day; the infusion lasted 10 h and was repeated for 3 days (total dose 750 mg/kg), according to the manufacturer's indications.

Collected data included the demographic characteristics of the patients (age and sex), the type of admission (surgical or medical admission), the diagnosis at admission, the SOFA score calculated the first day of administration of ivIgGAM (SOFA D1), the SAPS II score, the Murray Lung Injury Score (LIS), the site of occurrence of septic shock, which was considered ICU-acquired when it occurred $\geq$ 48 h after the admission, the primary site of infection, the antibiotics administered and their adequacy, the microorganisms isolated within 12 h from the diagnosis, the interval elapsing from the ICU admission and the first administration of ivIgGAM, the LOS_{ICU} and the outcome at the ICU discharge. The goal of the study was to estimate the effect of the timing of administration of ivIgGAM on in-ICU mortality in patients with septic shock caused either by antibiotic-sensible or MDR pathogens. Since it was not aimed to compare the effectiveness of different treatments, it was not necessary to identify a control group.

To assess these relationships, initial descriptive comparisons between survivors and nonsurvivors at discharge from ICU were carried out. Continuous variables were described by median and interquartile range and compared with the Wilcoxon–Mann–Whitney test (and the ANOVA test in case of ivIgGAM delay, in order to compare also the means), whereas categorical variables were described by absolute and relative frequencies and compared with the χ^2 test and the z score for proportions. Then, univariable logistic regression models were estimated for each parameter and subsequently a multivariable logistic regression model was build; we selected the final subset of predictors by means of a backward conditional step-wise procedure starting from the list of variables that resulted to be significantly associated with the outcome at univariable analyses. The Hosmer–Lemeshow test was used to assess the goodness of fit of estimated models. A p value < 0.05 was considered significant. Finally, the prediction accuracy of the multivariable regression model was evaluated by means of a Receiver Operating Characteristic (ROC) curve and the Area Under the Curve (AUC) was compared with that of the ROC curves of any of the parameters used in the model using the De Long test. The same analyses were applied to the subset of patients with septic shock caused by MDR bacteria, considering at univariable analysis a significant p value < 0.10 due to the small sample size, but maintaining at multivariable analysis a cutoff of p value < 0.05. To evaluate whether the effect of the early administration of ivIgGAM on the outcome had significant interactions with some of the most relevant patient's characteristics, we performed further subgroup analyses. Variables considered were: the primary site of infection, the result of the cultures and the SOFA score, as a patient severity index.

All statistical computations were calculated using the R statistical package, software version 3.3.3.

Results

During the considered period 355 patients met the inclusion criteria: 107 of them (30%) died in ICU. All patients received the first dose of empirical antimicrobial therapy within 2 h from septic shock diagnosis. Cultures were positive in 264 patients (74%) (in particular 201 cases reported positive blood cultures) and negative in 58 (17%). In 33 patients (9%) cultures within 12 h from the diagnosis were not obtained. The most frequently isolated microorganisms were: Escherichia coli (91 cases), Enterococcus faecium (36), Klebsiella pneumoniae (27), methicillin-sensitive Staphylococcus aureus (26), Enterococcus faecalis (25), MRSA (22), Pseudomonas aeruginosa (18). The median of the delay in the administration of ivIgGAM from the admission in ICU was 12 h (interquartile range 3-39). Even if the median value of delay was not significantly different between survivors and nonsurvivors at the Wilcoxon–Mann–Whitney test, the mean value was different (respectively, 36 vs 66 h, $p = 0.002$, ANOVA test) indicating a higher mean delay in the nonsurvivor group. The survivors had significantly lower SAPS II, SOFA and LIS score at admission and a lower rate of MDR-related septic shock. The distribution per year of enrollment was similar in the two groups

(Table 1). The univariable logistic regression showed a statistically significant association between the timing in the administration of ivIgGAM and the outcome (Table 2). The other variables significantly related to a higher risk of dying in ICU were higher SAPS II, SOFA D1 and LIS and cultures positive for MDR bacteria or fungi. We verified that the year of enrollment was not a confounding factor because this variable did not influence the mortality (Table 2).

The multivariable analysis showed that the association between the delay in the administration of ivIgGAM and the outcome was independent from the other variables taken into account (for each 24-hour increase adjusted OR 1.15, CI 95% 1.05-1.27, $p=0.0005$) (Table 3), Hosmer and Lemeshow test p value $=0.20$. Put differently, in a patient with median SAPS II and median SOFA D1, without fungal infections, a 24-hour delay in ivIgGAM administration from the admission resulted in roughly a 2% increase in the probability of dying during his ICU stay. The estimated effect of delay in administration of ivIgGAM on the probability of in-ICU death is represented in Fig. 2 using the corresponding logit function

Table 1 Characteristics of the studied patients subdivided into Survivors and Nonsurvivors at discharge from ICU

	All patients (355)	Survivors (248)	Nonsurvivors (107)	*p* Value
Age (years)	68 (57-74)	68 (57–74)	70 (58–76)	0.27
Sex				0.197
Female	151 (42.54%)	111 (44.8%)	40 (37.4%)	
Male	204 (57.46%)	137 (55.2%)	67 (62.6%)	
SAPS II	53 (45–62)	51 (43–58)	57 (49–69)	<0.001
SOFA D1	11 (9–13)	10 (8–12)	12 (11–14)	<0.001
Murray Lung Injury Score	3 (1–5)	3 (1–5)	4 (3–6)	<0.001
Type of admission				0.052
Surgical	264 (74.8%)	192 (77.7%)	77 (67.9%)	
Medical	89 (25.2%)	55 (22.3%)	34 (32.1%)	
Onset of septic shock				0.08
Extra ICU	265 (75.07%)	179 (72.5%)	86 (81.1%)	
Intra-ICU	88 (24.93%)	68 (27.5%)	20 (18.9%)	
Primary site of infection				<0.001
Abdomen	198 (55.77%)	150 (60.5%)	48 (44.9%)	$p=0.006$
Skin	27 (7.61%)	15 (6.0%)	12 (11.2%)	
Bloodstream	11 (3.1%)	6 (2.4%)	5 (4.7%)	
Not identified	19 (5.35%)	11 (4.4%)	8 (7.5%)	
Lungs	64 (18.03%)	33 (13.3%)	31 (29.0%)	$p<0.001$
Urinary tract	31 (8.73%)	28 (11.3%)	3 (2.8%)	$p=0.018$
Central nervous system	5 (1.41%)	5 (2.0%)	0 (0.0%)	
Adequacy of antimicrobial therapy				0.26
No	45 (17%)	28 (15%)	17 (21%)	
Yes	219 (83%)	155 (84%)	64 (79%)	
MDR bacteria				0.01
Absent	277 (85.76%)	202 (89%)	75 (78.1%)	
Present	46 (14.24%)	25 (11%)	21 (21.9%)	
Fungi				0.014
Absent	262 (81.11%)	192 (84.6%)	70 (72.9%)	
Present	61 (18.89%)	35 (15.4%)	26 (27.1%)	
Length of stay (days)	10 (6–17)	11 (6–17)	9 (3–17)	0.019
Year of enrollment	2011 (2008–2013)	2011 (2008–2013)	2011 (2008–2013)	0.57
Delay in ivIgGAM administration from admission in ICU (hours)	12 (3–39)	12 (3–33)	14 (3–66)	0.22

Variables are medians (interquartile range) or absolute frequencies (relative frequencies)

ivIgGAM Intravenous IgM- and IgA-enriched immunoglobulins; *ICU* intensive care unit; *MDR* multidrug resistant; *SAPS II* Simplified Acute Physiology Score; *SOFA D1*, sequential organ failure assessment calculated the first day of administration of ivIgGAM

Table 2 Univariable logistic regression analyses of risk factors for in-ICU mortality

	OR	95% CI	*p* Value
Age	1.004	0.98–1.02	0.62
Sex (male)	1.36	0.86–2.17	0.198
SAPS II	1.046	1.028–1.065	< 0.001
SOFA D1	1.24	1.15–1.35	< 0.001
Murray Lung Injury Score	1.14	1.04–1.24	0.003
Onset of septic shock (Intra-ICU)	0.61	0.34–1.06	0.08
Type of admission (Surgical)	0.607	0.37–1.006	0.053
MDR bacteria	2.26	1.18–4.28	0.01
Fungi	2.037	1.14–3.62	0.01
Year of enrollment	0.97	0.91–1.023	0.253
Adequacy of antimicrobial therapy	0.68	0.348–1.328	0.259
Delay in ivIgGAM administration from admission in ICU	1.0039	1.0013–1.0066	0.0035

ivIgGAM Intravenous IgM- and IgA-enriched immunoglobulins; *ICU* intensive care unit; *MDR* multidrug resistant; *SAPS II* Simplified Acute Physiology Score; *SOFA D1* sequential organ failure assessment calculated the first day of administration of ivIgGAM

Table 3 Multivariable logistic regression analysis of risk factors for in-ICU mortality

	OR	95% CI	*p* Value
SAPS II	1.04	1.018–1.06	< 0.001
SOFA D1	1.15	1.052–1.27	0.003
Fungi	2.21	1.17–4.18	0.015
Delay in ivIgGAM administration from admission in ICU	1.006	1.003–1.009	< 0.001

ivIgGAM Intravenous IgM- and IgA-enriched immunoglobulins; *ICU* intensive care unit; *SAPS II* Simplified Acute Physiology Score; *SOFA D1* sequential organ failure assessment calculated the first day of administration of ivIgGAM

estimated from the multivariable logistic regression model, adjusted to median value of SAPS II, SOFA D1 and without fungal infection (these values were chosen as the most representative values in this population). As shown in Fig. 2, since the relationship between the delay in drug administration and the risk of death in ICU appeared linear, it is not possible to identify an optimal cutoff, as survival progressively increases with the precociousness of drug administration.

The ROC curve obtained from the model showed an AUC of 0.75 with 95% CI 0.69–0.81, significantly higher than the univariable logistic models considering SAPS II, SOFA D1 and fungal infection ($p < 0.001$) (Fig. 3).

During the study period only 46 patients (14%) met the diagnosis of septic shock due to MDR bacteria and 21 of them (46%) died in ICU (Additional file 1). The most frequently isolated MDR microorganisms were: MRSA (45.6%) and Escherichia coli ESBL (21.7%). In this group of patients also an earlier administration of ivIgGAM was associated with a better outcome (see Additional file 1).

Finally, we evaluated the effect of the timing of administration of ivIgGAM on death in ICU in different subgroups. In the subgroup with pulmonary infection (64 patients), univariable analysis did not show a statistically significant association between delay in ivIgGAM administration and mortality ($p = 0.557$). In the remaining cases the correlation was significant ($p = 0.001$). We also analyzed the subgroup of patients with abdominal infection (198 patients): in this group the relationship between the delay of ivIgGAM administration and the risk of death in ICU was statistically significant ($p = 0.008$).

Considering the results of the cultures, the sample was divided into two subgroups: patients with positive cultures within 12 h from the diagnosis of septic shock (264) and patients with negative cultures (58). In this analysis, patients in whom the cultures were not performed within 12 h (33) were not taken into consideration. In the subgroup of patients with positive cultures, the delay in administration of ivIgGAM from admission in ICU remained significantly correlated with the risk of death at both univariable ($p = 0.001$) and multivariable analysis ($p < 0.001$). In the subgroup of patients with negative cultures, this correlation was not confirmed ($p = 0.994$), but the small size of the sample should be taken into account.

To assess if the relationship between the timing of ivIgGAM administration and death in ICU depended on severity, the sample was divided into two subgroups according to the median value of the SOFA score of the first day of administration of ivIgGAM (SOFA score median value = 11, see Table 1).

At univariable analyses, the relationship was less statistically significant in the subgroup with SOFA score greater than the median (OR 1.004, $p = 0.05$), while it was highly significant in the subgroup with SOFA score lower than the median (OR 1.005, $p = 0.01$). At multivariable analyses the significance of the effect of early ivIgGAM administration was similar in the two subgroups (in both cases, $p <= 0.02$), even if the estimated effect was stronger in the less severe patients (see Additional file 1).

No adverse effects attributable to the ivIgGAM were observed.

Discussion

In septic shock the dysregulation of both arms of the immune system accounts for both the initial hyperinflammatory phase and for the subsequent shift toward a more advanced stage in which an immunoparalysis can dominate the clinical course, leading to secondary infections by MDR germs and to the reactivation of latent viruses [1, 25]. This cycle can recur several times during the ICU stay, thus leading to a chronic critical illness,

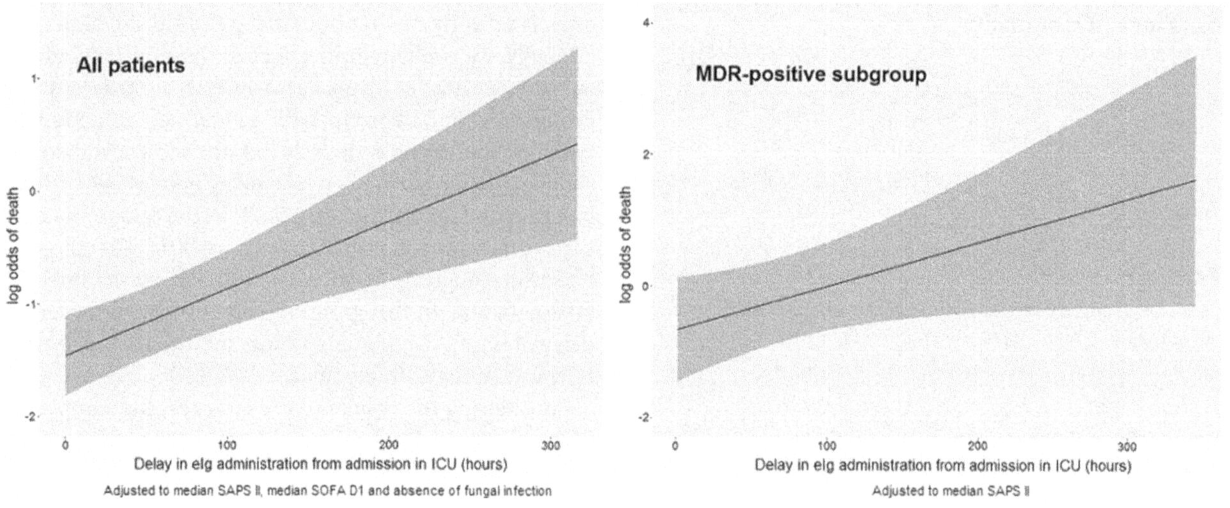

Fig. 2 Logit function from the multivariable logistic regression model in the group of all patients (right) showing the effect of delay in administration of IgM-enriched immunoglobulins on the probability of in-ICU death (solid line) with 95% confidence interval (gray area) adjusted to median value of SAPS II, SOFA D1 and without fungal infection. Comparison with logit functions from the multivariable logistic regression model for MDR-positive patients adjusted for median value of SAPS II (left). ivIgGAM, intravenous IgM- and IgA-enriched immunoglobulins; ICU, intensive care unit; MDR, multidrug resistant; SAPS II, Simplified Acute Physiology Score; SOFA D1, sequential organ failure assessment calculated the first day of administration of ivIgGAM

which is rather common among elderly patients affected by preexistent co-morbidities as well as in debilitated subjects of all ages [26, 27].

Currently, steroids and ivIg are the only immunomodulatory agents available, pending the results of several clinical trials with more innovative agents [28, 29]. However, it appears that what can be relatively beneficial in the initial stage of sepsis and septic shock, such as steroids, could be harmful in the following one [1, 29]; conversely, the ivIgGAM are suitable both in its early and in the advanced phase, due to their combined antibacterial and immunomodulatory properties [14–21]. The biological rationale for their administration can be found in the results of some studies demonstrating that not only low levels of IgG, IgM and IgA measured at the admission but also their failed increase during the ICU stay were associated with both the transition from severe sepsis to septic shock and with a reduced survival [30–32]; yet, despite these evidences, the role of ivIgGAM in the treatment of septic shock remains controversial notwithstanding their use began several decades ago.

Basically, supporters of ivIgGAM claim that (a) their dual action on the immune response make them valuable throughout the whole clinical course of sepsis and septic shock and that (b) their positive effect on the outcome has been confirmed by a number of meta-analyses [7–10]. On the other front, opponents reply that the clinical studies published so far suffer from such an elevated heterogeneity of patients and of preparations used, so that it is impossible to draw definite conclusion from their results [13]. Despite these biases, the ivIgGAM are widely used and the German guidelines for the treatment of sepsis [33] suggest considering their administration in septic shock patients while they discourage the use of ivIg. Therefore, it appears that more data about the clinical use of ivIgGAM are keenly needed. The results of this study not only confirm some investigations but also add further information.

First, although there was a small difference in the timing of administration of ivIgGAM between S and NS, their early administration influenced the outcome; actually, a time effect has been demonstrated previously by Berlot et al. [23] who reported a 3% increase in mortality for every 24 h of delay and by Cavazzuti et al. [34] who demonstrated a reduced mortality rate in septic shock patients treated with ivIgGAM within 24 h after shock onset. This finding recalls what has been reported in other investigations, which demonstrated an increase in mortality for each hour of delay in the administration of antibiotic [35–37]. The positive effect of ivIgGAM on the outcome persisted across the whole period of the study and was independent of other variations of the overall treatment. As shown by subgroup analyses, the benefit of early ivIgGAM administration appears to be more intense in clinically less severe patients, as already reported in the literature [38] and greater for abdominal primary site of infection. This time effect appears to be independent from the adequacy of the antibiotic therapy

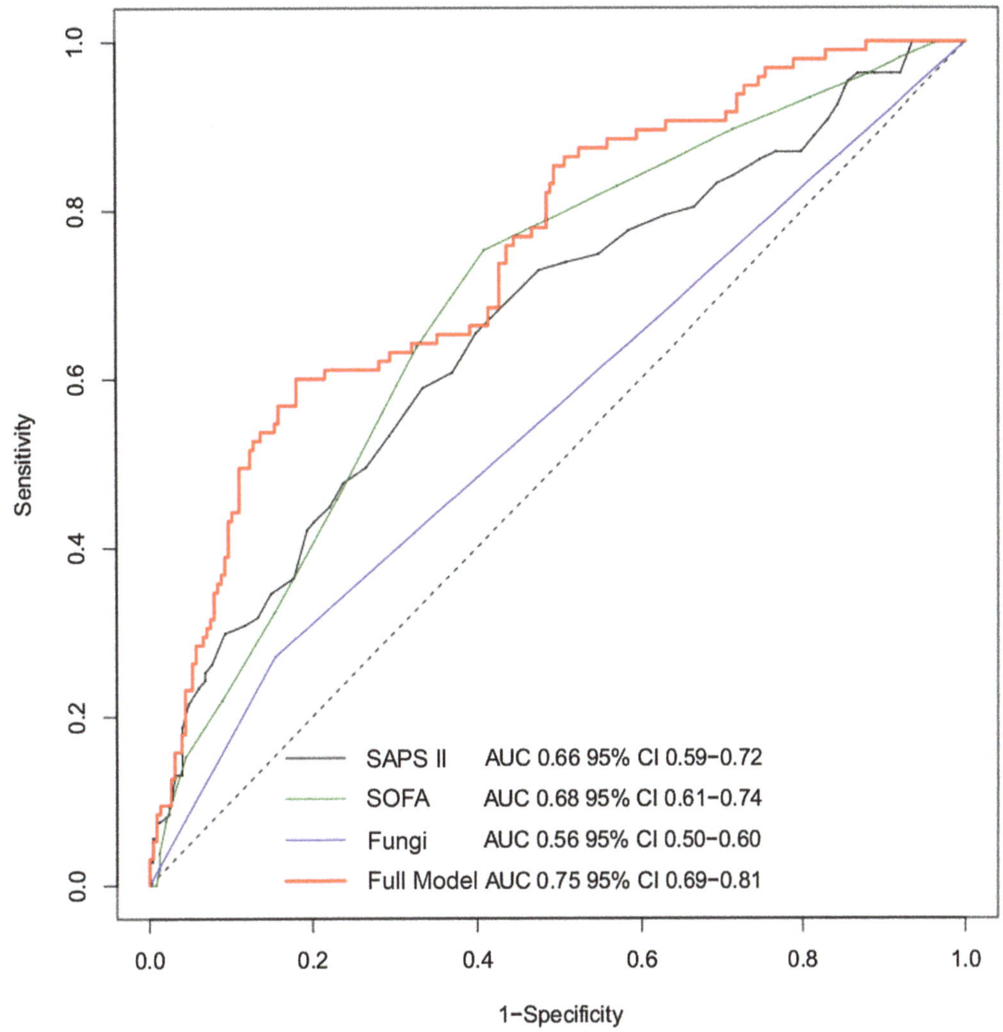

Fig. 3 ROC curves comparing the predictive accuracy of the multivariable regression model (red curve) for all patients with each parameter used in the model: SAPS II (gray curve), SOFA D1 (green curve) and fungal infection (blue curve). SAPS II, Simplified Acute Physiology Score; SOFA, sequential organ failure assessment calculated the first day of administration of ivIgGAM

since this latter variable did not differ among the two groups.

Second, this "time window effect" was present also in the group of patients whose infections were caused by a wide array of MDR pathogens. Although the timing of ivIgGAM administration was not specifically addressed in their studies, also Busani [39] and Giamarellos [40] demonstrated an increased survival in MDR germs-related septic shock treated with ivIgGAM as compared with the control group. However, it is worthwhile to remark that (a) the rate of MDR infections in our population was considerably lower than the one reported in these studies and that (b) since only 1 out of 3 cases of MDR-related septic shock was ICU-acquired, it is possible that the administration of ivIgGAM in patients already admitted to the ICU prevented their colonization and subsequent infection with these germs. Then, it is hypothesizable that in the acute phase the ivIgGAM could act by increasing the bacterial clearance and reducing the hyperinflammatory reaction while in the later one they could contribute to restore the compromised immune capabilities by replenishing the IgM and IgA stores.

Our study has some limitations, including (a) the absence of the EBM criteria such as the randomization of the patients and their prolonged time of enrollment and lack of validation of the results in an independent cohort; however, as stated by some authors [29, 41] the past issues of the SSC guidelines contained several recommendations derived from the results of EBM- based

RCTs that were not confirmed by subsequent studies and were removed later on; (b) the lack of a biological marker, such as the measurement of the blood levels of CRP and PCT and/or IgG, IgM and IgA suited to trigger the administration of ivIgGAM; actually, this reflects the real-world scenario because the results of these and other tests evaluating the immune capability are not universally available and, more important, what is a "safe" concentration of endogenous IgM and IgA in septic shock patients is not clear [13]; (c) due to the wide time span of the study, we could not establish precisely the rate of the appropriate antimicrobial treatment; however, as antibiotics were given according to the yearly updated hospital guidelines based on the local microbiological findings, we guess that it was evenly distributed among survivors and deceased patients.

Conclusions

In our experience, the administration of ivIgGAM was safe and well tolerated. Overall, survivors were treated earlier than nonsurvivors and this finding was present also in patients with MDR-associated septic shock, a specific sepsis population with high mortality risk.

In the perspective of personalized medicine, further studies and particularly RCTs are needed to identify the characteristics of the best septic shock candidate to receive ivIgGAM as adjunctive treatment. Our study contributes by showing the potential effect of the time factor on the effectiveness of ivIgGAM.

Abbreviations

AUC: area under the curve; ICU: intensive care unit; ivIg: polyclonal intravenous immunoglobulins; ivIgGAM: intravenous IgM- and IgA-enriched immunoglobulins; Ig: immunoglobulins; LIS: Murray Lung Injury Score; MDR: multidrug resistant; MRSA: methicillin-resistant *Staphylococcus aureus*; MRSE: methicillin-resistant *Staphylococcus epidermidis*; SBL: extended-spectrum beta-lactamase; VRE: vancomycin-resistant Enterococci; SAPS II: Simplified Acute Physiology Score; SDD: selective digestive tract decontamination; SOFA: sequential organ failure assessment; ROC: receiver operating characteristic.

Authors' contributions

GB (the corresponding author) contributed substantially to the conception and design of the study, wrote the manuscript and provided reference articles. MCV, NB, MNY, TI, MB, RD, IL, AC, AS, FI and AT participated in the data collection. SB and GQ participated in the data collection and contributed to the writing of the manuscript. GB made the statistical analysis and contributed to the drafting of the statistical section of the article. All authors read and approved the final manuscript.

Author details

[1] Department of Anesthesia, Resuscitation and Pain Therapy, Cattinara Hospital, University of Trieste, Strada di Fiume 447, 34149 Trieste, Italy. [2] Department of Anesthesia and Intensive Care, San Martino Hospital, Largo Rosanna Benzi 10, 16132 Genoa, Italy. [3] Biostatistics Unit, Department of Medicine, Surgery and Health Sciences, Cattinara Hospital, University of Trieste, Strada di Fiume 447, 34149 Trieste, Italy.

Acknowledgements

Not applicable.

Competing interests

The authors declare that they have no competing interests.

Funding

No source of funding for the research reported has to be declared.

References

1. Boomer JS, Green JM, Hotchkiss RS. The changing immune system in sepsis: is individualized immuno-modulatory therapy the answer? Virulence. 2014;5:45–56.
2. van Vught LA, Klein Klouwenberg PM, Spitoni C, et al. Incidence, risk factors, and attributable mortality of secondary infections in the intensive care unit after admission for sepsis. JAMA. 2016;315:1469–79.
3. Venet F, Gebeile R, Bancel J, et al. Assessment of plasmatic immunoglobulin G, A and M levels in septic shock patients. Int Immunopharmacol. 2011;11:2086–90.
4. Taccone FS, Stordeur P, De Backer D, et al. Gamma-globulin levels in patients with community-acquired septic shock. Shock. 2009;32:379–85.
5. Myrianthefs PM, Boutzouka E, Baltopoulos GJ. Gamma-globulin levels in patients with community-acquired septic shock. Shock. 2010;33:556–7.
6. Späth PJ. Structure and Function of Immunoglobulins. Sepsis. 1999;3:197–218.
7. Pildal J, Gøtzsche PC. Polyclonal immunoglobulin for treatment of bacterial sepsis: a systematic review. Clin Infect Dis. 2004;39:38–46.
8. Laupland KB, Kirkpatrick AW, Delaney A. Polyclonal intravenous immunoglobulin for the treatment of severe sepsis and septic shock in critically ill adults: a systematic review and meta-analysis. Crit Care Med. 2007;35:2686–92.
9. Turgeon AF, Hutton B, Fergusson DA, et al. Meta-analysis: intravenous immunoglobulin in critically ill adult patients with sepsis. Ann Intern Med. 2007;146:193–203.
10. Kreymann KG, de Heer G, Nierhaus A, et al. Use of polyclonal immunoglobulins as adjunctive therapy for sepsis or septic shock. Crit Care Med. 2007;35:2677–8.
11. Rhodes A, Evans LE, Alhazzani W, et al. Surviving sepsis campaign: international guidelines for management of sepsis and septic shock: 2016. Crit Care Med. 2017;45:486–552.
12. Welte T, Dellinger RP, Ebelt H, et al. Efficacy and safety of trimodulin, a novel polyclonal antibody preparation, in patients with severe community-acquired pneumonia: a randomized, placebo-controlled, double-blind, multicenter, phase II trial (CIGMA study). Intens Care Med. 2018;44:438–48.
13. Almansa R, Tamayo E, Andaluz-Ojeda D, et al. The original sins of clinical trials with intravenous immunoglobulins in sepsis. Crit Care. 2015;19:90.
14. Esen F, Tugrul S. IgM-enriched Immunoglobulins in Sepsis. In: Vincent JL, editor. Intensive Care Medicine, vol. 2009., Annual UpdateNY: New York; 2009. p. 102–10.
15. Trautmann M, Held TK, Susa M, et al. Bacterial lipopolysaccharide (LPS)-specific antibodies in commercial human immunoglobulin preparations: superior antibody content of an IgM-enriched product. Clin Exp Immunol. 1998;111:81–90.
16. Garbett ND, Munro CS, Cole PJ. Opsonic activity of a new intravenous immunoglobulin preparation: pentaglobin compared with Sandoglobulin. Clin Exp Immunol. 1989;76:8–12.

17. Walpen AJ, Laumonier T, Aebi C, et al. Immunoglobulin M-enriched intravenous immunoglobulin inhibits classical pathway complement activation, but not bactericidal activity of human serum. Xenotransplantation. 2004;11:141–8.
18. Ehrenstein MR, Notley CA. The importance of natural IgM: scavenger, protector and regulator. Nat Rev Immunol. 2010;10:778–86.
19. Shankar-Hari M, Spencer J, Sewell WA, et al. Bench-to-bedside review: immunoglobulin therapy for sepsis–biological plausibility from a critical care perspective. Crit Care. 2012;16:206.
20. Rossmann FS, Kropec A, Laverde D, et al. In vitro and in vivo activity of hyperimmune globulin preparations against multiresistant nosocomial pathogens. Infection. 2015;43:169–75.
21. Stehr SN, Knels L, Weissflog C, et al. Effects of IgM-enriched solution on polymorphonuclear neutrophil function, bacterial clearance, and lung histology in endotoxemia. Shock. 2008;29:167–72.
22. Rieben R, Roos A, Muizert Y, et al. Immunoglobulin M-enriched human intravenous immunoglobulin prevents complement activation in vitro and in vivo in a rat model of acute inflammation. Blood. 1999;93:942–51.
23. Berlot G, Vassallo MC, Busetto N, et al. Relationship between the timing of administration of IgM and IgA enriched immunoglobulins in patients with severe sepsis and septic shock and the outcome: a retrospective analysis. J Crit Care. 2012;27:167–71.
24. Singer M, Deutschmann CS, Seymour CW, et al. The 3rd international consensus definitions for sepsis and septic shock. JAMA. 2016;315:801–10.
25. Hotchkiss RS, Monneret G, Payen D. Sepsis-induced immunosuppression: from cellular dysfunctions to immunotherapy. Nat Rev Immunol. 2013;13:862–74.
26. Mira JC, Gentile LF, Mathias BJ, et al. Sepsis pathophysiology, chronic critical illness, and persistent inflammation-immunosuppression and catabolism syndrome. Crit Care Med. 2017;45:253–62.
27. Gentile LF, Cuenca AG, Efron PA, et al. Persistent inflammation and immunosuppression: a common syndrome and new horizon for surgical intensive care. J Trauma Acute Care Surg. 2012;72:1491–501.
28. Cohen J, Vincent JL, Adhikari NK, et al. Sepsis: a roadmap for future research. Lancet Infect Dis. 2015;15:581–614.
29. Vincent JL. Individual gene expression and personalised medicine in sepsis. Lancet Respir Med. 2016;4:242–3.
30. Giamarellos-Bourboulis EJ, Apostolidou E, Lada M, et al. Kinetics of circulating immunoglobulin M in sepsis: relationship with final outcome. Crit Care. 2013;17:R247.
31. Bermejo-Martin JF, Giamarellos-Bourboulis EJ. Endogenous immunoglobulins and sepsis: new perspectives for guiding replacement therapies. Int J Antimicrob Agents. 2015;46:S25–8.
32. Bermejo-Martín JF, Rodriguez-Fernandez A, Herrán-Monge R, et al. Immunoglobulins IgG1, IgM and IgA: a synergistic team influencing survival in sepsis. J Intern Med. 2014;276:404–12.
33. Reinhart K, Brunkhorst FM, Bone HG, et al. Prevention, diagnosis, therapy and follow-up care of sepsis: 1st revision of S-2k guidelines of the German Sepsis Society (Deutsche Sepsis-Gesellschaft e.V. (DSG)) and the German Interdisciplinary Association of Intensive Care and Emergency Medicine (Deutsche Interdisziplinäre Vereinigung für Intensiv- und Notfallmedizin (DIVI)). Ger Med Sci. 2010;8:Doc14.
34. Cavazzuti I, Serafini G, Busani S, et al. Early therapy with IgM-enriched polyclonal immunoglobulin in patients with septic shock. Intensive Care Med. 2014;40:1888–96.
35. Kumar A, Roberts D, Wood KE, et al. Duration of hypotension before initiation of effective antimicrobial therapy is the critical determinant of survival in human septic shock. Crit Care Med. 2006;34:1589–96.
36. Ferrer R, Martin-Loeches I, Phillips G, et al. Empiric antibiotic treatment reduces mortality in severe sepsis and septic shock from the first hour: results from a guideline-based performance improvement program. Crit Care Med. 2014;42:1749–55.
37. Seymour CW, Kahn JM, Martin-Gill C, et al. Delays From First Medical Contact to Antibiotic Administration for Sepsis. Crit Care Med. 2017;45:759–65.
38. Martin-Loeches I, Muriel-Bombìn A, Ferrer R, et al. The protective association of endogenous immunoglobulins against sepsis mortality is restricted to patients with moderate organ failure. Ann Intensive Care. 2017;7(1):44.
39. Busani S, Serafini G, Mantovani E, et al. Mortality in patients with septic shock by multidrug resistant bacteria: risk factors and impact of sepsis treatments. J Intensive Care Med. 2017.
40. Giamarellos-Bourboulis EJ, Tziolos N, Routsi C, et al. Improving outcomes of severe infections by multidrug-resistant pathogens with polyclonal IgM-enriched immunoglobulins. Clin Microbiol Infect. 2016;22:499–506.
41. Perner A, Myburgh J. Ten 'short-lived' beliefs in intensive care medicine. Intensive Care Med. 2015;41:1703–6.

Impact of individualized target mean arterial pressure for septic shock resuscitation on the incidence of acute kidney injury

Rajat N. Moman[1,2], Stuart A. Ostby[1,3], Abbasali Akhoundi[1,4], Rahul Kashyap[1,5] and Kianoush Kashani[1,4,6*]

Abstract

Background: To examine the relationship between delta mean arterial pressure (ΔMAP; MAP change between pre-admission minus post-resuscitation) and acute kidney injury (AKI) among patients with septic shock. In this retrospective, single-center cohort study of adult patients pre-admission MAP is defined as the median MAP recorded from 365 to 7 days before admission. Post-resuscitation MAP was median MAP during the 7th hour after initiating resuscitation.

Results: In our cohort ($N = 233$; 55% male), the median (interquartile range [IQR]) age was 71 (58–81) years and the median (IQR) acute physiology, age, chronic health evaluation (APACHE) III score was 81 (66–97). Although those in the lowest ΔMAP quartile (−24.5 to 3.9 mmHg) had no demographic differences compared with the rest of the cohort, the odds ratio for AKI was 0.26 (95% CI 0.11–0.57) after adjustment for other known AKI risk factors. Among patients with a history of hypertension, the lowest quartile had an odds ratio for AKI of 0.12 (95% CI 0.04–0.37) after adjusting for risk factors for AKI in this cohort.

Conclusions: The incidence of AKI was lowest among those whose post-resuscitation MAP was closest to or higher than their pre-admission MAP. Further study regarding the effect of targeting the pre-admission MAP for post-resuscitation on the incidence of AKI is warranted.

Keywords: Blood pressure target, Early goal-directed therapy, Fluid resuscitation, Hypertension, Severe sepsis

Background

Acute kidney injury (AKI) is a devastating sequela of critical illnesses [1]. Sepsis is a common pathway to AKI. The Surviving Sepsis Campaign Guidelines [2] recommend a mean arterial pressure (MAP) of 65 mmHg or higher as the goal of resuscitation (Grade 1C recommendation) to minimize the risk of death and end-organ failure. However, this recommendation is not supported by substantial evidence, and whether a goal MAP of 65 mmHg is adequate for all patients remains controversial [3, 4].

*Correspondence: kashani.kianoush@mayo.edu
[1] Multidisciplinary Epidemiology and Translational Research in Intensive Care (METRIC), Division of Pulmonary and Critical Care Medicine, Department of Medicine, Mayo Clinic, 200 First Street SW, Rochester, MN 55905, USA
Full list of author information is available at the end of the article

Sepsis-associated AKI (SA-AKI) is a common and clinically significant condition. Sepsis is associated with AKI in 42–48% of cases in the intensive care unit (ICU) [1, 5, 6]. Compared with other non-sepsis causes of AKI, SA-AKI is associated with higher ICU and in-hospital mortality rates [5]. Patients with severe sepsis and AKI had higher 90-day mortality rates than those with severe sepsis alone [7]. Patients with even a modest increase in serum creatinine (sCR) have markedly higher health care costs, hospital length of stay, and risk of death [8]. A critical need exists to determine optimal resuscitation strategies that prevent SA-AKI or its progression in patients with septic shock.

In a recent investigation, Asfar et al. [4] randomized patients with septic shock to high (80–85 mmHg) or low (65–70 mmHg) MAP targets and observed no difference in 28-day mortality rates between groups. A subset of 167 patients with chronic arterial hypertension had a lower incidence of sCR doubling and required less renal replacement therapy when randomized to the high MAP target group. However, the higher MAP target group also had a higher incidence of atrial fibrillation. Chronic arterial hypertension results in a rightward shift of the autoregulatory pressure-organ perfusion curve [9, 10]. Therefore, an increased MAP target may improve organ perfusion for patients with higher pre-admission MAP [3, 4, 11]. Given the results of previous studies, the pre-admission blood pressure of patients in septic shock may need to be considered when defining an appropriate MAP goal for optimal resuscitation [3, 4, 11–13].

Appropriate MAP targets for resuscitation are controversial, and previous studies suggest that the pre-admission blood pressure may help determine the optimal resuscitation MAP target. To date, no published studies have assessed whether patients would benefit from a specific post-resuscitation MAP target that is similar to or higher than the pre-admission MAP. We conducted a retrospective cohort study of patients who were treated for severe sepsis and septic shock. We examined the association between the achieved MAP target and the pre-admission MAP, and AKI incidence was the primary outcome.

Methods

Approval of study design

This retrospective cohort study was reviewed and approved by the Mayo Clinic Institutional Review Board (protocol number 14-002109). Informed consent was waived for patients who provided research authorization.

Participants

We conducted a study of adult patients (≥ 18 years old) who received care at a tertiary care academic hospital for severe sepsis or septic shock. Consecutive adult patients admitted to the Medical ICU from January 2007 through January 2009 were included in the study if their records included a history of noninvasive blood pressure monitoring. We excluded patients who developed AKI before sepsis and those with end-stage renal disease or receiving hemodialysis before sepsis. We also excluded patients who never had urine output measured with a Foley catheter, had a ureteral stent, were in the ICU for fewer than 6 h, or did not have sufficient clinical information available. In order to evaluate the impact ΔMAP on the AKI incidence, we excluded patients who met AKI criteria by oliguria during first 6 h of resuscitation.

Data collection

Patient demographics, pre-admission and post-resuscitation MAP, body mass index (BMI), baseline sCR from 6 months to 7 days prior to hospitalization, sCR during hospitalization, use of inotropic and vasoactive agents, fluid balance, preexisting conditions, and urine output were abstracted from the electronic health record. Charlson comorbidity index (CCI) [14], sequential organ failure assessment (SOFA) score [15], and acute physiology, age, chronic health evaluation (APACHE) III [16] scores at 24 h were calculated.

Study definitions

The pre-admission MAP was defined as the median of all MAPs recorded from 365 to 7 days before ICU admission. We chose the median because it was less likely to be skewed by an outlier MAP measurement compared to a mean value. By comparing the median and mean pre-admission MAPs of the cohort, we found the mean pre-admission MAP had a mean of 82.2 mmHg and standard deviation of 10.5 mmHg; the median pre-admission MAP had a mean of 81.5 mmHg and standard deviation of 10.8 mmHg (R^2 0.97, $p < .0001$). Post-resuscitation MAP was defined as the median of all MAPs during the 7th hour after initiation of sepsis resuscitation. This definition of post-resuscitation MAP was chosen because the goal of resuscitation is to have a stable blood pressure at the end of 6 h of treatment. The ΔMAP, as an independent variable, was defined as the pre-admission MAP minus the post-resuscitation MAP. Therefore, if the value of a patient's post-resuscitation MAP is higher than their pre-admission MAP, the ΔMAP would be negative. Conversely, if the value of their post-resuscitation MAP is lower than their pre-admission MAP, the ΔMAP would be positive. All MAPs before admission were determined from noninvasive blood pressure measures. The primary outcome, AKI, was defined by Kidney Disease Improving Global Outcomes criteria [17]. sCR and urine output (UOP) were used where: stage 1 was defined as sCR 1.5–1.9 times baseline or greater than or equal to 0.3 mg/dl increase, UOP < 0.5 cc/kg/h for 6–12 h; stage 2 defined as sCR 2.0–2.9 times baseline, UOP < 0.5 cc/kg/h for greater than or equal to 12 h; and stage 3 defined as sCR 3.0 times baseline or increase to greater than or equal to 4.0 or initiation of renal replacement therapy, UOP < 0.3 cc/kg/h for greater than or equal to 24 h or anuria for greater than or equal to 12 h.

Statistical analysis

Demographic data are shown as frequency count and percentage for categorical variables and median and interquartile range (IQR) for continuous variables.

Categorical variables were analyzed with the χ^2 test. ΔMAP was examined as a continuous variable and also by quartiles as a categorical variable, with comparisons made between the ΔMAP quartiles. Backward stepwise logistic regression analyses were performed. Odds ratios (ORs) and c-statistics were calculated. All p values $<.05$ in a 2-sided hypothesis were considered statistically significant. Statistical analyses were conducted with JMP software (version 10.0.0; SAS Institute Inc).

Results

We identified 651 patients with severe sepsis or septic shock during the study period. After exclusions, 233 patients were included in the final analysis (Fig. 1); the median (IQR) age was 71 (58–81) years, 55% of patients were male, and the median (IQR) APACHE III score was 81 (66–97). One hundred sixty patients (69%) had AKI developed during treatment for severe sepsis or septic shock. Table 1 shows patient characteristics, stratified by presence or absence of AKI.

Regression analysis of ΔMAP as a continuous variable was not significantly associated with the rate of AKI (OR 0.99 [95% CI 0.97–1.01]; $p=.31$). The relationship of ΔMAP and AKI did not become significant with the addition of fluid balance to the model. Regression analysis of post-resuscitation MAP ≥ 65 mmHg was not significantly associated with AKI (OR 0.9 [95% CI 0.27–3.74]). When patients were categorized into quartiles on the basis of ΔMAP values (first quartile, −24.5 to 3.9 mmHg; second quartile, 4.0–12.4 mmHg; third quartile, 12.5–19.9 mmHg; fourth quartile, 20.0–43.8 mmHg), in terms of age, sex, BMI, history of hypertension, CCI, APACHE III score, SOFA score, and fluid balance, patients in quartile 1 were similar to patients in quartiles 2 through 4. Patients in the first quartile had a lower percentage and odds of AKI compared with the other the third quartiles ([56.9% vs. 72.6%, respectively; $p=.03$] and [OR 0.50, 95% CI 0.27–0.93], respectively) (Additional file 1: Fig. S1 and Additional file 2: Fig. S2). Patients in the first quartile had a lower pre- ($p<.01$) and higher post-resuscitation MAP ($p<.01$) (Table 2). Rates of AKI for patients in second, third and fourth quartiles ($p=.11$, $p=.51$, $p=.87$, respectively) were not significantly different when compared with the rest of the cohort. In addition, following adjusting for history of hypertension, being within the

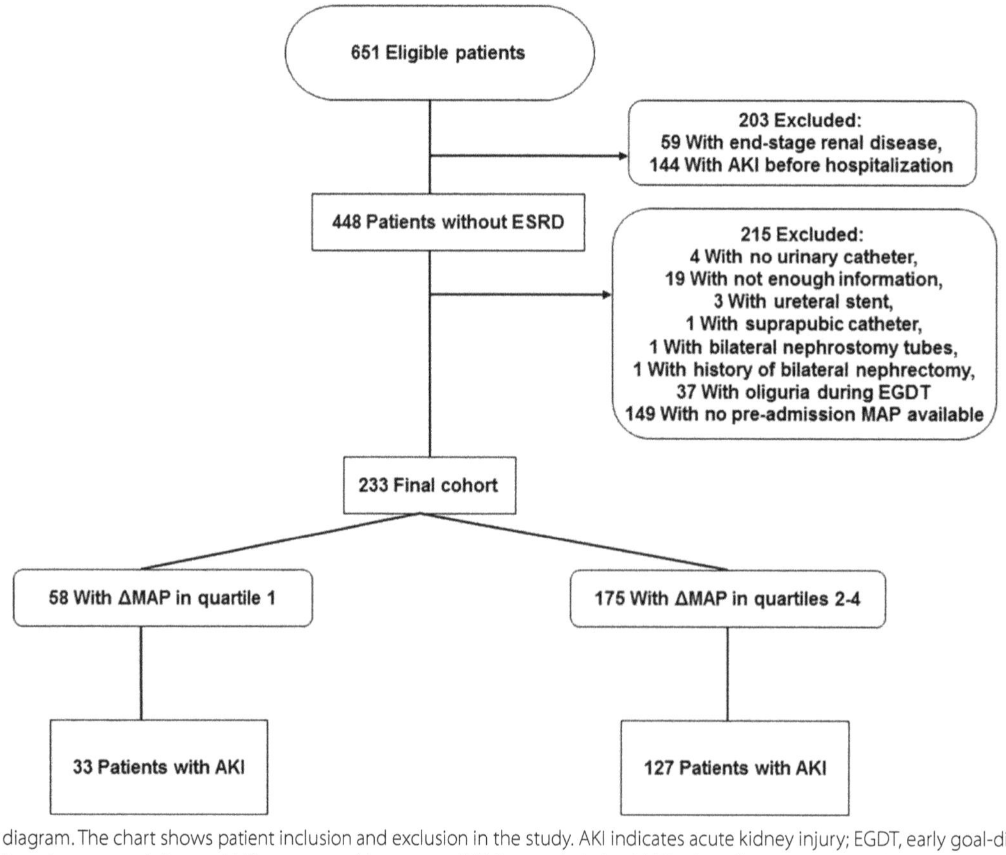

Fig. 1 Flow diagram. The chart shows patient inclusion and exclusion in the study. AKI indicates acute kidney injury; EGDT, early goal-directed therapy; ESRD, end-stage renal disease; MAP, mean arterial pressure; ΔMAP, pre-admission MAP minus the post-resuscitation

Table 1 Patient characteristics, stratified by acute kidney injury status ($N=233$)

Patient characteristics	No AKI ($n=73$)	AKI ($n=160$)	*p* value
Age, median (IQR), year	66.8 (56.0–80.8)	72.8 (59.7–81.6)	.21
Body mass index, median (IQR), kg/m^2	25.2 (21.8–28.6)	27.9 (23.2–33.1)	.01
Male sex, No. (%)	45 (61.6)	83 (51.9)	.20
Pre-admission MAP, median (IQR), mmHg[a]	83.8 (76.0–91.5)	78.5 (73.4–87.6)	.05
MAP at first hour of admission, median (IQR), mmHg	67.5 (59.0–78.0)	65.0 (57.0–73.3)	.1
MAP at first hour of resuscitation, median (IQR), mmHg	62.3 (57.0–73.3)	63.0 (55.8–70.9)	.2
Post-resuscitation MAP, median (IQR), mmHg[b]	71.0 (66.0–79.0)	66.0 (61.0–73.0)	.01
ΔMAP from Baseline to 7th hour of resuscitation, median (IQR), mmHg[c]	11.0 (0.5–20.3)	12.4 (5.7–19.8)	.31
Charlson comorbidity index, median (IQR)	6 (4–8.5)	7 (5–11)	.02
APACHE III score, 24 h, median (IQR)	67 (55.5–79)	88 (72–103)	.01
SOFA score, day 1, median (IQR)	5 (3–7)	7 (5–10.8)	.01
Culture positive septic shock (%)	31 (42)	85 (53)	.2
Positive culture source			.7
Blood (%)	7 (10)	20 (13)	
Urine (%)	5 (7)	19 (12)	
Respiratory (%)	16 (22)	33 (20)	
Wound (%)	1 (1)	6 (4)	
Other (%)	2 (2)	7 (4)	
Culture negative septic shock (%)	42 (58)	75 (47)	.2
Preexisting condition, No. (%)			
Hypertension	38 (52.1)	115 (71.9)	.01
Myocardial infarction	10 (13.7)	39 (24.4)	.08
Congestive heart failure	8 (11.0)	37 (23.1)	.03
Peripheral vascular disease	3 (4.1)	25 (15.6)	.02
Dementia	5 (6.8)	7 (4.4)	.52
Cerebrovascular accident	6 (8.2)	34 (21.3)	.01
Chronic pulmonary disease	16 (21.9)	54 (33.8)	.09
Rheumatic heart disease	8 (11.0)	15 (9.4)	.81
Diabetes mellitus	15 (20.5)	61 (38.1)	.01
Peptic ulcer disease	6 (8.2)	20 (12.5)	.38
Cirrhosis	4 (5.5)	10 (6.3)	>.99
Hemiplegia	4 (5.5)	3 (1.9)	.21
Kidney disease	10 (13.7)	45 (28.1)	.02
Brittle diabetes mellitus	4 (5.5)	26 (16.3)	.02
Cancer	28 (38.4)	49 (30.6)	.29
Leukemia	1 (1.4)	9 (5.6)	.18
Lymphoma	2 (2.7)	8 (5.0)	.73
Moderate or severe liver disease	3 (4.1)	5 (3.1)	.71
Metastatic cancer	7 (9.6)	14 (8.8)	.81
Any inotropic agent, No. (%)	4 (5.5)	28 (17.5)	.01
Any vasoactive agent, No. (%)	32 (43.8)	108 (67.5)	.01
Fluid balance, median (IQR), mL	4945 (2019–8282)	6948 (3658–10,810)	.01

APACHE acute physiology, age, chronic health evaluation, *MAP* mean arterial pressure, *SOFA* sequential organ failure assessment

[a] From noninvasive blood pressure monitoring

[b] Seventh hour of early goal-directed therapy

[c] Defined as pre-admission minus post-resuscitation MAP

Table 2 Comparison of patients in quartile 1 versus quartiles 2–4 of delta mean arterial pressure ($N = 233$)

Characteristic	Quartile 1 ($n = 58$)	Quartiles 2–4 ($n = 175$)	p value
Age, median (IQR), year	66.3 (55.7–79.9)	72.1 (59.4–81.7)	.60
Body mass index, median (IQR), kg/m^2	27.8 (23.7–32.8)	26.8 (22.2–31.6)	.23
Male sex, No. (%)	32 (55.2)	96 (54.9)	>.99
Pre-admission MAP, median (IQR), mmHg[a]	73.9 (67.8–81.9)	82.0 (76.3–91.0)	.01
Post-resuscitation MAP, median (IQR), mmHg[b]	79.0 (70.5–87.1)	66.0 (61.0–71.0)	.01
Acute kidney injury, No. (%)	33 (56.9)	127 (72.6)	.03
Stage 1	13 (17.8)	60 (82.2)	
Stage 2	14 (26.0)	40 (74.1)	
Stage 3	6 (18.2)	27 (81.8)	
Charlson comorbidity index, median (IQR)	7 (4.8–10.3)	7 (5.0–10.0)	.55
APACHE III score, 24 h, median (IQR)	78 (64.8–97.3)	82 (66–97)	.66
SOFA score, day 1, median (IQR)	6 (4–9)	7 (4–10)	.76
Culture positive septic shock (%)	29 (50)	87 (50)	.96
Positive culture source			.5
Blood (%)	5 (9)	22 (13)	
Urine (%)	5 (9)	19 (11)	
Respiratory (%)	16 (28)	33 (19)	
Wound (%)	2 (3)	5 (3)	
Other (%)	1 (1)	8 (4)	
Culture negative septic shock (%)	29 (50)	88 (50)	.96
Preexisting condition, No. (%)			
Hypertension	36 (62.1)	117 (66.9)	.53
Myocardial infarction	11 (19.0)	38 (21.7)	.71
Congestive heart failure	16 (27.6)	29 (16.6)	.08
Peripheral vascular disease	5 (8.6)	23 (13.1)	.49
Dementia	0 (0)	12 (6.9)	.04
Cerebrovascular accident	9 (15.5)	31 (17.7)	.84
Chronic pulmonary disease	16 (27.6)	54 (30.9)	.74
Rheumatic heart disease	7 (12.1)	16 (9.1)	.61
Diabetes mellitus	22 (37.9)	54 (30.9)	.34
Peptic ulcer disease	7 (12.1)	19 (10.9)	.81
Cirrhosis	2 (3.4)	12 (6.9)	.53
Hemiplegia	5 (8.6)	2 (1.1)	.01
Kidney disease	14 (24.1)	41 (23.4)	>.99
Brittle diabetes mellitus	7 (12.1)	23 (13.1)	>.99
Cancer	19 (32.8)	58 (33.1)	>.99
Leukemia	3 (5.2)	7 (4.0)	.71
Lymphoma	7 (12.1)	3 (1.7)	.01
Moderate or severe liver disease	2 (3.4)	6 (3.4)	>.99
Metastatic cancer	6 (10.3)	15 (8.6)	.79
Any inotropic agent, No. (%)	5 (8.6)	27 (15.4)	.27
Any vasoactive agent, No. (%)	35 (60.3)	105 (60.0)	>.99
Fluid balance, median (IQR), mL	6405 (2141–9723)	6102 (3210–9742)	.31

APACHE acute physiology, age, chronic health evaluation, *MAP* mean arterial pressure, *SOFA* Sequential organ failure assessment

[a] From noninvasive blood pressure monitoring

[b] Seventh hour of early goal-directed therapy

first quartile was significantly associated with a lower rate of AKI ($p = .04$).

We used backward stepwise regression analysis of all relevant variables with 25% probability to enter and 10% probability to leave the model. The final model included being in the first quartile, CCI, APACHE III score, SOFA score, comorbidities, vasoactive agents, inotropic agents, pre-admission MAP, and post-resuscitation MAP. BMI, pre-admission MAP, inclusion in quartiles 2 through 4, and APACHE III scores were significant predictors of AKI, and these were entered into a nominal logistic regression analysis (Table 3). Compared with patients in quartiles 2 through 4 combined, those in quartile 1 had decreased odds of AKI (OR 0.26 [95% CI 0.11–0.57]) in a multivariate analysis controlling for all significant predictors. The c-statistic of this model was 0.80 for AKI, and Hosmer–Lemeshow test for goodness of fit showed excellent calibration (Chi-squared 3.6 and p value 0.9). When this same nominal logistic regression analysis was run with the addition of the history of hypertension variable, all four variables listed in Table 3 remained significant, and history of hypertension was not a significant predictor of AKI ($p = 0.28$).

Hypertension subgroup analysis

One hundred fifty-three patients (66.0%) had a history of high blood pressure. When comparing those who did and did not have a history of hypertension, age ($p = .01$), BMI ($p = .01$), incidence of AKI (75.2% and 56.3%, respectively; $p = .01$), CCI ($p = .01$), and APACHE III score ($p = .01$) were significantly different (Table 4).

In the subgroup analysis of patients with a history of hypertension, the ΔMAP values that fell into each quartile did not change significantly from the entire cohort (as described above). The ΔMAP in the first quartile ranged from −24.5 to 4 mmHg; quartile 2, from 4.1 to 12.7 mmHg; quartile 3, from 13 to 21 mmHg; and quartile 4, from 21.1 to 43.8 mmHg. Patients in the first quartile had similar risk factors for AKI as those in quartiles 2 through 4. AKI was less common for patients in the first quartile than the other 3 quartiles combined (62% vs. 80%, respectively; $p = .03$) (Table 5). Similarly, the odds of AKI was lowest for those in quartile 1 vs. quartiles 2 through 4 (OR 0.40 [95% CI 0.18–0.90]).

In the subgroup analysis of patients with a history of hypertension, backward stepwise regression analysis with all variables entered, as described above, showed that BMI, pre-admission MAP, APACHE III score, the presence of brittle diabetes mellitus, inclusion in quartiles 2 through 4, and norepinephrine use were statistically significant predictors of AKI (Table 6). Compared with the patients in quartiles 2 through 4 combined, patients in quartile 1 had lower odds of AKI (OR 0.12 [95% CI 0.04–0.37]) in multivariate analysis after controlling for significant predictors (Table 6). The c-statistic for this model of AKI was 0.87.

Table 3 Regression model for prediction of acute kidney injury for all patients

Characteristic	Odds ratio	95% confidence interval	p value
Being in the first quartile[a]	0.26	0.11–0.57	.01
Body mass index	0.92	0.87–0.96	.01
APACHE III score, 24 h	0.96	0.94–0.97	.01
Pre-admission MAP	1.04	1.01–1.08	.01

APACHE acute physiology, age, chronic health evaluation, *MAP* mean arterial pressure

[a] Patients had ΔMAP values in the lowest quartile

Table 4 Patient characteristics, stratified by history of hypertension ($N = 233$)

Characteristic	No hypertension ($n = 80$)	History of hypertension ($n = 153$)	p value
Age, median (IQR), year	62.5 (50.6–78.0)	74.5 (63.4–82.6)	.01
Body mass index, median (IQR), kg/m^2	25.0 (21.2–28.7)	28.0 (23.3–33.6)	.01
Male sex, No. (%)	45 (56.3)	83 (54.2)	.78
Pre-admission MAP, median (IQR), mmHg[a]	77.3 (72.1–87.3)	81.3 (75.0–90.5)	.13
Post-resuscitation MAP, median (IQR), mmHg[b]	68.0 (62.2–76.5)	68.0 (62.0–74.4)	.98
ΔMAP, median (IQR), mmHg[c]	11.3 (3.0–17.9)	12.7 (4.0–21.0)	.18
Acute kidney injury, No. (%)	45 (56.3)	115 (75.2)	.01
Stage 1	25 (34.3)	48 (65.8)	
Stage 2	12 (22.2)	42 (77.8)	
Stage 3	8 (24.2)	25 (75.8)	
Charlson comorbidity index, median (IQR)	5 (3–7)	8 (6–11)	.01
APACHE III score, 24 h, median (IQR)	71 (61.3–88.8)	86 (69.5–103)	.01
SOFA score, day 1, median (IQR)	6 (4–9)	7 (4–10)	.40
Any inotropic agent, No. (%)	8 (10.0)	24 (15.7)	.32
Any vasoactive agent, No. (%)	46 (57.5)	94 (61.4)	.58
Fluid balance, median (IQR), mL	6419 (3334–8953)	6073 (2398–10,225)	.43

APACHE acute physiology, age, chronic health evaluation, *MAP* mean arterial pressure, *SOFA* Sequential organ failure assessment

[a] From noninvasive blood pressure monitoring

[b] Seventh hour of early goal-directed therapy

[c] Defined as pre-admission minus post-resuscitation MAP

Table 5 Comparison of patients with hypertension in quartile 1 versus quartiles 2–4 of delta mean arterial pressure (*n* = 153)

Characteristic	First quartile (*n* = 39)	Second to fourth quartiles (*n* = 114)	*p* value
Age, median (IQR), year	73.7 (55.9–80.7)	74.8 (64.2–83.1)	.14
Body mass index, median (IQR), kg/m^2	28.6 (23.9–34.1)	27.9 (23.3–33.6)	.39
Male sex, No. (%)	22 (56.4)	61 (53.5)	.85
Pre-admission MAP, median (IQR), mmHg[a]	75.0 (69.0–84.0)	83.5 (76.7–91.3)	.01
Post-resuscitation MAP, median (IQR), mmHg[b]	79.0 (71.5–86.0)	65.0 (61.0–70.3)	.01
Acute kidney injury, No. (%)	24 (61.5)	91 (79.8)	.03
Stage 1	9 (18.8)	39 (81.3)	
Stage 2	10 (23.8)	32 (76.2)	
Stage 3	5 (20.0)	20 (80.0)	
Charlson comorbidity index, median (IQR)	9 (6–12)	7.5 (6–11)	.62
APACHE III score, day 1, median (IQR)	88 (72–99)	85.5 (68.8–104.3)	.51
SOFA score, day 1, median (IQR)	6 (4–8)	7 (4–10)	.28
Preexisting condition, No. (%)			
Myocardial infarction	10 (25.6)	31 (27.2)	>.99
Congestive heart failure	14 (35.9)	25 (21.9)	.09
Peripheral vascular disease	5 (12.8)	22 (19.3)	.47
Dementia	0 (0)	10 (8.8)	.07
Cerebrovascular accident	8 (20.5)	28 (24.6)	.67
Chronic pulmonary disease	12 (30.8)	40 (35.1)	.70
Rheumatic heart disease	6 (15.4)	10 (8.8)	.24
Diabetes mellitus	18 (46.2)	48 (42.1)	.71
Peptic ulcer disease	6 (15.4)	18 (15.8)	>.99
Cirrhosis	0 (0)	8 (7.0)	.20
Hemiplegia	5 (12.8)	2 (1.8)	.01
Kidney disease	13 (33.3)	35 (30.7)	.84
Brittle diabetes mellitus	7 (17.9)	20 (17.5)	>.99
Cancer	15 (38.5)	36 (31.6)	.44
Leukemia	2 (5.1)	4 (3.5)	.65
Lymphoma	4 (10.3)	3 (2.6)	.07
Moderate or severe liver disease	0 (0)	4 (3.5)	.57
Metastatic cancer	5 (12.8)	10 (8.8)	.53
Any inotropic agent, No. (%)	3 (7.7)	21 (18.4)	.13
Any vasoactive agent, No. (%)	24 (61.5)	70 (61.4)	>.99
Fluid balance, median (IQR), mL	7193 (1349–10,280)	5733 (2820–10,220)	.32

ΔMAP is defined as pre-admission minus post-resuscitation MAP

APACHE acute physiology, age, chronic health evaluation, *MAP* mean arterial pressure, *SOFA* sequential organ failure assessment

[a] From noninvasive blood pressure monitoring

[b] Seventh hour of early goal-directed therapy

Discussion

In this report, we identified a hemodynamic variable that was associated with AKI among patients with septic shock. When stratifying patients by ΔMAP, those in the first quartile of MAP change (−24.5 to 3.9 mmHg, i.e., patients with post-resuscitation MAP higher than or equal to their pre-admission MAP) had a significantly lower incidence of AKI. Being in the second to fourth delta-MAP quartiles, body mass index, APACHE III score, and pre-admission MAP were independently associated with risk of AKI.

These results suggest that having a ΔMAP value within the first quartile could be a modifiable risk factor that is associated with a lower risk of AKI in patients with severe sepsis and septic shock. Thus, pre-admission MAP values could be used to guide post-resuscitation MAP

Table 6 Regression model for prediction of acute kidney injury for all patients with hypertension history

Characteristic	Odds ratio	95% confidence interval	*p* value
Being in the first quartile[a]	0.12	0.04–0.37	.01
Body mass index	0.90	0.84–0.96	.01
APACHE III score, 24 h	0.97	0.95–0.99	.01
Pre-admission MAP	1.07	1.01–1.12	.01
Brittle diabetes mellitus	6.03	1.36–44.19	.04
Norepinephrine use	3.72	1.42–10.54	.01

APACHE acute physiology, age, chronic health evaluation, *MAP* mean arterial pressure

[a] Patients had ΔMAP values in the lowest quartile

targets. In other words, our report suggests that a post-resuscitation MAP that is no more than 4 mmHg lower than pre-admission MAP may be protective against the development of AKI in this cohort. This guideline could potentially provide a specific, individualized MAP target for each patient with severe sepsis or septic shock. While our results provide a new hypothesis, the lack of a clear dose-response relationship between ΔMAP quartiles 2–4 and AKI could mean another variable plays a role in the development of SA-AKI. In either case, this deserves further attention in terms of prospective study.

The concept of ΔMAP itself is not quite novel. ΔMAP previously was investigated in high-risk patients undergoing cardiopulmonary bypass [18]. The authors reported a higher rate of AKI when MAP was at least 26 mmHg lower than baseline during cardiopulmonary bypass. We note that the ΔMAP targets described in that study specifically pertained to patients undergoing cardiac surgery and is not applicable to SA-AKI.

In a previous study of SA-AKI, Badin et al. [11] found that the time-averaged MAP in the early phase of acute circulatory failure was lower in patients who had septic shock, prior renal function impairment, and AKI. Our results confirm those of Badin et al. and go a step further; the decrement of post-resuscitation MAP relative to pre-admission MAP seems to be associated with the incidence of AKI. Having ΔMAP values in quartile 1 (i.e., patients with post-resuscitation MAP mostly higher than their pre-admission MAP) was significantly associated with a lower incidence of AKI for the total cohort. Additionally, the association of ΔMAP values in quartile 1 was independent of a history of hypertension. Our results further suggest that ΔMAP values may help better define an individualized goal MAP for each patient by taking into consideration pre-admission blood pressures and preexisting conditions such as chronic hypertension. Our results are similar to those of the SEPSISPAM (Sepsis and Mean Arterial Pressure) investigators' trial [4], which reported an association between patients with a history of hypertension and a need for a higher goal MAP.

In our study, the non-AKI group had a median (IQR) post-resuscitation MAP of 71 (66–79) mmHg, whereas, among the AKI group, it was 66 (61–73) mmHg. These values were consistent with the findings of other reports [11, 12]. The mean post-resuscitation MAP of the group without AKI was lower than that suggested by the FINNAKI (Finnish Acute Kidney Injury) study [13]. Although Asfar et al. [4] proposed a lower MAP to avoid adverse effects of resuscitation, their low-target MAP group had an actual MAP of 75 mmHg, which is similar to our non-AKI group's post-resuscitation MAP and the findings of other studies [4, 11, 13].

Our study has some limitations, including its retrospective and observational nature and that it was restricted to a single center. We could not control for interventions, including patients' resuscitation MAP goals. While our investigation focused on the association of ΔMAP with an important renal outcome, effects on other organ systems were not included in this investigation and are unknown. The retrospective collection of noninvasive blood pressure readings from the electronic health record was not ideal since these blood pressures are collected in the hospital setting and may not reflect patients "healthy" blood pressure; we attempted to mitigate this problem by using the median of MAPs to prevent an outlier from skewing the patients' pre-admission MAP values. As the main focus of this retrospective analysis was generating hypothesis for targeted AKI preventive interventions for future prospective study, we did not report the impact of delta-MAP on other organs including the cardiovascular system. Further, a retrospective collection of noninvasive blood pressure readings may have limited the number of patients in our analysis and may have inadvertently included more patients with preexisting hypertension or other comorbidities associated with regular blood pressure monitoring. We corrected for the higher prevalence of hypertension by including it in our multivariate model and confirming that it does not account for our findings. Indeed, our results were independent of a history of hypertension. Due to these limitations, this study may have limited generalizability. The strengths of this study include the detailed characterization of enrolled patients.

Conclusions

Our study is the first to analyze ΔMAP, defined as pre-admission MAP minus post-resuscitation MAP, as a risk factor for SA-AKI. Patients with ΔMAP values in the lowest quartile (i.e., patients with post-resuscitation MAP mostly higher than their pre-admission MAP) had a significantly lower incidence of AKI independent of a history of hypertension. Analysis of the subgroup of patients with hypertension showed the same relationship. Our results are hypothesis generating and suggest that, for patients with severe sepsis or septic shock, clinicians may better define an individualized target MAP for the resuscitation phase goals by considering the patient's pre-admission MAP. We recommend future studies to further explore the usefulness of this hemodynamic target for sepsis resuscitation.

Abbreviations

AKI: acute kidney injury; APACHE: acute physiology, age, chronic health evaluation; BMI: body mass index; CCI: Charlson comorbidity index; EGDT: early goal-directed therapy; ICU: intensive care unit; IQR: interquartile range; MAP: mean arterial pressure; OR: odds ratio; SA-AKI: sepsis-associated acute kidney injury; sCR: serum creatinine; SOFA: sequential organ failure assessment; UOP: urine output.

Authors' contributions

RNM helped in study design, data collection, data interpretation, and preparation of the manuscript; SAO and AA contributed to data collection; RK helped in study design, data collection, data interpretation, and preparation of the manuscript; KK served the principal role and supervisor in study design, data interpretation, and preparation of the paper. Dr. Kianoush Kashani had full access to all the data in the study and took responsibility for the integrity of the data and the accuracy of the data analysis. All authors read and approved the final manuscript.

Author details

[1] Multidisciplinary Epidemiology and Translational Research in Intensive Care (METRIC), Division of Pulmonary and Critical Care Medicine, Department of Medicine, Mayo Clinic, 200 First Street SW, Rochester, MN 55905, USA. [2] Department of Anesthesiology and Perioperative Medicine, Mayo Clinic, Rochester, MN, USA. [3] Department of Obstetrics and Gynecology, University of Alabama Birmingham, Birmingham, AL, USA. [4] Division of Pulmonary and Critical Care Medicine, Department of Medicine, Mayo Clinic, Rochester, MN, USA. [5] Anesthesia Clinical Research Unit, Department of Anesthesiology and Perioperative Medicine, Mayo Clinic, Rochester, MN, USA. [6] Division of Nephrology and Hypertension, Department of Medicine, Mayo Clinic, Rochester, MN, USA.

Acknowledgements

This work was supported by the National Center for Advancing Translational Sciences (NCATS) [Grant Number UL1 TR000135]. Its contents are solely the responsibility of the authors and do not necessarily represent the official views of the NIH. The sponsor had no role in the development of the research and manuscript.

Competing interests

The authors declare that they have no competing interests.

Funding

This publication was supported by Grant Number UL1 TR000135 from the National Center for Advancing Translational Sciences (NCATS). Its contents are solely the responsibility of the authors and do not necessarily represent the official views of the NIH.

References

1. Uchino S, Kellum JA, Bellomo R, Doig GS, Morimatsu H, Morgera S, Schetz M, Tan I, Bouman C, Macedo E, et al. Acute renal failure in critically Ill patients: a multinational, multicenter study. JAMA. 2005;294(7):813–8.
2. Rhodes A, Evans LE, Alhazzani W, Levy MM, Antonelli M, Ferrer R, Kumar A, Sevransky JE, Sprung CL, Nunnally ME, et al. Surviving sepsis campaign: international guidelines for management of sepsis and septic shock. Intensive Care Med. 2016;2017:1–74.
3. Russell JA. Is there a good map for septic shock? N Engl J Med. 2014;370(17):1649–51.
4. Asfar P, Meziani F, Hamel J-F, Grelon F, Megarbane B, Anguel N, Mira J-P, Dequin P-F, Gergaud S, Weiss N, et al. High versus low blood-pressure target in patients with septic shock. N Engl J Med. 2014;370(17):1583–93.
5. Bagshaw SM, George C, Bellomo R, Committee ADM. Early acute kidney injury and sepsis: a multicentre evaluation. Crit Care (London, England). 2008;12(2):R47.
6. Bagshaw SM, Uchino S, Bellomo R, Morimatsu H, Morgera S, Schetz M, Tan I, Bouman C, Macedo E, Gibney N, et al. Septic acute kidney injury in critically Ill patients: clinical characteristics and outcomes. Clin J Am Soc Nephrol CJASN. 2007;2(3):431–9.
7. Poukkanen M, Vaara ST, PettilÄ V, Kaukonen KM, Korhonen AM, Hovilehto S, Inkinen O, Laru-Sompa R, Kaminski T, Reinikainen M, et al. Acute kidney injury in patients with severe sepsis in Finnish Intensive Care Units. Acta Anaesthesiol Scand. 2013;57(7):863–72.
8. Chertow GM, Burdick E, Honour M, Bonventre JV, Bates DW. Acute kidney injury, mortality, length of stay, and costs in hospitalized patients. J Am Soc Nephrol. 2005;16(11):3365–70.
9. Hill JV, Findon G, Appelhoff RJ, Endre ZH. Renal autoregulation and passive pressure-flow relationships in diabetes and hypertension. Am J Physiol Renal Physiol. 2010;299(4):F837–44.
10. Iversen BM, Sekse I, Ofstad J. Resetting of renal blood flow autoregulation in spontaneously hypertensive rats. Am J Physiol. 1987;252(3 Pt 2):F480–6.
11. Badin J, Boulain T, Ehrmann S, Skarzynski M, Bretagnol A, Buret J, Benzekri-Lefevre D, Mercier E, Runge I, Garot D, et al. Relation between mean arterial pressure and renal function in the early phase of shock: a prospective, explorative cohort study. Crit Care. 2011;15(3):R135.
12. Deruddre S, Cheisson G, Mazoit JX, Vicaut E, Benhamou D, Duranteau J. Renal arterial resistance in septic shock: effects of increasing mean arterial pressure with norepinephrine on the renal resistive index assessed with Doppler ultrasonography. Intensive Care Med. 2007;33(9):1557–62.
13. Poukkanen M, Wilkman E, Vaara ST, Pettila V, Kaukonen KM, Korhonen AM, Uusaro A, Hovilehto S, Inkinen O, Laru-Sompa R, et al. Hemodynamic variables and progression of acute kidney injury in critically ill patients with severe sepsis: data from the prospective observational FINNAKI study. Crit Care. 2013;17(6):R295.
14. Charlson M, Szatrowski TP, Peterson J, Gold J. Validation of a combined comorbidity index. J Clin Epidemiol. 1994;47(11):1245–51.
15. Vincent JL, Moreno R, Takala J, Willatts S, De Mendonça A, Bruining H, Reinhart CK, Suter PM, Thijs LG. The SOFA (Sepsis-related Organ Failure Assessment) score to describe organ dysfunction/failure. Intensive Care Med. 1996;22(7):707–10.
16. Knaus WA, Wagner DP, Draper EA, Zimmerman JE, Bergner M, Bastos PG, Sirio CA, Murphy DJ, Lotring T, Damiano A, et al. The APACHE III prognostic system. Risk prediction of hospital mortality for critically ill hospitalized adults. Chest. 1991;100(6):1619–36.
17. Section 2: AKI Definition. Kidney inter, Suppl 2012;2(1):19–36.
18. Kanji HD, Schulze CJ, Hervas-Malo M, Wang P, Ross DB, Zibdawi M, Bagshaw SM. Difference between pre-operative and cardiopulmonary bypass mean arterial pressure is independently associated with early cardiac surgery-associated acute kidney injury. J Cardiothorac Surg. 2010;5:71.

Polymyxin-B hemoperfusion in septic patients: analysis of a multicenter registry

Salvatore Lucio Cutuli[1*], Antonio Artigas[2], Roberto Fumagalli[3], Gianpaola Monti[3], Vito Marco Ranieri[4], Claudio Ronco[5], Massimo Antonelli[1] and The EUPHAS 2 Collaborative Group

Abstract

Background: In 2010, the EUPHAS 2 collaborative group created a registry with the purpose of recording data from critically ill patients suffering from severe sepsis and septic shock treated with polymyxin-B hemoperfusion (PMX-HP) for endotoxin removal. The aim of the registry was to verify the application of PMX-HP in the daily clinical practice.

Methods: The EUPHAS 2 registry involved 57 centers between January 2010 and December 2014, collecting retrospective data of 357 patients (297 in Europe and 60 in Asia) suffering from severe sepsis and septic shock caused by proved or suspected infection related to Gram negative bacteria. All patients received atleast one cycle of extracorporeal endotoxin removal by PMX-HP.

Results: Septic shock was diagnosed in 305 (85.4 %) patients. The most common source of infection was abdominal (44.0 %) followed by pulmonary (17.6 %). Gram negative bacteria represented 60.6 % of the pathogens responsible of infection. After 72 h from the first cycle of PMX-HP, some of the SOFA score components significantly improved with respect to baseline: cardiovascular (2.16 ± 1.77 from 3.32 ± 1.29, $p < 0.0001$), respiratory (1.95 ± 0.95 from 2.40 ± 1.06, $p < 0.001$) and renal (1.84 ± 1.77 from 2.23 ± 1.62, $p = 0.013$). Overall 28-day survival rate was 54.5 % (60.4 % in abdominal and 47.5 % in pulmonary infection). Patients with abdominal infection treated with PMX-HP within 24 h from the diagnosis of septic shock had a 28-day survival rate of 64.5 %. Patients showing a significantly cardiovascular improvement after PMX-HP had a 28-survival rate of 75 % in comparison to the 39 % of patients who did not ($p < 0.001$). Cox regression analysis found the variation of cardiovascular, respiratory and coagulation SOFA to be independent covariates for 28-day survival. In European patients were observed a higher 28-day (58.8 vs. 34.5 %, $p = 0.003$), ICU (59 vs. 36.7 %, $p = 0.006$) and hospital survival rate (53.2 vs. 35 %, $p = 0.02$) than in Asian patients. However, the two populations were highly heterogeneous in terms of source of infection and severity scores at admission.

Conclusion: The EUPHAS 2 is the largest registry conducted outside Japan on the clinical use of PMX-HP in septic patients. Data analysis confirmed the feasibility of PMX-HP to treat septic patients in daily clinical practice, showing clinical benefits associated with endotoxin removal without significant adverse events related to the extracorporeal technique.

Keywords: Sepsis, Septic shock, Infection, EAA, Extracorporeal endotoxin removal, Polymyxin-B hemoperfusion

Background

Polymyxin-B hemoperfusion (PMX-HP) [1] is a blood purification technique designed to bind and neutralize circulating endotoxins by extracorporeal removal, inhibiting the progression of the septic cascade mediated by lipopolysaccharide (LPS) [2–16], the core lipid portion of the Gram negative bacterial wall. Endotoxin is removed from the blood by extracorporeal hemoperfusion with a polymyxin-B-adsorbing cartridge that binds endotoxin through covalent and ionic bonds. This therapy was first introduced in Japan in 1994 and 10 years later it was introduced in Europe.

*Correspondence: sl.cutuli@gmail.com
[1] Department of Intensive Care and Anaesthesiology, Agostino Gemelli University Hospital, Catholic University of the Sacred Heart, Largo A. Gemelli, 8, 00168 Rome, Italy
Full list of author information is available at the end of the article

The most common indication for PMX-HP has been septic shock due to abdominal infections. In case of impairment of the intestinal mucosa, LPS can translocate into the bloodstream. The consequent huge activation of the immune system can lead to the dysfunction of multiple organs until the loss of their function (MOF). The importance of endotoxin to determine the unfavorable evolution of sepsis related to Gram negative bacteria has been clearly demonstrated [2–15].

Several trials have been carried out to verify the hypothesis that removing circulating endotoxin from the blood of patients suffering from abdominal septic shock could improve their clinical outcome, in terms of organ dysfunction and mortality [4–15].

The Italian nationwide Early Use of Polymyxin B Hemoperfusion in Abdominal Septic Shock (EUPHAS) Randomized Control Trial (RCT) [15], demonstrated a significant improvement in cardiovascular response and outcome of patients treated by PMX-HP for severe sepsis and septic shock due to abdominal infections. On the other hand, the French ABDOMIX RCT [16] failed to demonstrate clinical benefits of PMX-HP application in a cohort of patients suffering from peritonitis-induced septic shock after emergency surgery.

Furthermore, PMX-HP has been applied in septic patients with source of infection different from the abdomen as respiratory system [17].

Due to the conflicting evidence given by EUPHAS and ABDOMIX RCTs in sepsis sustained by abdominal source of infection and new potential indication highlighted by case report on respiratory infections, the real application of PMX-HP in daily clinical practice is unclear.

In 2010, the EUPHAS 2 project [18] was launched, to create an international registry with the purpose of recording data from patients affected by Gram negative related severe sepsis and septic shock treated with PMX-HP. The aim of the project was to evaluate the application of PMX-HP in the daily clinical practice, both in order to verify the reproducibility of data currently available in the literature and to evaluate the population actually elected for the therapy.

The EUPHAS 2 project is divided into two phases. The first retrospective phase aimed to collect data from at least 250 patients. The analysis of the data from this phase was used to optimize the data collection for the second prospective phase, which aims to collect data from a much larger patient population. The results from the second phase will be used to identify subpopulations of patients who may benefit from this treatment more than others.

A preliminary analysis of EUPHAS 2 retrospective phase [19] confirmed the results of EUPHAS RCT in abdominal septic patients. In the current paper are presented the full results from the first retrospective phase of EUPHAS 2.

Methods

The EUPHAS 2 project was a voluntary registry specifically conceived for the evaluation and analysis of PMX-HP application in the real clinical life.

All the patients admitted to the 57 participating centers with suspected Gram negative related severe sepsis and septic shock unresponsive to standard care [20] were included in the registry. Forty-six centers were located in Europe (Italy, Spain and Switzerland), and eleven centers in Asia (India). Data collection started in January 2010 and ended in December 2014.

The definition of severe sepsis and septic shock followed the consensus guideline enounced by Surviving Sepsis Campaign [20].

The Gram negative etiology of sepsis was suspected in relation to the source of infection (the abdomen is colonized by Gram negative species) or proven by microbiological tests. In 24 out of 57 centers involved in the registry, LPS might be assessed on peripheral blood sample by the neutrophil-dependent chemiluminescence-based endotoxin activity assay (EAA) [24]. EAA quantifies endotoxin levels through a relative scale ranking from 0 to 1. EAA is characterized by a sensitivity of 85.3 %, a specificity of 44 %, a negative predictive value of 98.6 % for the exclusion of Gram negative infection and 94.8 % for the exclusion of all infection [21]. Marshall et al. [21] demonstrated a progressive mortality increase related to endotoxin activity (EA) rising value. Highest mortality rate was observed for EA greater than 0.6, whereby it is considered the threshold to start the LPS removal.

PMX-HP is not ruled by specific guidelines and this therapy is recommended in severe sepsis and septic shock unresponsive to standard care [20], caused by proved or suspected infection related to Gram negative bacteria. All patients received fluid infusion and vasopressor therapy if needed [20] and independently to PMX-HP.

In all patients, PMX-HP was performed using Toraymyxin® cartridge (Toray Medical Company, Tokyo, Japan) connected to the patient through a 10–12 French veno-venous catheter inserted into the right or left femoral or internal jugular vein and the pump flow rate was 80–120 mL/min.

Each session of PMX-HP lasted 2 h. In relation to clinical condition of the patient and EA (where available), the clinician decided to perform a second cycle of PMX-HP with a delay of 24 h from the first treatment.

Heparin intravenous administration as anticoagulant was set starting from a bolus of 3000 UI before the beginning of PMX-HP with a continuous infusion of 20 UI/

kg/h during the treatment. The recommended dose of heparin could be modified in relation to the hemorrhagic risk of the patient.

Main data collection included: timing of diagnosis of severe sepsis/septic shock and treatment with PMX-HP; hemodynamic status; septic organ function impairment; outcome at 28 days, ICU and hospital discharge. Septic progressive organ function impairment was monitored with SOFA score [22–25], hemodynamic status was evaluated with mean arterial pressure (MAP), lactates concentration in the blood and vasopressor load expressed as the inotropic core [(dopamine dose x 1) + (dobutamine dose x 1) + (adrenaline dose x 100) + (noradrenaline dose x 100) + (phenylephrine dose x 100), wherein all doses are expressed as μg/kg/min]. SOFA score, inotropic score and lactates concentration in the blood were assessed at the time of the first PMX-HP (t_0) and every 24 h until 72 h (t_{72}) from t_0.

Patients showing with a reduction of at least one point in cardiovascular SOFA between t_0 and t_{72} were considered "cardiovascular responders"; otherwise, they were "cardiovascular non-responders".

Adverse events associated with PMX-HP were recorded and defined as tachycardia-heart rate (HR) >100 bpm or HR increase >10 % HR pre-treatment during 10′ from the beginning of PMX-HP, hypotension-MAP <70 mmHg or PAM reduction >10 % MAP pre-treatment during 10′ from the beginning of PMX-HP, bleeding-every type of hemorrhagic complication, cartridge clotting-coagulation of polymyxin-B fiber cartridge. Clotting of the PMX cartridge is an adverse event because it causes a premature interruption of the treatment (limiting its benefit) and blood lost for the patient.

IRBs and Ethical Committee of all centers approved data collection and the study.

Statistical analysis

Normality tests were performed using the Kolmogorov–Smirnov test. Quantitative normally distributed variables (APACHE II, SAPS II, SOFA score and body temperature) were presented as mean ± standard deviation (SD) and non-normally distributed variables (age, time to treatment, vasopressors, EAA and biochemical data) as medians and the 25th–75th quartiles range. Univariate comparison was performed to compare variables between two groups. The organ dysfunction scores were compared using the unpaired t test. Categorical variables were expressed as actual numbers and percentages. In all comparisons, $p < 0.05$ was considered statistically significant.

Analysis was performed using R statistical software. Student's t test, Wilcoxon test and Mann–Whitney test were used to compare means in case of normal paired or unpaired samples, non-normal paired samples and non-normal unpaired samples, respectively. Fisher's exact test was carried out to evaluate significance in contingency tables. Multiple logistic regression was performed to evaluate the dependence of categorical variables on one or more predictors, and linear multiple regression was used to model the dependence of scalar variables on one

Table 1 Demographic characteristics of patients treated with PMX-HP

Demographic characteristics	*N* 357
Age, years, mean ± SD	63 (51–72)
Gender, male	240 (67.2)
SAPS II at admission, mean ± SD	50.3 ± 19.2
APACHE II at admission, mean ± SD	21.8 ± 7.2
SOFA at admission, mean ± SD	10.9 ± 3.5
Incidence of shock	305 (85.4)
Source of sepsis	
Abdominal	157 (44)
Pulmonary	63 (17.6)
Urinary	16 (4.5)
Cardiac	23 (6.4)
Trauma	19 (5.3)
Other[a]	79 (22)
Patients without microbiological cultures *N* (%)	139 (38.9)
Patients with microbiological cultures	218 (61.1)
Negative microbiological cultures	41 (18.8)
Positive microbiological cultures	177 (81.1)
Gram positive only	17 (7.8)
Gram negative only	81 (37.2)
Fungi only	13 (6.0)
Mixed including gram negatives	51 (23.4)
Mixed not including gram negatives	8 (3.7)
Patients with endotoxin activity assay, *N* (%)	132 (37)
Abdominal	47 (35.6)
Non-abdominal	85 (64.4)
Without microbiology data	33 (25)
Negative cultures	12 (9)
Gram positive only	7 (5.3)
Gram negative only	43 (32.6)
Fungi only	14 (10.6)
Mixed including gram negatives	21 (15.9)
Mixed not including gram negatives	3 (2.2)
Patients with 2 treatments, *N* (%)	219 (61)
Patients with 1 treatment, *N* (%)	138 (39)
28 days survival	180 (54.5)
ICU survival	192 (55.2)
Hospital survival	172 (50)

Data are expressed as *N* (%) apart from otherwise indicated

[a] Other includes soft tissue infections, CVC-related infections, meningitides

or more explanatory variables. Cox proportional hazard model was used to relate time-to-death to multiple covariates. For all of the statistics tests and models, a 0.05 significance level was considered.

Results

Demographic and clinical data of the 357 patients treated with PMX-HP are reported in Table 1. Data were recorded by 35 out of 57 centers with a median of patients per center of 9 [3–13] in Europe and 4.5 (2.7–11) in Asia.

Septic shock was diagnosed in 305 patients and severe sepsis in 52 patients. Eight patients had not data about vasopressor infused and they were considered presumably affected by severe sepsis. Main sources of infection were the abdomen (44 %) and the lung (17.6 %).

EA was recorded in 18 out of 24 centers in which the assay was available. EAA was measured in 132 out of 357 patients (37.0 %) with a median value of 0.77 (0.69–0.90) at t_0. EAA was $\geq$0.6 in 120 patients and <0.6 in 12 patients, but the small number did not allowed any comparison between two groups.

Microbiological evidence of infection was documented in 174 (49.5 %) patients. Gram negative bacteria were isolated in 60.6 % of the microbiological samples (37.2 % mono-microbial and 23.4 % poly-microbial). In 139 patients, microbiological results were either not or partly reported.

Each session of PMX-HP theoretically lasted 2 h. No data about reason (except cartridge clotting) and timing of its premature interruption were recorded in the registry.

The majority of patients (73.8 %) were treated within 24 h from the onset of severe sepsis and septic shock; 13.2 % of patients received the PMX-HP between 24 and 48 h after the diagnosis of severe sepsis and septic shock, while 12.9 % of patients had a delay of more than 2 days.

Safety of Polymyxin-B hemoperfusion

Two cycles of PMX-HP were performed in 219 patients; 138 patients received only one treatment.

Twenty-six adverse events were recorded (two tachycardias, ten hypotensions, one bleeding, thirteen cartridge clottings) (Additional file 1: Table S12).

Among the PMX-HP clotted cartridge, in eight patients was not administered heparin bolus at the beginning of the treatment and a lower amount of continuous heparin infusion was prescribed as compared to the recommended standard dose. No information about heparin dosage was reported for the remaining five clotted cartridges.

None of these adverse events caused clinical worsening or death of the patients.

Table 2 Variables changes 72 h after PMX-HP

Patients	t_0 $N = 357$	t_{72} $N = 299$	*p* (Wilcoxon)
SOFA score	12.4 ± 4.2	10.5 ± 5.3	*<0.001*
Cardiovascular SOFA	3.32 ± 1.29	2.16 ± 1.77	*<0.001*
Renal SOFA	2.23 ± 1.62	1.84 ± 1.77	*0.013*
Hepatic SOFA	1.22 ± 1.28	1.19 ± 1.30	0.80
Respiratory SOFA	2.40 ± 1.06	1.95 ± 0.95	*<0.001*
Coagulation SOFA	1.33 ± 1.29	1.67 ± 1.38	*0.004*
Inotropic score	30 (11.9–72.5)	6.0 (0.0–22)	*<0.001*
Lactate, mmol/L	3.4 (1.9–6.0)	1.9 (1.3–2.9)	*<0.001*
Platelets, 10^3/μL	117 (56–220)	86 (40–163)	*<0.001*

Normally distributed data are expressed as mean ± SD and non-normally distributed data as median (interquartile range)

Italics indicates significant *p* values

Effect of PMX-HP on organ dysfunction

SAPS II score was 48.0 ± 16.6 in patients suffering from severe sepsis versus 50.5 ± 19.5 in patients suffering from septic shock patients. SOFA score at t_0 was 8.1 ± 2.9 in patients suffering from severe sepsis versus 12.9 ± 4.1 in patients suffering from septic shock patients; 72 h from the beginning of PMX-HP, SOFA score decreased in patients suffering from septic shock, but not in patients suffering from severe sepsis (10.7 ± 5.4 vs 8.9 ± 4.3, respectively).

Table 2 shows the variations of each SOFA component between t_0 and t_{72}.

A significant improvement of cardiovascular ($t_0 = 3.32 \pm 1.29$ vs. $t_{72} = 2.16 \pm 1.77$; $p < 0.001$), respiratory ($t_0 = 2.40 \pm 1.06$ vs. $t_{72} = 1.95 \pm 0.95$; $p < 0.001$) and renal ($t_0 = 2.23 \pm 1.62$ vs. $t_{72} = 1.84 \pm 1.77$; $p = 0.013$) scores with a reduction of inotropic score [$t_0 = 30.0$ (11.9–72.5) vs. $t_{72} = 6.0$ (0.0–22.0); $p < 0.001$] and lactate levels [$t_0 = 3.4$ (1.9–6.0) vs. $t_{72} = 1.9$ (1.3–2.9); $p < 0.001$] were observed after a follow-up of 72 h. Only the coagulation score significantly increased ($t_0 = 1.33 \pm 1.29$ vs. $t_{72} = 1.67 \pm 1.38$; $p = 0.004$) together with platelet reduction [$t_0 = 117$ (56–220) vs. $t_{72} = 86$ (40–163); $p < 0.001$]; both were not responsible of meaningful clinical worsening. These results were confirmed excluding patients dead at 72 h except for renal SOFA improvement (Additional file 1: Table S1).

Length of stay and mortality

Median ICU and hospital length of stay (LoS) were 16 days (8–29) and 28 days (16–49), respectively. Overall 28-day survival after PMX-HP was 54.5 %. Patients with abdominal sepsis treated within 24 h from the diagnosis of septic shock had a survival rate of 64.5 %.

A Cox regression model, stratified by age, was carried out to identify the independent covariates affecting

Table 3 Cox regression on mortality stratified by age

	Univariate		*p*	Multivariate		*p*
	HR	95 % CI		HR	95 % CI	
Septic source						
Abdominal versus respiratory	1.56	0.93–2.63	0.09	0.99	0.25–3.97	0.99
Abdominal versus urinary	0.47	0.14–1.61	0.23	0.86	0.04–16.75	0.92
Cardiovascular SOFA at t_0	1.17	0.98–1.41	0.09	1.61	0.98–2.67	0.06
Coagulation SOFA at t_0	1.10	0.95–1.28	0.21	0.96	0.68–1.36	0.83
Respiratory SOFA at t_0	1.14	0.94–1.39	0.17	1.42	0.83–2.44	0.20
Renal SOFA at t_0	0.97	0.81–1.17	0.75	0.85	0.53–1.38	0.52
Liver SOFA at t_0	1.17	0.98–1.39	0.08	1.38	0.89–2.14	0.15
Δ Cardiovascular SOFA	1.39	1.20–1.62	*<0.001*	1.68	1.21–2.32	*0.002*
Δ Coagulation SOFA	1.46	1.13–1.90	*0.004*	1.64	1.07–2.50	*0.022*
Δ Respiratory SOFA	1.26	1.01–1.56	*0.04*	1.68	0.99–2.84	*0.05*
Δ Renal SOFA	1.29	0.94–1.76	0.11	0.83	0.47–1.47	0.51
Δ Liver SOFA	1.74	1.20–2.52	0.003	1.66	0.93–2.94	0.08
Timing[a]	0.99	0.96–1.02	0.61	0.95	0.88–1.01	0.20
European versus asiatic	0.53	0.33–0.86	*0.001*	2.51	0.29–22.03	0.41

Italics indicates significant *p* values

[a] Time between the diagnosis of severe sepsis/septic shock and PMX-HP

Table 4 Factors influencing the lack of cardiovascular response

All patients	Odds ratio	95 % CI	*p*
Age	0.99	0.97–1.02	0.82
Cardiovascular SOFA at t_0	1.51	1.07–2.13	*<0.019*
Coagulative SOFA at t_0	0.96	0.75–1.24	0.78
Liver SOFA at t_0	1.09	0.83–1.42	0.54
Renal SOFA at t_0	1.17	0.88–1.55	0.28
Respiratory SOFA at t_0	0.54	0.39–0.75	*<0.001*
European versus Asian	1.38	0.43–4.42	0.59

Italics indicates significant *p* values

28-day overall survival (Table 3). The variation of cardiovascular, respiratory and coagulation SOFA were identified as independent covariates for 28-day survival. No significant difference in survival was observed between patients receiving one or two treatments ($p = 0.44$).

Factors influencing the lack of cardiovascular response have been evaluated by a logistic regression (Table 4).

Cardiovascular and respiratory SOFA at t_0 were independent factors influencing cardiovascular response. Cardiovascular response was positively associated with the former [OR 1.51 (1.07–2.13, 95 % CI with $p < 0.019$)] and negatively with the latter [OR 0.54 (0.39–0.75, 95 % CI with $p < 0.001$)].

Cardiovascular SOFA at baseline between responders and non-responders (3.7 ± 0.7 vs. 3.2 ± 1.4, $p \leq 0.001$) was significantly different. Survival rates between cardiovascular responders and non-responders were 74.6 and 41.9 %, respectively ($p < 0.001$, Additional file 2: Figure S1). No significant differences in terms of age and SAPS II (48.6 ± 19.2 vs 51.2 ± 19.2, $p = 0.32$) were detected between the two subgroups (Additional file 1: Table S3).

The univariate Cox regression model identified the geographical origin as a factor influencing the mortality.

The characteristics of European and Asian patients are reported in Table 5.

Europeans were older [66 (54–74) years vs. 54 (41.3–62), $p < 0.001$], their SOFA score at enrollment was lower (11.8 ± 3.9 vs. 15.6 ± 4.7, $p < 0.001$), the length of ICU and hospital stay was shorter [ICU LoS 11 (1–123) days vs. 17 (1–213), $p < 0.001$; hospital LoS 14.5 (2–140) days vs. 34 (2–407), $p < 0.001$], and they had a higher survival rate at 28-day than Asian (Additional file 3: Figure S2), both in the ICU (59 vs. 36.7 %, $p = 0.006$) and in the hospital (53.2 vs. 35.0 %, $p = 0.02$).

The degree of cardiovascular response to PMX-HP treatment was similar between the two populations (47.4 % in European compared to 50 % in Asian patients), as well as the time between the diagnosis and start of the treatment.

Discussion

The EUPHAS 2 data collection represents the largest database on PMX-HP application describing its utilization in the real clinical life. EUPHAS 2 registry was created to describe the actual use of the PMX-HP in the

Table 5 Characteristics of enrolled patients by geographical origin

Characteristics of enrolled patients by origin	$N = 297$ European	$N = 60$ Asian	p
Age, years	66 (54–74)	54 (41.3–62)	*<0.001*
SOFA score at admission	10.8 ± 3.5	12.3 ± 3.4	0.16
SAPS II at admission	49.6 ± 18.0	53.8 ± 25.2	0.21
Incidence of shock N (%)	257 (86.5)	48 (80)	0.31
Septic source N (%)			
Abdominal	142 (47.8)	15 (25)	*0.002*
Pulmonary	42 (14.1)	21 (35)	*<0.001*
Urinary	13 (4.4)	3 (5)	0.90
Postoperative cardiac surgery	22 (7.4)	1 (1.7)	0.17
Trauma	19 (6.4)	0	–
Other	59 (19.9)	20 (33.3)	*0.03*
Days from diagnosis to enrollment N (range)	1 (0–2.0)	1.0 (0.0–1.0)	0.45
SOFA score at enrollment	11.8 ± 3.9	15.6 ± 4.7	*<0.001*
Cardiovascular SOFA at t_0	3.4 ± 1.2	3.2 ± 1.5	0.38
Renal SOFA at t_0	2.2 ± 1.6	2.6 ± 1.6	0.08
Hepatic SOFA at t_0	1.1 ± 1.2	1.9 ± 1.6	*<0.001*
Respiratory SOFA at t_0	2.3 ± 1.0	2.8 ± 1.1	*0.002*
Coagulation SOFA at t_0	1.3 ± 1.3	1.5 ± 1.3	0.17
Inotropic score at t_0	6.0 (0.0–20.3)	5.0 (0.0–49.3)	0.15
Lactate at t_0, mmol/L	1.9 (1.2–2.8)	2.7 (1.5–5.2)	0.18
Platelets at t_0, $10^3/\mu L$	84 (35.3–166.8)	90 (55.0–129.0)	0.12
SOFA score at t_{72}	10.2 ± 5.1	13.3 ± 6.4	*<0.001*
Cardiovascular SOFA at t_{72}	2.2 ± 1.8	2.0 ± 1.9	0.64
Renal SOFA at t_{72}	1.8 ± 1.8	2.2 ± 1.8	0.92
Hepatic SOFA at t_{72}	1.1 ± 1.3	2.0 ± 1.5	*0.006*
Respiratory SOFA at t_{72}	1.9 ± 0.9	2.0 ± 1.1	0.92
Coagulation SOFA at t_{72}	1.7 ± 1.4	1.7 ± 1.2	0.72
Inotropic Score at t_{72}	6.0 (0.0–20.3)	5.0 (0.0–49.3)	0.76
Lactates at t_{72}, mmol/L	1.9 (1.2–2.8)	2.7 (1.5–5.2)	0.09
Platelets at t_{72}, $10^3/\mu L$	84 (35.3–166.8)	90 (55.0–129.0)	0.63
28-day survival, N (%)	160 (58.8)	20 (34.5)	*0.003*
ICU survival, N (%)	170 (59)	22 (36.7)	*0.006*
Hospital survival, N (%)	158 (53.2)	21 (35)	*0.02*

Normally distributed data are expressed as mean ± SD and non-normally distributed data as median (interquartile range)

Italics indicates significant p values

real life collecting data from unselected populations of septic patiens. PMX-HP is a complementary retreatment applied to patients affected by severe sepsis and septic shock that not respond to standard care.

The registry lacked of data about fluid load administered and hemodynamic monitor directing fluid resuscitation. However, each center performed PMX-HP only after the application of international consensus recommendation for sepsis, as strategy of resuscitation.

Surprisingly, in 142 patients (42 %) with clinical diagnosis of severe sepsis or septic shock, microbiological culture results were not reported that, if not performed, indicates a poor compliance to the bundles recommendations [20].

In 68 patients, EA was high although microbiological analysis did not reveal the presence of Gram negative germs. We can only suspect that the measured EA came from a Gram negative component of infection, which was either not revealed in microbiological tests or it was caused by direct translocation of endotoxin due to sepsis-induced permeability of the gut.

PMX-HP seemed to be safe: no major adverse events were reported. Data analysis showed a significant platelet count reduction at t_{72} without clinical worsening of the patients. The phenomenon observed could be a manifestation of the septic cascade evolution, which could alter platelet count and function, otherwise a complication of the extracorporeal technique. Data collected in the registry did not permit to establish a relationship between platelet decline and PMX-HP or other causes. The majority of patients who experienced a severe decline in platelet numbers were also receiving Renal Replacement Therapy.

Despite the retrospective nature of EUPHAS 2 data collection and the lack of a control group, the relevant number of patients allowed a reliable statistical analysis of PMX-HP feasibility in a real clinical context.

Recently published epidemiologic studies reported a 48.7 % in-hospital mortality for septic shock in France [26], as well as a 44 % hospital mortality for severe sepsis in Asian countries [27], having both the same period of time of EUPHAS 2. The comparison between EUPHAS 2 and epidemiologic studies in France [26] and Asia [27] showed a trend to clinical improvement without significant adverse event associated with endotoxin removal. Patients with abdominal infections treated within 24 h from the diagnosis of septic shock, had a 28-day survival of 64.5 %, which was comparable with 68 % observed in EUPHAS [15].

Recently, Zhou et al. [28] extended the analysis of effectiveness to all types of extracorporeal therapies in sepsis RCTs and concluded that the effect on mortality was mainly driven by studies using PMX-HP.

Iwagami et al. [29] published a retrospective analysis on 590 patients treated with PMX-HP matched through a propensity score to 590 patients treated with standard care who had open abdominal surgery on the day of admission for perforation of lower gastrointestinal tract, requiring the infusion of vasopressors. The authors showed a 28-day mortality of 17.1 % (101 of 590) in the PMX-HP group and 16.3 % (96 of 590) in the control group ($p = 0.696$). Data came from a nationwide inpatient database in Japan, showing no benefit of PMX-HP in a less severe population characterized by a low mortality rate. However, Payen et al. in the ABDOMIX randomized controlled trial [16] observed an absence of benefit from the use of PMX membranes to treat peritonitis-induced septic shock after emergency surgery.

In ABDOMIX, the 28-day mortality rate was close to recent clinical RCTs on selected patient population affected by septic shock [30] unlike EUPHAS 2, which is a registry without specific inclusion criteria. ABDOMIX excluded patients affected by life-threatening abdominal diseases included in EUPHAS 2 as ischemia, obstruction, inflammatory colitis and trauma. In ABDOMIX, only 81 over the 119 treated patients had completed two sessions of PMX-HP unlike EUPHAS [15], in which all patients enrolled had completed the two PMX-HP planned with a definitely higher mortality in the control group. In ABDOMIX, the isolation of yeasts from peritoneum was more frequent in PMX-treated group than in controls: this kind of disease represents a severe life-threatening condition not susceptible to improve by the endotoxin-adsorption blood purification techniques.

EUPHAS 2 confirmed that PMX-HP is often used to treat non-abdominal infection. The respiratory source was in fact the second clinical condition most frequently observed in the study and in this context the efficacy of the PMX-HP seemed less efficient. ICU and hospital survival were quite similar between patients with abdominal and respiratory sepsis, but patients with respiratory infections showed a trend toward a higher mortality rate at 28 days (Additional file 1: Table S2).

Lower respiratory tract infections might have some differences compared to abdominal or urinary sepsis. Pulmonary sepsis seems to respond less to the two sessions of endotoxin removal because source control is substantially achieved through the antibiotic action and the resolution needs a longer time. Differently in patients with intra-abdominal sepsis, the source control is obtained through surgery and the concomitant PMX treatment, achieving a more rapid resolution.

Another limitation of EUPHAS 2 is the lack of information about patients comorbidities and early antibiotic therapy appropriately applied, which cannot be obtained from the phase 1 of the registry. The phase 2 will clarify the implication of these important factors related to the outcome.

The database included both 297 European and 60 Asian patients. Even if baseline characteristics of patients at admission were similar between the two groups except for the age (Asian were younger than European, respectively 51.6 ± 14.7 vs 62.1 ± 14.8 years, $p < 0.001$), there was a significant difference at the enrollment to PMX-HP in terms of SOFA score and septic source. European and Asiatic population were not comparable for the septic source identified: Abdominal sepsis was prevalent in European patients, and pulmonary sepsis was most frequent in Asian patients.

Asiatic patients had a SOFA score higher than European patients (15.6 ± 4.7 vs 12.4 ± 4.2 respectively, $p < 0.001$), especially for respiratory and hepatic components. Phua et al. [27] reported a lower compliance with surviving sepsis campaign bundles in Asian ICUs, particularly during the first 24 h. A lower adherence to bundles correlated with worsening clinical condition and higher mortality.

Both European and Asian patients showed a similar clinical effect of PMX-HP treatment on organ dysfunction, that is mainly a significant reduction of vasopressor dependence and an improvement in gas exchange.

Published papers have underlined the positive effect of endotoxin removal by PMX-HP on cardiovascular dysfunction both increasing the arterial pressure and reducing the need of vasopressors.

In EUPHAS 2 registry, the cardiovascular component of SOFA represented 26.7 % of the overall score when the treatment was started. This means that enrolled patients were likely to have a high vasopressor load. Several studies showed that a higher vasopressor load is related to a higher risk of death in septic shock. A recent publication by Monti et al. [31] analyzed the response to PMX-HP of patients affected by refractory septic shock. They concluded that an early hemodynamic improvement highlighted by a vasopressor load reduction, potentially attenuates the mortality rate. The Cox regression analysis of 28-day mortality recognized the variation between baseline and 72 h of cardiovascular and coagulation components of SOFA score as independent covariates.

The similar degree of cardiovascular response to the PMX-HP treatment did not reflect a similar effect on mortality in Europe and Asia (Additional file 4: Figure S3, Additional file 5: Figure S4). Asian patients showed a lower survival rate and a higher length of stay than European patients, both justified by the worse organ dysfunction at the beginning of PMX-HP despite a cardiovascular response similar to European patients. The worse outcome of Asian patients could be related to the lower adherence to sepsis guideline and the higher incidence of respiratory infection than European patients.

In conclusion, notwithstanding the retrospective nature of the present data collection and the lack of a control group, these data confirmed the feasibility of the PMX-HP application in the usual clinical context without life-threatening adverse events related to its application, as already described in previous RCTs and observational studies. The ongoing EUPHRATES RCT [32] will clarify the effective clinical collocation of PMX-HP in patients suffering from endotoxin-mediated septic shock.

Abbreviations
EAA: endotoxin activity assay; EA: endotoxin activity; ICU: intensive care units; LPS: lipopolysaccharide; MOF: multiple organ failure; PMX-HP: polymyxin-B hemoperfusion; RCT: randomized controlled trial; SS: severe sepsis; SSh: septic shock; HR: heart rate; MAP: mean arterial pressure.

Authors' contributions
All authors contributed in each part of the paper, from the drafting of the protocol, to the collection and analysis of data, up to the drafting of the manuscript. All authors read and approved the final manuscript.

Author details
[1] Department of Intensive Care and Anaesthesiology, Agostino Gemelli University Hospital, Catholic University of the Sacred Heart, Largo A. Gemelli, 8, 00168 Rome, Italy. [2] Critical Care Center, Sabadell Hospital, CIBER Enfermedades Respiratorias, Corporació Sanitària Universitària Parc Taulí, Universitat Autònoma de Barcelona, Sabadell, Spain. [3] Department of Anaesthesia and Intensive Care Medicine, Niguarda Ca' Granda Hospital, University of Milan-Bicocca, Milan, Italy. [4] Department of Anaesthesia and Intensive Care Medicine, University of Rome "La Sapienza", Rome, Italy. [5] Department of Nephrology, Dialysis and Transplantation, International Renal Research Institute of Vicenza (IRRIV), San Bortolo Hospital, Vicenza, Italy.

Acknowledgements
The Early Use of Polymyxin B Hemoperfusion in the Abdominal Sepsis 2 Collaborative Group: Riccardo Maviglia, Sandra Cicconi, Davide Silvestri, Giuseppe Bello, Alessandra Brendolan, Federico Nalesso, Gianluca Villa, Pasquale Piccinni, Erica Martin, Vincenzo Cantaluppi, Sergio Vesconi, Giampaolo Casella, Egidio Fasanella, Michele Debitonto, Gianmario Monza, Angelo Blasetti, Rosaria Coletta, Michele D'Ambrosio, Gilda Cinnella, Patrizia Murino, Eugenio Piscitelli, Gaetano Centonze, Marco Cucurachi, Giuseppe Altieri, Vincenzo Leonardo, Anna Sara Idra, Goffredo Del Rosso, Maria Polidoro, Nicola Stigliano, Giuseppe Pittella, Gianluca Paternoster, Giuseppe Pulito, Daniela Puscio, Diego Cingolani, Gabriele Falzetti, Pietro Vecchiarelli, Francesco Giunta, Francesco Forfori, Giacomo Castiglione, Stefano Greco, Carlo Capra, Luciano Crema, Leonor Tamayo, Cristina Urbano, Brunello Pezza, Nadia Zarrillo, Pasquale Di Monaco, Giuseppe Climaco, Pasquale De Negri, Pasqualina Modano, Riccardo Pagliarulo, Claudio Petrillo, Tania Stripoli, Roberto Oggioni, Laura Campiglia, Anna Rita Valletta, Manuela Lugano, Domenico Milella, Laura Micucci, Ursula Reist, Rolf Ensner, Christian Gianbarba, Lukas Brander, Rajib Paul, Rajesh Crawla, Sanjeev Jasujia, Rajesh Pande, Pratibha Dileep, Sankaran Sundar, Raju Ganesan, Sandeep Dewan, Vivek Nangia, Raj Kumar Mani, Omender Singh, Pracee Sathe, Gupta Sachin, Pradeep M. D'Costa, Samavedam Srivanas, Yogendra Pal Singh, Kent Doi, Fumika Taki, Ricard Ferrer Roca, Eduardo Romay Medina, Josè Gernacho, Francisco Martí, Alberto Martinez-Ruiz, Fernando Martinez-Sagasti, Rafael Zaragoza Crespo, Paola Torti, Valeria Terzi.

Competing interests
The authors MA, SLC, VMR received an unrestricted research grant from ESTOR s.p.a. that funded part of the EUPHAS study published in the JAMA; AM is a member of the steering committee of the Euphrates study; AA received an unrestricted research grant from Ferrer Pharma, Grifols, Rubio, AM Pharma; CR received an unrestricted research grant from Toray, GE, Asahi, Astute.

Funding
The study was partially supported by ESTOR s.p.a.

References
1. Shoji H. Extracorporeal endotoxin removal for the treatment of sepsis: endotoxin adsorption cartridge (Toraymyxin). Ther Apher Dial. 2003;7:108–14.
2. Opal SM, Gluck T. Endotoxin as a drug target. Crit Care Med. 2003;31:S57–64.
3. Kellum JA. A targeted extracorporeal therapy for endotoxemia: the time has come. Crit Care. 2007;11:137.
4. Marshall JC, Foster D, Vincent JL, Cook DJ, Cohen J, Dellinger RP, Opal S, Abraham E, Brett SJ, Smith T, Mehta S, Derzko A, Romaschin A. Diagnostic and prognostic implications of endotoxemia in critical illness: results of the MEDIC study. J Infect Dis. 2004;190:527–34.
5. Perego AF, Morabito S, Graziani G, Casella GP, Parodi O. Polymyxin-B direct hemoperfusion (PMX-DHP) in gram negative sepsis. G Ital Nefrol. 2006;23(Suppl 36):S94–102.
6. Nakamura T, Ebihara I, Shoji H, Ushiyama C, Suzuki S, Koide H. Treatment with polymyxin B-immobilized fiber reduces platelet activation in septic

shock patients: decrease in plasma levels of soluble P-selectin, platelet factor 4 and beta-thromboglobulin. Inflamm Res. 1999;48:171–5.
7. Cantaluppi V, Assenzio B, Pasero D, Romanazzi GM, Pacitti A, Lanfranco G, Puntorieri V, Martin EL, Mascia L, Monti G, Casella G, Segoloni GP, Camussi G, Ranieri VM. Polymyxin-B hemoperfusion inactivates circulating proapoptotic factors. Intensive Care Med. 2008;34:1638–45.
8. Kushi H, Miki T, Okamaoto K, Nakahara J, Saito T, Tanjoh K. Early hemoperfusion with an immobilized polymyxin B fiber column eliminates humoral mediators and improves pulmonary oxygenation. Crit Care. 2005;9:R653–61.
9. Suzuki H, Nemoto H, Nakamoto H, Okada H, Sugahara S, Kanno Y, Moriwaki K. Continuous hemodiafiltration with Polymyxin-B immobilized fiber is effective in patients with sepsis syndrome and acute renal failure. Ther Apher. 2002;6:234–40.
10. Uriu K, Osajima A, Hiroshige K, Watanabe H, Aibara K, Inada Y, Segawa K, Anai H, Takagi I, Ito A, Kamochi M, Kaizu K. Endotoxin removal by direct hemoperfusion with an adsorbent column using polymyxin B-immobilized fiber ameliorates systemic circulatory disturbance in patients with septic shock. Am J Kidney Dis. 2002;39:937–47.
11. Nemoto H, Nakamoto H, Okada H, Sugahara S, Moriwaki K, Arai M, Kanno Y, Suzuki H. Newly developed immobilized polymyxin B fibers improve the survival of patients with sepsis. Blood Purif. 2001;19:361–8.
12. Nakamura H, Matsuda K, Suzuki Y, Shoji H, Koide H. Polymyxin B-immobilized fiber hemoperfusion in patients with sepsis. Dial Transplant. 2003;32:602–7.
13. Ruberto F, Pugliese F, D'Alio A, Martelli S, Bruno K, Marcellino V, Summonti D, Celli P, Perrella S, Cappannoli A, Pietropaoli C, Tosi A, Diana B, Novelli G, Rossi M, Ginanni-Corradini S, Ferretti G, Berloco PB, Pietropaoli P. Clinical effects of direct hemoperfusion using a polymyxin-B immobilized column in solid organ transplanted patients with signs of severe sepsis and septic shock. A pilot study. Int J Artif Org. 2007;30:915–22.
14. Cruz DN, Perazella MA, Bellomo R, de Cal M, Polanco N, Corradi V, Lentini P, Nalesso F, Ueno T, Ranieri VM, Ronco C. Effectiveness of polymyxin B-immobilized fiber column in sepsis: a systematic review. Crit Care. 2007;11:R47.
15. Cruz DN, Antonelli M, Fumagalli R, Foltran F, Brienza N, Donati A, Malcangi V, Petrini F, Volta G, Bobbio Pallavicini FM, Rottoli F, Giunta F, Ronco C. Early use of polymyxin B hemoperfusion in abdominal septic shock: the EUPHAS randomized controlled trial. JAMA. 2009;301:2445–52.
16. Payen DM, Guilhot J, Launey Y, Lukaszewicz AC, Kaaki M, Veber B, Pottecher J, Joannes-Boyau O, Martin-Lefevre L, Jabaudon M, Mimoz O, Coudroy R, Ferrandiere M, Kipnis E, Vela C, Chevallier S, Mallat J, Robert R. Early use of polymyxin B hemoperfusion in patients with septic shock due to peritonitis: a multicenter randomized control trial. Intensive Care Med. 2015;41(6):975–84.
17. Tsushima K, Kubo K, Yoshikawa S, Koizumi T, Yasuo M, Furuya S, Hora K. Effects of PMX-DHP treatment for patients with directly induced acute respiratory distress syndrome. Ther Apher Dial. 2007;11(2):138–45.
18. Martin EL, Cruz DN, Monti G, Casella G, Vesconi S, Ranieri VM, Ronco C, Antonelli M. Endotoxin removal: how far from the evidence? The EUPHAS 2 Project. Contrib Nephrol. 2010;167:119–25.
19. Early Use of Polymyxin B Hemoperfusion in the Abdominal Sepsis 2 Collaborative Group. Polymyxin B hemoperfusion in clinical practice: the picture from an unbound collaborative registry. Blood Purif. 2014;37(Suppl 1):22–5.
20. Dellinger RP, Levy MM, Rhodes A, Annane D, Gerlach H, Opal SM, Sevransky JE, Sprung CL, Douglas IS, Jaeschke R, Osborn TM, Nunnally ME, Townsend SR, Reinhart K, Kleinpell RM, Angus DC, Deutschman CS, Machado FR, Rubenfeld GD, Webb SA, Beale RJ, Vincent JL, Moreno R. Surviving sepsis campaign: international guidelines for management of severe sepsis and septic shock: 2012. Crit Care Med. 2013;41:580–637.
21. Marshall JC, Walker PM, Foster DM, Harris D, Ribeiro M, Paice J, Romaschin AD, Derzko AN. Measurement of endotoxin activity in critically ill patients using whole blood neutrophil dependent chemiluminescence. Crit Care. 2002;6:342–8.
22. Vincent JL, Moreno R, Takala J, Willatts S, De Mendonca A, Bruining H, Reinhart CK, Suter PM, Thijs LG. The SOFA (Sepsis-related Organ Failure Assessment) score to describe organ dysfunction/failure. On behalf of the Working Group on Sepsis-Related Problems of the European Society of Intensive Care Medicine. Intensive Care Med. 1996;22:707–10.
23. Ferreira FL, Bota DP, Bross A, Melot C, Vincent JL. Serial evaluation of the SOFA score to predict outcome in critically ill patients. JAMA. 2001;286:1754–8.
24. Moreno R, Vincent JL, Matos R, Mendonca A, Cantraine F, Thijs L, Takala J, Sprung C, Antonelli M, Bruining H, Willatts S. The use of maximum SOFA score to quantify organ dysfunction/failure in intensive care. Results of a prospective, multicentre study. Working Group on Sepsis related Problems of the ESICM. Intensive Care Med. 1999;25:686–96.
25. Jones AE, Trzeciak S, Kline JA. The Sequential Organ Failure Assessment score for predicting outcome in patients with severe sepsis and evidence of hypoperfusion at the time of emergency department presentation. Crit Care Med. 2009;37:1649–54.
26. Quenot JP, Binquet C, Kara F, Martinet O, Ganster F, Navellou JC, Castelain V, Barraud D, Cousson J, Louis G, Perez P, Kuteifan K, Noirot A, Badie J, Mezher C, Lessire H, Pavon A. The epidemiology of septic shock in French intensive care units: the prospective multicenter cohort EPISS study. Crit Care. 2013;17:R65.
27. Phua J, Koh Y, Du B, Tang YQ, Divatia JV, Tan CC, Gomersall CD, Faruq MO, Shrestha BR, Gia Binh N, Arabi YM, Salahuddin N, Wahyuprajitno B, Tu ML, Wahab AY, Hameed AA, Nishimura M, Procyshyn M, Chan YH. Management of severe sepsis in patients admitted to Asian intensive care units: prospective cohort study. BMJ. 2011;342:d3245.
28. Zhou F, Peng Z, Murugan R, Kellum JA. Blood purification and mortality in sepsis: a meta-analysis of randomized trials. Crit Care Med. 2013;41:2209–20.
29. Iwagami M, Yasunaga H, Doi K, Horiguchi H, Fushimi K, Matsubara T, Yahagi N, Noiri E. Postoperative polymyxin B hemoperfusion and mortality in patients with abdominal septic shock: a propensity-matched analysis. Crit Care Med. 2014;42(5):1187–93.
30. Angus DC, Barnato AE, Bell D, Bellomo R, Chong CR, Coats TJ, Davies A, Delaney A, Harrison DA, Holdgate A, Howe B, Huang DT, Iwashyna T, Kellum JA, Peake SL, Pike F, Reade MC, Rowan KM, Singer M, Webb SA, Weissfeld LA, Yealy DM, Young JD. A systematic review and meta-analysis of early goal-directed therapy for septic shock: the ARISE, ProCESS and ProMISe Investigators. Intensive Care Med. 2015;41(9):1549–60.
31. Monti G, Terzi V, Calini A, Di Marco F, Cruz D, Pulici M, Brioschi P, Vesconi S, Fumagalli R, Casella G. Rescue therapy with polymyxin B hemoperfusion in high-dose vasopressor therapy refractory septic shock. Miner Anestesiol. 2015;81:516–25.
32. Klein DJ, Foster D, Schorr CA, Kazempour K, Walker PM, Dellinger RP. The EUPHRATES trial (Evaluating the Use of Polymyxin B Hemoperfusion in a Randomized controlled trial of Adults Treated for Endotoxemia and Septic shock): study protocol for a randomized controlled trial. Trials. 2014;11(15):218. doi:10.1186/1745-6215-15-218.

22

Combination of C-reactive protein, procalcitonin and sepsis-related organ failure score for the diagnosis of sepsis in critical patients

Yi Yang[1†], Jianfeng Xie[1†], Fengmei Guo[1], Federico Longhini[1,2], Zhiwei Gao[1], Yingzi Huang[1] and Haibo Qiu[1*]

Abstract

Objective: To measure the ability of a new bioscore to diagnose sepsis in a general critical care population.

Methods: The study was done at an intensive care unit (ICU) from April to December 2012. Demographic and clinical patient information were recorded on admission to the ICU with blood samples taken for C-reactive protein (CRP), procalcitonin (PCT), interleukin-6, white blood cell count, as well as body temperature, age and the sepsis-related organ failure (SOFA) score. These parameters were used to create a scoring system. The scoring system then underwent analysis by univariate analysis and multivariate logistic regression analysis to identify which of these clinical parameters were statistically different in septic versus non-septic patients. The bioscore was then tested in a receiver operator characteristic curve to determine statistical significance of the scoring systems ability to predict sepsis. Finally, a bioscore cutoff value was defined to provide a level for sepsis diagnosis.

Results: Three hundred patients were enrolled, of which 107 patients were septic and 193 patients were non-septic. Univariate logistic regression showed that age, gender, CRP, PCT and SOFA were risk factors for occurrence of sepsis. Multivariate analysis revealed CRP (AUC 0.729, 95 % CI 0.671–0.787, $P < 0.001$), PCT (AUC 0.711, 95 % CI 0.652–0.770, $P < 0.001$) and SOFA (AUC 0.670, 95 % CI 0.607–0.733, $P < 0.001$) to be statistically significant. The combination of these values in the bioscore had an AUC of 0.790 (95 % CI 0.739–0.834, $P < 0.001$). A bioscore of $\geq$2.65 was considered to be statistically significant in making a positive diagnosis of sepsis.

Conclusions: This bioscore using CRP, PCT and SOFA score may potentially be used in the future to help identify septic patients earlier, improving their access to timely treatment modalities.

Keywords: C-reactive protein, Procalcitonin, Interleukin-6, Sepsis, Bioscore

Background

Sepsis and septic shock are pathological conditions impacting a large proportion of patients admitted to the ICU, and these patients unfortunately have poor outcomes [1]. Sepsis results from a dysregulated host response to infection leading to uncontrolled inflammation and organ dysfunction and potentially a hypotensive state known as septic shock [2]. This clinical scenario falls under the multiple organ dysfunction syndrome [3].

Early diagnosis and direct appropriate therapy within the first hours of hospital admission has been shown to have beneficial effects with respect to patient outcome [4]. Furthermore, diagnostic and treatment delay prolongs hospital length of stay and increases healthcare costs [5, 6]. As a result, the availability of an efficient biomarker/evaluation system would be crucial to help diagnose sepsis quickly. To be useful, a biomarker should be characterized by its "capacity to provide timely

*Correspondence: haiboq2000@163.com
†Yi Yang and Jianfeng Xie contributed equally to this work
[1] Department of Critical Care Medicine, Nanjing Zhong-Da Hospital, School of Medicine, Southeast University, Nanjing 210009, Jiangsu, China
Full list of author information is available at the end of the article

information beyond that which is readily available from routine physiologic data and clinical examination" [7].

Several bloodstream biomarkers in sepsis have been previously investigated [8], including PCT and CRP [9]. Sepsis-induced cytokines promote the production of PCT, which is typically secreted by C cells of the thyroid in response to hypercalcemia. Similarly, CRP is an acute-phase reactant, synthesized by the liver, mainly in response to IL-6. IL-6 is a cytokine that generates an initial response to injury or infection; its levels rise significantly during early sepsis, and for this reason, it has been used for sepsis diagnosis and patient outcome prediction [10, 11]. Despite their common use, all these biomarkers suffer individual applicability limitations, including lack of sepsis specificity [12]. Another approach has been to consider a combination of markers and clinical parameters, known as a bioscore. Recently, Gibot et al. [13] demonstrated high diagnostic performance by a bioscore that combined the intensity of CD64 expression on polymorphonuclear cells (PMN CD64 index) together with PCT and the soluble triggering receptor expressed on myeloid cells-1 (sTREM-1) serum levels. However, while PCT measurement is widely and easily performed, sTREM-1 determination (by an ELISA assay) and CD64 assessment (by flow cytometery) is not routinely available in all hospitals, giving some limitations to this approach.

We hypothesized that by combining the common clinical biomarkers CRP, PCT and IL-6 with other clinical information, such as WBC, body temperature, age and gender, and the SOFA score in an extended bioscore (e-BS), we might be able to increase sensitivity and specificity of the combination of these tools for sepsis diagnosis. The aim of this investigation was to evaluate the value of these individual markers and to investigate whether an e-BS might have potential to improve early sepsis diagnosis.

Methods

Study design

This prospective study was performed in the ICU of a Nanjing Zhong-Da Hospital from April to December 2012. The protocol was approved by the local Institutional Ethics Committee (Approval Number: 2012ZD11KY08.0) in accordance with the ethical standards of the Declaration of Helsinki. Patients admitted into the ICU were enrolled in this study following informed consent from the patient or their guardian.

Patients

Inclusion criteria were: (1) ICU admission; (2) signed informed consent from the patient or their guardian; (3) $\geq$18 years of age. Patients were excluded from enrollment if they had been hospitalized or received antibiotics in the preceding 2 weeks, or if it was an ICU re-admission.

All eligible patients were treated by the attending physician according to normal clinical practice. If an infection was suspected or documented, samples of organic fluids were collected for microbiologic cultural tests and antimicrobial therapy was prescribed according to the ICU practice and guidelines [14] without any intervention by the researchers.

Sepsis was clinically defined as a diagnosed infection and at least two of four systemic inflammatory response syndrome (SIRS) criteria [15] which include: (a) body temperature >38 or <36 °C, (b) heart rate >90 beats/min, (c) respiratory rate >20 breaths/min or an arterial partial pressure of carbon dioxide < 4.3 kPa (32 mmHg), (d) white blood cell count >12,000 or <4000/mm^3, or the presence of >10 % immature neutrophils. The infection was defined on the basis of infection sites, clinical features, clinical microbiology and imaging tests. Two intensive care physicians were asked to retrospectively and independently analyze the clinical documentation for each patient, signs, symptoms and recent medical history to make the diagnosis of sepsis.

Data collection

The acquired dataset included the patients' demographic information, reason for admission, department of origin, infection site, blood culture results and laboratory characteristics. The patients were subsequently followed for 28 days for mortality.

Acute physiology and chronic health evaluation II (APACHE II) and sepsis-related organ failure assessment (SOFA) scores were calculated using data from the first 24 h after admission. Clinically significant WBC count was defined as WBC <4000 cells/μL (leukopenia) or >12,000 cells/μL (leukocytosis). Clinically significant body temperature was defined as <36 °C (hypothermia) or >38 °C (hyperthermia) [14, 15]. We also recorded the ICU and hospital length of stay.

Measurement of CRP, PCT and IL-6

Within 12 h after ICU admission, 5–10 mL of blood was sampled for CRP, PCT and IL-6 measurements. CRP concentrations were measured in a serum sample, using a turbidimetric immunoassay test (BNII, Siemens Healthcare Diagnostic, Germany). PCT concentrations were assessed in a serum sample, using an immunoassay with a sandwich technique and a chemiluminescent detection system, while IL-6 concentrations using a turbidimetric immunoassay test (Roche Elecsys® and MODULAR® E170, Switzerland). CRP, PCT and IL-6 were transformed into categorical score values (Additional file 1: Table S1).

Statistics and the scoring system

Normality distribution for quantitative variables was tested by the Kolmogorov–Smirnov test ($P > 0.10$). For categorical variables, Chi-square test, Fisher's exact test or McNemar test were applied as appropriate. Comparison of continuous variables between the two groups was conducted with Student's t test or Mann–Whitney U test depending on Gaussian distribution. To compare data from three or more patient groups, we applied the one-way analysis of variance (ANOVA), and, when indicated, the Student–Newmann–Keuls method was used as a post hoc test. Sensitivity and specificity were computed for all biomarker assays.

Logistic regression was used according to the presence or absence of sepsis and death as dependent variables to calculate the corresponding regression coefficients (using round numbers). The bioscore system was analyzed for the area under the curve, and the subsequent ROC curves were used to evaluate the prognostic value. The Youden index was applied to set the cutoffs and compared between the combined evaluation method and single evaluation methods.

Normally distributed data are expressed as mean ± SD, while non-normal distributed as median [25th–75th IQR]. All statistical analyses were performed using SPSS 19.0 software (IBM SPSS, USA); two-tailed P values <0.05 were considered statistically significant.

Results

Baseline data

Three hundred consecutive patients were included. The entire population characteristics including infection and organism findings of septic populations are shown in Table 1 and Additional file 1: Table S2. Specifically, we

Table 1 Whole population characteristics and difference between septic and non-septic patients

Characteristics	Total 300	Septic patients 107 (36 %)	Non-septic patients 193 (64 %)	*P* value
Age (years)	64 ± 18	69 ± 15	61 ± 19	<0.001
Male sex, *n* (%)	173 (58)	74 (69)	99 (51)	<0.001
Body temperature, *n* (%)				0.03
<36 or >38 °C	97 (32.3 %)	43 (40.2)	54 (28.0)	
36–38 °C	203 (67.7 %)	64 (59.8)	139 (72.0)	
APACHE II score	17 ± 8	19 ± 7	16 ± 8	0.002
SOFA score	6.8 ± 3.5	8.2 ± 3.5	6.1 ± 3.2	<0.001
Admission department—no. (%)				
Emergency room	86 (28.7)	39 (36.4)	47 (24.4)	0.026
Surgical wards	164 (54.7)	32 (29.9)	132 (68.4)	<0.001
Without surgical procedure	5 (1.7)	3 (2.8)	2 (1.0)	0.252
With surgical procedure	159 (53)	29 (27.1)	130 (67.3)	<0.001
Medical wards	50 (16.7)	36 (33.6)	14 (7.2)	<0.001
Pathology of admission—no. (%)				
Acute pancreatitis	2 (0.7)	1 (0.9)	1 (0.5)	1.0
Intracerebral hemorrhage	32 (10.7)	8 (7.5)	24 (12.4)	0.183
Cardiac arrest	8 (2.7)	2 (1.9)	6 (3.1)	0.519
Trauma	17 (5.7)	3 (2.8)	15 (7.8)	<0.001
Acute myocardial infarction	10 (33.3)	4 (3.7)	6 (3.1)	0.777
High-risk surgery	130 (43.3)	0	130 (67.4)	
Cardiac surgery	51 (17.0)	0	51 (26.4)	
Non-cardiac surgery	79 (26.3)	0	79 (40.9)	
Sever sepsis	79 (26.3)	79 (73.8)	0	
Other	22 (7.3)	10 (9.3)	12 (6.1)	0.296
CRP	37.25 (8.79–87.13)	63.8 (32.3–114)	21.8 (5.20–60.55)	<0.001
PCT	0.66 (0.16–3.13)	1.79 (0.57–8.95)	0.38 (0.11–1.54)	<0.001
IL-6	125.2 (52.5–463.3)	124.8 (43.9–418.3)	125.6 (54.5–479.9)	0.97
Length of ICU stay—no. of days	5 [2–10]	8 [4–14]	3 [1–8]	<0.001
Length of hospital stay—no. of days	19 [10–28]	23 [13–32]	18 [9–26]	0.005
28-day mortality—no. (%)	75 (25)	32 (30)	43 (22)	0.144

collected data on age, gender, core body temperature, WBC, PCT, CRP, IL-6 and calculated a SOFA score. Of note, 107 (35.7 %) patients (septic population) were septic, which included the subgroups of sepsis ($n = 28$, 9.3 %), severe sepsis ($n = 41$, 13.7 %) or septic shock ($n = 38$, 12.7 %) patients. The other 193 patients were not septic.

Diagnostic value of the scoring system

Univariate analysis of the measured raw patient parameters using a ROC curve showed that CRP, PCT and SOFA were significant for the diagnosis of sepsis (Fig. 1a). The AUCs were 0.729, 0.737 and 0.671, respectively (Table 2). The analysis revealed that clinical laboratory values of 21.1, 0.4475 and 6, respectively, were cutoff points that helped make the diagnosis of sepsis. However, given that the AUC values were low, we felt using the raw laboratory values would not accurately be able to predict a sepsis diagnosis. Therefore, we used the measured parameters to define a categorical-based scoring system in an attempt to better delineate syndrome clusters.

In order to define the scoring system (bioscore), each measured clinical variable (using a rounded number) was converted into categorical values as a final weighted value, as shown in Additional file 1: Table S3. Subsequent univariate analysis of these ordinal values indicated that age, gender, PCT, CRP and SOFA were significantly correlated with occurrence of sepsis according to the score in Additional file 1: Table S1 (Table 3). However, we did not find WBC, body temperature and IL-6 had diagnostic value in recognizing sepsis. Then, multivariate analysis by logistic regression using the presence or absence of sepsis as a dependent variable and the parameters identified by univariate analysis found statistical significance of age, gender, CRP, PCT and SOFA (Table 3).

To further refine the scoring system, we eliminated age and gender as we felt these parameters were less specific to predicting when a patient was truly septic. Therefore, we analyzed the total bioscore of each patient (using only CRP, PCT and SOFA score) on a ROC. When the bioscore was plotted for analysis by ROC curve (Fig. 1b), the AUC was 0.790 (95 % CI 0.739–0.834, $P < 0.001$) with a cutoff value of 2.65 suggesting a diagnosis of sepsis above this value. The sensitivity and specificity of the scoring system were 78.5 and 70 %, respectively, with a positive likelihood ratio of 2.61 and negative likelihood ratio of 0.31, respectively (Table 2).

Diagnostic value of the scoring system in subgroup populations

Surgical procedures impact physiologic parameters and, therefore, sought to evaluate the predictive ability of this

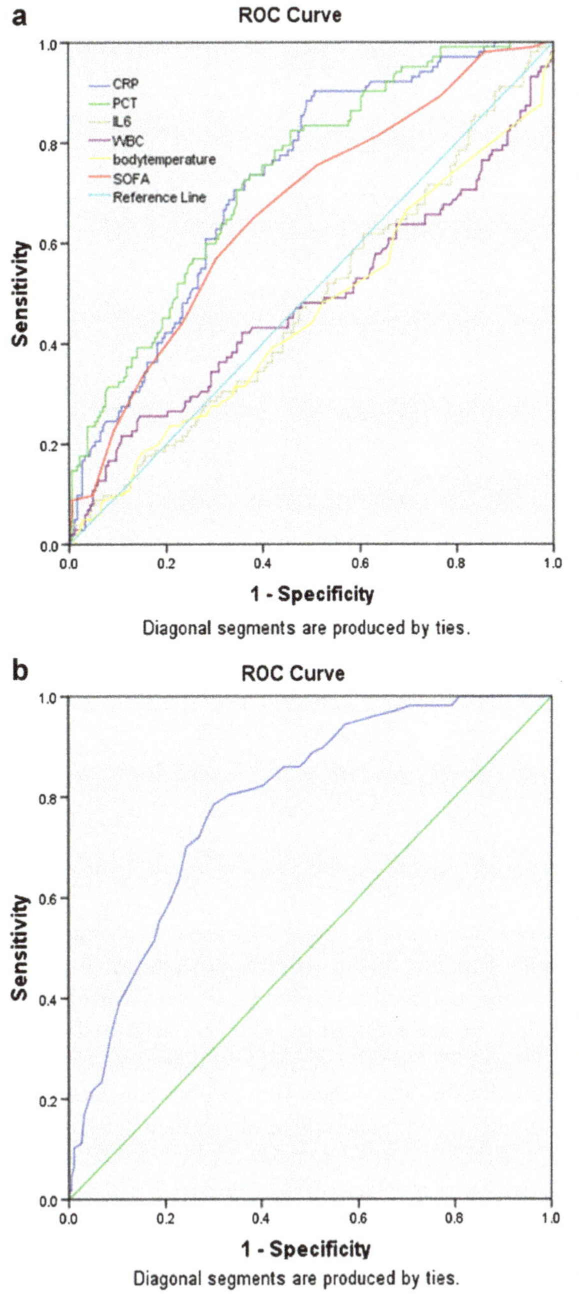

Fig. 1 Diagnostic values for sepsis of clinical variables estimated by receiver operating curve (ROC) analysis. **a** Area under the curve (AUC) for a null hypothesis was 0.5. AUC for C-reactive protein (CRP) was 0.729 (95 % CI 0.675–0.779, $P < 0.001$), procalcitonin (PCT) 0.737 (95 % CI 0.683–0.786, $P < 0.001$), interleukin-6 (IL-6) 0.511 (95 % CI 0.452–0.570, $P = 0.760$), white blood cells (WBC) 0.472 (95 % CI 0.400–0.545, $P = 0.426$), body temperature 0.468 (95 % CI 0.398–0.539, $P = 0.362$) and sepsis-related organ failure assessment (SOFA) 0.671 (95 % CI 0.615–0.714, $P < 0.001$). **b** For calculated score: Area under the curve (AUC) for a null hypothesis was 0.5. AUC for calculated score was 0.790 (95 % CI 0.739–0.834, $P < 0.001$)

Table 2 Diagnostic value of each parameter in sepsis

Variables	AUC	*P* value	Sensitivity	Specificity	+LR	−LR
All patients						
SOFA	0.671	<0.001	66.4	61.7	1.73	0.55
CRP	0.729	<0.001	90.7	49.7	1.80	0.19
PCT	0.737	<0.001	82.9	53.9	1.80	0.32
IL-6	0.511	0.760	28.2	78.7	1.32	0.91
Score	0.790	<0.001	78.5	70.0	2.61	0.31
Surgical patients						
SOFA	0.587	0.150	51.7	62.6	1.38	0.77
CRP	0.697	<0.001	89.7	45.0	1.63	0.23
PCT	0.698	<0.001	65.5	71.0	2.26	0.49
IL-6	0.522	0.713	75.9	36.4	1.19	0.66
Score	0.745	<0.001	82.8	63.4	2.26	0.27
Non-surgical patients						
SOFA	0.684	<0.001	71.8	59.7	1.78	0.47
CRP	0.762	<0.001	91.0	59.7	2.26	0.15
PCT	0.810	<0.001	75.0	77.4	3.32	0.32
IL-6	0.503	0.953	68.1	43.3	1.20	0.74
Score	0.836	<0.001	78.2	77.4	3.46	0.28
Newly hospitalized patients						
SOFA	0.781	<0.001	84.6	66.0	2.49	0.23
CRP	0.805	<0.001	89.7	66.0	2.64	0.16
PCT	0.868	<0.001	84.6	80.9	4.42	0.19
IL-6	0.601	0.101	82.1	44.7	1.48	0.40
Score	0.896	<0.001	84.6	83.0	4.97	0.19

bioscore in a subset of surgical patients. In a subgroup of patients that underwent surgical procedures ($n = 160$), univariate analysis determined significance for only CRP and PCT in sepsis diagnosis (Fig. 2a; Table 2). The AUC of CRP and PCT was 0.697 and 0.698, respectively. When the previously determined bioscore system was evaluated by ROC curve analysis in this patient subgroup, the AUC was 0.745 (95 % CI 0.670–0.810, $P < 0.001$) with a sensitivity and specificity of 82.8 and 63.4 %, respectively. The scoring system, which contained more contributing measurable data points, was higher than any of the individual parameters (Fig. 2b; Table 2).

In the non-surgically treated patients ($n = 140$), CRP, PCT and SOFA score had significant diagnostic value in diagnosing sepsis (Fig. 2c; Table 2). When the scoring system was evaluated by ROC curve analysis in this patient subgroup, the AUC was 0.836 (95 % CI 0.764–0.893, $P < 0.001$), which was better at identifying sepsis than any of the individual parameters (Fig. 2d; Table 2).

In the newly hospitalized patient subgroup ($n = 86$), univariate analysis revealed that CRP, PCT and SOFA were statistically significant in diagnosing sepsis (Fig. 2e; Table 2). Bioscores in this subgroup gave an AUC of 0.896 (95 % CI 0.812–0.952, $P < 0.001$) also showing a greater ability at identifying sepsis than any individual parameter (Fig. 2f; Table 2).

Risk factors for the 28-day mortality

Univariate analysis detected age, body temperature, SOFA score and IL-6 demonstrating significance association with the 28-day mortality (OR 1.017, 95 % CI 1.001–1.033, $P = 0.038$; OR 1.214, 95 % CI 1.002–1.471, $P = 0.048$; OR 1.261, 95 % CI 1.160–1.371, $P < 0.001$; OR 1.010, 95 % CI 1.001–1.017, $P = 0.045$, respectively). Multivariate logistic regression analysis showed that only age and SOFA were independently associated with 28-day mortality (OR 1.022, 95 % CI 1.003–1.041, $P = 0.024$; OR 1.263, 95 % CI 1.148–1.389, $P < 0.001$) (Table 4). Cox and Snell R^2 was 0.144, and Nagelkerke R^2 was 0.215.

Table 3 Univariate and multivariate associations of PCT, CRP, SOFA score with sepsis

Marker	Univariate		Multivariate	
	OR (95 % CI)	*P*	OR (95 % CI)	*P*
Age[a]	3.171 (1.833, 5.485)	<0.001	2.662 (1.382, 5.127)	0.003
Gender[a]	0.470 (0.285, 0.773)	0.003	0.377 (0.203, 0.701)	0.002
WBC	0.871 (0.540, 1.405)	0.571	0.704 (0.378, 1.311)	0.268
PCT				
0	1.0 (Reference)		1.0 (Reference)	
1[a]	4.169 (2.158, 8.055)	<0.001	3.485 (1.561, 7.780)	0.008
2	4.345 (2.155, 8.761)	<0.001	3.550 (1.467, 8.593)	0.074
3[a]	8.369 (3.815, 18.359)	<0.001	6.501 (2.326, 18.173)	0.001
CRP				
0	1.0 (Reference)		1.0 (Reference)	
1	3.191 (1.453, 7.011)	0.004	2.491 (0.958, 6.477)	0.061
2[a]	7.700 (3.138, 18.894)	<0.001	6.795 (2.188, 21.096)	0.001
3[a]	8.800 (3.964, 19.537)	<0.001	6.593 (2.395, 18.125)	<0.001
SOFA	1.204 (1.117, 1.297)	<0.001	2.314 (1.260, 14.251)	0.007
IL-6				
0	1.0 (Reference)		1.0 (Reference)	
1	1.691 (0.586, 4.877)	0.331	1.380 (0.343, 5.559)	0.651
2	1.364 (0.468, 3.976)	0.569	0.639 (0.152, 2.678)	0.540
3	1.524 (0.526, 4.415)	0.438	0. 576 (0.146, 2.278)	0.432
4	1.227 (0.425, 3.542)	0.706	0. 422 (0.106, 1.681)	0.221

[a] Cox and Snell R^2 was 0.282, and Nagelkerke R^2 was 0.389

Discussion

It is now generally agreed that a single clinical biomarker is not acceptable for accurately diagnosing and predicting prognosis during sepsis. The aim of this investigation was to evaluate the ability of an enhanced bioscore, where common clinical biomarkers are combined with other clinical laboratory information, to provide a more reliable diagnosis and prediction tool for sepsis patients. The study combined the most common clinical biomarkers for sepsis at ICU admission and clinical scoring methods to evaluate the possibility of increasing the accuracy of sepsis diagnosis in a general population of a Chinese ICU. The results of this study show that when threshold values of CRP, PCT and SOFA were taken into consideration by calculation of a bioscore value, this could be considered a statistically significant predictor for sepsis diagnosis. In these cases, the AUC values for the combined parameter score were more predictive than any one individual marker. Therefore, we consider these methods to have value in predicting sepsis.

CRP, PCT and IL-6 are used widely in attempting to clinically diagnose sepsis. In keeping with previous published data, our results confirm a low diagnostic value of CRP in a general ICU population [16]. However, when evaluating our entire study population, the accuracy of PCT was relatively low compared to previous studies and improved only slightly after selecting out surgical patients. In addition, we found that IL-6 suffered low diagnostic significance. There have also been contrasting results of IL-6 in diagnosing sepsis in the previous work, which may have been a result of different baseline patient characteristics [17–19].

Since CRP, PCT and IL-6 had been demonstrated to be elevated by various conditions without infection, i.e., trauma, surgery, burn, pancreatitis [20–22], we decided to analyze the subgroup populations [13]. We found a low diagnostic value of CRP and PCT in surgical patients and a high diagnostic value in non-surgical patients, especially in newly admitted patients. Our population was similar to the one described by Gibot et al. [13], and the diagnostic value of the previously mentioned biomarkers was comparable in their subgroup patients. However, we found the value of IL-6 in diagnosing sepsis did not change in the subgroup population, indicating IL-6 may not be a valuable biomarker for our cohort of patients.

(See figure on next page.)
Fig. 2 Diagnostic values for sepsis patients estimated by receiver operating curve (ROC) analysis. **a** For clinical variables in non-surgically treated patients: Area under the curve (AUC) for a null hypothesis was 0.5. AUC for C-reactive protein (CRP) was 0.697 (95 % CI 0.620–0.767, $P < 0.001$), procalcitonin (PCT) 0.698 (95 % CI 0.620–0.768, $P < 0.001$), interleukin-6 (IL-6) 0.522 (95 % CI 0.441–0.602, $P = 0.713$), white blood cells (WBC) 0.525 (95 % CI 0.445–0.604, $P = 0.676$), body temperature 0.511 (95 % CI 0.431–0.591, $P = 0.851$) and sepsis-related organ failure assessment (SOFA) 0.587 (95 % CI 0.507–0.664, $P < 0.001$). **b** For calculated score in non-surgically treated patients: Area under the curve (AUC) for a null hypothesis was 0.5. AUC for calculated score was 0.745 (95 % CI 0.670–0.810, $P < 0.001$). **c** For clinical variables in non-surgically treated patients: Area under the curve (AUC) for a null hypothesis was 0.5. AUC for C-reactive protein (CRP) was 0.762 (95 % CI 0.683–0.830, $P < 0.001$), procalcitonin (PCT) 0.810 (95 % CI 0.734–0.871, $P < 0.001$), interleukin-6 (IL-6) 0.503 (95 % CI 0.415–0.591, $P = 0.953$), white blood cells (WBC) 0.486 (95 % CI 0.390–0.582, $P = 0.775$), body temperature 0.478 (95 % CI 0.382–0.575, $P = 0.659$) and sepsis-related organ failure assessment (SOFA) 0.684 (95 % CI 0.600–0.769, $P < 0.001$). **d** For calculated score in non-surgically treated patients: Area under the curve (AUC) for a null hypothesis was 0.5. AUC for calculated score was 0.836 (95 % CI 0.764–0.893, $P < 0.001$). **e** For clinical variables in newly hospitalized sepsis patients: Area under the curve (AUC) for a null hypothesis was 0.5. AUC for C-reactive protein (CRP) was 0.805 (95 % CI 0.705–0.882, $P < 0.001$), procalcitonin (PCT) 0.868 (95 % CI 0.778, 0.931, $P < 0.001$), interleukin-6 (IL-6) 0.601 (95 % CI 0.490–0.705, $P = 0.102$), white blood cells (WBC) 0.482 (95 % CI 0.354–0.610, $P = 0.774$), body temperature 0.505 (95 % CI 0.378–0.632, $P = 0.940$) and sepsis-related organ failure assessment (SOFA) 0.781 (95 % CI 0.679–0.863, $P < 0.001$). **f** For calculated score in newly hospitalized sepsis patients: Area under the curve (AUC) for a null hypothesis was 0.5. AUC for calculated score was 0.896 (95 % CI 0.812–0.952, $P < 0.001$)

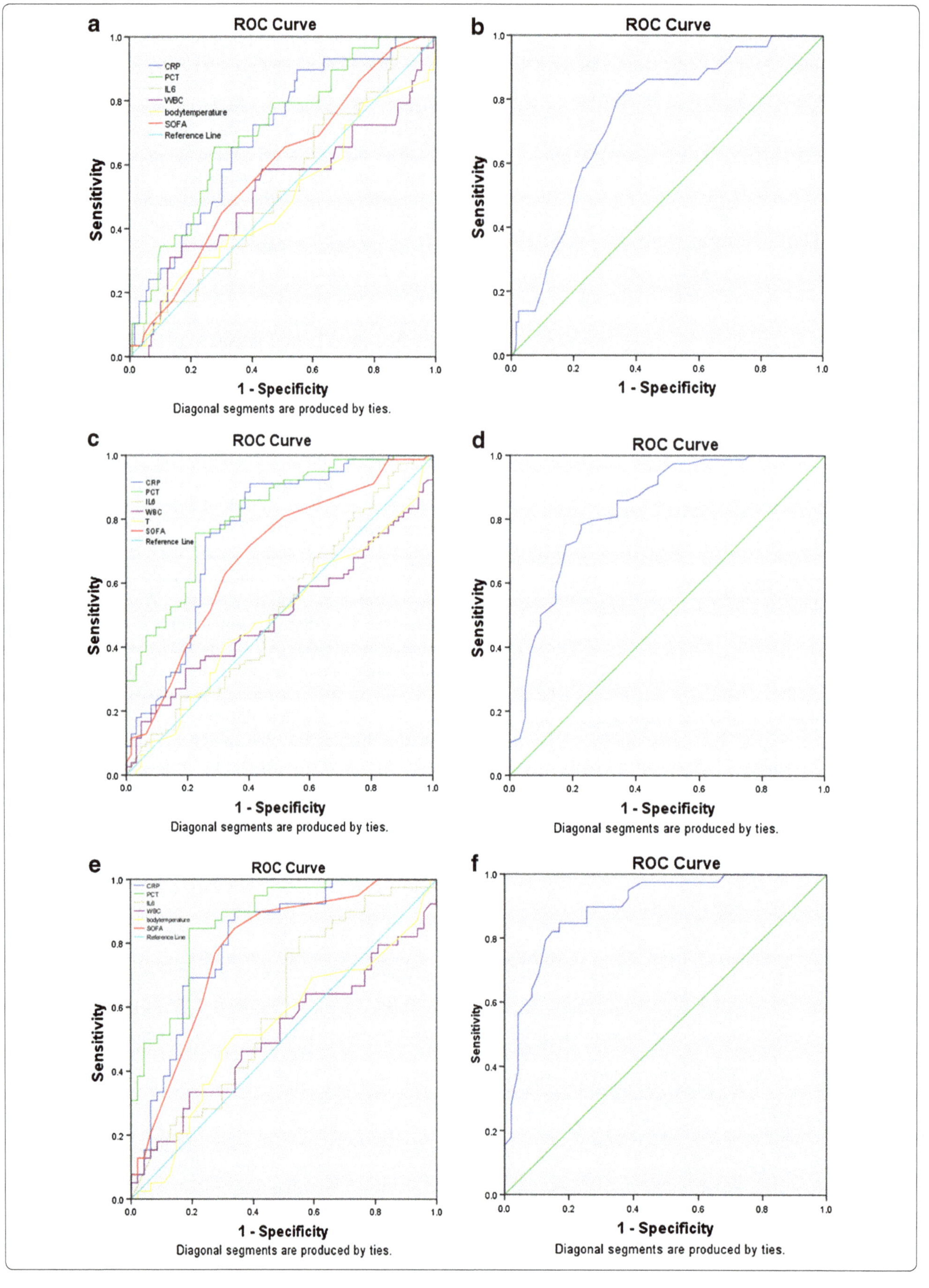
a
ROC Curve
CRP
PCT
IL6
WBC
bodytemperature
SOFA
Reference Line
Sensitivity
1 - Specificity
Diagonal segments are produced by ties.
b
ROC Curve
Sensitivity
1 - Specificity
c
ROC Curve
CRP
PCT
IL6
WBC
T
SOFA
Reference Line
Sensitivity
1 - Specificity
Diagonal segments are produced by ties.
d
ROC Curve
Sensitivity
1 - Specificity
Diagonal segments are produced by ties.
e
ROC Curve
Sensitivity
1 - Specificity
Diagonal segments are produced by ties.
f
ROC Curve
Sensitivity
1 - Specificity
Diagonal segments are produced by ties.

Table 4 Univariate and multivariate analysis of 28-day mortality

Marker	Univariate		Multivariate	
	OR (95 % CI)	*P*	OR (95 % CI)	*P*
Age[a]	1.017 (1.001, 1.033)	0.038	1.022 (1.003, 1.041)	0.024
Gender	0.670 (0.389, 1.156)	0.150	0.805 (0.437, 1.485)	0.488
PCT (ng/mL)	0.999 (0.996, 1.003)	0.671	0.997 (0.982, 1.013)	0.720
CRP (mg/L)	1.001 (0.997, 1.005)	0.606	0.999(0.994, 1.004)	0.718
SOFA[a]	1.261 (1.160, 1.371)	<0.001	1.263 (1.148, 1.389)	<0.001
IL-6	1.010 (1.001, 1.017)	0.045	1.000 (1.000, 1.001)	0.128
WBC	1.007 (0.997, 1.018)	0.179	1.005 (0.994, 1.004)	0.392
Body temperature	1.214 (1.002, 1.471)	0.048	1.100 (0.876, 1.381)	0.413

[a] Cox and Snell R^2 was 0.144, and Nagelkerke R^2 was 0.215

Other factors widely assessed in the diagnosis of sepsis and determining prognosis are body temperature and WBC count. However, these factors have repeatedly being shown to have poor sensitivity and specificity for sepsis diagnosis [23, 24]. Similarly, we found a low diagnostic value of body temperature and WBC count in our analysis.

Single parameter measurement had a relatively low diagnostic value in sepsis. Therefore, we combined multiple clinical parameters to build a scoring system to improve diagnostic abilities. Recently, Gibot and colleagues reported that some relatively new biomarkers (PCT, sTREM-1 and PMN CD64 index) were useful for diagnosing sepsis and that the combination of them in a score had an impressive diagnostic accuracy [13]. However, as the authors stated, these measurements may not be routinely available in all hospitals, limiting the scoring systems applicability. In contrast, CRP, PCT and IL-6 are available in most of the hospital laboratories, and their combination in an easily computable score could improve the accuracy of sepsis diagnosis. By analyzing ROC curves in this study, we were able to select a cutoff value for the bioscore for diagnosis prediction. In each population of patients, including the total ICU population, the non-surgical subpopulation and the newly hospitalized subpopulation, this method provided a better prediction of diagnosis than any of the other biomarkers in isolation that were assessed in this study, which was similar to previous published information [13].

The present study has its limitations. First, this is a single-center study and the numbers of patients studied are limited. A larger population would add more power, making the results more generalizable. Different studies have described different ROC and AUC for the same biomarkers. This can be explained by different studied populations and laboratory techniques, all of which can impact the diagnostic and prognostic power of these tests. However, our measurements are consistent with the previous literature, validating our results. Second, we considered values only at ICU admission and we did not analyze trends during the course of stay. For example, temperature pattern can be more useful than a single value at admission [25, 26]. Moreover, other studies show how the trend and modification of biomarkers could be helpful to manage antibiotic usage [27], to monitor the patient's recovery from sepsis and to predict the outcome. Given our aim to measure the value of a composite of clinical and laboratory data to assist the clinician toward making the correct and timely diagnosis of sepsis, in order to increase accuracy, we limited our evaluations to those at patient admission.

Conclusions

The present study shows a combined PCT, CRP and SOFA score, used to calculate a patient bioscore, may be a valuable predictive tool to accurately diagnose sepsis.

Authors' contributions

YY contributed to study conception and design, data analysis, statistical analysis, and drafting the manuscript. JX contributed to study conception and design, and data analysis, statistical analysis, and drafting the manuscript. FG contributed to study design, statistical analysis, and revision of the manuscript for important intellectual content. FL contributed to data analysis, revision of manuscript for important intellectual content. ZG and YH contributed to data analysis. HQ contributed to study conception and design, data analysis, statistical analysis, and revision of the manuscript for important intellectual content. All authors read and approved the final manuscript.

Author details

[1] Department of Critical Care Medicine, Nanjing Zhong-Da Hospital, School of Medicine, Southeast University, Nanjing 210009, Jiangsu, China. [2] Department of Translational Medicine, Eastern Piedmont University "A. Avogadro", Novara, Italy.

Acknowledgements

We thank all patients for participation in the study and the healthcare professionals of the Intensive Care Unit of Zhong-Da Hospital (Nanjing, China) for their helpful and continuous support. We also thank Dr. Nathan J. Klingensmith (Department of Surgery, Emory University, Atlanta, GA, USA) to help us to modify the language of this paper.

Competing interests

The authors declare that they have no competing interests.

Source of funding

The protocol was financially supported by funds of the Ministry of Health of China and of Jiangsu Province.

References

1. Vincent JL, Rello J, Marshall J, Silva E, Anzueto A, Martin CD, Moreno R, Lipman J, Gomersall C, Sakr Y, Reinhart K. International study of the prevalence and outcomes of infection in intensive care units. JAMA. 2009;302:2323–9.
2. Coelho FR, Martins JO. Diagnostic methods in sepsis: the need of speed. Rev Assoc Med Bras. 2012;58:498–504.
3. Nee PA. Critical care in the emergency department: severe sepsis and septic shock. Emerg Med J. 2006;23:713–7.
4. Rivers E, Nguyen B, Havstad S, Ressler J, Muzzin A, Knoblich B, Peterson E, Tomlanovich M. Early goal-directed therapy in the treatment of severe sepsis and septic shock. N Engl J Med. 2001;345:1368–77.
5. Garnacho-Montero J, Ortiz-Leyba C, Herrera-Melero I, Aldabo-Pallas T, Cayuela-Dominguez A, Marquez-Vacaro JA, Carbajal-Guerrero J, Garcia-Garmendia JL. Mortality and morbidity attributable to inadequate empirical antimicrobial therapy in patients admitted to the ICU with sepsis: a matched cohort study. J Antimicrob Chemother. 2008;61:436–41.
6. Kumar G, Kumar N, Taneja A, Kaleekal T, Tarima S, McGinley E, Jimenez E, Mohan A, Khan RA, Whittle J, Jacobs E, Nanchal R. Nationwide trends of severe sepsis in the 21st century (2000–2007). Chest. 2011;140:1223–31.
7. Marshall JC, Reinhart K. Biomarkers of sepsis. Crit Care Med. 2009;37:2290–8.
8. Marshall JC, Vincent JL, Fink MP, Cook DJ, Rubenfeld G, Foster D, Fisher CJ Jr, Faist E, Reinhart K. Measures, markers, and mediators: toward a staging system for clinical sepsis. A report of the Fifth Toronto Sepsis Roundtable, Toronto, Ontario, Canada, October 25–26, 2000. Crit Care Med. 2003;31:1560–7.
9. Simon L, Saint-Louis P, Amre DK, Lacroix J, Gauvin F. Procalcitonin and C-reactive protein as markers of bacterial infection in critically ill children at onset of systemic inflammatory response syndrome. Pediatr Crit Care Med. 2008;9:407–13.
10. Bozza FA, Salluh JI, Japiassu AM, Soares M, Assis EF, Gomes RN, Bozza MT, Castro-Faria-Neto HC, Bozza PT. Cytokine profiles as markers of disease severity in sepsis: a multiplex analysis. Crit Care. 2007;11:R49.
11. Yende S, D'Angelo G, Kellum JA, Weissfeld L, Fine J, Welch RD, Kong L, Carter M, Angus DC. Inflammatory markers at hospital discharge predict subsequent mortality after pneumonia and sepsis. Am J Respir Crit Care Med. 2008;177:1242–7.
12. Chan T, Gu F. Early diagnosis of sepsis using serum biomarkers. Expert Rev Mol Diagn. 2011;11:487–96.
13. Gibot S, Bene MC, Noel R, Massin F, Guy J, Cravoisy A, Barraud D, De Carvalho Bittencourt M, Quenot JP, Bollaert PE, Faure G, Charles PE. Combination biomarkers to diagnose sepsis in the critically ill patient. Am J Respir Crit Care Med. 2012;186:65–71.
14. Dellinger RP, Levy MM, Carlet JM, Bion J, Parker MM, Jaeschke R, Reinhart K, Angus DC, Brun-Buisson C, Beale R, Calandra T, Dhainaut JF, Gerlach H, Harvey M, Marini JJ, Marshall J, Ranieri M, Ramsay G, Sevransky J, Thompson BT, Townsend S, Vender JS, Zimmerman JL, Vincent JL. Surviving sepsis campaign: international guidelines for management of severe sepsis and septic shock: 2008. Crit Care Med. 2008;36:296–327.
15. American College of Chest Physicians/Society of Critical Care Medicine Consensus Conference. Definitions for sepsis and organ failure and guidelines for the use of innovative therapies in sepsis. Crit Care Med. 1992;20:864–74.
16. Su L, Han B, Liu C, Liang L, Jiang Z, Deng J, Yan P, Jia Y, Feng D, Xie L. Value of soluble TREM-1, procalcitonin, and C-reactive protein serum levels as biomarkers for detecting bacteremia among sepsis patients with new fever in intensive care units: a prospective cohort study. BMC Infect Dis. 2012;12:157.
17. Tsalik EL, Jaggers LB, Glickman SW, Langley RJ, van Velkinburgh JC, Park LP, Fowler VG, Cairns CB, Kingsmore SF, Woods CW. Discriminative value of inflammatory biomarkers for suspected sepsis. J Emerg Med. 2012;43:97–106.
18. Bloos F, Reinhart K. Rapid diagnosis of sepsis. Virulence. 2014;5:154–60.
19. Lin S, Huang Z, Wang M, Weng Z, Zeng D, Zhang Y, Zhu Y, Jiang J. Interleukin-6 as an early diagnostic marker for bacterial sepsis in patients with liver cirrhosis. J Crit Care. 2015;30: 732–8.
20. Hegazy MA, Omar AS, Samir N, Moharram A, Weber S, Radwan WA. Amalgamation of procalcitonin, C-reactive protein, and sequential organ failure scoring system in predicting sepsis survival. Anesth Essays Res. 2014;8:296–301.
21. Rowland T, Hilliard H, Barlow G. Procalcitonin: potential role in diagnosis and management of sepsis. Adv Clin Chem. 2015;68:71–86.
22. Castelli GP, Pognani C, Cita M, Stuani A, Sgarbi L, Paladini R. Procalcitonin, C-reactive protein, white blood cells and SOFA score in ICU: diagnosis and monitoring of sepsis. Minerva Anestesiol. 2006;72:69–80.
23. Seigel TA, Cocchi MN, Salciccioli J, Shapiro NI, Howell M, Tang A, Donnino MW. Inadequacy of temperature and white blood cell count in predicting bacteremia in patients with suspected infection. J Emerg Med. 2012;42:254–9.
24. Laupland KB, Shahpori R, Kirkpatrick AW, Ross T, Gregson DB, Stelfox HT. Occurrence and outcome of fever in critically ill adults. Crit Care Med. 2008;36:1531–5.
25. Cuesta D, Varela M, Miro P, Galdos P, Abasolo D, Hornero R, Aboy M. Predicting survival in critical patients by use of body temperature regularity measurement based on approximate entropy. Med Biol Eng Comput. 2007;45:671–8.
26. Papaioannou VE, Chouvarda IG, Maglaveras NK, Pneumatikos IA. Temperature variability analysis using wavelets and multiscale entropy in patients with systemic inflammatory response syndrome, sepsis, and septic shock. Crit Care. 2012;16:R51.
27. Oliveira CF, Botoni FA, Oliveira CR, Silva CB, Pereira HA, Serufo JC, Nobre V. Procalcitonin versus C-reactive protein for guiding antibiotic therapy in sepsis: a randomized trial. Crit Care Med. 2013;41:2336–43.

Fluorescence imaging of ATP in neutrophils from patients with sepsis using organelle-localizable fluorescent chemosensors

Koichiro Sueyoshi[1*], Yuka Sumi[1], Yoshiaki Inoue[1], Yoko Kuroda[1], Kumiko Ishii[2], Hitoshi Nakayama[3], Kazuhisa Iwabuchi[3], Yasutaka Kurishita[4], Hajime Shigemitsu[4], Itaru Hamachi[4] and Hiroshi Tanaka[1]

Abstract

Background: The activation of polymorphonuclear neutrophils (PMNs) plays an important role in sepsis. Previously, we showed that ATP release and feedback via ATP receptors are essential for PMN activation; however, the dynamics remain poorly understood. Two new fluorescent chemosensors, PMAP-1 and MitoAP-1, were developed to detect ATP in the plasma membrane and mitochondria of living cells, respectively. In this study, we aimed to evaluate ATP localization using these chemosensors in PMNs of sepsis patients.

Methods: Live PMNs isolated from 16 sepsis patients and healthy controls (HCs) were stained with these chemosensors and observed by confocal microscopy, and their mean fluorescence intensities (MFIs) were evaluated using flow cytometry. CD11b expression in PMNs was also evaluated.

Results: The MFIs of PMAP-1 and MitoAP-1 and CD11b expression in PMNs from sepsis patients on days 0–1 were significantly higher than those of HCs. The MFI of PMAP-1 and CD11b expression on days 3–4 decreased significantly compared to those observed at days 0–1, whereas MitoAP-1 MFI was maintained at a high level. The PMAP-1 MFI was significantly positively correlated with CD11b expression, white blood cell counts, neutrophil counts, and C-reactive protein levels in patients.

Conclusions: The higher MFIs of PMAP-1 and MitoAP-1 in sepsis patients suggest a pivotal role of ATP for PMN activation. The temporal difference in ATP levels suggests that ATP plays different roles in the mitochondria and on the cell surface. These data should contribute to the understanding of the dynamics of ATP in PMNs and help to develop a novel therapy for sepsis.

Keywords: Polymorphonuclear neutrophils (PMNs), PMAP-1, MitoAP-1, Plasma membrane, Mitochondria, Flow cytometry

Background

ATP is well known as the energy currency of cells and is involved in both intracellular signaling and extracellular signaling. Although polymorphonuclear neutrophils (PMNs) are one of the most important phagocytic cell types in defending against invading pathogens and play a pivotal role in inflammation, their activation can be a double-edged sword. In particular, their pathophysiological processes can damage the host tissue when activated during sepsis, trauma, ischemia–reperfusion injury, and inflammatory diseases [1]. PMNs can migrate to compromised tissues in response to chemotactic gradients. The activation of PMNs is triggered by the recognition of bacterial peptides and innate inflammatory mediators. Although a signal amplification system is crucial for the activation of PMNs, the underlying mechanisms remain obscure [2–4]. We previously found that ATP was released extracellularly by PMNs through pannexin-1 (PANX1) hemichannels and that autocrine feedback

*Correspondence: ksueyoshi@juntendo-urayasu.jp
[1] Department of Emergency and Critical Care Medicine, Juntendo University, Urayasu Hospital, 2-1-1 Tomioka, Urayasu, Chiba 279-0021, Japan
Full list of author information is available at the end of the article

through the P2Y2 receptor, one of eight P2Y G protein-coupled receptors, is an essential mechanism for activating PMNs [5, 6]. We also reported that plasma ATP levels were correlated with PMN activation and were significantly higher in mouse models of cecal ligation and puncture (CLP) [7].

In recent decades, much effort has been dedicated to developing fluorescent chemosensors for ATP to study its diverse functions [8, 9]. Consequently, two new fluorescent chemosensors were developed (PMAP-1 and MitoAP-1), which can detect ATP and its derivatives in specific regions of living cells [10]. PMAP-1 and MitoAP-1 are also referred to as 2-2Zn(II) and 3-2Zn(II), respectively [10]. PMAP-1 can localize to the plasma membrane and detect the extracellular release of ATP. In contrast, MitoAP-1 can spontaneously localize in the mitochondria and detect local ATP.

Sepsis is the major cause of death in critically ill patients and is the predominant cause of multiple organ dysfunction syndrome [11, 12]. In spite of progress in intensive care medicine and strict adherence to established treatment protocols such as the "Surviving Sepsis Campaign" guidelines [13], mortality in sepsis patients remains high. Millions of patients worldwide are afflicted each year, resulting in the death of one in three patients [11]. Multiple organ failure in sepsis is the prevailing cause of death, and mitochondrial dysfunction has been suggested to contribute to the development of organ dysfunction and failure in sepsis [14]. However, the associated pathogenic mechanisms remain unclear.

In this study, we evaluated a new approach to quantify ATP release on the cell surface and ATP production in the mitochondria of PMNs by flow cytometry. As described above, ATP is known to play a key role in the activation of PMNs; thus, we hypothesized that ATP levels on the plasma membrane and in the mitochondria of PMNs could serve as an informative biomarker for sepsis. Here, we report the correlation between ATP levels and the clinical conditions of sepsis patients.

Methods

Patients

After obtaining approval from the ethics committee of Juntendo University, Urayasu Hospital (25–47), 16 sepsis patients admitted to our critical care center between October 2013 and April 2015 were enrolled in the study. All patients met the diagnostic criteria for sepsis determined by the American College of Chest Physicians and Society of Critical Care Medicine [15], and all patients (or their legal representatives) provided informed consent for participation in the research. Patients with malignant disease or chronic administration of steroids were excluded. The patients comprised nine males and seven females, with a mean ± SD age of 67 ± 9 years, a serum C-reactive protein (CRP) level of 27.0 ± 12.1 mg/dL, a white blood cell (WBC) count of 13.3 ± 9.1 × 10^3/μL, an Acute Physiology and Chronic Health Evaluation (APACHE) II score [16] of 22.1 ± 7.8, a Sequential Organ Failure Assessment (SOFA) score [17] of 7.9 ± 4.6, and a Japanese Association for Acute Medicine (JAAM) disseminated intravascular coagulation (DIC) score [18] of 3.8 ± 1.7. The cause of sepsis was urinary tract infection in five patients; burn in three patients; pneumonia in three patients; and necrotic cholecystitis, cellulitis, gas gangrene, cervical abscess, and peritonitis in one patient each. Two patients died during hospitalization (Table 1). The healthy control (HC) group consisted of six males and three females, with a mean ± SD age of 37 ± 5 years.

Blood samples

A 10-mL heparinized blood sample was collected via the peripheral vein of each healthy volunteer and via arterial lines in sepsis patients. Blood collection for all sepsis patients was performed within 24 h after the patients were diagnosed with sepsis (days 0–1) and at days 3–4 of sepsis.

Isolation of PMNs

Human PMNs were isolated from the heparinized whole blood of healthy volunteers and sepsis patients using Polymorphprep™ centrifugation (Alere Technologies AS, Oslo, Norway). The neutrophil population was >95 % pure, as determined by Wright–Giemsa staining.

PMAP-1 and MitoAP-1

Both PMAP-1 and MitoAP-1 were designed on the basis of a fluorescent ATP probe containing a xanthene fluorophore [10]. PMAP-1 selectively localizes on the plasma membrane via a biocompatible anchor for the membrane, which possesses a hydrophobic oleyl moiety at the end of a long ethylene glycol linker [10]. MitoAP-1 selectively localizes to the mitochondria via a positively charged pyronin ring [10].

Imaging of PMNs with confocal microscopy

Isolated human PMNs (2.0 × 10^6 cells/mL) were plated on a 35-mm glass-bottomed dish (IWAKI, Tokyo, Japan), coated with 100 μL of poly-L-lysine solution (Sigma-Aldrich, St. Louis, MO, USA), and incubated for 10 min. All incubations were performed under a humidified atmosphere of 5 % CO_2 at 37 °C in the dark. Cells were treated with 400 nM (final concentration) of MitoTracker® Green FM (Invitrogen, Carlsbad, CA, USA), followed by incubation with 1 μM MitoAP-1 (final concentration) for 20 min. Cells were incubated with 5 μM PMAP-1 (final concentration) for 10 min. After

Table 1 Characteristics of sepsis patients

Patients	Cause of sepsis	APACHE II score	SOFA score	JAAM DIC score	WBC (/μL)	CRP (mg/dL)	Mortality
1.	Necrotic cholecystitis	31	15	7	4600	27.9	Alive
2.	Pneumonia	18	3	4	18,600	48.8	Alive
3.	Burn	12	2	2	10,600	23.9	Alive
4.	Pneumonia	24	7	3	17,900	35.8	Dead
5.	Cellulitis	11	3	3	19,300	54.0	Alive
6.	Burn	29	12	4	4100	14.2	Dead
7.	UTI	36	14	8	13,900	17.9	Alive
8.	UTI	26	11	3	16,400	15.5	Alive
9.	UTI	14	6	3	20,700	10.4	Alive
10.	Burn	29	13	4	4600	25.5	Alive
11.	UTI	20	8	6	31,900	25.8	Alive
12.	Gas gangrene	17	2	2	17,100	15.6	Alive
13.	Cervical abscess	20	5	3	5000	29.4	Alive
14.	UTI	11	4	3	800	29.7	Alive
15.	Peritonitis	29	9	3	23,700	21.8	Alive
16.	Pneumonia	27	13	3	900	36.0	Alive

APACHE Acute Physiology and Chronic Health Evaluation, *SOFA* Sequential Organ Failure Assessment, *JAAM* Japanese Association for Acute Medicine, *DIC* disseminated intravascular coagulation, *WBC* white blood cell counts, *CRP* C-reactive protein, *UTI* urinary tract infection

washing twice with 37 °C Hanks' balanced salt solution (HBSS, Sigma-Aldrich), stained cells were examined with a TCS SP5 Leica confocal laser-scanning microscope equipped with a Plan-Apochromat 100× oil-immersion objective lens at 37 °C, under a 5 % CO_2 humidified atmosphere.

Fluorescence quantification by flow cytometry

Isolated PMNs were washed with HBSS and incubated at 37 °C for 10 min with or without *N*-formyl-met-leu-phe (fMLP, ScyTek Laboratories, Logan, UT, USA) stimulation before staining. Cells were incubated with 1 μM (final concentration) of MitoAP-1 and allophycocyanin-conjugated anti-CD11b antibodies (BD Biosciences, San Jose, CA, USA) at 37 °C for 20 min, followed by incubation with 5 μM PMAP-1 (final concentration) at 37 °C for 10 min. The cells were placed on ice for 10 min and centrifuged at 1500 rpm for 5 min at 4 °C. After washing twice with HBSS, cells were fixed with fluorescence-activated cell sorting (FACS) sheath fluid (BD Biosciences) and then analyzed by flow cytometry (FACSCalibur, BD Bioscience).

Statistical analysis

The data are expressed as the mean ± SEM unless stated otherwise. Statistical analyses were performed using GraphPad Prism version 6.0 (GraphPad, San Diego, CA, USA). The data were analyzed for significant differences by a paired *t* test or Wilcoxon signed-rank test for comparisons of paired groups. One-way analysis of variance (ANOVA) and the Kruskal–Wallis test were used for comparisons of three groups. Spearman's rank correlation was performed as indicated. Differences were considered statistically significant at $p < 0.05$.

Results

Successful establishment of a staining protocol for human PMNs with MitoAP-1

Imaging studies using PMAP-1 and MitoAP-1 were limited to cultured cells [10] and T cells [19] until Bao et al. [20] first reported imaging studies of human PMNs using PMAP-1. As in their study, the bright green fluorescence emitted by PMAP-1 was predominantly observed on the plasma membrane of PMNs (Fig. 1a). However, there has been no previous report of the successful staining of human PMNs with MitoAP-1. We observed a punctate pattern of bright red fluorescence emitted by MitoAP-1 within the cells. MitoAP-1 fluorescence overlapped well with that of MitoTracker® Green FM, a typical dye used to stain the mitochondria, indicating that MitoAP-1 selectively and spontaneously localized to the mitochondria (Fig. 1b). Thus, we successfully established a method for staining human PMNs with MitoAP-1.

ATP release on the plasma membrane of HC PMNs increased with fMLP stimulation

Stimulation of the formyl peptide receptor was previously found to cause ATP release from PMNs through maxi-anion channels and PANX1 hemichannels [6]. To confirm this finding, the MFI of PMAP-1 on the plasma

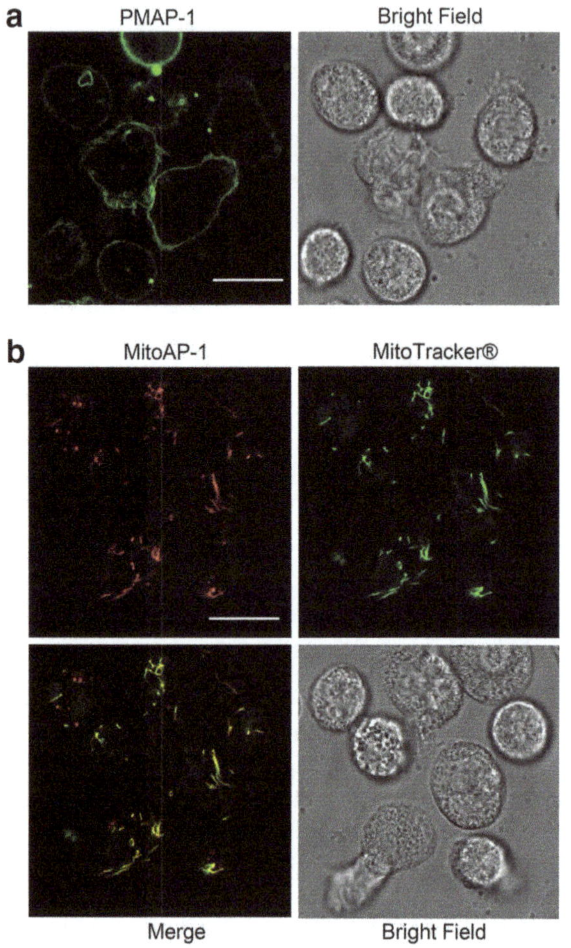

Fig. 1 Confocal micrographs of human polymorphonuclear neutrophils (PMNs) stained with PMAP-1 and MitoAP-1. **a** ATP on the plasma membrane was stained with PMAP-1. The *bright green* fluorescence observed on the plasma membrane of PMNs resulted from PMAP-1 conjugation to ATP (×100 oil objective, NA 1.4). *Scale bar* 10 µm. **b** ATP in the mitochondria was stained with MitoAP-1 (*red*) and MitoTracker® Green FM (*green*), and they colocalized well (×100 oil objective, NA 1.4). *Scale bar* 10 µm

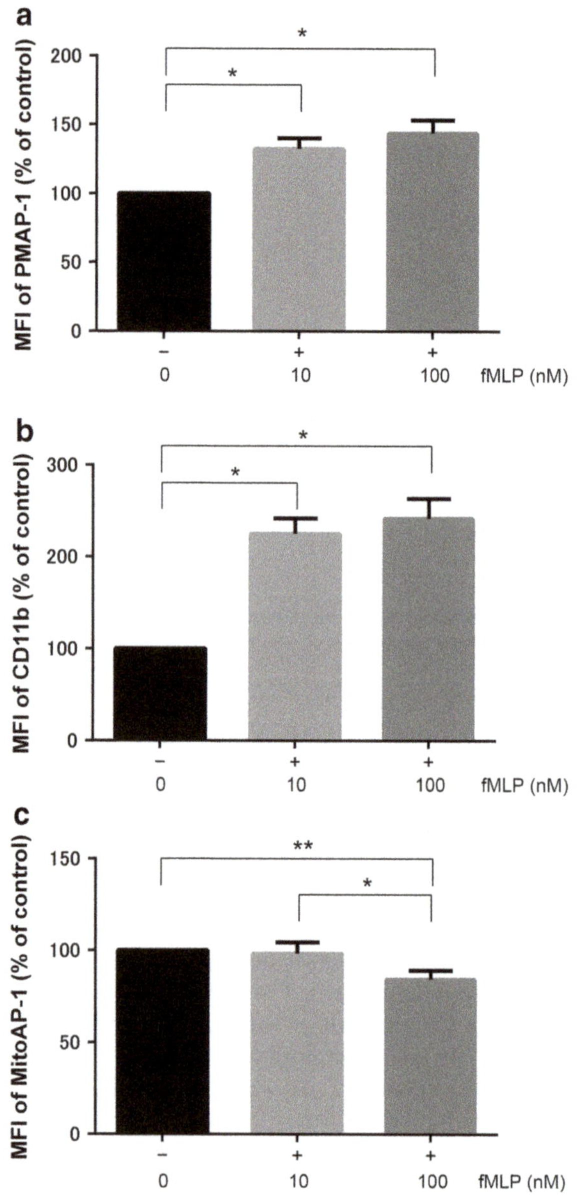

Fig. 2 ATP level and CD11b expression after fMLP stimulation in healthy control subjects. **a** Changes in the mean fluorescence intensity (MFI) of PMAP-1 after stimulation with the indicated fMLP concentrations; MFI values were normalized to those of controls (no fMLP) ($n = 8$ per group). The data shown are the mean ± SEM, and groups were compared with one-way ANOVA and Tukey's post hoc test (*$p < 0.01$). **b** Changes in CD11b expression of polymorphonuclear neutrophils after fMLP stimulation; expression levels were normalized to those of controls (no fMLP) ($n = 8$ per group). The data shown are the mean ± SEM, and groups were compared with one-way ANOVA with Tukey's post hoc test (*$p < 0.01$). **c** Changes in MFI of MitoAP-1 after stimulation with the indicated fMLP concentrations; MFI values were normalized to those of controls (no fMLP) ($n = 8$ per group). The data shown are the mean ± SEM, and groups were compared with one-way ANOVA with Tukey's post hoc test (*$p < 0.01$, **$p < 0.05$)

membrane of HC PMNs was quantified by flow cytometry after stimulation with the indicated concentrations of fMLP (Fig. 2a). The MFI of PMAP-1 following fMLP stimulation increased in a dose-dependent manner. CD11b expression on the plasma membrane of PMNs was also measured as a marker of PMN activation. Cell surface CD11b expression in PMNs stimulated with fMLP also increased in a dose-dependent manner (Fig. 2b).

Mitochondrial ATP levels in the HC group decreased with fMLP stimulation

Mitochondria are often referred to as the powerhouse of the cells, as they generate ATP by oxidative phosphorylation. To our knowledge, changes in mitochondrial ATP levels in PMNs have not been reported. The MFI of MitoAP-1 following fMLP stimulation decreased significantly in a dose-dependent manner (Fig. 2c).

ATP release on the plasma membrane and mitochondrial ATP levels in PMNs were higher in sepsis patients than in HC subjects

The MFIs of PMAP-1 and MitoAP-1 in sepsis patients were evaluated by flow cytometry within 24 h after diagnosis of sepsis (days 0–1). Both values were significantly higher than those of the HC group (Fig. 3a, b). CD11b expression on the plasma membrane was also upregulated in sepsis patients (Fig. 3c). Activated PMNs in sepsis patients appeared to cause a burst of extracellular ATP release and to increase ATP synthesis by oxidative phosphorylation in the mitochondria. The same experiments were conducted at days 3–4 as the patients' clinical conditions improved, which revealed that the MFIs of PMAP-1 and CD11b expression decreased significantly compared to those at days 0–1 (Fig. 3a, c), whereas a high MitoAP-1 MFI was maintained (Fig. 3b). Namely, the temporal changes of ATP release and CD11b expression on the plasma membrane were similar, but ATP production showed distinct behavior in the mitochondria.

ATP release on the plasma membrane correlated with PMN activation

As described above, ATP release and CD11b expression decreased as the clinical conditions of the patients improved. Furthermore, the MFIs of PMAP-1 and CD11b expression showed a significant positive correlation in the sepsis patients (Fig. 4).

ATP release on the plasma membrane correlated with WBC counts, neutrophil counts, and CRP levels

To determine relationships between ATP release on the plasma membrane or ATP production in the mitochondria and clinical conditions (WBC counts, neutrophil counts, CRP levels, SOFA scores, APACHE II scores, and JAAM DIC scores), their correlation coefficients were investigated. The MFI of PMAP-1 was significantly positively correlated with WBC counts, neutrophil counts, and CRP levels (Fig. 5), but not with SOFA scores, APACHE II scores, and JAAM DIC scores. No correlation was found between the MFI of MitoAP-1 of PMNs and any clinical variable.

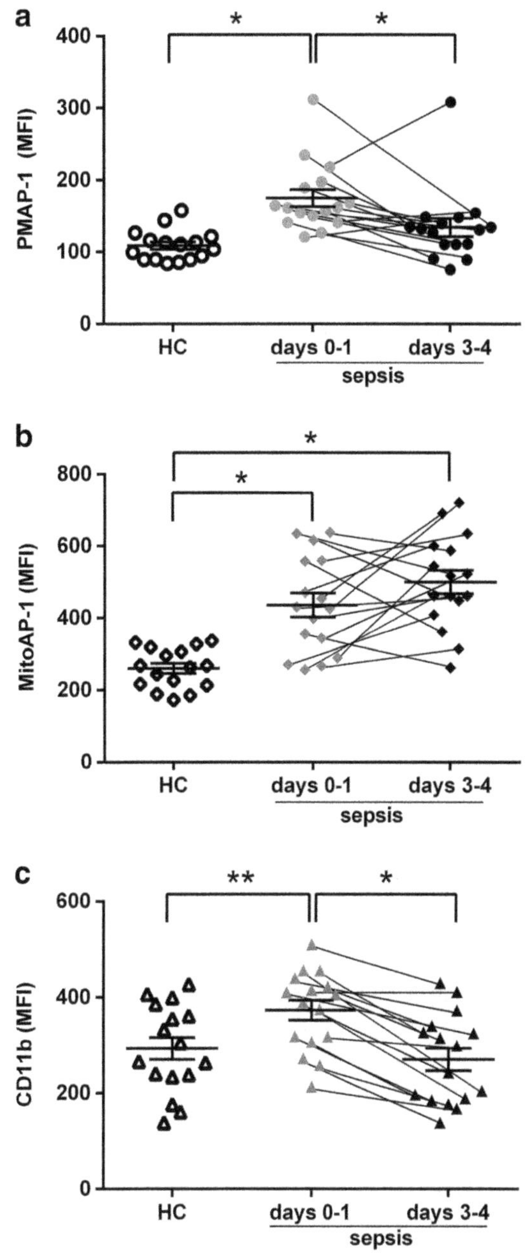

Fig. 3 Mean fluorescent intensity (MFI) of PMAP-1, MitoAP-1, and CD11b expression in PMNs in sepsis patients and healthy control (HC) subjects. **a** MFI of PMAP-1 in sepsis patients (days 0–1 postdiagnosis) was significantly higher than that of HCs and decreased significantly on days 3–4 (mean ± SEM, Kruskal–Wallis test with Dunn's post hoc test, *$p < 0.01$). **b** The MFI of MitoAP-1 in sepsis patients (days 0–1) was significantly higher than that of HCs and did not decrease significantly on days 3–4 (mean ± SEM, Kruskal–Wallis test with Dunn's post hoc test, *$p < 0.01$). **c** CD11b expression in sepsis patients (days 0–1) was significantly higher than that of HCs and decreased significantly on days 3–4 (mean ± SEM, one-way ANOVA with Tukey's post hoc test, *$p < 0.01$, **$p < 0.05$)

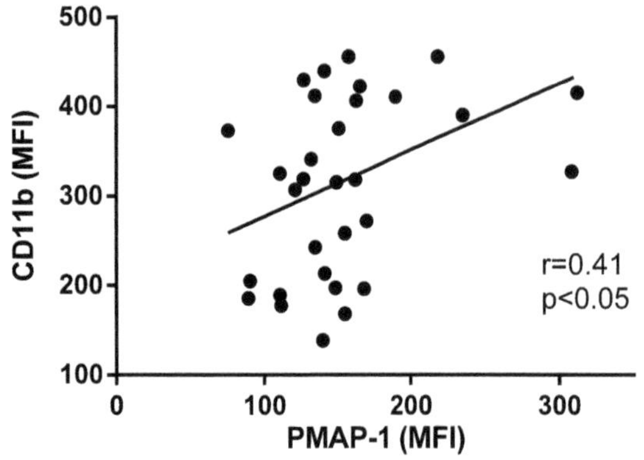

Fig. 4 Correlation between the mean fluorescent intensity (MFI) of PMAP-1 and polymorphonuclear neutrophil (PMN) activation (CD11b expression). Comparison of PMAP-1 and CD11b expression on the plasma membrane showed a significant positive correlation in sepsis patients ($n = 16$, Spearman's rank correlation coefficient, $p < 0.05$). The 32 data points shown consist of samples from both days 0–1 and days 3–4 following sepsis diagnosis

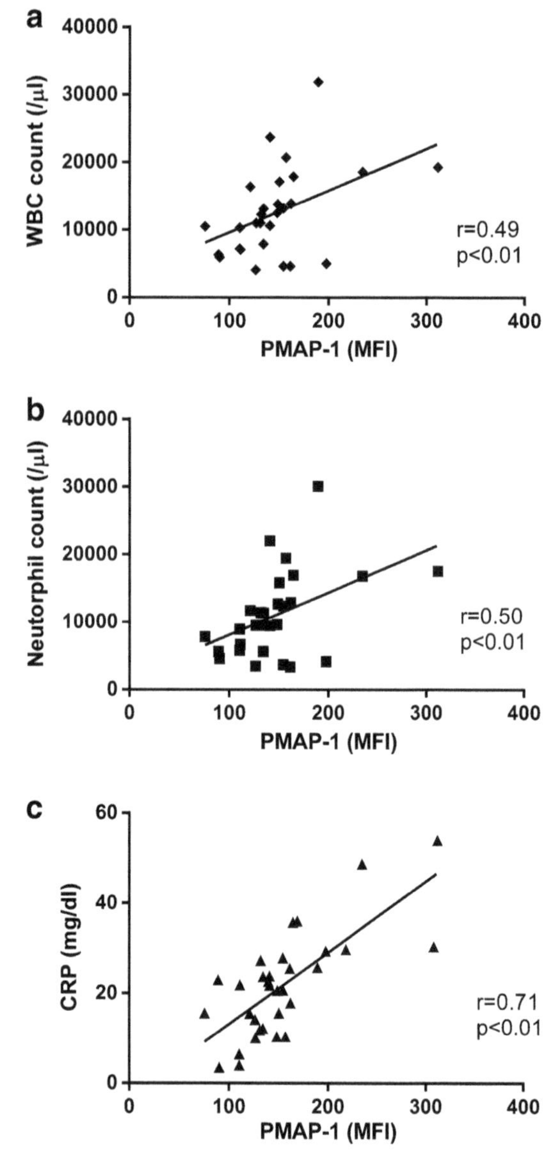

Fig. 5 Correlation of PMAP-1 MFI with white blood cell (WBC) counts, neutrophil counts, and C-reactive protein (CRP) levels in sepsis patients. **a**, **b** Spearman's rank correlation coefficient, $p < 0.01$ ($n = 14$). Two patients with leukopenia were excluded. The 28 data points shown consist of samples from both days 0–1 and days 3–4 following sepsis diagnosis. **c** Spearman's rank correlation coefficient, $p < 0.01$ ($n = 16$). The 32 data points shown consist of samples from both days 0–1 and days 3–4 of sepsis

Discussion

To our knowledge, this is the first report of the visualization of mitochondrial ATP in the PMNs of sepsis patients with fluorescent chemosensors. PMNs are the major leukocytes recruited to inflamed sites in response to infection. Although PMNs play a central role in protecting the host from infection, their pathophysiological processes can also cause tissue damage in the host [1, 21]. To develop therapies that can reduce PMN-induced tissue damage, it is crucial to elucidate the mechanisms underlying the activation of PMNs.

ATP, which is well known as the "molecular unit of currency" of intracellular energy transfer, is released extracellularly by physiological stimulation and acts as a signaling molecule. Burnstock et al. [22] first reported that healthy neurons can release cellular ATP, which then serves as an intercellular messenger. Recently, neurons and many other types of cells have been shown to release ATP under physiological stimulation, including PMNs [23–33]. Previously, we showed that ATP release and purinergic signaling are essential for PMN activation. Extracellular ATP is released by PANX1 hemichannels and controls the chemotaxis of PMNs through P2Y2 receptors [5, 6]. The autocrine feedback through P2Y2 receptors is essential for PMN activation [6].

Substantial effort has been dedicated to developing fluorescent chemosensors for ATP to elucidate its diverse physiological functions [8–10, 34, 35]. To date, a few imaging studies using genetically encoded fluorescence ATP probes have been reported for this purpose [34, 35]. These probes are posttranslationally conjugated to a protein anchored to a certain organelle through genetically encoded localization signals. Although successful, these techniques are not convenient, because they require cumbersome and time-consuming processes for protein expression and maturation. Therefore, Kurishita et al. [10] developed two new types of fluorescent chemosensors, PMAP-1 and MitoAP-1, which can spontaneously and selectively localize in a specific cellular region [10].

For example, PMAP-1 localizes to the plasma membrane and can be used to detect the extracellular release of ATP, whereas MitoAP-1 localizes to the mitochondria and senses mitochondrial ATP. Thus, these fluorescent chemosensors are highly suited for investigating the dynamics of ATP in biological events occurring in target cellular regions [10].

The finding that cell surface ATP release and CD11b expression in the HC group increased dose-dependently following fMLP stimulation is consistent with our previous finding that ATP is released by fMLP stimulation via PANX1 hemichannels [6]. In sepsis patients, extracellular ATP release in PMNs was elevated on days 0–1, corroborating our previous work in mouse sepsis models, wherein plasma ATP levels were elevated and contributed to PMN activation [7]. Collectively, these findings indicate that PMNs may be a main source of elevated circulating ATP levels. Furthermore, ATP release on the plasma membrane was correlated with CD11b expression, WBC counts, neutrophil counts, and CRP levels in sepsis patients; thus, ATP release on the plasma membrane may reflect PMN activation and could potentially serve as an activation marker for sepsis. Given that excessive activation of PMNs can damage host organs, inhibition of purinergic signaling could serve as a potential therapeutic strategy for treating sepsis. Previously, we reported that the P2 receptor antagonist suramin reduced PMN activation in a mouse CLP model [7]. Thus, suramin may potentially be used as an effective therapeutic strategy for sepsis patients. In contrast to the complications mediated by an overactive neutrophil compartment, severe systemic inflammation is a risk factor for the development of immune suppression. The circulating neutrophil pool displays a paradoxical phenotype, exhibiting characteristics of both activated and suppressed functionality. Therefore, further investigations are required to resolve this paradox of the role of PMNs in sepsis [36].

Mitochondria play an essential role in the activation of PMNs by producing ATP, which triggers the purinergic signaling processes [20]. During this process, mitochondria generate ATP and release ATP extracellularly following fMLP stimulation. However, in the HC group, the mitochondrial ATP levels in PMNs decreased with fMLP stimulation in a dose-dependent manner, demonstrating that the mitochondrial ATP was consumed in this process in healthy PMNs. Mitochondrial ATP levels in PMNs from sepsis patients were significantly higher than those of the HC group. Although further investigations are required to determine the definite cause for this difference, it is intriguing to speculate that pathways other than fMLP stimulation may be essential for ATP elevation in the mitochondria. Evaluation of mitochondrial function in various cells has been previously reported in the context of sepsis [37, 38]. For example, Adrie et al. [37] demonstrated reduced mitochondrial membrane potential in peripheral blood monocytes from patients with severe sepsis. On the other hand, Belikova et al. [38] showed peripheral blood mononuclear cells from patients with severe sepsis had a significantly higher baseline value of oxygen consumption compared with healthy volunteer cells. This report supports our study that mitochondrial ATP production in PMNs from sepsis patients was increased. Therefore, understanding the interaction among cells is essential to elucidate the mechanism of sepsis. Our method shows potential to clarify the mechanism of sepsis from the point of view of mitochondrial function.

Furthermore, although the PMAP-1 MFI on days 3–4 of sepsis decreased in parallel with CD11b downregulation, the MFI of MitoAP-1 did not change. These findings suggest that ATP serves different functions on the cell surface and in the mitochondria of PMNs in sepsis patients.

Conclusions

In conclusion, we developed a novel approach for quantifying ATP release on the cell surface and mitochondrial ATP production in PMNs with two new types of fluorescent chemosensors, which was applied to the study of sepsis patients. ATP release on the plasma membrane of PMNs was demonstrated to be a potentially valuable biomarker for sepsis. Taken together with our previous studies, our current findings suggest that PMN responses can be regulated by therapeutic strategies that target the purinergic signaling mechanisms of PMNs. Additional studies are needed to determine whether and how these purinergic signaling mechanisms can be targeted in order to best benefit sepsis patients.

Abbreviations

ANOVA: analysis of variance; APACHE: Acute Physiology and Chronic Health Evaluation; CLP: cecal ligation and puncture; CRP: C-reactive protein; DIC: disseminated intravascular coagulation; FACS: fluorescence-activated cell sorting; fMLP: *N*-formyl-met-leu-phe; HBSS: Hanks' balanced salt solution; HC: healthy controls; JAAM: Japanese Association for Acute Medicine; MFI: mean fluorescence intensity; PMN: polymorphonuclear neutrophil; SOFA: Sequential Organ Failure Assessment; WBC: white blood cell.

Authors' contributions

KS and YS designed and performed the experiments. KS and YS analyzed the data and prepared the manuscript. YK performed the experiments with FACS. KI supervised and carried out the experiments with confocal microscopy. HN and KI supervised the isolation of PMNs. YK, HS, and IH synthesized PMAP-1 and MitoAP-1 and supervised the usage of PMAP-1 and MitoAP-1. YI and HT conceived the idea, reviewed the manuscript, and supervised the whole project. All authors read and approved the final manuscript.

Author details
[1] Department of Emergency and Critical Care Medicine, Juntendo University, Urayasu Hospital, 2-1-1 Tomioka, Urayasu, Chiba 279-0021, Japan. [2] Lipid Biology Laboratory, Riken Advanced Science Institute, Wako, Saitama, Japan. [3] Institute for Environmental and Gender Specific Medicine, Juntendo University, Urayasu, Chiba, Japan. [4] Department of Synthetic Chemistry and Biological Chemistry, Graduate School of Engineering, Kyoto University, Kyoto, Japan.

Acknowledgements
This study was supported in part by the Japan Society for the Promotion of Science (23792086, 25462830, to Y.S.), a Grant-in-Aid (S1311011) from the Foundation of Strategic Research Projects in Private Universities from the Ministry of Education, Culture, Sports, Science, and Technology (MEXT), Japan (to K.S.), and Juntendo University Young Investigator Award 2013 (K1310, to K.S).

Competing interests
The authors declare that they have no competing interests.

References

1. Nussler AK, Wittel UA, Nussler NC, Beger HG. Leukocytes, the Janus cells in inflammatory disease. Langenbecks Arch Surg. 1999;384:222–32.
2. Ridley AJ, Schwartz MA, Burridge K, Firtel RA, Ginsberg MH, Borisy G, et al. Cell migration: integrating signals from front to back. Science. 2003;302:1704–9.
3. Van Haastert PJ, Devreotes PN. Chemotaxis: signalling the way forward. Nat Rev Mol Cell Biol. 2004;5:626–34.
4. Zigmond SH. Ability of polymorphonuclear leukocytes to orient in gradients of chemotactic factors. J Cell Biol. 1977;75:606–16.
5. Chen Y, Corriden R, Inoue Y, Yip L, Hashiguchi N, Zinkernagel A, et al. ATP release guides neutrophil chemotaxis via P2Y2 and A3 receptors. Science. 2006;314:1792–5.
6. Chen Y, Yao Y, Sumi Y, Li A, To UK, Elkhal A, et al. Purinergic signaling: a fundamental mechanism in neutrophil activation. Sci Signal. 2010;3:ra45.
7. Sumi Y, Woehrle T, Chen Y, Bao Y, Li X, Yao Y, et al. Plasma ATP is required for neutrophil activation in a mouse sepsis model. Shock. 2014;42:142–7.
8. Ojida A, Takashima I, Kohira T, Nonaka H, Hamachi I. Turn-on fluorescence sensing of nucleoside polyphosphates using a xanthene-based Zn(II) complex chemosensor. J Am Chem Soc. 2008;130:12095–101.
9. Kurishita Y, Kohira T, Ojida A, Hamachi I. Rational design of FRET-based ratiometric chemosensors for in vitro and in cell fluorescence analyses of nucleoside polyphosphates. J Am Chem Soc. 2010;132:13290–9.
10. Kurishita Y, Kohira T, Ojida A, Hamachi I. Organelle-localizable fluorescent chemosensors for site-specific multicolor imaging of nucleoside polyphosphate dynamics in living cells. J Am Chem Soc. 2012;134:18779–89.
11. Angus DC, van der Poll T. Severe sepsis and septic shock. N Engl J Med. 2013;369:840–51.
12. Hotchkiss RS, Karl IE. The pathophysiology and treatment of sepsis. N Engl J Med. 2003;348:138–50.
13. Dellinger RP, Levy MM, Rhodes A, Annane D, Gerlach H, Opal SM, et al. Surviving sepsis campaign: international guidelines for management of severe sepsis and septic shock: 2012. Crit Care Med. 2013;41:580–637.
14. Jeger V, Djafarzadeh S, Jakob SM, Takala J. Mitochondrial function in sepsis. Eur J Clin Invest. 2013;43:532–42.
15. Levy MM, Fink MP, Marshall JC, Abraham E, Angus D, Cook D, et al. 2001 SCCM/ESICM/ACCP/ATS/SIS international sepsis definitions conference. Crit Care Med. 2003;31:1250–6.
16. Knaus WA, Draper EA, Wagner DP, Zimmerman JE. APACHE II: a severity of disease classification system. Crit Care Med. 1985;13:818–29.
17. Vincent JL, Moreno R, Takala J, Willatts S, De Mendonca A, Bruining H, On behalf of the Working Group on Sepsis-Related Problems of the European Society of Intensive Care Medicine, et al. The SOFA (Sepsis-related Organ Failure Assessment) score to describe organ dysfunction/failure. Intensive Care Med. 1996;22:707–10.
18. Gando S, Iba T, Eguchi Y, Ohtomo Y, Okamoto K, Koseki K, et al. A multicenter, prospective validation of disseminated intravascular coagulation diagnostic criteria for critically ill patients: comparing current criteria. Crit Care Med. 2006;34:625–31.
19. Ledderose C, Bao Y, Lidicky M, Zipperle J, Li L, Strasser K, et al. Mitochondria are gate-keepers of T cell function by producing the ATP that drives purinergic signaling. J Biol Chem. 2014;289:25936–45.
20. Bao Y, Ledderose C, Seier T, Graf AF, Brix B, Chong E, et al. Mitochondria regulate neutrophil activation by generating ATP for autocrine purinergic signaling. J Biol Chem. 2014;289:26794–803.
21. Weiss SJ. Tissue destruction by neutrophils. N Engl J Med. 1989;320:365–76.
22. Burnstock G. Historical review: ATP as a neurotransmitter. Trends Pharmacol Sci. 2006;27:166–76.
23. Bodin P, Burnstock G. Evidence that release of adenosine triphosphate from endothelial cells during increased shear stress is vesicular. J Cardiovasc Pharmacol. 2001;38:900–8.
24. Buxton IL, Kaiser RA, Oxhorn BC, Cheek DJ. Evidence supporting the Nucleotide Axis Hypothesis: ATP release and metabolism by coronary endothelium. Am J Physiol Heart Circ Physiol. 2001;281:H1657–66.
25. Eltzschig HK, Eckle T, Mager A, Kuper N, Karcher C, Weissmuller T, et al. ATP release from activated neutrophils occurs via connexin 43 and modulates adenosine-dependent endothelial cell function. Circ Res. 2006;99:1100–8.
26. Fabre AC, Vantourout P, Champagne E, Terce F, Rolland C, Perret B, et al. Cell surface adenylate kinase activity regulates the F(1)-ATPase/P2Y (13)-mediated HDL endocytosis pathway on human hepatocytes. Cell Mol Life Sci. 2006;63:2829–37.
27. Gerasimovskaya EV, Ahmad S, White CW, Jones PL, Carpenter TC, Stenmark KR. Extracellular ATP is an autocrine/paracrine regulator of hypoxia-induced adventitial fibroblast growth. Signaling through extracellular signal-regulated kinase-1/2 and the Egr-1 transcription factor. J Biol Chem. 2002;277:44638–50.
28. Homolya L, Steinberg TH, Boucher RC. Cell to cell communication in response to mechanical stress via bilateral release of ATP and UTP in polarized epithelia. J Cell Biol. 2000;150:1349–60.
29. Roman RM, Fitz JG. Emerging roles of purinergic signaling in gastrointestinal epithelial secretion and hepatobiliary function. Gastroenterology. 1999;116:964–79.
30. Schwiebert EM, Zsembery A. Extracellular ATP as a signaling molecule for epithelial cells. Biochim Biophys Acta. 2003;1615:7–32.
31. Sorensen CE, Novak I. Visualization of ATP release in pancreatic acini in response to cholinergic stimulus. Use of fluorescent probes and confocal microscopy. J Biol Chem. 2001;276:32925–32.
32. Sprague RS, Stephenson AH, Ellsworth ML. Red not dead: signaling in and from erythrocytes. Trends Endocrinol Metab. 2007;18:350–5.
33. Yegutkin G, Bodin P, Burnstock G. Effect of shear stress on the release of soluble ecto-enzymes ATPase and 5′-nucleotidase along with endogenous ATP from vascular endothelial cells. Br J Pharmacol. 2000;129:921–6.
34. Berg J, Hung YP, Yellen G. A genetically encoded fluorescent reporter of ATP:ADP ratio. Nat Methods. 2009;6:161–6.
35. Imamura H, Nhat KP, Togawa H, Saito K, Iino R, Kato-Yamada Y, et al. Visualization of ATP levels inside single living cells with fluorescence resonance energy transfer-based genetically encoded indicators. Proc Natl Acad Sci USA. 2009;106:15651–6.
36. Pillay J, Ramakers BP, Kamp VM, Loi AL, Lam SW, Hietbrink F, et al. Functional heterogeneity and differential priming of circulating neutrophils in human experimental endotoxemia. J Leukoc Biol. 2010;88:211–20.
37. Adrie C, Bachelet M, Vayssier-Taussat M, Russo-Marie F, Bouchaert I, Adib-Conquy M, et al. Mitochondrial membrane potential and apoptosis peripheral blood monocytes in severe human sepsis. Am J Respir Crit Care Med. 2001;164:389–95.
38. Belikova I, Lukaszewicz AC, Faivre V, Damoisel C, Singer M, Payen D. Oxygen consumption of human peripheral blood mononuclear cells in severe human sepsis. Crit Care Med. 2007;35:2702–8.

Design and conduct of the activated protein C and corticosteroids for human septic shock (APROCCHSS) trial

Djillali Annane[1*], Christian Brun Buisson[2], Alain Cariou[3], Claude Martin[4], Benoit Misset[5], Alain Renault[6], Blandine Lehmann[7], Valérie Millul[8], Virginie Maxime[1], Eric Bellissant[6] and The APROCCHSS Investigators for the TRIGGERSEP Network

Abstract

Background: We aimed at assessing the benefit-to-risk ratio of activated protein C (drotrecogin-alfa activated, DAA) and corticosteroids, given alone or in combination, in patients with septic shock.

Methods: We implemented an investigator-led, publicly funded, multicenter, randomized according to a 2 × 2 factorial design, placebo-controlled, double-blind trial in four parallel groups in which adults with persistent septic shock and no contraindication to DAA were assigned to either DAA alone (24 mg/kg/h for 96 h), or hydrocortisone (50 mg intravenous bolus q6 for 7 days) and fludrocortisone (50 μg once daily through the nasogastric tube for 7 days) alone, or their respective combinations, or their respective placebos. Primary endpoint was 90-day mortality rate. Follow-up duration was 6 months. Statistical analysis was planned to be performed in intent-to-treat once after all participants completed 180-day follow-up and according to the 2 × 2 factorial design.

Results: The first patient was recruited in September 2008. The trial was suspended on October 25, 2011, owing to the withdrawal from the market of DAA. At this time, 411 patients had been enrolled. On May 17, 2012, the continuation of the trial on two parallel groups was approved by all legal authorities with the aim of investigating the benefit-to-risk ratio of corticosteroids. On June 30, 2014, the trial was suspended again by the study sponsor upon request of the independent data and safety monitoring board. Recruitment restarted on October 7, 2014, after any safety concern was ruled out. Finally, the trial was completed on June 23, 2015, with the recruitment of 1241 patients.

Conclusions: This report details the design, statistical plan and conduct of a randomized controlled trial of hydrocortisone and fludrocortisone in septic shock.

Trial registration The trial was registered at ClinicalTrials.gov under NCT00625209

Keywords: Septic shock, Clinical trial, Design, Ethics, Corticosteroids

Background

Septic shock is now defined by a vasopressor requirement to maintain a mean arterial pressure $\geq$65 mmHg and serum lactate >2 mmol/l in the absence of hypovolemia [1] (it was defined by the need for vasopressors to restore cardiovascular homeostasis [2] at the time the protocol was planned). Its mortality and sequalae remain unacceptably high with roughly one out of two patients dying within 1 year and half of survivors suffering from cognitive decline [3]. International guidelines recommend immediate source control and antibiotics, fluid resuscitation and norepinephrine [4].

Drotrecogin-alfa activated (DAA) was the only marketed therapy for sepsis after promising early findings [5].

*Correspondence: djillali.annane@aphp.fr
[1] General ICU, Service de Réanimation, Hôpital Raymond Poincaré, Laboratory of Infection and Inflammation, U1173, AP-HP, University of Versailles SQY and INSERM, 104 Boulevard Raymond Poincaré, 92380 Garches, France
Full list of author information is available at the end of the article

Subsequent investigations failed to reproduce survival benefit from this drug in sepsis [6] or in septic shock [7, 8].

Corticosteroids have been used for more than 60 years, mainly in inflammatory conditions, autoimmune diseases or cancer. They have also been used in infectious diseases and sepsis. Corticosteroids have pleiotropic effects including immune modulation, metabolic and cardiovascular effects. So far, sepsis trials have failed to rule in or out survival benefit from corticosteroids. Most physicians and researchers would agree against using short course (<3 days) of high dose (>400 mg per day of hydrocortisone or equivalent) in sepsis [4]. Treatment with ≤400 mg per day of hydrocortisone (or equivalent) for ≥3 days has variably been associated with survival benefit [9]. The two largest trials of corticosteroids for septic shock with 300 [10] and 500 [11] patients, respectively, reported treatment benefits in terms of hemodynamics and organ functions. One trial showed survival benefit in septic shock and blunted cortisol response to corticotrophin [10]. There were remarkable differences in trials' design (Table 1). Current guidelines suggest restricting hydrocortisone to patients who are poorly responsive to vasopressors, not using fludrocortisone and not based on Synacthen test [4].

Description of the study design

Clinical question and trial objectives

On the one hand, there was a strong rationale for using DAA or corticosteroids in sepsis [12]. DAA may act via direct immunomodulation and by counteracting sepsis-induced hypercoagulopathy [12, 13]. It was associated with survival benefit in a phase III trial in severe sepsis [5]. The hypothalamic–pituitary–adrenal (HPA) axis was identified as the main endogenous counter-regulator of inflammation [14]. Then, disrupted HPA axis and exaggerated inflammation may favor multiple organ failure and death in sepsis [15]. Corticosteroids were associated in Ger-Inf-05 [10], a phase III trial of hydrocortisone plus fludrocortisone, with survival benefit in septic shock and post-corticotrophin increase in cortisol levels ≤9 μg/dl, so-called non-responders [16].

On the other hand, there was equipoise among physicians about routine use of DAA and corticosteroids [17, 18]. Although DAA was approved for sepsis, failure to confirm its benefit in mild sepsis [6] yielded controversy about its benefits and risks with limited use in routine practice. Likewise, CORTICUS cast doubt about the benefit of hydrocortisone [11].

Therefore, the activated protein C and corticosteroids for human septic shock (APROCCHSS) trial aimed at evaluating in septic shock the benefit-to-risk ratio of DAA and corticosteroids, given alone or in combination, and any interaction between response to corticosteroids and non-responder status.

Study design

We designed an investigator-led, publicly funded, multicenter, randomized, 2 × 2 factorial, placebo-controlled, double-blind trial in four parallel groups.

Selection of study population

Evidence suggested greater benefit from DAA or corticosteroids in septic shock than in sepsis, in adults than in children, and when administered within 24 h [12]. In routine practice, physicians may consider adjunct therapy after optimal management of sepsis source and of organs function [2].

Therefore, were eligible in the trial, adults admitted to the intensive care unit (ICU) for <7 days and with indisputable or probable septic shock [2] for <24 h. Septic shock was defined by (1) clinically or microbiologically documented infection, (2) Sequential Organ Failure Assessment (SOFA) [19] score ≥3 for ≥2 organs for ≥6 consecutive hours, (3) treatment for ≥6 h with catecholamines (≥0.25 μg/kg/min or ≥1 mg/h of norepinephrine, epinephrine or any other vasopressor) to maintain systolic (SBP) ≥90 mmHg or mean blood pressure (MBP) ≥65 mmHg. Patient's informed consent or next of kin assent was obtained before inclusion whenever possible. Otherwise, deferred consent from patients was recorded [20].

Owing to the risk of bleeding with DAA [21], non-inclusion criteria were (1) surgical procedure ≤7 days; (2) gastrointestinal bleeding ≤6 weeks; (3) chronic liver disease; (4) trauma ≤3 months; (5) any intracranial mass, stroke or head injury ≤3 months; (6) thrombocytopenia <30,000/mm^3; (7) formal indication for anticoagulation except venous thromboembolism prophylaxis which should be continued whenever indicated; (8) any other condition with increased risk of bleeding, as per patient's physician. Owing to uncertainty of effects of DAA or corticosteroids in pregnant women and in newborns, patients were not included in case of pregnancy or lactation. Additional non-inclusion criteria were (1) patients with palliative goals, (2) underlying fatal (≤1 month) condition, (3) patients currently taking corticosteroids (30 mg prednisone equivalent ≥1 month), (4) known hypersensitivity to DAA, (5) no affiliation to social security.

A priori defined subgroups of interest to explore survival benefits from corticosteroids were: (1) non-responders, i.e., patients who increase their cortisol levels by 9 μg/dl or less at 30 and 60 min following 250 μg intravenous bolus of corticotrophin; (2) community-acquired pneumonia; (3) acute respiratory distress syndrome

Table 1 Comparison of (a) targeted population, (b) experimental treatments of four trials on corticosteroids for septic shock

	Ger-Inf-05	CORTICUS	APROCCHSS	ADRENALS
(a)				
Expected sample size	300	800	1240	3800
Actual sample size	300	500	1241	?
Time window for inclusion since onset of shock	3 h then protocol amended for 8 h	72 h	24 h	24 h
Age	≥18 years	≥18 years	≥18 years	≥18 years
Shock criteria	SBP < 90 mm Hg for at least 1 h despite adequate fluid replacement and >5 µg/kg/h of dopamine or epinephrine or norepinephrine; Arterial lactate >2 mmol/l	SBP < 90 mmHg or decrease >50 mmHg in SBP in previous hypertensive patients despite adequate fluid replacement or need for vasopressors to maintain SBP ≥ 90 mmHg Administration of vasopressor for ≥1 h	Norepinephrine or epinephrine at a rate ≥0.25 µg/kg/min or ≥1 mg/h) or any other vasopressor to maintain SBP ≥ 90 mmHg or MBP ≥ 65 mmHg Administration of vasopressors for ≥6 h	Vasopressors or inotropes to maintain a SBP > 90 mmHg, or MBP > 60 mmHg, or a MBP target set by the treating clinician for maintaining perfusion Administration of vasopressors or inotropes for =4 h
Mechanical ventilation as a mandatory entry criteria	Yes	No	No	Yes
Organ failure	Urinary output of <0.5 ml/kg for ≥1 h Or $PaO_2/FIO_2 < 280$ mmHg	Urine output <0.5 ml/kg/h for ≥1 h Or pH < 7.3, or arterial base deficit ≥5.0 mmol/l, or arterial lactate >2 mmol/l Or $PaO_2/FIO_2 < 280$ in the absence of pneumonia, and <200 in the presence of pneumonia Or platelet count ≤100,000 cells/mm^3 Or Glasgow Coma Scale <14 or acute change from baseline)	Sequential Organ Failure Assessment (SOFA) score ≥3 for ≥2 organs for ≥6 consecutive hours	Not mentioned
Non-responders to the Synacthen test as the primary subgroup of interest	Yes	Yes	Yes	No
(b)				
Type of corticosteroids	Hydrocortisone hemisuccinate and 9-α-fludrocortisone	Hydrocortisone hemisuccinate	Hydrocortisone hemisuccinate and 9-α-fludrocortisone	Hydrocortisone
Dose per day	Hydrocortisone 200 mg Fludrocortisone 50 µg	200 mg	Hydrocortisone 200 mg Fludrocortisone 50 µg	200 mg
Route of administration	Hydrocortisone: four intravenous bolus of 50 mg Fludrocortisone: 50 µg via the nasogastric tube	Four intravenous bolus of 50 mg	Hydrocortisone: four intravenous bolus of 50 mg Fludrocortisone: 50 µg via the nasogastric tube	Intravenous continuous infusion rate without loading dose
Duration	Seven days at full dose	Five days at full dose then tapered to 50 mg intravenously every 12 h for days 6 to 8, 50 mg every 24 h for days 9 to 11, and then stopped	Seven days at full dose	Seven days at full dose, while in the ICU

(ARDS). Indeed, it was expected that non-responders, patients with community-acquired pneumonia or ARDS may be more likely to draw survival benefit from corticosteroids [9].

Study interventions

DAA was infused intravenously at 24 μg/kg/h from foil-wrapped bags for 96 h. Infusion was interrupted 2 h before any percutaneous procedure or major surgery and resumed 1 or 12 h later, respectively, in the absence of bleeding complication. Identical blinded volume of 0.9 % saline was used as placebo for DAA.

Type, dose and duration (7 days) of corticosteroids were determined according to Ger-Inf-05 [10] and not to CORTICUS [11]. Hydrocortisone was administered as 50 mg intravenous bolus every 6 h, and 50 μg tablet of fludrocortisone was given via the nasogastric tube once daily in the morning. Placebos of French commercial forms of hydrocortisone and fludrocortisone were manufactured for the requirements of the trial. Active and placebo drugs had similar aspects (checked and certified by qualified persons for each batch), i.e., vials of white, freeze-dried powder for parenteral use of hydrocortisone hemisuccinate 100 mg or placebo, and tablets for oral fludrocortisone 50 μg or placebo in blisters of ten.

Co-interventions were harmonized across centers according to 2008 Surviving Sepsis Campaign guidelines [22]. Blood glucose levels were monitored at least every 4 h and maintained at ≤150 mg/dl by intravenous infusion of insulin. Intravenous broad-spectrum antibiotics were given after drawing specimen from all potential sites of infection and adjusted to actual pathogens whenever needed. Investigators followed guidelines for the prevention of superinfection [23]. Open-labeled corticosteroids and non-steroidal anti-inflammatory drugs, open-labeled DAA, anti-thrombin III and any anticoagulant (except venous thromboembolism prophylaxis) were discouraged. The use of antiplatelet agents was left at physicians' discretion. Neuromuscular blockade agents were discouraged, except in the first 24 h of refractory hypoxia. The investigators were provided with published guidelines for the management of septic shock. We systematically recorded, on a daily basis during the first week post-randomization, in the case report form, blood glucose levels and dose and duration of insulin, source and pathogens identification and dose and duration of any antibiotic administered to the patients, type and dose of fluid therapy and of vasopressor therapy, score of sedation and delirium and use of any sedation or neuromuscular blocking drug, dose and duration of any anticoagulant, and type, dose and reason for use of any open-labeled corticosteroids. These data will allow careful examination of the adherence of investigators to guidelines for co-interventions. In addition, at each investigators meeting, these guidelines were systematically discussed to reinforce compliance.

Randomization and blinding

Randomization was centralized, through a secured Web site, and stratified according to center, using permutation blocks where size was unknown by investigators. Patients were randomly allocated to receive DAA and hydrocortisone plus fludrocortisone, placebo of DAA and hydrocortisone plus fludrocortisone, or DAA and placebos of hydrocortisone and fludrocortisone, or all placebos. The day of randomization was considered as study day 0. The system printed prefilled prescriptions and, during the first part of the trial, individual infusion tables of DAA/placebo for care unit and pharmacy.

Treatment boxes were coded and masked centrally. Corticosteroids or placebos were sealed in sequentially numbered, identical boxes containing 30 vials of lyophilized hydrocortisone and 30 ampoules of injectable water, and a blister package with 10 tablets of fludrocortisone or its placebo. Each box has a detachable sticker for traceability of dispensing by hospital pharmacy and for administration by nurses.

Numbered boxes of DAA/placebo were also prepared on site. One patient received one corticosteroid/placebo box and one DAA/placebo box with the same randomization number. All study drugs were shipped to participating sites by AGEPS, AP-HP, Paris, France. The sequence was concealed from patients, staff members, investigators, members of independent data safety monitoring board (DSMB), sponsor and local pharmacists for corticosteroids.

Definitions

Organ system failure was defined for each of the 6 major organ systems as a SOFA score of 3 or 4 points (on a scale of 0–4 for each organ system, for an aggregate score of 0–24, with higher scores indicating more severe organ dysfunction) [19]. *Reversal of shock* was defined as MBP ≥ 60 mmHg for ≥24 h after cessation of vasopressor. *Superinfection* was defined using standard criteria [23], as a new infection occurring ≥48 h after randomization. *New sepsis* was defined as a new episode with microbiologic confirmation. *New septic shock* was defined as a new episode of septic shock after reversal of the initial episode.

Investigated parameters and follow-up

Baseline data

We systematically recorded (1) demographic and anthropometric data; (2) time of hospital and ICU admissions; (3) location prior to ICU admission (community, hospital, long-term care facility); (4) co-morbidities using Acute Physiology and Chronic Health Evaluation (APACHE) disability scale [24] and McCabe class [25]; (5) severity of illness using vital signs, Simplified Acute Physiology Score (SAPS) II [26] and SAPS III [27] and SOFA score [19]; (6) core temperature; (7) type and dose of any antibiotics in the week before randomization; (8) type and dose of vasopressors and inotropic drugs; (9) time from shock onset; (10) hematologic, chemical data, blood gas analyses and arterial lactate levels; (11) Gram examination and cultures of samples from any suspected site of infection; (12) plasma cortisol levels before, 30 and 60 min after 250 μg intravenous bolus of corticotrophin.

Follow-up

Patients were followed up for 180 days. We recorded daily from randomization to study day 7, at day 10, day 14, day 21 and day 28 or at ICU discharge (depending on which occurred first): (1) vital signs; (2) muscular disability rating score (MDRS) ranging from 1 to 5 with 1 meaning no deficit, 2 minimal deficit or atrophy, 3 mild-to-moderate distal deficit, 4 mild-to-moderate proximal deficit and 5 severe proximal deficit or atrophy [28]; (3) CAM-ICU scale [29]; (4) any bleeding; (5) results from standard laboratory tests; (6) cultures of specimens from any new suspected site of infection; (7) cumulated doses of intravenous insulin (UI/L/24 h), minimal and maximal infusion rates (μg/h; given for at least 1 h) of catecholamine, blood product transfusion, mode of ventilation (spontaneous breathing, noninvasive or invasive mechanical ventilation), need for and mode of renal replacement therapy and treatment with statins; (8) SOFA scores. If the patient was sedated, MDRS score and CAM-ICU were assessed ≥6 h after interruption of sedation. In case of abnormal neurological status, brain imaging (CT scan or magnetic resonance imaging) was performed.

Mid-term sequalae were assessed at day 90 and day 180 post-randomization, by means of the Short-Form General Health Survey [30], the Impact of Events scale [31] and Hospital Anxiety and Depression scale [32].

Biobanking

Fifteen milliliters of blood was sampled at baseline, day 1, day 4 and day 7. Then, aliquots of serum and plasma were stored at −80 °C, and DNA was stored at +4 °C at each participating hospital. On a regularly basis, samples were shipped to a core laboratory.

Study endpoints

Ninety-day mortality was the primary endpoint. Although most of sepsis-related deaths occur within 28 days, increasing evidence suggests that sepsis continues to kill patients beyond day 28. In previous sepsis trials, significant number of 28-day survivors died during the same hospital stay [33].

Secondary endpoints included (1) death rates at ICU and hospital discharge, at day 28 and day 180; (2) proportion of patients with decision to withhold/withdraw care; (3) time to wean off vasopressors, i.e., shock reversal; (4) number of days alive (up to 28 and 90 days) and free of vasopressors; (5) time to SOFA score <6; (6) number of days alive (up to 28 and 90 days) and with SOFA score <6; (7) time to wean off mechanical ventilation; (8) number of days alive (up to 28 and 90 days) and free of mechanical ventilation; (9) length of ICU and hospital stay in all patients and in survivors.

Safety outcomes included occurrence up to 90 days of superinfection, new sepsis, new septic shock, gastrointestinal bleeding and neurological sequalae (cognitive impairment and muscles weakness) at ICU and hospital discharge, at day 90 and at day 180.

Sample size calculation and statistical analysis plan

We anticipated a 90-day mortality rate among patients with septic shock of 45 % [10]. Using 2 × 2 factorial design with a bilateral formulation, 320 patients per group (i.e., total of 1280 patients) were needed to detect an absolute reduction of 10 % of 90-day mortality ($\alpha = 0.05$ and power at 95 %) with either DAA or corticosteroids.

After DAA withdrawal from the market, we analyzed the effects of DAA in patients included before trial suspension without analyzing the effects of corticosteroids [8].

As initially planned in the protocol, statistical analyses will be performed in intent-to-treat after all participants have completed 180-day follow-up and according to the 2 × 2 factorial design. This analysis will allow assessing the interaction between DAA and corticosteroids and corticosteroids effect (on the basis of a comparison of 2 groups of approximately 620 patients) with the initially planned power. The effect of DAA will be reanalyzed on the basis of a comparison including 208 patients with DAA and 1033 patients without DAA with a statistical power of 76 %.

For continuous variables, means and SD or median (IQR), in case of non-normality of distribution, will be reported. For categorical variables, number of patients in each category and corresponding percentages will be given. Missing data will not be replaced.

The effects of treatments on frequency of fatal events (mortality rates at day 28, at day 90, at discharge from ICU or from hospital and at day 180) will be compared using a logistic regression. The same analysis will be used for the proportion of patients with decision to withhold/withdraw care and safety outcomes. An analysis of variance will be used to compare continuous variables as length of stay. Cumulative event curves (censored endpoints) will be estimated with Kaplan–Meier procedure, and Cox model will be used to compare treatments effects (time to death, time to wean off vasopressors and mechanical ventilation, time to a SOFA score <6). Analysis of variance will be used to compare number of days alive and free of vasopressors, mechanical ventilation, and with a SOFA score <6.

The same analyses will be conducted for subgroups unless the numbers of patients are insufficient. In this case, statistical methods will be adapted according to sample sizes.

The statistical analysis plan will be revised after blind review of data and before access to randomization list. All analyses will be conducted with SAS statistical software (version 9.4; Cary, NC, USA).

Study Organization and Funding

The protocol was approved by all investigators on June 2007. It was independently approved for scientific and financial aspects by the national jury of the Clinical Research Hospital Program on October 2007, and the Ministry of Health confirmed funding under contract number P 070128. The protocol and qualification of all investigators were approved by the Ethics Committee (*Comité de Protection des Personnes, CPP*) of Saint-Germain-en-Laye, France, on November 22, 2007. The CPP allowed for waiver of consent and deferred consent.

DSMB was set up prior to recruitment of the first patient, included experts in critical care medicine, infectious diseases, pharmacology and statistics, had full access to raw data and met on a regular basis.

Data monitoring was performed by the sponsor (*AP-HP; Délégation à la Recherche Clinique d'Ile de France, DRRC*). AP-HP had full access to patients' charts and checked all data recorded onto the electronic case report form (CRF) against original chart. The trial used a Web-based electronic CRF (Telemedecine Technology, France).

Data management and statistical analysis were performed independently of the sponsor and of investigators by specialized Biometry unit (*Unité de Biométrie, INSERM 1414 Clinical Investigation Centre, Rennes University Hospital, Rennes 1 University, Rennes France*).

Institutional pharmacists (AGEPS) were responsible for obtaining corticosteroids and their placebos, shipping study drugs to participating sites and getting back unused drugs. They were responsible for accurateness of blinding and pharmaceutical organization of the trial.

Vials of lyophilizate for parenteral use of hydrocortisone hemisuccinate 100 mg or placebo and diluent ampoules were obtained from Serb pharmaceutical company. Active and placebo tablets for oral route of fludrocortisone 50 µg were supplied from French commercial market under responsibility of AGEPS. Due to the study length, fludrocortisone shelf-life and commercial changes, different companies were involved: EP-HP AP-HP, Genopharm and HAC pharma company. No change in formulation, specifications or quality controls occurred. This was approved by National Agency for Drug Safety (ANSM, Saint-Denis, France). Anticipation of manufacturing campaigns avoided any supply disruption.

Several documents were provided to caregivers and pharmacists to ensure safety, compliance and good use of study drugs: prefilled prescriptions (with patient ID, weight, treatment number, DAA/placebo infusions description when required), DAA/placebo personalized administration table (number of perfusions, dose/perfusion, durations, etc.), DAA/placebo preparation sheet for hospital pharmacists, nurse tracking administration file, pharmacy dispensing and return book. All documents were revised after DAA withdrawal from the market.

A total of 65 ICU were authorized to recruit patients, 19 at university hospitals and 46 at community hospitals. Among them 34 participated actively in recruiting patients in this trial.

Trial registration

The trial was registered on February 19, 2008, before inclusion of the first patient, at ClinicalTrials.gov under the number NCT00625209.

Study conduct

Study suspension and completion

The first patient was recruited on September 2, 2008, and the last patient on June 23, 2015. The study was suspended twice. Study sponsor, Steering committee, investigators, pharmacists and study statisticians always remained blinded to study treatments.

On October 25, 2011, while the trial was still recruiting, Lilly announced DAA withdrawal from the market [34]. Since DAA was no longer available and Lilly refused to provide the drug for our study, AP-HP immediately suspended the study. The Steering committee, while remaining blinded to study treatments, proposed to analyze effects of DAA in the 411 patients included before trial suspension without analyzing effects of corticosteroids as there was no interaction between the two treatments. There was no benefit from

DAA [8]. The Steering committee recommended trial's continuation to assess effects of corticosteroids. These recommendations were approved by ethics committee on February 10, 2012, and by ANSM on April 18, 2012. Inclusions into the study restarted on May 18, 2012. On June 24, 2013, additional funding was granted from Ministry of Health (contract P 12-002-0030; AOM 07008).

On July 22, 2014, AP-HP decided to suspend the trial after DSMB requested careful examination of serious adverse events and checking study drugs quality. Subsequently, detailed description of all serious adverse events was provided for all patients. Meanwhile, independent investigations confirmed study drugs quality. DSMB advised on October 1, 2014, AP-HP to restart the trial. The trial continuation was approved on October 7, 2014 by ANSM and on November 13, 2014 by CPP. The trial was completed by December 23, 2015, after the last patient reached 180 day post-randomization. Figure 1 shows the actual recruitment curve.

In April 2014, ANSM announced a shortage of Synacthen 0.25 in Europe. The trial was not suspended. Investigators and sites' pharmacists asked to continue sampling for random cortisol measurement whenever Synacthen was not available at their hospital.

Study protocol amendments

There were 29 amendments to study protocol (Table 2). They were approved by investigators, study statistician, AP-HP, CPP and ANSM.

The main substantial modification to the protocol was approved in October 2011, following DAA withdrawal from the market. Two study arms, i.e., active DAA and its placebo, were stopped, and the design was modified to a two parallel groups. As sample size was originally computed to show a 10 % absolute reduction in 90-day mortality between corticosteroids versus placebo-treated patients, or DAA versus placebo-treated patients, there was no need to modify it. DAA-related exclusion criteria were no longer justified and withdrawn (Table 2). This last amendment to the protocol was associated with a significant ($p < 0.001$) rise in recruitment rate into the study. There were 0.42 ± 0.89 (range 0–9, median 0 [0;1]) and 0.89 ± 1.46 (range 0–11, median 0 [0;1]) patients per site per month, before and after study amendment, respectively.

Study monitoring

The Steering committee had monthly conference calls. The study site coordinator (Raymond Poincaré hospital) provided on-demand 24/7 services via phone calls or

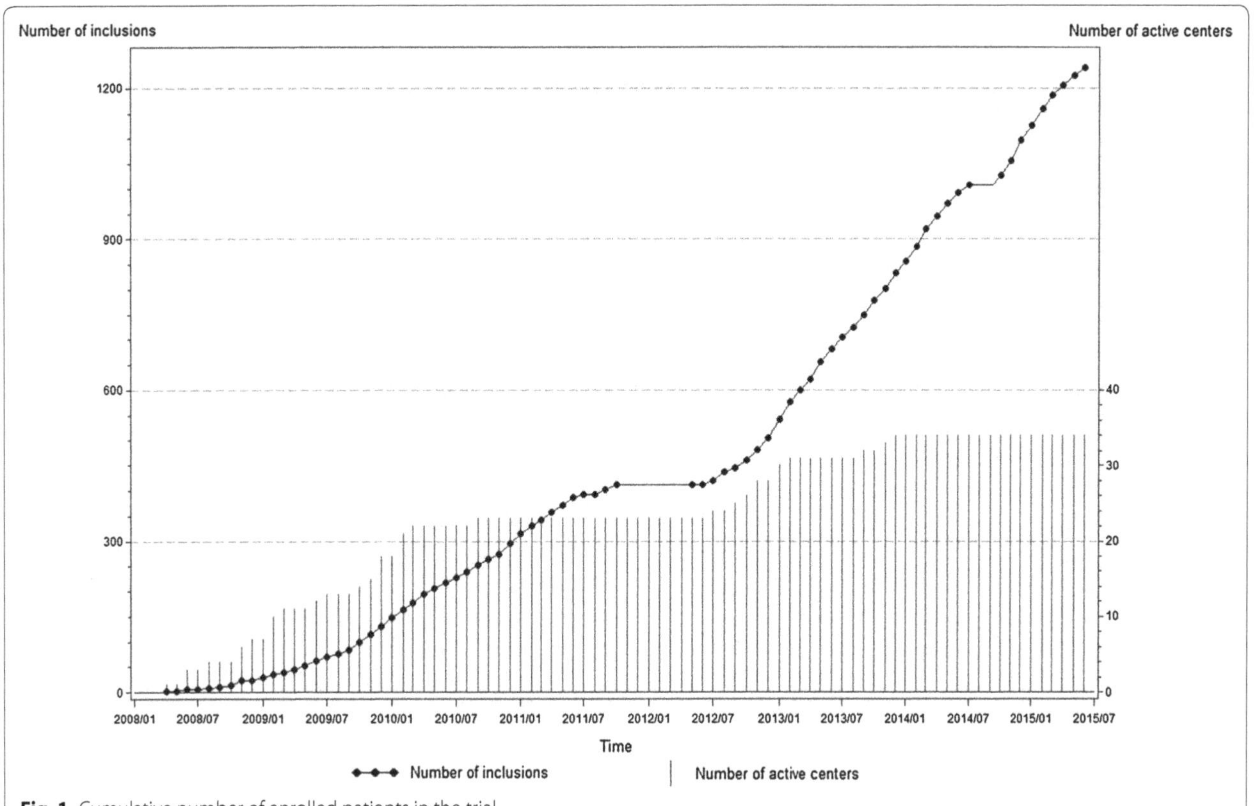

Fig. 1 Cumulative number of enrolled patients in the trial

emails to advise investigators about patients' eligibility or any other issues that may have risen between randomization and 180-day follow-up. There were a total of 28 face-to-face investigators meeting in which trial protocol and procedures were systematically recalled and investigators adherence and compliance to them discussed. A monthly electronic newsletter informed investigators on trial conduct and on any new information from sepsis literature.

DSMB met 5 times. DRRC organized data monitoring and quality audits. Baseline characteristics, eligibility criteria, primary outcome and serious adverse events reported in the CRF were systematically checked against original chart for all research participants. In addition, for one-third of study population, all data reported in CRF were validated against patient's original chart. Serious adverse events and major protocol violations were reported to DRRC, ANSM and CPP.

The study coordinator had quarterly face-to-face meeting with DRRC, AP-HP, independent pharmacists to monitor trial conduct according to highest standard for protection of research participants.

All randomized patients completed follow-up for the primary outcome and 180-day mortality data.

Discussion

This trial was designed to assess the role of DAA and corticosteroids in adult septic shock. Evaluation of DAA was terminated early owing to its withdrawal from the market by Lilly [34]. We found no evidence for any benefit from DAA [8]. Owing to the lack of interaction between DAA and corticosteroids, the trial continued to allow evaluation of corticosteroids. The study was suspended on request of DSMB to check safety issues. The two trial suspensions had no impact on its conduct, except delaying its completion. There were several amendments to the protocol mainly related to DAA. In particular, after DAA withdrawal from the market, corresponding exclusion criteria were removed and trial design changed for a two-parallel groups' design. This amendment accelerated the recruitment rate into the trial. Then, we will explore any interaction between this change in the protocol and response to corticosteroids.

This trial replicated as much as possible Ger-Inf-05 [10] contrasting with CORTICUS [11] and ADRENAL [35] trials (Tables 1, 2). APROCCHSS trial has investigated the effects of hydrocortisone and fludrocortisone at the same doses, durations and routes of administration than for Ger-Inf-05 [10]. Likewise, it focused on patients with persistent vasopressor dependency and organ failure. Finally, non-responders [16] were an a priori defined subgroup in analyzing corticosteroids effects.

Risk of bias assessment

First, selection biases were minimized. Allocating interventions to research participants used a random list which sequence was computer-generated by an independent statistician. To prevent forth knowledge of forth allocation, randomization was centralized through a secured Web site and used permutation blocks where size was not known by patients, nurses and physicians, investigators, pharmacists, and study sponsor. Thus, the allocation sequence was adequately concealed. Second, to minimize performance biases, we used a centralized procedure for masking corticosteroids and their placebos. Sites pharmacists received sealed boxes containing either active drugs or placebos in identical forms. Blood glucose levels were kept of $\leq$150 mg/dl. Previous experiences from this group of investigators [10, 36] as from others [11] demonstrated that nurses, physicians and investigators can remain appropriately blinded to corticosteroids administration. Third, to prevent detection biases, for short-term and long-term outcomes, hospital staff, investigators, pharmacists and outcome assessors will remain blinded until public release of trial findings. Finally, there were no obvious attrition biases. There was no lost-to-follow-up for mortality data up to 180 days. According to French regulation, vital status of any citizen is publicly available at city hall of the town the citizen was born.

Other potential sources of bias may include the fact that the study design and statistical analysis plan were reported after all patients have been enrolled. This was done deliberately to also report the way the trial was conducted, in particular any amendment to the protocol. We did not plan any interim analysis and did not perform any. In fact, after the withdrawal of DAA from the market, we reported the analysis of the effects of this drug after checking for the absence of interaction with low-dose steroids. The code was never broken for corticosteroids, and all the parties involved in the trial remained fully blinded. Therefore, it is unlikely that the lack of reporting of the trial protocol before completion of recruitment may be a source of bias.

In conclusion, APROCCHSS trial is the only trial replicating Ger-Inf-05. Its design and conduct allowed appropriate minimization of risk of bias. It will provide sufficient reliable data to inform routine practice for management of adult septic shock. At the present time, the analysis is still pending, and all parties involved in this trial remain blinded.

Table 2 List of amendments to the protocol

Amendments number	Changes in protocol	CPP approval date	ANSM approval date	Official version of trial protocol
1	Changes in following exclusion criteria: "surgical procedure in the past 7 days" was changed for "surgical procedure within 72 h, or any surgery associated with high risk of bleeding, or a planned surgery within 24 h" "chronic liver disease" was clarified as "chronic liver disease with Child score C" "severe thrombopenia" was clarified" as severe thrombopenia (<30,000/mm^3, before transfusion) Minor wording modifications in title, study acronym, randomization paragraph Recruitment of 4 additional centers	14/02/2008	27/03/2008	Protocol V2 dated 28/01/2008
2	Recruitment of 1 additional center Withdrawal of 1 center	12/06/2008	Not applicable	Protocol V2 dated 28/01/2008 unchanged
3	Recruitment of 9 additional centers	03/07/2008	Not applicable	Protocol V2 dated 28/01/2008 unchanged
4	Recruitment of 1 additional center	13/11/2008	Not applicable	Protocol V2 dated 28/01/2008 unchanged
5	The time window for the use of a prepared (i.e., ready for infusion) infusion bag of Xigris and of its placebo was increased from 14 h to 24 h	12/02/2009	26/12/2008	Protocol V3 dated 11/12/2008
6	Recruitment of 1 additional center Change in contact details of 3 centers	15/01/2009	Not applicable	Protocol V3 dated 11/12/2008 unchanged
7	Recruitment of 1 additional center	9/04/2009	Not applicable	Protocol V3 dated 11/12/2008 unchanged
8	Recruitment of 2 additional centers	18/06/2009	Not applicable	Protocol V3 dated 11/12/2008 unchanged
9	The exclusion criteria: surgical procedure within 72 h, or any surgery associated with high risk of bleeding, or a planned surgery within 24 h "was changed for" surgical procedure within 12 h, or any surgery associated with high risk of bleeding	17/09/2009	25/08/2009	Protocol V3.0 dated 20/07/2009
10	Recruitment of 1 additional center	12/11/2009	Not applicable	Protocol V3.0 dated 20/07/2009 unchanged
11	Recruitment of 1 additional center	10/12/2009	Not applicable	Protocol V3.0 dated 20/07/2009 unchanged
12	Recruitment of 1 additional center	11/03/2010	Not applicable	Protocol V3.0 dated 20/07/2009 unchanged
13	Inclusion criteria: admitted to the ICU for <7 days was removed. New exclusion criteria: patients who had a previous episode of sepsis during the same hospital stay Prolongation of the recruitment period Recruitment of 3 additional centers Withdrawal of 11 inactive centers	10/06/2010	11/06/2010	Protocol V4 dated 10/05/2010
14	Withdrawal of 4 inactive centers	09/09/2010	Not applicable	Protocol V4 dated 10/05/2010 unchanged
15	Recruitment of 1 additional center	23/11/2010	Not applicable	Protocol V4 dated 10/05/2010 unchanged
16	Recruitment of 1 additional center Implementation of biobanking: serum, plasma, DNA Change in informed consent sheet	23/11/2010	09/11/2010	Protocol V6 dated 03/11/2010 Informed consent sheet V1.1 dated 26/10/2010
17	Recruitment of 1 additional center	13/10/2010	Not applicable	Protocol V6 dated 03/11/2010 unchanged
18	Recruitment of 7 additional centers	13/01/2011	Not applicable	Protocol V6 dated 03/11/2010 unchanged
19	Recruitment of 1 additional center	7/04/2011	Not applicable	Protocol V6 dated 03/11/2010 unchanged

Table 2 continued

Amendments number	Changes in protocol	CPP approval date	ANSM approval date	Official version of trial protocol
20	Recruitment of 1 additional center	12/05/2011	Not applicable	Protocol V6 dated 03/11/2010 unchanged
20 BIS	Following the withdrawal of DAA from the market: Study design was modified from a 2 × 2 factorial to a two-parallel groups' trial Withdrawal of following exclusion criteria: (1) any surgery in the past 12 h, or any surgery associated with high risk of bleeding; (2) chronic liver disease with a Child score C; (3) recent trauma; (4) any intracranial mass, or stroke or head injury in the past 3 months; (5) severe thrombocytopenia (<30,000/mm^3, before platelet transfusion); (6) formal indication for anticoagulation, or any other condition associated with increased risk of bleeding, as appreciated by the patient's physician Change in informed consent form	10/02/2012	18/04/2012	Protocol V7 du 30/11/2011 Informed consent sheet V3.0 dated 05/01/2012
21	Prolongation of recruitment period	05/07/2012	Not applicable	Protocol V8 dated 27/06/2012 Informed consent form V3.1 dated 21/09/2012
22	Recruitment of 2 additional centers	13/09/2012	Not applicable	Protocol V9 dated 27/08/2012
23	Recruitment of 2 additional centers Withdrawal of 4 centers	13/12/2012	Not applicable	Protocol V10 dated 04/12/2012
24	Recruitment of 2 additional centers Removal of exclusion criteria related to XIGRIS Withdrawal of 5 centers	21/03/2013	22/03/2013	Protocol V11.0 dated 20/02/2013 Protocol V11.1 dated 18/03/2013
25	Minor edits to the informed consent form upon CPP request	24/04/2014	Not applicable	Protocol V12 du 15/10/2013 Informed consent form V3.2 dated 21 01 2014
26	Suspension of inclusions upon DSMB request Changes in DSMB members	18/09/2014	29/08/2014	Protocol V13 dated 24/07/2014
27	Request to restart inclusion following: (1) demonstration of the quality of study active drugs and placebos (2) advice from DSMB	13/11/2014	07/10/2014	Protocol V13 dated 24/07/2014, unchanged
28	Prolongation of trial duration	11/06/2015	Not applicable	Protocol V14.0 dated 12/05/2015

CPP comité de protection des personnes, *ANSM* Agence nationale de sécurité des médicaments et produits de santé

Authors' contributions

DA took the responsibility to coordinate the project, DA, CBB, AC, CM, BM and EB designed the protocol, AR and EB were responsible for the statistical plan, BL was responsible for the pharmaceutical aspects and study drug management, and VM was responsible for the regulatory and administrative management of the study. All authors read and approved the final manuscript.

Author details

[1] General ICU, Service de Réanimation, Hôpital Raymond Poincaré, Laboratory of Infection and Inflammation, U1173, AP-HP, University of Versailles SQY and INSERM, 104 Boulevard Raymond Poincaré, 92380 Garches, France. [2] Service de Réanimation Médicale, Hôpital Henri Mondor, AP-HP, Créteil, France. [3] Service de Réanimation Médicale, Hôpital Cochin, AP-HP, Paris, France. [4] Service d'Anesthésie Réanimation, Hôpital Nord, AP-HM, Marseille, France. [5] Service de Médecine Intensive et Réanimation, Hôpital Saint-Joseph, AP-HP, Université Paris Descartes, Paris Sorbonne Cité, Paris, France. [6] Service de Pharmacologie, Centre d'Investigation Clinique INSERM 1414, CHU de Rennes, Université de Rennes 1, Rennes, France. [7] Département des Essais Cliniques, AGEPS, Paris, France. [8] Délégation à la Recherche Clinique, Hôpital Saint-Louis, AP-HP, Paris, France.

Funding

The study was publicly funded by a grant from the Ministry of Health contract number P090902 and contract P 12-002-0030.

Appendix: Study organization

Study chairs: Djillali Annane (Principal Investigator) and Eric Bellissant (Methodologist).

Statistics and data management: Eric Bellissant and Alain Renault.

Steering committee: Djillali Annane (chair), Eric Bellissant, Alain Cariou, Christian Brun Buisson, Claude Martin, Benoit Misset.

Monitor: Valérie Millul: Délégation à la Recherche Clinique, Hôpital Saint-Louis, Paris.

Monitoring: Layide Meaude: URC Paris Ouest, Délégation à la Recherche Clinique, Hôpital Saint-Louis, Paris.

Quality Assurance: Délégation à la Recherche Clinique, Hôpital Saint-Louis, Paris.
Data safety and Monitoring Board: Gérard Nitenberg (chair) Jacques Bénichou, Didier Dreyfuss.
Pharmacists: Blandine Lehmann: Département Essais Cliniques, AGEPS, AP-HP, Paris.

Study centers and investigators

Surname and name of sites principal investigator	Study sites details
Annane, Djillali Fadel, Fouad Polito, Andrea Clair, Bernard Maxime, Virginie Luis, David	Service de Réanimation médicale HOPITAL RAYMOND POINCARE 104 BD RAYMOND POINCARE 92380 GARCHES
Quenot, Jean-Pierre	Service de réanimation 14 RUE GAFFAREL BP 77908 21079 DIJON CEDEX HÔPITAL F. MITTERRAND CHU DE DIJON
Megarbane, Bruno	Service de Réanimation Médicale et Toxicologique Hôpital LARIBOISIERE 2 rue AMBROISE PARE 75010 PARIS
Siami, Shidasp Percheron, Stéphanie	Service d' Anesthésie-réanimation du Dr. Lorenzo CENTRE HOSPITALIER D'ETAMPES 26 AV CHARLES DE GAULLE 91150 ETAMPES
Mignon, Alexandre Baudin, Francois Antona, Marion Meghenem, Alia Demesmay, Marine	Service d' Anesthésie Réanimation Hôpital COCHIN 27 R FAUBOURG ST-JACQUES 75014 PARIS
Forceville, Xavier Kuba-Kusuti, Jean-Kamiena Touati, Samia	Service de Réanimation Polyvalente CENTRE HOSPITALIER DE MEAUX 6 R SAINT FIACRE 77100 MEAUX
Reignier, Jean Colin, Gwenhaël Martin-Lefevre, Laurent Bachoumas, Konstantinos Henry-Lagarrigue, Matthieu Yehia, Aihem Lascarrou, Jean-baptiste Lebert, Christine Lacherade, Jean-claude	Service de réanimation CENTRE HOSPITALIER DEPARTEMENTAL SITE DE LA ROCHE-SUR-YONLES OUDAIRIES 85925 LA ROCHE SUR YON CEDEX 9
Asehnoune, Karim Loutrel, Olivier Dumont, Romain Roquilly, Antoine Mahe, Pierre-Joachim Demeure Dit Latte, Dominique Champin, Philippe Arnould, Jean François Cinotti, Raphaël Le Floch, Ronan	Service d'Anesthésie Réanimation chirurgicale, CHU DE NANTES 19 RUE GENERAL MARGUERITTE, 44000 NANTES

Surname and name of sites principal investigator	Study sites details
Mercier, Emmanuelle Garot, Denis Dequin, Pierre François Perrotin, Dominique Legras, Annick Mankikian, Julie Talec, Patrice Ehrmann, Stephan Joret, Aurélie Lhommet, Claire Joret, Aurélie Lhommet, Claire Rouve, Emmanuelle Bodet-Contentin, Laetitia Jouan, Youenn Salmon-Gandonniere, Charlotte	Service de réanimation polyvalente, CHU BRETONNEAU, 2, BOULEVARD TONNELLE, 37044 TOURS
Antonini, François Martin, Claude Denis Ragonnet, Benoît	Service d' Anesthésie Réanimation HOPITAL NORD Chemin des BOURRELY 13015 MARSEILLE
Brun Buisson, Christian Razazi, Keyvan De Prost, Nicolas Carteaux, Guillaume	Service de Réanimation Médicale Hôpital HENRI MONDOR 51 AV DE LATTRE DE TASSIGNY 94010 CRETEIL
Wolff, Michel Mourvillier, Bruno Timsit, Jean françois	Service de Réanimation - Maladies Infectieuses Hôpital BICHAT CLAUDE BERNARD 46 Rue HENRI HUCHARD 75018 PARIS
Chagnon, Jean-Luc Ali Ben Ali, Mohamed	Service de Réanimation Polyvalente C.H. DE VALENCIENNES 114 AV DESANDROUINS BP 479 59322 VALENCIENNES
Chimot, Loic Delour, Pierre Dessalles, Pierre Henri Monseau, Yannick Saint-Leger, Mélanie Bedon-Carte, Sandrine	Service de Réanimation CENTRE HOSPITALIER PERIGUEUX 80, AVENUE GEORGES POMPIDOU CS 61205 24019 PERIGUEUX CEDEX
Boulain, Thierry Mathonnet, Armelle Bretagnol, Anne Runge, Isabelle Barbier, François Muller, Gregoire	Service de réanimation polyvalente CHR D'ORLEANS 1, RUE PORTE-MADELEINE – 45000ORLEANS
Francois, Bruno Clavel, Marc Vignon, Philippe Pichon, Nicolas Fedou, Anne-Laure Chapellas, Catherine Galy, Antoine	Service de réanimation polyvalente CHU LIMOGES 2, AVENUE MARTIN LUTHER KING 87042 LIMOGES
Timsit, Jean-Francois	Service de Réanimation médicale CHU DE GRENOBLE Avenue du Maquis du Gresivaudan, Pavillon Dauphiné BP 217 38043 GRENOBLE

Surname and name of sites principal investigator	Study sites details
Misset, Benoit Garrouste Orgeas, Maité Philippart, François	Service de Réanimation médicale polyvalente HOPITAL SAINT-JOSEPH 185 R RAYMOND LOSSERAND 75674 PARIS
Souweine, Bertrand Ait-Hssain, Ali	Service de Réanimation CHU CLERMONT-FERRAND 58 RUE MONTALEMBERT BP69 63003 CLERMONT FERRAND
Charpentier, Claire	Service de Réanimation chirurgicale HOPITAL CENTRAL 29 AVENUE DU MARECHAL DE LATTRE DE TASSIGNY 54037 NANCY
Mignon, Alexandre Baudin, Francois Antona, Marion Meghenem, Alia Demesmay, Marine	Service d'Anesthésie Réanimation Hôpital COCHIN 27 R FAUBOURG ST-JACQUES 75014 PARIS
Petitpas, Franck Mimoz, Olivier Nanadoumgar, Hodanou	Service de Réanimation Chirurgicale HÔPITAL DE LA MILETRIE 2 RUE DE LA MILETRIE B. P. 577 86021 POITIERS
Chastre, Jean Combes, Alain Nieszkowska, Ania	Service de Réanimation Médicale C.H.U. PITIE SALPETRIERE 47 BOULEVARD DE L'HOPITAL 75013 PARIS
Amathieu, Roland Levesque, Eric	Réanimations et surveillance continue chirurgicales HOPITAL HENRI MONDOR 51 AV DE LATTRE DE TASSIGNY 94010 CRETEIL
Cook, Fabrice	Réanimations et surveillance continue chirurgicales HOPITAL HENRI MONDOR 51 AV DE LATTRE DE TASSIGNY 94010 CRETEIL
Constantin, Jean-Michel Chartier, Christian Jabaudon, Mathieu Perbet, Sébatien	Service d'Anesthésie et réanimation HÔPITAL HOTEL DIEU Boulevard Léon Malfreyt 63058 CLERMONT FERRAND CEDEX 1

References

1. Singer M, Deutschman CS, Seymour CW, Shankar-Hari M, Annane D, Bauer M, et al. The third international consensus definitions for sepsis and septic shock (Sepsis-3). JAMA. 2016;315(8):801–10.
2. Annane D, Bellissant E, Cavaillon JM. Septic shock. Lancet. 2005;365:63–78.
3. Annane D, Sharshar T. Cognitive decline after sepsis. Lancet Respir Med. 2015;3:61–9.
4. Dellinger RP, Levy MM, Rhodes A, Annane D, Gerlach H, Opal SM, et al. Surviving Sepsis Campaign Guidelines Committee including The Pediatric Subgroup. Surviving Sepsis Campaign: international guidelines for management of severe sepsis and septic shock, 2012. Intensive Care Med. 2013;39:165–228.
5. Bernard GR, Vincent JL, Laterre PF, LaRosa SP, Dhainaut JF, Lopez-Rodriguez A, Steingrub JS, Recombinant human protein C Worldwide Evaluation in Severe Sepsis (PROWESS) study group, Garber GE, Helterbrand JD, Ely EW, Fisher CJ Jr. Efficacy and safety of recombinant human activated protein C for severe sepsis. N Engl J Med. 2001;344:699–709.
6. Abraham E, Laterre PF, Garg R, Levy H, Talwar D, Trzaskoma BL, Francois B, Guy JS, Bruckmann M, Rea-Neto A, Rossaint R, Perrotin D, Sablotzki A, Arkins N, Utterback BG, Macias WL, Administration of Drotrecogin Alfa (Activated) in Early Stage Severe Sepsis (ADDRESS) Study Group. Drotrecogin alfa (activated) for adults with severe sepsis and a low risk of death. N Engl J Med. 2005;353:1332–41.
7. Ranieri VM, Thompson BT, Barie PS, Dhainaut JF, Douglas IS, Finfer S, Gardlund B, Marshall JC, Rhodes A, Artigas A, Payen D, Tenhunen J, Al-Khalidi HR, Thompson V, Janes J, Macias WL, Vangerow B. Williams MD; PROWESS-SHOCK Study Group. Drotrecogin alfa (Activated) in Adults with Septic Shock. N Engl J Med. 2012;366:2055–64.
8. Annane D, Timsit JF, Megarbane B, Martin C, Misset B, Mourvillier B, Siami S, Chagnon JL, Constantin JM, Petitpas F, Souweine B, Amathieu R, Forceville X, Charpentier C, Tesnière A, Chastre J, Bohe J, Colin G, Cariou A, Renault A, Brun-Buisson C, Bellissant E, APROCCHSS Trial Investigators. Recombinant human activated protein C for adults with septic shock: a randomized controlled trial. Am J Respir Crit Care Med. 2013;187(10):1091–7.
9. Annane D, Bellissant E, Bollaert PE, Briegel J, Keh D, Kupfer Y. Corticosteroids for treating sepsis. Cochrane Database Syst Rev. 2015;12:CD002243.
10. Annane D, Sebille V, Charpentier C, Bollaert PE, François B, Korach JM, et al. Effect of treatment with low doses of hydrocortisone and fludrocortisone on mortality in patients with septic shock. JAMA. 2002;288:862–71.
11. Sprung C, Annane D, Keh D, Moreno R, Singer M, Freivogel K, et al. The CORTICUS randomized, double-blind, placebo-controlled study of hydrocortisone therapy in patients with septic shock. N Engl J Med. 2008;358:111–24.
12. Annane D. Adjunct therapy for sepsis: how early? current infectious disease reports. Curr Infect Dis Rep. 2010;12:361–7.
13. Yuksel M, Okajima K, Uchiba M, Horiuchi S, Okabe H. Activated protein C inhibits lipopolysaccharide-induced tumor necrosis factor-alfa production by inhibiting activation of both nuclear factor-kappa B and activator protein-1 in human monocytes. Thromb Haemost. 2002;88:267–73.
14. Silverman MN, Sternberg EM. Glucocorticoid regulation of inflammation and its functional correlates: from HPA axis to glucocorticoid receptor dysfunction. Ann N Y Acad Sci. 2012;1261:55–63.
15. Annane D. Corticosteroids for severe sepsis: an evidence-based guide for physicians. Ann Intensive Care. 2011;1(1):7.
16. Annane D, Sébille V, Troché G, Raphael JC, Gajdos P, Bellissant E. A 3-level prognostic classification in septic shock based on cortisol levels and cortisol response to corticotropin. JAMA. 2000;283(8):1038–45.
17. Lagu T, Rothberg MB, Nathanson BH, Pekow PS, Steingrub JS, Lindenauer PK. Variation in the care of septic shock: the impact of patient and hospital characteristics. J Crit Care. 2012;27:329–36.
18. Stoneking L, Denninghoff K, Deluca L, Keim SM, Munger B. Sepsis bundles and compliance with clinical guidelines. J Intensive Care Med. 2011;26:172–82.
19. Vincent JL, de Mendonca A, Cantraine F, et al. Use of the SOFA score to assess the incidence of organ dysfunction/failure in intensive care units: results of a multicenter, prospective study. Crit Care Med. 1998;26:1793–800.
20. http://www.legifrance.gouv.fr/affichTexte.do?cidTexte=JORFTEXT000000787078&dateTexte. Accessed 2 Nov 2015.
21. Marti-Carvajal AJ, Sola I, Lathyris D, Cardona AF. Human recombinant activated protein C for severe sepsis. Cochrane Database Syst Rev. 2012;3:CD004388.
22. Dellinger RP, Levy MM, Carlet JM, et al. Surviving Sepsis Campaign: international guidelines for management of severe sepsis and septic shock. Crit Care Med. 2008;36:296–327.
23. Guide "100 recommandations pour la surveillance et la préventions des infections nosocomiales". Bulletin épidémiologique hebdomadaire du 30 novembre 1992. http://www.invs.sante.fr/beh/1992/48/beh_48_1992.pdf. Accessed 3 Nov 2015.
24. Knaus WA, Zimmerman JE, Wagner DP, Draper EA, Lawrence DE. APACHE-acute physiology and chronic health evaluation: a physiologically based classification system. Crit Care Med. 1981;9:591–7.

25. McCabe WR, Jackson GG. Gram-negative bacteremia: I. Etiology and ecology. Arch Intern Med. 1962;110:847–55.
26. Le Gall JR, Lemeshow S, Saulnier F. A new Simplified Acute Physiology Score (SAPSII) based on a European/North American multicenter study. JAMA. 1993;270:2957–63 **(Erratum in: JAMA 1994; 271:1321)**.
27. Moreno RP, Metnitz PG, Almeida E, Jordan B, Bauer P, Campos RA, Iapichino G, Edbrooke D, Capuzzo M, Le Gall JR. From evaluation of the patient to evaluation of the intensive care unit. Part 2: Development of a prognostic model for hospital mortality at ICU admission. Intensive Care Med. 2005;31:1345–55.
28. Mathieu J, DeBraekeleer M, Prévost C, Boily C. Myotonic dystrophy: clinical assessment of muscular disability in an isolated population with presumed homogeneous mutation. Neurology. 1992;42:203–8.
29. Ely EW, Inouye SK, Bernard GR, Gordon S, Francis J, May L, Truman B, Speroff T, Gautam S, Margolin R, Hart RP, Dittus R. Delirium in mechanically ventilated patients: validity and reliability of the confusion assessment method for the intensive care unit (CAM-ICU). JAMA. 2001;286:2703–10.
30. Leplege A, Ecosse E, Verdier A, Perneger TV. The French SF-36 Health Survey: translation, cultural adaptation and preliminary psychometric evaluation. J Clin Epidemiol. 1998;51:1013–23.
31. Sundin EC, Horowitz MJ. Impact of event scale: psychometric properties. Br J Psychiatry. 2002;180:205–9.
32. Zigmond AS, Snaith RP. The hospital anxiety and depression scale. Acta Psychiatr Scand. 1983;67:361–70.
33. Annane D. Improving clinical trials in the critically ill: unique challenge—sepsis. Crit Care Med. 2009;37:S117–28.
34. Lilly Announces Withdrawal of Xigris (R) Following Recent Clinical Trial Results. http://pi.lilly.com/us/xigris.pdf. Accessed on 25 Oct 2011.
35. Venkatesh B, Myburgh J, Finfer S, Webb SA, Cohen J, Bellomo R, ANZICS CTG Investigators, et al. The ADRENAL study protocol: adjunctive corticosteroid treatment in critically ill patients with septic shock. Critical Care Resusc. 2013;15:83–8.
36. COIITSS Study Investigators. Corticosteroid treatment and intensive insulin therapy for septic shock in adults: a randomised controlled trial. JAMA. 2010;303(4):341–8.

Permissions

All chapters in this book were first published in AIC, by Springer; hereby published with permission under the Creative Commons Attribution License or equivalent. Every chapter published in this book has been scrutinized by our experts. Their significance has been extensively debated. The topics covered herein carry significant findings which will fuel the growth of the discipline. They may even be implemented as practical applications or may be referred to as a beginning point for another development.

The contributors of this book come from diverse backgrounds, making this book a truly international effort. This book will bring forth new frontiers with its revolutionizing research information and detailed analysis of the nascent developments around the world.

We would like to thank all the contributing authors for lending their expertise to make the book truly unique. They have played a crucial role in the development of this book. Without their invaluable contributions this book wouldn't have been possible. They have made vital efforts to compile up to date information on the varied aspects of this subject to make this book a valuable addition to the collection of many professionals and students.

This book was conceptualized with the vision of imparting up-to-date information and advanced data in this field. To ensure the same, a matchless editorial board was set up. Every individual on the board went through rigorous rounds of assessment to prove their worth. After which they invested a large part of their time researching and compiling the most relevant data for our readers.

The editorial board has been involved in producing this book since its inception. They have spent rigorous hours researching and exploring the diverse topics which have resulted in the successful publishing of this book. They have passed on their knowledge of decades through this book. To expedite this challenging task, the publisher supported the team at every step. A small team of assistant editors was also appointed to further simplify the editing procedure and attain best results for the readers.

Apart from the editorial board, the designing team has also invested a significant amount of their time in understanding the subject and creating the most relevant covers. They scrutinized every image to scout for the most suitable representation of the subject and create an appropriate cover for the book.

The publishing team has been an ardent support to the editorial, designing and production team. Their endless efforts to recruit the best for this project, has resulted in the accomplishment of this book. They are a veteran in the field of academics and their pool of knowledge is as vast as their experience in printing. Their expertise and guidance has proved useful at every step. Their uncompromising quality standards have made this book an exceptional effort. Their encouragement from time to time has been an inspiration for everyone.

The publisher and the editorial board hope that this book will prove to be a valuable piece of knowledge for researchers, students, practitioners and scholars across the globe.

List of Contributors

Nicolas Peschanski, Rémy Lucas and Vianney Aquilina
Department of Emergency Medicine, Centre Hospitalo-universitaire de Rouen, 1 rue de Germont, 76000 Rouen, France

Camille Chenevier-Gobeaux
Department of Automated Biological Diagnosis, Hôpitaux Universitaires Paris Centre (HUPC) – Hôpital Cochin, Assistance Publique des Hôpitaux de Paris (AP-HP), Paris, France

Lynda Mzabi
Department of Emergency Medicine, Hôpitaux Universitaires Est Parisien - Hôpital Tenon, Assistance Publique des Hôpitaux de Paris (AP-HP), 4 rue de la Chine, 75020 Paris, France

Patrick Ray
Department of Emergency Medicine, Hôpitaux Universitaires Est Parisien - Hôpital Tenon, Assistance Publique des Hôpitaux de Paris (AP-HP), 4 rue de la Chine, 75020 Paris, France
Sorbonne Universités UMPC Université Paris 06, DHU Fighting Aging and Stress (FAST), Paris, France

Siham Ouahabi and Guillaume Lefevre
Department of Biochemistry and Hormonology, Hôpitaux Universitaires Est Parisien - Hôpital Tenon, Assistance Publique des Hôpitaux de Paris (AP-HP), 4 rue de la Chine, 75020 Paris, France

Valéry Brunel
Department of Biochemistry, Clinical Biology Institut, Centre Hospitalo-universitaire de Rouen, 1 rue de Germont, 76000 Rouen, France

Nara Aline Costa, Ana Lúcia Gut, Paula Schmidt Azevedo, Suzana Erico Tanni, Natália Baraldi Cunha, Eloá Siqueira Magalhães, Bertha Furlan Polegato, Leonardo Antonio Mamede Zornoff, Sergio Alberto Rupp de Paiva, André Luís Balbi, Daniela Ponce and Marcos Ferreira Minicucci
Department of Internal Medicine, Botucatu Medical School, UNESP – Univ Estadual Paulista, Rubião Júnior s/n, Botucatu, SP CEP: 18618-970, Brazil

Graziela Biude Silva
Department of Food and Experimental Nutrition, Faculty of Pharmaceutical Science, University of São Paulo, São Paulo, SP, Brazil

Nicolas Allou, Jérôme Allyn, Dorothée Valance, Julien Jabot, Bruno Bouchet, Richard Galliot and Laure Corradi
Réanimation polyvalente, Hôpital Felix Guyon, Centre Hospitalier Universitaire Felix Guyon, Allée des Topazes, Bellepierre, 97405 Saint Denis, France

Aurélie Snauwaert, Astrid Bouteau, Philippe Montravers and Pascal Augustin
Département d'Anesthésie Réanimation, AP-HP, Centre Hospitalier Universitaire Bichat-Claude-Bernard, 46, rue Henri-Huchard, 75018 Paris, France

Imoigele P. Aisiku
Division of Emergency Critical Care Medicine, Department of Emergency Medicine, Brigham and Women's Hospital, 75 Francis St., Neville House, Boston, MA 02115, USA

Raghu R. Seethala and Peter C. Hou
Division of Emergency Critical Care Medicine, Department of Emergency Medicine, Brigham and Women's Hospital, 75 Francis St., Neville House, Boston, MA 02115, USA
Surgical ICU Translational Research (STAR) Center, Brigham and Women's Hospital, Boston, MA, USA

Gyorgy Frendl
Surgical ICU Translational Research (STAR) Center, Brigham and Women's Hospital, Boston, MA, USA
Department of Anesthesiology, Perioperative and Pain Medicine, Brigham and Women's Hospital, Boston, MA, USA

Pauline K. Park
Division of Acute Care Surgery, Department of Surgery, University of Michigan Health System, Ann Arbor, MI, USA

Mark E. Mikkelsen
Division of Pulmonary, Allergy, and Critical Care Medicine, Department of Medicine, Perelman School of Medicine, University of Pennsylvania, Philadelphia, PA, USA

Steven Y. Chang
Division of Pulmonary and Critical Care, Department of Medicine, UCLA, Los Angeles, CA, USA

Ognjen Gajic
Division of Pulmonary and Critical Care Medicine, Department of Medicine, Mayo Clinic, Rochester, MN, USA

Jonathan Sevransky
Division of Pulmonary and Critical Care Medicine, Department of Medicine, Mayo Clinic, Rochester, MN, USA
Division of Pulmonary, Allergy and Critical Care, Department of Medicine, Emory University, Atlanta, GA, USA

David Andaluz-Ojeda, Ramón Cicuéndez, Francisco Gandía and Leonor Nogales
Servicio de Medicina Intensiva, Hospital Clínico Universitario, Avda Ramón y Cajal 3, 47005 Valladolid, Spain
Group for Biomedical Research in Sepsis(Bio·Sepsis), Hospital Clínico Universitario, Avda Ramón y Cajal 3, 47005 Valladolid, Spain

Jesús F. Bermejo-Martín
Group for Biomedical Research in Sepsis(Bio·Sepsis), Hospital Clínico Universitario, Avda Ramón y Cajal 3, 47005 Valladolid, Spain

Eduardo Tamay
Group for Biomedical Research in Sepsis(Bio·Sepsis), Hospital Clínico Universitario, Avda Ramón y Cajal 3, 47005 Valladolid, Spain
Servicio de Anestesiología y Reanimación, Hospital Clínico Universitario, Avda/Ramón y Cajal 3, 47005 Valladolid, Spain

H. Bryant Nguyen
Division of Pulmonary and Critical Care Medicine, Department of Medicine, Loma Linda University, Loma Linda, CA, USA

Nicolas Meunier-Beillard, Jean-Pierre Quenot, Auguste Dargent and Pierre Emmanuel Charles
Service de Réanimation Médicale, Hôpital Bocage Central, C.H.U. DIJON, 14 rue Gaffarel, B.P. 77908-21079, Dijon Cedex, France

Dolores Calvo, Esther Zarca and Cristina Andrés
Servicio de Análisis Clínicos, Hospital Clínico Universitario, Avda Ramón y Cajal 3, 47005 Valladolid, Spain

Jose María Eiros
Departmento de Microbiología, Facultad de Medicina, Universidad de Valladolid, Avda/ Ramón y Cajal 7, 47005 Valladolid, Spain

Juan Carlos Yébenes
Critical Care Department, Hospital de Mataró, Mataró, Spain
Grup de Recerca en Sepsis, Imflamació i Seguretat (AGAUR 2014-SGR926), Barcelona, Spain
Escola Superior de Ciencies de la Salut, Universitat Pompeu Fabra, Mataró, Spain
Servei de Medicina Intensiva, Hospital de Mataró, Carretera de Cirera s/n, 08304 Mataró, Spain

Juan Carlos Ruiz-Rodriguez
Critical Care Department, Vall d'Hebron University Hospital, Barcelona, Spain
Shock, Organ Dysfunction and Resuscitation (SODIR) Research Group, Vall d' Hebron Research Institut, Universitat Autònoma de Barcelona, Barcelona, Spain

Ricard Ferrer
Critical Care Department, Vall d'Hebron University Hospital, Barcelona, Spain
Shock, Organ Dysfunction and Resuscitation (SODIR) Research Group, Vall d' Hebron Research Institut, Universitat Autònoma de Barcelona, Barcelona, Spain
CIBER Enfermedades Respiratorias, Madrid, Spain

Montserrat Clèries and Anna Bosch
Divisió d'Anàlisi de la Demanda i l'Activitat, Servei Català de la Salut (CatSalut), Barcelona, Spain

Carol Lorencio
Critical Care Department, Hospital Universitari Dr. Josep Trueta, Girona, Spain

Alejandro Rodriguez
Grup de Recerca en Sepsis, Imflamació i Seguretat (AGAUR 2014-SGR926), Barcelona, Spain
Critical Care Department, Hospital Universitari Joan XXIII, Tarragona, Spain
IISPV/URV, Tarragona, Spain

Xavier Nuvials
Critical Care Department, Hospital Universitari Arnau de Vilanova, Lleida, Spain
Institut de Recerca Biomèdica (IRB), Lleida, Spain

Ignacio Martin-Loeches
Multidisciplinary Intensive Care Research Organization (MICRO), St James's University Hospital, Trinity Centre for Health Sciences, Dublin, Ireland

Antoni Artigas
CIBER Enfermedades Respiratorias, Madrid, Spain
Critical Care Center, Sabadell Hospital, Corporació Sanitaria Universitaria Parc Tauli, Sabadell, Spain
Universitat Autonoma de Barcelona, Sabadell, Spain

Leyla Alegría, Magdalena Vera, Jorge Dreyse, Ricardo Castro, David Carpio, Carolina Henriquez, Daniela Gajardo, Sebastian Bravo, Felipe Araneda, Eduardo Kattan and Glenn Hernández
Departamento de Medicina Intensiva, Facultad de Medicina, Pontificia Universidad Católica de Chile, Marcoleta 367, Santiago 8320000, Chile

Pedro Torres
Hospital San Francisco, Quito, Ecuador

Gustavo Ospina-Tascón
Intensive Care Medicine Department, Fundación Valle del Lili - Universidad ICESI, Cali, Colombia

Jean-Louis Teboul
Assistance Publique-Hôpitaux de Paris, Hôpitaux universitaires Paris-Sud, Hôpital de Bicêtre, Service de Réanimation Médicale, Le Kremlin-Bicêtre, France

Jan Bakker
Departamento de Medicina Intensiva, Facultad de Medicina, Ponti icia Universidad Católica de Chile, Marcoleta 367, Santiago 8320000, Chile
Department of Intensive Care Adults, Erasmus University Medical Center, Rotterdam, The Netherlands

Yaseen M. Arabi
Intensive Care Department, MC-1425, Respiratory Services, College of Medicine, King Abdullah International Medical Research Center, King Saud bin Abdulaziz University for Health Sciences, Riyadh 11426, Kingdom of Saudi Arabia

Hasan M. Al-Dorzi, Ahmed Alamry, Ra'ed Hijazi, Sami Alsolamy, Majid Al Salamah, Saad Al-Qahtani, Abdulaziz Al-Dawood, Abdellatif M. Marini, Fatimah H. Al Ehnidi, Shihab Mundekkadan, Amal Matroud, Mohamed S. Mohamed and Saadi Taher
King Abdullah International Medical Research Center, King Saud bin Abdulaziz University for Health Sciences, Riyadh, Kingdom of Saudi Arabia

Hani M. Tamim
King Abdullah International Medical Research Center, King Saud bin Abdulaziz University for Health Sciences, Riyadh, Kingdom of Saudi Arabia
Department of Internal Medicine, American University of Beirut- Medical Center, Beirut, Lebanon

Adrien Mirouse and Frédéric Pène
Réanimation médicale, hôpital Cochin, Assistance Publique-Hôpitaux de Paris (AP-HP) and Université Paris Descartes, 27 rue du Faubourg Saint-Jacques, 75014 Paris, France

Matthieu Resche-Rigon
Département de biostatistiques, Hôpital Saint-Louis, APHP and Université Paris Diderot, Paris, France

Virginie Lemiale and Elie Azoulay
Réanimation médicale, Hôpital Saint-Louis, AP-HP and Université Paris Diderot, Paris, France

Djamel Mokart
Département d'anesthésie-réanimation, Institut Paoli-Calmettes, Marseille, France

Achille Kouatchet
Réanimation médicale et médecine hyperbare, CHU d'Angers, Angers, France

Julien Mayaux
Réanimation médicale, Hôpital de la Pitié-Salpêtrière, AP-HP and Université Pierre et Marie Curie, Paris, France

François Vincent
Réanimation polyvalente, Centre Hospitalier Intercommunal, Montfermeil, France

Martine Nyunga
Centre Hospitalier de Roubaix, Roubaix, France

Fabrice Bruneel
Réanimation polyvalente, Hôpital André Mignot, Le Chesnay, France

Antoine Rabbat
Unité de soins intensifs respiratoires, Hôpital Cochin, AP-HP and Université Paris Descartes, Paris, France

Christine Lebert
Réanimation polyvalente, Centre Hospitalier Départemental, La Roche-sur-Yon, France

Pierre Perez
Réanimation médicale, Hôpital Brabois, Nancy, France

Anne Renault
Réanimation médicale, Centre Hospitalier de Brest, Brest, France

Anne-Pascale Meert
Service des soins intensifs et urgencies oncologiques, Institut Jules Bordet, Brussels, Belgium

Dominique Benoit
Ghent University Hospital, Ghent, Belgium

Rebecca Hamidfar
Réanimation médicale, CHU Grenoble-Alpes, Grenoble, France

Mercé Jourdain
Université de Lille and Réanimation Polyvalente, CHU de Lille, Lille, France

Michaël Darmon
Réanimation médicale, Centre Hospitalier de Saint-Etienne, Saint-Etienne, France

Georg Franz Lehner, Ulrich Harler, Viktoria Maria Haller, Julia Hasslacher, Romuald Bellmann and Michael Joannidis
Division of Intensive Care and Emergency Medicine, Department of Internal Medicine, Medical University Innsbruck, Anichstrasse 35, 6020 Innsbruck, Austria

Clemens Feistritzer
Department of Internal Medicine V - Haematology and Oncology, Medical University Innsbruck, Anichstrasse 35, 6020 Innsbruck, Austria

Chin-Chieh Wu, Gerald N. Blaney III and Zhen-Ying Liu
Department of Emergency Medicine, Chang Gung Memorial Hospital, Keelung, Taiwan

Hao-Min Lan
School of Medicine, Chang Gung University, Taoyuan, Taiwan

Shih-Tsung Han, Chung-Hsien Chaou and Chih-Huang Li
Department of Emergency Medicine, Chang Gung Memorial Hospital, Linkou, Taiwan

Chun-Fu Yeh
Division of Infectious Diseases, Department of Internal Medicine, Chang Gung Memorial Hospital at Linkou, Chang Gung University College of Medicine, Taoyuan, Taiwan

Su-Hsun Liu
School of Medicine, Chang Gung University, Taoyuan, Taiwan
Department of Family Medicine, Chang Gung Memorial Hospital, Linkou, Taiwan

Kuan-Fu Chen
Department of Emergency Medicine, Chang Gung Memorial Hospital, Keelung, Taiwan
Department of Emergency Medicine, Chang Gung Memorial Hospital, Linkou, Taiwan
Clinical Informatics and Medical Statistics Research Center, Chang Gung University, 5 Fu-Shin Street, Gueishan Village, Taoyuan 333, Taiwan
Community Medicine Research Center, Chang Gung Memorial Hospital, Keelung, Taiwan

M. Cuartero and A. J. Betbesé
Intensive Care Department and Institut d'Investigacions Biomèdiques, Hospital de la Santa Creu i Sant Pau, Universitat Autònoma de Barcelona, Sant Quintí 89, 08041 Barcelona, Spain

J. Ballús, J. Sabater and X. Pérez
Intensive Care Department, Hospital Universitari Bellvitge, Hospitalet de Llobregat, Universitat de Barcelona, Feixa Llarga, 08907 L'Hospitalet de Llobregat, Barcelona, Spain

N. Nin
Intensive Care Department, Hospital Universitario de Getafe, Km 12500 Madrid - Toledo Road, 28905 Getafe, Madrid, Spain

J. Ordonez-Llanos
Biochemistry Department and Institut d'Investigacions Biomèdiques, Hospital de la Santa Creu i Sant Pau, Universitat Autònoma de Barcelona, Sant Quintí 89, 08041 Barcelona, Spain

Tuanny Teixeira Pinheiro, Flávio Geraldo Rezende de Freitas, Karla Tuanny Fiorese Coimbra, Vanessa Marques Ferreira Mendez, Heloísa Baccaro Rossetti, Paulo Vinicius Talma, Antônio Tonete Bafi and Flávia Ribeiro Machado
Anesthesiology, Pain and Intensive Care Department, Federal University of Sao Paulo, Napoleão de Barros 737, Sao Paulo, SP 04024002, Brazil

Toshiaki Iba
Department of Emergency and Disaster Medicine, Juntendo University Graduate School of Medicine, 2-1-1 Hongo Bunkyo-ku, Tokyo 113-8421, Japan

Akiyoshi Hagiwara
National Center for Global Health and Medicine, Emergency Medicine and Critical Care, Tokyo, Japan

Daizoh Saitoh
Division of Traumatology, Research Institute, National Defense Medical College, Tokyo, Japan

Hideaki Anan
Emergency Medical Center, Fujisawa City Hospital, Fujisawa, Japan

Yutaka Ueki
Department of Acute Critical Care and Disaster Medicine, Tokyo Medical and Dental University, Tokyo, Japan

Koichi Sato
Department of Surgery, Juntendo Shizuoka Hospital, Juntendo University Graduate School of Medicine, Izunokuni-shi, Japan

Satoshi Gando
Division of Acute and Critical Care Medicine, Department of Anesthesiology and Critical Care Medicine, Hokkaido University Graduate School of Medicine, Sapporo, Japan

Djillali Annane
Service de Reanimation Medicale, Hopital R. Poincare, 104 Bd Raymond Poincare, 92380 Garches, France

Jean-Paul Mira
Sorbonne Paris Cité, Cochin Hotel-Dieu University Hospital Medical Intensive Care Unit, AP-HP, Université Paris Descartes, 75014 Paris, France

Lorraine B. Ware
Departments of Medicine and Pathology, Microbiology and Immunology, Vanderbilt University School of Medicine, 1161 21st Avenue South T1218 MCN, Nashville, TN 37232-2650, USA

Anthony C. Gordon
Section of Anaesthetics, Pain Medicine, and Intensive Care, Charing Cross Hospital, Imperial College London, Fulham Palace Road, London W6 8RF, UK

Charles J. Hinds
Barts and The London School of Medicine, Queen Mary University of London, London, UK

David C. Christiani
Harvard Medical School and School of Public Health, 665 Huntington Avenue, Building I Room 1401, Boston, MA 02115, USA

Jonathan Sevransky and Timothy G. Buchman
Emory Center for Critical Care, Woodruff Health Sciences Center, Emory University, Atlanta, GA, USA

Kathleen Barnes
Division of Allergy and Clinical Immunology, Department of Medicine, Johns Hopkins University, Baltimore, MD, USA

Patrick J. Heagerty
Department of Biostatistics, University of Washington, F-600, Health Sciences Building, Office: H-665D HSB, Seattle, WA 98195-7232, USA

Robert Balshaw, Nadia Lesnikova and Karen de Nobrega
Syreon Corporation, Vancouver, BC, Canada

Hugh F. Wellman, Mauricio Neira and Alexandra D. J. Mancini
Formerly with Sirius Genomics Inc, Vancouver, BC, Canada

Keith R. Walley and James A. Russell
Critical Care Research Laboratories, Centre for Heart Lung Innovation, St. Paul's Hospital, University of British Columbia, Burrard Building, Rm 166 - 1081 Burrard St, Vancouver, BC V6Z 1Y6, Canada

Gretchen L. Sacha, Simon W. Lam, Heather Torbic, Stephanie N. Bass, Sarah C. Welch and Seth R. Bauer
Department of Pharmacy, Cleveland Clinic, 9500 Euclid Avenue (Hb-105), Cleveland, OH 44195, USA

Abhijit Duggal
Respiratory Institute, Cleveland Clinic, Cleveland, OH, USA

Robert S. Butler
Department of Quantitative Health Sciences, Cleveland Clinic, Cleveland, OH, USA

Solenn Remy, Karine Kolev-Descamps and Etienne Javouhey
Hospices Civils de Lyon, Paediatric Intensive Care Unit, Mother and Children University Hospital, 59 Boulevard Pinel, 69500 Bron, France

Morgane Gossez and Julie Demaret
Hospices Civils de Lyon, Immunology Laboratory, E. Herriot Hospital, 69003 Lyon, France

Fabienne Venet and Guillaume Monneret
Hospices Civils de Lyon, Immunology Laboratory, E. Herriot Hospital, 69003 Lyon, France
EA 7426, Pathophysiology of Injury-Induced Immunosuppression, University Claude Bernard Lyon 1, BioMérieux Hospices Civils de Lyon, E. Herriot Hospital, 69003 Lyon, France

Jacob C. Jentzer
Department of Cardiovascular Medicine, Mayo Clinic, 200 First Street SW, Rochester, MN 55905, USA
Division of Pulmonary and Critical Care Medicine, Department of Medicine, Mayo Clinic, Rochester, MN, USA

Saraschandra Vallabhajosyula
Department of Cardiovascular Medicine, Mayo Clinic, 200 First Street SW, Rochester, MN 55905, USA
Division of Pulmonary and Critical Care Medicine, Department of Medicine, Mayo Clinic, Rochester, MN, USA
Multidisciplinary Epidemiology and Translational Research in Intensive Care (METRIC) Laboratory, Mayo Clinic, Rochester, MN, USA

Vivek N. Iyer
Division of Pulmonary and Critical Care Medicine, Department of Medicine, Mayo Clinic, Rochester, MN, USA
Multidisciplinary Epidemiology and Translational Research in Intensive Care (METRIC) Laboratory, Mayo Clinic, Rochester, MN, USA

Aditya A. Kotecha
Multidisciplinary Epidemiology and Translational Research in Intensive Care (METRIC) Laboratory, Mayo Clinic, Rochester, MN, USA
Division of Pulmonary and Critical Care Medicine, Department of Medicine, Henry Ford Hospital/ Wayne State University, Detroit, MI, USA

Dennis H. Murphree Jr.
Department of Health Sciences Research, Robert D. and Patricia E. Kern Center for the Science of Health Care Delivery, Mayo Clinic, Rochester, MN, USA

Erin F. Barreto
Multidisciplinary Epidemiology and Translational Research in Intensive Care (METRIC) Laboratory, Mayo Clinic, Rochester, MN, USA
Department of Health Sciences Research, Robert D. and Patricia E. Kern Center for the Science of Health Care Delivery, Mayo Clinic, Rochester, MN, USA
Department of Pharmacy, Mayo Clinic, Rochester, MN, USA

Ashish K. Khanna
Center for Critical Care, Anesthesiology Institute, Cleveland Clinic, Cleveland, OH, USA
Department of Outcomes Research, Cleveland Clinic, Cleveland, OH, USA

Giorgio Berlot, Nicola Busetto, Margarita Nieto Yabar, Tatiana Istrati, Silvia Baronio, Giada Quarantotto, Roberto Dattola, Irene Longo, Antonino Chillemi, Alice Scamperle, Fulvio Iscra and Ariella Tomasini
Department of Anesthesia, Resuscitation and Pain Therapy, Cattinara Hospital, University of Trieste, Strada di Fiume 447, 34149 Trieste, Italy

Mattia Bixio and Michele Claudio Vassallo
Department of Anesthesia and Intensive Care, San Martino Hospital, Largo Rosanna Benzi 10, 16132 Genoa, Italy

Giulia Barbati
Biostatistics Unit, Department of Medicine, Surgery and Health Sciences, Cattinara Hospital, University of Trieste, Strada di Fiume 447, 34149 Trieste, Italy

Rajat N. Moman
Multidisciplinary Epidemiology and Translational Research in Intensive Care (METRIC), Division of Pulmonary and Critical Care Medicine, Department of Medicine, Mayo Clinic, 200 First Street SW, Rochester, MN 55905, USA
Department of Anesthesiology and Perioperative Medicine, Mayo Clinic, Rochester, MN, USA

Stuart A. Ostby
Multidisciplinary Epidemiology and Translational Research in Intensive Care (METRIC), Division of Pulmonary and Critical Care Medicine, Department of Medicine, Mayo Clinic, 200 First Street SW, Rochester, MN 55905, USA
Department of Obstetrics and Gynecology, University of Alabama Birmingham, Birmingham, AL, USA

Abbasali Akhoundi
Multidisciplinary Epidemiology and Translational Research in Intensive Care (METRIC), Division of Pulmonary and Critical Care Medicine, Department of Medicine, Mayo Clinic, 200 First Street SW, Rochester, MN 55905, USA
Division of Pulmonary and Critical Care Medicine, Department of Medicine, Mayo Clinic, Rochester, MN, USA

Rahul Kashyap
Multidisciplinary Epidemiology and Translational Research in Intensive Care (METRIC), Division of Pulmonary and Critical Care Medicine, Department of Medicine, Mayo Clinic, 200 First Street SW, Rochester, MN 55905, USA
Anesthesia Clinical Research Unit, Department of Anesthesiology and Perioperative Medicine, Mayo Clinic, Rochester, MN, USA

Kianoush Kashani
Multidisciplinary Epidemiology and Translational Research in Intensive Care (METRIC), Division of Pulmonary and Critical Care Medicine, Department of Medicine, Mayo Clinic, 200 First Street SW, Rochester, MN 55905, USA
Division of Pulmonary and Critical Care Medicine, Department of Medicine, Mayo Clinic, Rochester, MN, USA
Division of Nephrology and Hypertension, Department of Medicine, Mayo Clinic, Rochester, MN, USA

Salvatore Lucio Cutuli and Massimo Antonelli
Department of Intensive Care and Anaesthesiology, Agostino Gemelli University Hospital, Catholic University of the Sacred Heart, Largo A. Gemelli, 8, 00168 Rome, Italy

Antonio Artigas
Critical Care Center, Sabadell Hospital, CIBER Enfermedades Respiratorias, Corporació Sanitària Universitària Parc Taulí, Universitat Autònoma de Barcelona, Sabadell, Spain

Roberto Fumagalli and Gianpaola Monti
Department of Anaesthesia and Intensive Care Medicine, Niguarda Ca' Granda Hospital, University of Milan-Bicocca, Milan, Italy

Vito Marco Ranieri
Department of Anaesthesia and Intensive Care Medicine, University of Rome "La Sapienza", Rome, Italy

Claudio Ronco
Department of Nephrology, Dialysis and Transplantation, International Renal Research Institute of Vicenza (IRRIV), San Bortolo Hospital, Vicenza, Italy

Yi Yang, Jianfeng Xie, Fengmei Guo, Zhiwei Gao, Yingzi Huang and Haibo Qiu
Department of Critical Care Medicine, Nanjing Zhong-Da Hospital, School of Medicine, Southeast University, Nanjing 210009, Jiangsu, China

Federico Longhini
Department of Critical Care Medicine, Nanjing Zhong-Da Hospital, School of Medicine, Southeast University, Nanjing 210009, Jiangsu, China
Department of Translational Medicine, Eastern Piedmont University "A. Avogadro", Novara, Italy

Koichiro Sueyoshi, Yuka Sumi, Yoshiaki Inoue, Yoko Kuroda and Hiroshi Tanaka
Department of Emergency and Critical Care Medicine, Juntendo University, Urayasu Hospital, 2-1-1 Tomioka, Urayasu, Chiba 279-0021, Japan

Kumiko Ishii
Lipid Biology Laboratory, Riken Advanced Science Institute, Wako, Saitama, Japan

Hitoshi Nakayamav and Kazuhisa Iwabuchi
Institute for Environmental and Gender Specific Medicine, Juntendo University, Urayasu, Chiba, Japan

Yasutaka Kurishita, Hajime Shigemitsu and Itaru Hamachi
Department of Synthetic Chemistry and Biological Chemistry, Graduate School of Engineering, Kyoto University, Kyoto, Japan

Djillali Annane and Virginie Maxime
General ICU, Service de Réanimation, Hôpital Raymond Poincaré, Laboratory of Infection and Inflammation, U1173, AP-HP, University of Versailles SQY and INSERM, 104 Boulevard Raymond Poincaré, 92380 Garches, France

Christian Brun Buisson
Service de Réanimation Médicale, Hôpital Henri Mondor, AP-HP, Créteil, France

Alain Cariou
Service de Réanimation Médicale, Hôpital Cochin, AP-HP, Paris, France

Claude Martin
Service d'Anesthésie Réanimation, Hôpital Nord, AP-HM, Marseille, France

Benoit Misset
Service de Médecine Intensive et Réanimation, Hôpital Saint-Joseph, AP-HP, Université Paris Descartes, Paris Sorbonne Cité, Paris, France

Alain Renault and Eric Bellissant
Service de Pharmacologie, Centre d'Investigation Clinique INSERM 1414, CHU de Rennes, Université de Rennes 1, Rennes, France

Blandine Lehmann
Département des Essais Cliniques, AGEPS, Paris, France

Valérie Millul
Délégation à la Recherche Clinique, Hôpital Saint-Louis, AP-HP, Paris, France

Index

CPSIA information can be obtained
at www.ICGtesting.com
Printed in the USA
LVHW011947261221
707171LV00003B/188

9 781639 271078